RECENT ADVANCES
IN MEDICINE

RECENT ADVANCES IN MEDICINE

SIXTEENTH EDITION

EDITORS

D. N. BARON

M.D., D.Sc., F.R.C.P., F.R.C.Path.

*Professor of Chemical Pathology, The Royal Free Hospital
School of Medicine, London*

NIGEL COMPSTON

M.A., M.D., F.R.C.P.

*Physician, Royal Free Hospital Group, St. Stephen's Hospital,
Royal Masonic Hospital, and King Edward VII's Hospital for Officers*

A. M. DAWSON

M.D., F.R.C.P.

*Physician, St. Bartholomew's Hospital, London and King Edward VII's
Hospital for Officers*

CHURCHILL LIVINGSTONE

Edinburgh and London

1973

First Edition	.	.	.	.	1924
Second Edition	.	.	.	.	1925
Third Edition	.	.	.	.	1926
Fourth Edition		.	.	.	1928
Fifth Edition	.	.	.	.	1929
Sixth Edition	.	.	.	.	1931
Seventh Edition		.	.	.	1934
Eighth Edition	.	.	.	.	1936
Ninth Edition	.	.	.	.	1939
Tenth Edition	.	.	.	.	1941
Eleventh Edition		.	.	.	1943
Reprinted	.	.	.	.	1944
Reprinted	.	.	.	.	1945
Twelfth Edition	.	.	.	.	1947
Reprinted	.	.	.	.	1948
Thirteenth Edition		.	.	.	1952
Fourteenth Edition		.	.	.	1964
Reprinted	.	.	.	.	1965
Fifteenth Edition	.	.	.	.	1968
Reprinted	.	.	.	.	1969
Sixteenth Edition		.	.	.	1973

ISBN

0 443 00990 2

© Longman Group Limited 1973

Any communication relating to this publication should be directed to the publishers at 15–17 Teviot Place, Edinburgh, EHI 2XX.

Printed in Great Britain

PREFACE

In this edition the editors have sought to continue the successful pattern of the two previous editions. As before, there has been a complete change of subjects and writers. Topics have been selected from the important advances which have taken place in the last five years, and authors have been chosen who are actively involved in the development of their subject. 'Medicine' has been interpreted in the widest sense, to include environmental, clinical, and laboratory aspects of the subject.

This book is primarily intended for the postgraduate student and medical consultant to acquaint them with advances in other than their own speciality. It is hoped that the surveys of thirteen important subjects are both critical and readable, and will be of interest and value for both the undergraduate student and the general medical reader.

The editors wish to thank Churchill Livingstone for their patient and constant collaboration.

D. N. Baron
Nigel Compston
A. M. Dawson

November 1972

CONTRIBUTORS

E. G. ANDERSON, M.D., M.R.C.P.
Consultant Physician, Royal Gwent and Woolos Hospitals, Newport.

JOCELYN CHAMBERLAIN, M.B., B.S., M.R.C.S., L.R.C.P., D.C.H.
Senior Research Fellow, Chronic Disease Control Study Unit, Department of Public Health, London School of Hygiene.

M. L. CLARK, M.D., M.R.C.P.
Consultant Physician, St. Leonard's Hospital, London.

R. B. HEATH, M.D.
Reader in Virology, The Medical College of St. Bartholomew's Hospital, London.

B. D. HORE, B.SC., PHYSIOL., M.B., B.S., M.PHIL., M.R.C.P., M.R.C.PSYCH.
Consultant Psychiatrist, University Hospital of South Manchester, Withington; Consultant in charge of the Alcoholism Treatment Unit, Springfield Hospital, Manchester.

E. R. HUEHNS, PH.D., M.D., M.R.C.S., L.R.C.P., M.C.PATH.
Reader and Consultant in Haematology, University College Hospital Medical School, London.

D. N. S. KERR, M.S. (WISCONSIN), M.B., CH.B.
Professor in Medicine, University of Newcastle upon Tyne.

PAMELA M. LE QUESNE, B.SC., M.A., D.M., M.R.C.P., D.OBST., R.C.O.G.
Member M.R.C. Toxicological Unit; Honorary Consultant, The Middlesex Hospital, London.

R. H. S. MINDHAM, M.B., B.S., D.P.M., M.R.C.P.,, D.C.H.
Department of Psychiatry, General Hospital, Nottingham.

CELIA M. OAKLEY, M.D., F.R.C.P.
Consultant Physician, Hammersmith Hospital; Lecturer in Medicine (Clinical Cardiology), Royal Postgraduate Medical School, London.

W. G. REEVES, M.B., B.S., B.SC., M.R.C.P.
Lecturer in Immunology and Medicine, Royal Postgraduate Medical School, Hammersmith Hospital, London.

M. SHEPHERD, D.M., F.R.C.P., F.R.C.PSYCH., D.P.M.
Professor of Epidemiological Psychiatry, Institute of Psychiatry, University of London; Honorary Physician, Bethlem Royal and Maudsley Hospitals, London.

MARGARET TURNER-WARWICK, M.A., D.M., F.R.C.P., PH.D.
Professor of Medicine (Thoracic Medicine), University of London; Brompton Hospital and Cardiothoracic Institute, London.

H. S. WILLIAMS, M.SC., F.INST.P.
Chief Physicist, The Royal Free Hospital, London.

M. R. WILLS, M.D., M.R.C.PATH.
Reader in Chemical Pathology, Royal Free Hospital School of Medicine; Consultant Chemical Pathologist, Royal Free Hospital, London.

CONTENTS

CHAPTER 1

PARAMALIGNANT SYNDROMES

GERALD ANDERSON

Cancer frequently produces syndromes or generalised systemic effects which cannot be attributed to the mechanical effects of the tumour or its metastases. These paramalignant syndromes are clinically important since they may dominate the clinical picture or direct attention to a previously undiagnosed tumour. They are also of great theoretical importance in understanding the behaviour of malignant cells and of the host reaction to cancer. The paramalignant syndromes can be classified according to the particular tissue which is dominantly involved.

HORMONAL SYNDROMES

Tumours arising from non-endocrine tissues may give rise to endocrine disorders. In the majority of these syndromes there is evidence that the tumour secretes either normal body hormones or substances closely resembling them. The mechanism suppressing potential genetic information in normal cells is probably mediated by nuclear histones (Britten & Davidson, 1969). Tumour cells escape from suppression and it might be anticipated that ectopic hormones from these cells would resemble natural polypeptides which could be synthesised by enzymes and cytoplasmic ribose nucleic acid already in the cell rather than steroid hormones which require more complex biochemical mechanisms (Omenn, 1970). Most of the hormonal disorders of cancer have been shown to be due to polypeptide hormones.

Tumours arising from endocrine tissues will not be discussed.

The Ectopic-ACTH Syndrome

In 1928 Brown described a patient with Cushing's syndrome who was found at post-mortem to have bilateral adrenocortical hyperplasia and an oat cell bronchogenic carcinoma. This form of Cushing's syndrome with bilateral adrenocortical hyperplasia associated with a tumour is known as the 'Ectopic-ACTH syndrome' since it is due to release of an adrenocorticotrophic substance by the tumour. The associated tumour is usually bronchogenic or thymic. Azzopardi & Williams (1968) critically reviewed the previous reports of the Ectopic-ACTH syndrome and rejected many because of inadequate descriptions of the tumour histology or of the Cushing's syndrome. They divided the associated tumours into oat cell bronchial carcinomas, foregut tumours of endocrine origin, phaeochromocytomas and related tumours, and ovarian tumours. Except for oat cell carcinomas all the other tumours derive from endocrine tissue and Azzopardi & Williams suggested that the stem cell of oat cell carcinomas normally secreted ACTH or a related peptide since ACTH secretion by tumours was confined to such specific cell types that

1

it probably did not arise from random loss of ACTH suppression. In this respect it may differ from other normal syndromes.

Aetiology

In the Ectopic-ACTH syndrome the plasma contains an adrenal weight maintaining factor (Christy, 1961) and there is a high level of ACTH-like activity in plasma, tumour and metastases (Meador, Liddle, Island, Nicholas, Lucas, Nuckton & Leutscher, 1962). Tumour 'ACTH' and pituitary ACTH are indistinguishable in their biological reactions and give identical reactions with a fluorescent antibody (Jarrett, Lacy & Kipnis, 1964). In spite of this evidence the two compounds are not necessarily identical. ACTH contains 39 amino acids but adrenocorticotrophic activity is retained by molecules containing as few as 13 amino acids. The immunological activity of ACTH resides in the C-terminal portion of the molecule while the adrenocortical stimulating effect is in the N-terminal portion. Neurosecretory granules are a prominent feature of ACTH secreting tumours and may be the source of the hormone (Kay & Willson, 1970).

Hyperpigmentation is a feature of the Ectopic-ACTH syndrome and was originally attributed to the weak melanocyte stimulating action of ACTH. It was later shown that the pigmentary action of tumour extracts greatly exceeds that expected from the ACTH content. Melanocyte stimulating hormone and ACTH have been separately isolated from the same tumour. (Island, Shimizu, Nicholson, Abe, Ogata & Liddle (1965).) There is a close structural similarity between the molecules of ACTH and β melanocyte stimulating hormone and since the two compounds do not seem to occur separately in the pituitary or in tumours the same gene locus is probably responsible for their synthesis.

Clinical manifestations

In the majority of patients the syndrome is of very rapid onset. The clinical manifestations lag behind the biochemical features and the patients do not live long enough to develop clinical Cushing's syndrome. The ectopic-ACTH syndrome differs clinically from pituitary and adrenal forms of Cushing's syndrome since it is more common in men and occurs in an older age group. In addition diabetes mellitus, hyperpigmentation, oedema and the manifestations of hypokalaemia are all more prominent. The prognosis is poor and in one series the average survival time from first attendance was only 19 days (Friedman, Marshall-Jones & Ross, 1967). The reason for the poor prognosis is that these patients have hypokalaemia and often uncontrolled diabetes mellitus in addition to a malignant tumour.

Results of investigations

A striking feature is a hypokalaemic alkalosis which is less common in other forms of Cushing's syndrome (Bagshawe, 1960). The hypokalaemia is due to excessive renal potassium loss and is not corrected by oral potassium supplements. The serum cortisol level is raised with loss of the normal diurnal rhythm while urinary 17-oxogenic steroid excretion is elevated with normal excretion of 17-oxosteroids. Administration of exogenous ACTH usually fails to cause a rise in the serum cortisol level since the plasma ACTH normally exceeds the level at which maximal adrenal response occurs. The adrenal output of cortisol has escaped from pituitary control and is not suppressed by dexamethasone (Liddle, 1960). An elevated serum cortisol is commonly found in other cancer patients (Hatch, Segaloff & Ochsner, 1965) but is not associated with Cushing's syndrome, is suppressed by dexamethasone, rises further with administration of ACTH and is probably a non-specific stress effect of illness.

Treatment

The logical treatment is removal of the tumour, but this is rarely curative. Temporary remissions are sometimes obtained when the tumour is treated with radiotherapy or cytotoxic drugs. Bilateral total adrenalectomy may be a useful palliative measure but is often unjustified in a patient dying from a highly malignant tumour.

Hypokalaemia causes many of the unpleasant symptoms of the ectopic-ACTH syndrome and may be relieved by triamterene which reduces renal potassium loss (Meador, et al., 1962). Many other drugs have been used in this condition. Metyrapone inhibits the β-hydroxylase system responsible for the final step in cortisol synthesis. Occasional worthwhile palliation has been obtained using this drug (O'Riordan, Blanshard, Moxham & Nabarro, 1967), but most reports have been disappointing. The drug 2, 2bis (2-chlor-phenyl-4-chlorphenyl)-1, 1 dichlorethane (o, p-D.D.D.) and its derivate m, p-D.D.D. cause adrenal necrosis and atrophy in dogs, selectively affecting the zona fasciculata and reticularis. Both these drugs and aminoglutethimide which blocks corticosteroid synthesis have proved disappointing.

Non-Metastatic Hypercalcaemia

Hypercalcaemia in malignant disease may occur without bony metastases. A patient with a bronchogenic carcinoma without bone secondaries was described by Gutman, Tyson & Gutman (1936). Since then non-metastatic hypercalcaemia has frequently been described with a variety of tumours especially carcinoma of the breast, lung (squamous) and kidney. It was present in 32 per cent of cases of bronchogenic carcinoma coming to post-mortem (Azzopardi & Whittaker, 1969).

Aetiology

The parathyroid glands are not enlarged in non-metastatic hypercalcaemia, and immunoassay of a tumour and its metastases by Goldberg, Tashjian, Order & Dammin (1964) revealed a substance indistinguishable from para-thyroid hormone (PTH). This compound cross reacted with human and bovine PTH when treated with bovine parathyroid hormone antibody (Munson, Tashjian & Levine, 1965), but final proof has not been obtained that tumour 'PTH' is identical with the parathyroid hormone. There may be more than one form of non-metastatic hypercalcaemia since only 50 per cent of cases respond with a fall in serum calcium when given corticosteroids (Grimes, Fisher, Finn & Danowski, 1967).

Clinical manifestations

The clinical effects of hypercalcaemia are manifest in the kidney, gut and brain. The renal changes result in polyuria, thirst, dehydration and ultimately renal failure. The gastrointestinal effects are anorexia, nausea, vomiting, constipation and abdominal pain. The cerebral symptoms are headaches, psychosis, drowsiness and eventually coma. The association of headache, drowsiness and vomiting may lead to a mistaken diagnosis of cerebral metastases. Smaller elevations of serum calcium may be asymptomatic.

Results of investigations

The serum calcium may exceed 20 mg per 100 ml. Hypercalciuria is also present. The serum phosphorus is low and the alkaline phosphatase normal. Hypercalcaemia causes renal tubular damage and the resultant renal potassium leak may cause a hypokalaemic alkalosis. Non-metastatic hypercalcaemia closely resembles hyperparathyroidism with an increased renal phosphorous clearance and a decreased tubular reabsorbtion of phosphate. It may be distinguished from hyperparathyroidism by the more acute onset and a higher level of serum calcium. In non-metastatic hypercalcaemia, in addition, the changes of chronic hypercalcaemia are absent, hence renal stones, ectopic calcification or radiological evidence of hyperparathyroidism do not develop.

Treatment

Resection of the tumour results in a prompt return to normocalcaemia (Plimpton & Gellhorn, 1956). Following tumour irradiation the serum calcium is usually normal within a few days of initiating treatment. Cytotoxic drugs are less effective. The serum calcium may become elevated again when metastases appear but this is not invariable and presumably the metastases may lack ability to produce the hormone or produce only small amounts.

Patients with hypercalcaemia are dehydrated and require a high fluid intake, often intravenously. The dietary intake of calcium should be reduced. Corticosteroids relieve hypercalcaemia in about 50 per cent of cases (Grimes, et al., 1967). Corticosteroids should be given in doses as large as 100 mg of prednisone or 400 mg of hydrocortisone daily. Corticosteroids probably relieve hypercalcaemia by lowering tubular resorption of calcium. Oral phosphates are effective (Thalassinos & Joplin, 1968) by precipitating calcium in the gut, but may produce gastrointestinal symptoms. In emergency intravenous phosphate may be used but it may cause extraskeletal calcification (Breur & LeBauer, 1967). Intravenous sodium sulphate has been given but may cause dangerous hypernatraemia.

Syndrome of Inappropriate Secretion of Antidiuretic Hormone

The presence of hyponatraemia in cancer was first noted in a patient with bronchogenic carcinoma by Winkler & Crankshaw (1938), but these authors did not attribute the hyponatraemia to the presence of a substance with antidiuretic activity. The tumour most commonly associated with hyponatraemia is bronchogenic carcinoma, but hyponatraemia may also occur in non-malignant chest disease and in neurological disorders.

Aetiology

Schwartz, Bennett & Curelop (1957) described a patient with hyponatraemia and a bronchogenic carcinoma. They demonstrated release of an antidiuretic substance at a time when plasma osmolality was reduced so that its release was 'inappropriate'. Bioassay of the tumour showed the presence of a compound with antidiuretic activity. This syndrome could not result from pituitary release of ADH since it has been described in a patient whose posterior pituitary had been destroyed by a metastasis (Bower, Mason & Forsham, 1964). The hormone is chemically indistinguishable from arginine vasopressin. The tumour antidiuretic substance is inactivated by the vaso-pressinase system of normal human pregnancy plasma, while after exposure to a specific vasopressin antiserum the antidiuretic and milk-ejecting activity was lost (Vorherr, Massry, Utiger & Kleeman, 1968). Cell culture of tumour tissue showed that radioactive tyrosine is converted into vasopressin by the tumour (Klein, Rabson & Worksman, 1969). If the tumour ADH is assumed to be arginine vasopressin the level of urinary excretion is approximately ten times normal. In contrast to previous reports Whitelaw (1969) found that bioassay of a tumour from a patient with this syndrome showed oxytocic activity greater than that expected from arginine vasopressin, suggesting release of an abnormal ADH.

Where the syndrome occurs in non-malignant diseases, they can with a few exceptions, be classified into neurological and chest diseases. It has been suggested that in some neurological conditions there is reflex ADH secretion due to stimuli from damaged brain areas while in chest diseases there may be reflex pituitary ADH secretion from atrial or carotid body stimulation. (Olson, Buchan & Porter, 1969.)

Clinical manifestations

Hyponatraemia is sometimes asymptomatic but where the fall in serum sodium is more marked symptoms of water intoxication occur with weakness, lethargy, drowsiness, irritability, confusion, nausea and sometimes fits and coma. Oedema rarely occurs.

Results of investigations

Tumour ADH secretion results in an inability to dilute the urine or to excrete a free water load so that the urine is hyperosmolar to the plasma. The biochemical changes of this syndrome can be reproduced by giving ADH and water to normal subjects. The serum sodium is often reduced to less than 115 mmol per litre with relatively smaller reductions in serum potassium and chloride levels. Haemodilution leads to a low blood urea and haematocrit. The cause of the hyponatraemia is not fully understood. Hypervolaemia due to water retention would be expected to result in an increased glomerular filtration rate and natriuresis with depletional hypona-traemia. Hypervolaemia also leads to reduced aldosterone secretion resulting in dilutional hyponatraemia. This earlier concept of the pathogenesis of hyponatraemia is probably an oversimplification since the glomerular filtration rate in ADH may be normal (Fichman & Bethune, 1968) and some third factor seems to be involved possibly an intracellular shift of sodium (Kaye, 1966).

Patients with hyponatraemia and tumours sometimes show a functional defect of the proximal renal tubule with aminoaciduria, glycosuria, phos-phaturia, and an inability to acidify the urine (Rees, Rosalki & Maclean,

1960; Ross 1963), which results in excessive loss of urinary sodium, probably due to failure of sodium resorption in the proximal tubule. The cause of the tubular defect is unknown.

Treatment

The syndrome resolves with tumour resection and cure or relief may be obtained with treatment by radiotherapy or cytotoxic drugs. Oral or intravenous sodium chloride is promptly excreted and does not relieve the hyponatraemia. Water restriction is extremely effective and possibly acts by reducing the filtered sodium load. The syndrome may also respond to 9α-fluorohydrocortisone which has a potent sodium retaining effect.

Hyperthyroidism

Hyperthyroidism has been described in chorion carcinoma, hydatidiform mole, embryonal cell carcinoma of the testis, blood dyscrasias and carcinomas. In 300 cases of thyrotoxicosis Wanebo, Benua & Rawson (1966) found 83 had associated tumours although selection of cases may have been biased since the patients were attending a cancer clinic. In many reports there was no clinical evidence of thyrotoxicosis but unequivocally abnormal tests of thyroid function were present. This occult form of thyrotoxicosis was present in 7 of 93 patients with trophoblastic tumours (Odell, Bates, Rivlin, Lipsett & Hertz, 1963).

Assays of thyroid stimulating hormone (TSH) in paramalignant hyperthyroidism have shown raised levels unlike hyperthyroidism not associated with malignancy. A TSH-like substance extracted from a bronchogenic carcinoma, in a clinically euthyroid patient, was indistinguishable from pituitary TSH on bioassay and immunoassay (Hennen, 1967). The relatively high incidence of hyperthyroidism in trophoblastic tumours is probably related to the ability of normal placenta to produce TSH so that in these tumours the hormone production is probably not ectopic.

The clinical manifestations of paramalignant hyperthyroidism differ from other forms of thyrotoxicosis in the higher male incidence, later age of onset and the absence of goitre and eye signs. Lower levels of TSH are needed to release thyroxine than to produce goitre. Paramalignant hyperthyroidism is probably under-diagnosed because of the atypical clinical features and a tendency to attribute weakness and weight loss to the underlying tumour.

The syndrome responds to removal of the tumour and to antithyroid drugs.

Gynaecomastia and Gonadotrophin Secretion

Gynaecomastia has most frequently been described in lung cancer where it may be associated with hypertrophic pulmonary osteoarthropathy. Gynaecomastia has also been described in tumours of the liver, stomach, kidney, adrenal and retroperitoneal regions.

Four cases of anaplastic large cell bronchogenic carcinoma and gynaecomastia were studied by Fusco & Rosen (1966). In three where tumour tissue was available it contained gonadotrophic activity and the level of pituitary gonadotrophins was reduced. Preliminary characterisation of the hormone suggested it was luteinising hormone or chorionic gonadotrophin rather than follicle stimulating hormone (FSH). Subsequent reports have shown that gonadotrophin secretion occurs in other histological types of lung tumour and in hepatomas. In one case of lung cancer and gynaecomastia the venous blood from the tumour contained a higher level of FSH-like activity than the arterial blood, suggesting that the tumour secreted FSH which possibly stimulated the testes to produce oestrogen (Faiman, Colwell, Ryan, Hershman & Shields, 1967). An immunofluorescent method has been used to show that gonadotrophin is localised within tumour cells (Becker, Cottrell, Moore, Winnacker, Mathews & Katz, 1968).

Although gonadotrophins may sometimes be responsible for gynaecomastia there is no evidence that all cases of gynaecomastia can be attributed to this cause, since urine oestrogen levels have been normal in patients with gynaecomastia and tumours (Andrews, 1967). Starvation may cause gynaecomastia, but in cancer it frequently appears when the patient is well nourished.

Gynaecomastia is usually bilateral and may be painful. Galactorrhoea does not occur except in trophoblastic tumours. Testicular atrophy is sometimes present. The breasts show the histological changes of simple hyperplasia.

Tumour removal or radiotherapy relieves the condition. In a case of gynaecomastia and hypertrophic osteoarthropathy both conditions were relieved by vagotomy (Huckstep & Bodkin, 1958).

THE METABOLIC DISORDERS

Hyperglycaemia

Freund (1885) detected hyperglycaemia in 62 out of 70 patients with cancer. Following this report the association of cancer and hyperglycaemia was frequently noted so that a normal glucose tolerance test (GTT) was regarded as strong evidence against a diagnosis of cancer (Edwards, 1919).

Oral GTT's were performed in 628 cancer patients and 322 control subjects by Glicksman & Rawson (1956). No attempt was made to exclude those with hepatic metastases or with known diabetes mellitus. Diabetic levels were present in 37 per cent of cancer patients and in only 9 per cent of the normal subjects. Weisenfeld, Hecht & Goldner (1962) found impaired glucose tolerance in 32 per cent of a series of cancer patients but claimed it occurred in 37 per cent of a control series. The high incidence in the control subjects may have been because they were malnourished and ill since a diabetic GTT as a non-specific effect of illness has been described in tuberculosis, schizophrenia and multiple sclerosis. Impaired glucose tolerance does not mean diabetes mellitus and only represents an inability to deal with a non-physiological glucose intake. This impairment may be so gross that the patient becomes frankly diabetic. There is no evidence that this form of cancer hyperglycaemia is due to ectopic production of any hormone. In the case of lung cancer the serum cortisol is frequently elevated (Hatch, Segaloff & Ochsner, 1965) and possibly precipitates diabetes by its peripheral antagonism to insulin.

Hypoglycaemia

Hypoglycaemia in cancer is often classified as a hormonal syndrome, but since the mechanism of its production is obscure, this is unjustified.

The condition was first described by Doege (1930) in a patient with a mediastinal fibrosarcoma. The causative tumours are almost always large mesodermal tumours, mainly fibrosarcomas, or primary liver cell carcinomas.

Stimulation of the pancreatic β cells by tumour-produced trophic hormone seems an unlikely cause of hypoglycaemia since pancreatectomy does not improve the condition (Miller, Bolinger, Janigan, Crockett & Friesen, 1959). Most studies have attempted to determine whether the tumours produce insulin or a related substance or utilise excessive amounts of glucose. Tumour bioassays have sometimes shown the presence of an insulin-like material (August & Hiatt, 1958; Carey, Pretlow, Edzinli & Holland, 1966), and in one case the insulin-like activity was lost on adding beef insulin antibody to the tumour extract. In this patient there was a raised tumour vein lactate during glucose transfusion, although the serum insulin was normal and it was suggested that hypoglycaemia resulted from the insulin-like substance demonstrated in the tumour. Immunoreactive insulin was demonstrated in a tumour and its metastases by Shames, Dhurander & Blackard (1968). Tumour bioassay has demonstrated insulin in less than half of the recorded cases and immunoassay shows insulin-like activity even less frequently.

Tumours are known to show excessive glycolysis and it has been suggested that hypoglycaemia may be due to tumour uptake of glucose. Reliable reports of arterio-venous glucose differences across tumours are rare and even if correct the normal liver is capable of an enormous increase in glucose output which should compensate for any glucose utilisation by the tumour (Unger, 1966).

There is probably more than one mechanism of tumour hypoglycaemia including possibly a combination of insulin-like activity, defective hepatic glucose output, tumour trapping of glucose and ill defined insulin potentiators which may be released by the growth.

The clinical manifestations are episodic combinations of headache, visual disturbance, confusion, hallucinations, sometimes with focal neurological signs. Sweating, hunger and tachycardia are not marked.

The most effective treatment is tumour removal or radiotherapy (Ginsberg, 1964). The hypoglycaemia is not controlled by glucagon, diazoxide or corticosteroids.

Hyperuricaemia

The serum uric acid may be elevated in leukaemia, reticuloses and multiple myeloma because of the high turnover rate of malignant cells. Treatment of these diseases may result in an extremely high serum uric acid level and may cause an obstructive nephropathy (Kritzler, 1958) which may be prevented by treatment with allopurinol. In carcinomas a high uric acid level tends more often to be associated with metastases and hypercalcaemia is probably responsible for this. Clinical gout is rare in non-leukaemic malignancies. In a recent survey of 354 cases of gout, 2 had leukaemia but none, other tumours (Grahame and Scott, 1970).

Amyloidosis

Amyloidosis is a rare complication of malignancy and tends to be associated with multiple myeloma. In a post-mortem series of 93 patients with amyloidosis no cause was present apart from malignancy in 14 (Azzopardi & Lehner, 1966). Half of these 14 subjects had malignant reticuloses or myeloma. Paramalignant amyloidosis usually has features resembling secondary amyloidosis. In Hodgkin's disease radiotherapy and cytotoxic drugs have been claimed to accelerate deposition of amyloid. The frequent admixture of amyloid material and malignant cells suggests that amyloid is produced around the malignant cells as a local response to the tumour (Azzopardi & Lehner, 1966).

THE NEUROMYOPATHIES

Neuromyopathy is a collective term to describe the abnormalities of central nervous system, peripheral nerves, muscle and the autonomic nervous system occurring in malignancy. Bronchial carcinoma is the most commonly associated tumour since clinically detectable signs of neuromyopathy are present in 16 per cent of cases (Croft & Wilkinson, 1963). Nerve conduction studies and electromyography suggest that subclinical forms may be even more common (Moody, 1965).

It is a striking feature of the neuromyopathies that the progress of the neurological disorder bears an inconstant relation to the course of tumour growth. They precede the appearance of the tumour in most cases, often by many years, and in one-quarter of patients with lung cancer the neurological symptoms appear more than 3 years before the carcinoma (Morton, Itabashi & Grimes, 1966). Rarely they appear for the first time after successful resection of the growth. In general, treatment directed at the tumour does not influence the course of neuromyopathies.

Aetiology

Four theories have been advanced to explain the occurrence of neuromyopathies in cancer.

1. **Infection.** Cancer patients have an increased susceptibility to infections by bacteria, fungi and viruses. The histological features of progressive multifocal leukoencephalopathy are clearly different from the other neuromyopathies and have long been regarded as suggestive of viral infection. Zu Rheim & Chou (1965) recorded a patient with progressive multifocal leukoencephalopathy where the oligodendrocytes contained inclusion bodies indistinguishable from viruses of the *papova* group. These viruses cause cutaneous papillomata in man and this patient had many such lesions removed during the 6 years preceding his death. Probable *papova* virus inclusion bodies were also found in 4 cases of progressive multifocal leukoencephalopathy by Woodhouse, Dayan, Burston, Caldwell, Hume-Adams, Melcher & Urich (1967). It seems likely that this virus infects the oligodendrocytes which are then unable to maintain the normal myelin sheath. There is no evidence that any other form of neuromyopathy is due to infection.

2. **Toxic.** Tumours are known to secrete polypeptides and other substances and it is possible that they release an unknown toxin which causes neurological damage. This theory is unlikely in view of the observation that removal of the tumour does not usually improve the neurological lesion. Lambert & Rooke (1965) noted that the electromyographic (EMG) features of the myasthenic syndrome resembled those produced in normal muscle by neomycin, magnesium, and botulinus toxin which all interfere with acetycholine release at the neuromuscular junction. It is possible that the myasthenic syndrome is due to secretion by the tumour of a toxin with similar properties. This would explain the frequent symptomatic relief following tumour removal often found in the myasthenic syndrome.

3. **Autoimmune.** Organ specific antibodies against brain in 4 patients with sensory neuropathy were demonstrated by Wilkinson (1964), using a complement fixation technique. It was later shown (Wilkinson & Zeromski, 1965) that this antibody reacted with all parts of the central nervous system. Antibodies were absent in other types of neuromyopathy. The significance of these findings is difficult to assess since the antibodies may be produced as a secondary response to nerve cell damage rather than be causative. Tumours produce many types of specific antigen which evoke tumour antibodies. In some cases tumour and nervous tissue share common antigens resulting in an autoimmune antibrain response. Burnet (1965) postulated that in the neurological disease kuru. patients who were immunologically incompetent, tolerated persisting virus infections. The resultant release of brain antigens by damaged cells stimulated pathological clones of cells which caused further brain damage and antigen release. Once initiated such a process would perpetuate itself and if involved in the neuromyopathies

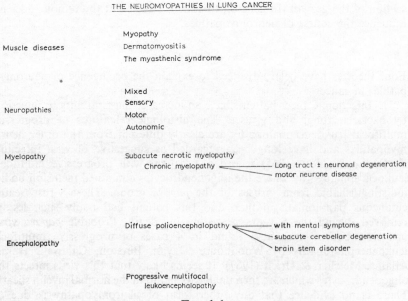

THE NEUROMYOPATHIES IN LUNG CANCER

Muscle diseases — Myopathy / Dermatomyositis / The myasthenic syndrome

Neuropathies — Mixed / Sensory / Motor / Autonomic

Myelopathy — Subacute necrotic myelopathy / Chronic myelopathy — Long tract ± neuronal degeneration / motor neurone disease

Encephalopathy — Diffuse polioencephalopathy — with mental symptoms / subacute cerebellar degeneration / brain stem disorder

Progressive multifocal leukoencephalopathy

FIG. 1.1

would explain their frequent progression after tumour removal. The spontaneous terminal remissions often seen could be due to the immunological incompetence of advanced cancer.

4. **Deficiency.** In experimental animal cancer the carcass fat may be reduced to 10 per cent of normal and large fat losses may be found with very small tumours. Marked loss of fat is often obvious clinically in human malignancy. Lipids comprise about half the dry weight of the brain and possibly such enormous losses of structural lipid may cause impaired neurological function (Costa & Holland, 1965). Earlier reports of the neuromyo-pathies often stressed the resemblance between these lesions and diseases produced by deficiencies of Vit. B_1 and B_{12} but the clinical and pathological features differ enormously. The peripheral neuropathy of carcinoma resembles that of B_1 and B_6 deficiency but does not respond to administration of these substances. The similarities between the two types of neuropathy merely seem to reflect the limited response of the peripheral nerve to a variety of abnormal stimuli.

Precise classification of the various forms of neuromyopathy is difficult and perhaps misleading as it may suggest that they exist as separate clear cut entities. These conditions very often co-exist and overlap. A suggested classification is a simplification of that proposed by Brain & Adams (1965) (Fig. 1.1). In 250 cases of lung cancer muscle disorders and neuromyopathy constituted about 80 per cent of cases and peripheral neuropathy 10 per cent; other syndromes were less common (Croft & Wilkinson, 1963).

Muscle Disorders

Understanding of these syndromes has been confused by the use of different names to describe the same condition.

Myopathy

This is the commonest type of neuromyopathy. The clinical course is subacute with symmetrical muscle weakness and wasting involving both girdles but more marked in the pelvic girdle and thighs so that difficulty in climbing stairs is usually an early symptom. The distal muscles are spared even where proximal weakness is severe. Peripheral neuropathy or the myasthenic syndrome are sometimes associated. In early or mild cases the diagnosis is frequently missed especially when the patient is confined to bed. The serum aldolase and creatine phosphokinase are raised when the process is active. The muscle histology is poorly described and may be normal even with gross muscle weakness. Where changes are present they are non-specific and possibly due to cachexia, and consist of patchy atrophy of individual fibres and areas of fibrosis. The EMG shows myopathic changes and motor conduction velocity is normal (Moody, 1965). It is difficult to judge the value of treatment since spontaneous remissions are common. Remissions are claimed to occur with corticosteroids using large initial doses (prednisone 40 mg to 80 mg daily), reducing to smaller maintenance doses (prednisone 5 mg to 15 mg daily). (Rose & Walton, 1966).

Dermatomyositis

The cutaneous changes in dermatomyositis will be discussed separately.

The myopathy is proximal. In the typical case it can be clearly differentiated from carcinomatous myopathy by the rash and other findings such as fever, arthralgia, dysphagia, dysarthria and Raynaud's phenomenon. Myopathy and dermatomyositis often overlap and precise diagnosis may be difficult. Some patients may not have a rash and the other features of dermatomyositis may be incomplete.

In dermatomyositis muscle biopsy shows fibre necrosis and infiltration by lymphocytes and the EMG shows myopathic changes. There is usually a good but incomplete response to corticosteroids.

The myasthenic syndrome

The myasthenic syndrome is almost always associated with intrathoracic tumours, usually oat cell carcinomas. The symptoms are muscle weakness and fatigability with delay in developing maximal strength on voluntary contraction. Muscle wasting is not prominent. Unlike myasthenia gravis there is loss or diminution of the tendon jerks, predominant involvement of the muscles of the shoulder and pelvic girdles, with relative or complete sparing of muscles supplied by the cranial nerves. The therapeutic test with edrophonium chloride (Tensilon) gives an incomplete response. Impotence, dryness of the mouth, peripheral neuropathy and myopathy may also be associated. In the myasthenic syndrome there is undue sensitivity to muscle relaxants of the competitive-inhibition type and to a lesser degree of the depolarising drugs. Use of muscle relaxants leads to prolonged paralysis and apnoea and may be fatal. Any patient with a carcinomatous myopathy or peripheral neuropathy should receive test doses of muscle relaxants before operation.

Muscle biopsy is unhelpful in confirming the diagnosis since normal muscle histology may accompany gross weakness (Lambert & Rooke, 1965). Where changes occur they are non-specific consisting of variations in fibre size, nuclear atrophy, loss of cross striations and fading of cellular outline. The EMG findings are usually characteristic and distinguish this condition from myasthenia gravis. In myasthenia gravis a single stimulus results in an action potential of normal amplitude but repeated rapid stimuli lead to a gradual fall in amplitude. In the myasthenic syndrome a single stimulus causes a reduced action potential even where the power of the muscle is normal. Repeated rapid stimuli result in facilitation with a temporary increase in amplitude followed by a progressive decline (Eaton & Lambert, 1957). Direct muscle stimulation gives a twitch of normal amplitude and conduction velocity in the peripheral nerves is normal. These findings show that the lesion is localised at the myoneural junction and the EMG characteristics indicate defective release of acetylcholine (Lambert & Rooke, 1965).

The myasthenic syndrome shows an incomplete response to anticholinesterases but guanidine hydrochloride is effective (Lambert & Rooke, 1965).

Neuropathies
Mixed neuropathy

A mixed neuropathy is the commonest type of neuropathy in cancer. It occurs with many different types of growth and may antedate appearance of the tumour by many years. The severity varies enormously. It may be asymptomatic and only diagnosed by finding absent tendon jerks and slowed nerve conduction. At the other extreme there may be a crippling sensorimotor defect. The clinical features are no different from mixed peripheral neuropathies due to other causes and remissions are fairly common and unrelated to tumour therapy.

On histological examination the muscles show the changes of denervation atrophy, while in the peripheral nerves there is a combination of axonal damage and segmental demyelination. (Victor, 1965.) These changes are more pronounced distally. Degenerative changes are also found in the anterior horn cells and neurones of the posterior root ganglion.

Sensory neuropathy

Sensory neuropathy is rare and almost invariably associated with bronchial carcinoma. It often precedes the appearance of the carcinoma.

The dominant feature is a progressive crippling sensory ataxia. All sensory modalities are lost with areflexia and paraesthesiae, while muscle power is normal. These abnormalities are more marked in the lower limbs. Nerve deafness is sometimes associated. Spontaneous remissions may occur but disability is always severe. The C.S.F. protein is often raised and sensory nerve action potentials are absent (Moody, 1965). The histological features are of sensory radiculitis. In the posterior root ganglion there is neuronal degeneration with perivascular lymphocytic cuffing. Secondary degeneration is present in the posterior columns and there is patchy degeneration of the peripheral nerves. Corticosteroids are claimed to produce occasional remissions.

Motor neuropathy

Motor neuropathy is poorly described. There may be great difficulty in distinguishing it from anterior horn cell disease, mixed peripheral neuropathy and myopathy especially, since these tend to occur together. The mixed form of peripheral neuropathy is sometimes dominantly motor and cases of motor neuropathy are possibly variants of this.

Autonomic neuropathy

Ivy (1961) recorded a patient with lung cancer and hyponatraemia who developed postural hypotension, anhidrosis and retention of urine without obstruction. A further case with postural hypotension, syncope, impotence and peripheral neuropathy was described by Siemsen and Meister (1963). The hypotension was reversed by angiotensin and adrenaline analogues. No necropsy was obtained.

Myelopathy

Myelopathy may occur in isolation or in association with sensory neuropathy.

Subacute necrotic myelopathy

Subacute necrotic myelopathy is usually but not invariably associated with malignancies. The syndrome was reviewed by Mancall & Rosales (1964). It is extremely rare. Clinically there is a rapidly progressive flaccid paraplegia with loss of all forms of sensation in the legs, areflexia and loss of sphincter control. Death occurs within 2 months of the onset. The C.S.F. may show an elevated protein and a pleiocytosis. The pathological changes are most marked in the thoracic cord with relative sparing of the lumbar region. There are large areas of necrosis and cavitation not limited to specific tracts and involving both grey and white matter. Secondary gliosis occurs and there are sometimes vascular changes which are probably a reaction to necrotic nerve tissue rather than a true vasculitis.

Chronic myelopathy

(a) **Long tract degeneration.** This produces a variable clinical picture depending on the relative amount of involvement of long tracts and neurones. Long tract involvement is usually associated with the various types of polio-encephalopathy, especially the cerebellar syndrome and is rarely isolated (Greenfield, 1934). Clinically there is a combination of pyramidal signs, loss of deep pain, position and vibration sense and a variable degree of motor weakness. Where neuronal damage also occurs there is again usually evidence of polio-encephalopathy although the cord signs may dominate the clinical picture. These patients have a combination of generalised sensory loss and sensory ataxia with motor weakness and loss of tendon jerks. Fasciculation is present; there may also be dementia. The findings resemble those of motor neurone disease with superadded sensory signs. At post-mortem there is long tract degeneration together with the findings of polio-encephalitis. There may also be loss of anterior horn cells in the cervical and upper thoracic cord with diffuse microglial activity and perivascular cuffing. Both anterior and posterior roots show demyelination and fibrosis.

(b) **Motor neurone disease (MND).** The maximum incidence of MND is between 50 and 70 years when the incidence of cancer is high so that co-existence of the two conditions may be fortuitous. Ten per cent of a group of 130 patients with amyotrophic lateral sclerosis had cancer, compared to 1·6 per cent of a control group with strokes (Norris & Engel, 1965). The apparent lower incidence in the controls may have been due to the shorter period of observation, failure to search for occult tumours and a lower necropsy incidence in this group. In another series (Shy & Silverstein, 1965) cancer was present in 4·6 per cent of patients with MND which was approximately the expected incidence in this age group.

Cases of cancer with MND have usually shown the typical findings of amyotrophic lateral sclerosis with mixed upper and lower motor neurone lesions. Progressive muscular atrophy with lower motor neurone signs alone is much less common. It has been suggested (Brain, Croft & Wilkinson, 1965) that carcinomatous MND pursues a slower course, but this impression may be erroneous since the number of patients studied was small.

The C.S.F. protein is sometimes raised. Electromyography reveals the typical findings of MND with fibrillation potential, reduction in the number of action potentials on maximal contraction and giant units. Motor conduction is normal. Fibre loss occurs both in the peripheral nerves and anterior roots. In the anterior horns and bulbar nuclei there is striking cell loss and the corticospinal fibres often degenerate. Brain *et al.* (1965) claimed the histological findings differed from typical MND since two of their series had histological evidence of sensory radiculitis. It is possible that these patients had a chance association of malignant sensory neuropathy and typical MND unrelated to the tumour.

In summary the evidence for the existence of a paramalignant form of MND is not totally convincing.

Encephalopathy

Diffuse polioencephalopathy

There is considerable overlap between the various forms of polio-encephalopathy and pure syndromes are uncommon. In spite of this a particular group of features usually dominates the clinical picture.

(a) Psychiatric manifestations. The most common finding is a toxic psychosis or a progressive dementia, but almost any psychosis or psycho-neurosis may occur, and patients often present at psychiatric units. Focal neurological signs are uncommon but pyramidal signs may be present. Spontaneous remissions are fairly common. The C.S.F. is usually normal and the EEG diffusely abnormal. Multiple cerebral metastases may give a similar picture, but signs of raised intracranial pressure and focal signs are usually present and the EEG and brain scan show focal lesions in most cases. The pathological findings are not well described. The changes may resemble those of limbic encephalitis with microglial nodules and lympho-cytic cuffing involving the hippocampus, amygdaloid nucleus and cingulate and orbital cortex (Henson, Hoffman & Urich, 1965). Gliosis is sometimes more diffuse and occasionally no abnormality is found. In general, the site and severity of the pathological lesions does not correlate well with the clinical findings.

(b) Subacute cerebellar degeneration. Brain & Wilkinson (1965) reviewed 19 personal cases and 20 others from the literature. The most common associated tumour was bronchial carcinoma but a large number were found with ovarian carcinoma. Cerebellar degeneration often precedes the appear-ance of the malignancy. The onset is subacute and the main feature is a rapidly progressive cerebellar ataxia involving all four limbs and sometimes the trunk. Dysarthria is usually present but nystagmus is inconstant and not marked. Extracerebellar lesions are usually present such as combinations of dementia, psychosis, pyramidal signs, sensory symptoms, diminished tendon reflexes or myopathy. Spontaneous remissions are common. The C.S.F. protein may be raised and the Lange colloidal gold curve is sometimes ab-normal. The striking pathological finding is degeneration of the Purkinje cells, the fibres leading from these cells to the dentate nucleus and the direct spinocerebellar tracts. Degenerative changes may be present in the posterior columns and less commonly in the cerebral cortex, subthalamic, dentate and occulomotor nuclei and in the anterior horn cells of the medulla and cord. There is patchy microglial activity in the white matter of the cerebellar and cerebral cortices. Perivascular cuffing is often found but is usually regarded as a reaction to rapidly degenerating nervous tissue rather than a primary phenomenon.

(c) Brain stem degeneration. This disorder is not sharply defined clinically or pathologically and is always associated with other forms of neuromyo-pathy. The lesions predominantly affect the lower pons and medulla leading to vertigo, dysarthria, ophthalmoplegia, bulbar palsy, nystagmus and extensor plantar responses. Death is often due to the neurological disability rather than the underlying carcinoma. The pathological changes are neuronal degeneration and perivascular cuffing involving the tegmentum and medulla.

Progressive multifocal leukoencephalopathy

This condition is usually associated with diseases characterised by immunological incompetence such as leukaemias, reticuloses and carcinomatosis. Progressive multifocal leukoencephalopathy is very rare. Forty-four cases were reviewed by Richardson (1965). The neurological signs are rapidly progressive and death usually occurs within 6 months of the onset. There are varying combinations of hemiparesis, quadriparesis, dementia, dysphasia, dysarthria, cerebellar ataxia, lower cranial nerve palsies, and sensory loss with a steady progression of signs. No treatment is available. The C.S.F. may show an elevated protein level and the EEG is diffusely abnormal. In the brain there are widely scattered areas of focal perivascular demyelination which later become confluent and involve both grey and white matter. The lesions are more marked in the posterior part of the cerebral hemispheres and may extend into the cord. Microscopically, in the focal lesions, the oligodendroglial nuclei are large and bizarre and contain inclusion bodies. Giant astrocytes are often present in the focal lesions and in the grey matter there is necrosis of nerve cells.

SKIN CHANGES

Abnormalities of the skin are a common finding in cancer patients and are often the first sign of a tumour. There are two groups of paramalignant skin disease. In the first the cause of the rashes is uncertain but they are secondary to malignancy. In the second congenital disorders of the skin are associated with an increased tendency to develop internal tumours, sometimes at particular sites.

Secondary Skin Disease
Dermatomyositis

Estimates of the frequency of cancer in dermatomyositis have varied considerably. There is a tendency to report those cases associated with tumours, and malignancy probably occurs in about 15 per cent of cases (Williams, 1959). In a case of breast carcinoma an aqueous tumour extract gave strongly positive immediate-type skin reactions in the same patient (Grace & Dao, 1959). Other authors have described complement-fixing antibodies in high titres which became lower following tumour removal. It is possible that dermatomyositis may result from tumour antibodies which cross react with skin and muscle.

The rash is violaceous and involves the nose, cheeks, ears, toes and dorsum of the hands. The non-cutaneous features which may accompany the rash have already been described. The tumour may not become apparent for many years after the first appearance of dermatomyositis and the condition usually improves after tumour resection.

Acanthosis nigricans

Acanthosis nigricans may occur as a congenital abnormality which is totally unrelated to cancer. Acquired acanthosis nigricans is almost invariably associated with internal carcinomas which are usually intra-abdominal and carry a poor prognosis. In about 75 per cent of cases the tumour is an adenocarcinoma (Curth, Hilberg & Machacek, 1962). The rash is warty and pigmented and involves mainly the axilla, groin and mouth.

Other rashes

Bowen's disease (intra-epidermal carcinoma of the skin) may appear many years before an internal tumour. It is not always accompanied by malignancy but in one series 5 of 9 patients with Bowen's disease developed tumours (Sneddon, 1963).

Erythema gyratum repens is a rare but characteristic rash which spreads in waves, giving the skin a woody appearance, and is associated with carcinoma of the bronchius.

Hypertrichosis lanuginosa is extremely rare but of such striking appearance that it can be immediately recognised. The entire hair bearing surface of the skin becomes covered with long red-blond hair giving an ape-like appearance. A congenital form is not associated with cancer but the acquired type always indicates a tumour, usually a small-cell bronchogenic carcinoma (Hensley & Glynn, 1969).

Many of the more common rashes seen in cancer patients are very non-specific and sometimes the association may be coincidental. Such non-specific rashes are generalised pigmentation, urticaria, erythema multiforme, periphigoid and ichthyosis. Generalised exfoliative dermatitis is sometimes seen in leukaemia and reticuloses. Pruritus is fairly common in all types of tumours.

Congenital Skin Disorders with Increased Incidence of Internal Malignancy

Such skin conditions are uncommon but it is important to appreciate their association with internal tumours.

Both Werner's syndrome (premature ageing) and the basal cell naevus syndrome are associated with a raised incidence of cancer. In the Peutz–Jeghers syndrome there is buccal pigmentation with gastrointestinal polypi which are usually benign but may become malignant. With adenoma sebaceum a cutaneous manifestation of tuberose sclerosis there may be neurogliomas and renal tumours. Neurofibromatosis is sometimes accompanied by phaeochromocytomas. Tylosis is a congenital hyperkeratosis of the palms and soles and although it is not usually related to malignancy in a single family there was an extremely high incidence of oesophageal carcinoma (Howel-Evans, McConnell, Clarke & Sheppard, 1958).

CARDIOVASCULAR ABNORMALITIES
Venous Thrombosis

Venous thrombosis occurs in all types of malignancy but is especially common in carcinoma of the body and tail of the pancreas, and in mucous secreting adenocarcinomas. The thrombus is bland with little reaction in the underlying vein wall and pulmonary embolisation is frequent. In patients with cancer and also in non-cancerous post-operative patients, the plasma may contain an increased concentration of a substance indistinguishable from antihaemo-philic-globulin (AHG) and the common factor predisposing to thrombo-embolism in both groups may be tissue injury resulting in a raised plasma AHG (Amunsden, Spittell, Thompson & Owen, 1963). Slight elevations of the platelet count are present in bronchial carcinoma (Levin & Conley, 1964) and paramalignant venous thrombosis may be due to combinations of a raised plasma AHG, thrombocythaemia and in some instances, a mucin-like compound secreted by adenocarcinomas which results in clotting.

The most striking clinical manifestation of venous thrombosis in cancer is the syndrome of thrombophlebitis migrans. This involves many veins often at unusual sites such as the upper extremities and superior vena cava, and venous gangrene may supervene. Thrombophlebitis migrans may be an early warning sign of malignancy. The condition does not respond to anticoagulants including heparin (De Matteis & Bonucci, 1964) but may respond to tumour removal (Fisher, Hochberg & Wilensky, 1951). The relation of cancer to a single typical episode of venous thrombosis is probably often indirect and due to immobility and surgery.

Non-bacterial Thrombotic Endocarditis

A form of endocarditis has long been recognised which is distinct from that due to infection, rheumatic fever and syphilis. This non-bacterial thrombotic endocarditis is not specifically related to malignancy and may be found at post-mortem in all types of chronic disease. Where this form of endocarditis is present at post-mortem, approximately 40 per cent of cases are found to have cancer (McDonald & Robbins, 1957; Eliakim & Pinchas, 1966). In some instances the endocarditis and thrombophlebitis migrans seem to be manifestations of the clotting tendency of cancer since they fre-quently occur in the same patient (Robbins & McDonald 1957; Rohner, Prior & Sipple, 1966).

The valve lesions are usually left-sided and the mitral valve is more often involved than the aortic although both may be affected. There are nodular friable vegetations of all sizes on the valve cusps. These vegetations may be single or multiple and consist of fibrin with enmeshed red cells, white cells and platelets. In the underlying valve there is a marked paucity of cellular reaction, but the valve contains swollen degenerated fibrin which merges imperceptibly with the thrombus (Rohner *et al.*, 1966). There is a predilection for valves scarred by previous rheumatic carditis and tiny ulcerated areas on the valve probably act as a nidus on which thrombus is deposited.

The presenting clinical features are those of arterial embolisation which may precede clinical appearance of the carcinoma by many months. Cerebral emboli can give rise to almost any neurological picture; hemiplegia is frequent and may be sudden or stuttering in onset. Extracerebral emboli are usually silent and only recognised at autopsy but splenic infarcts and splinter haemorrhages may be detected. Renal emboli may result in haema-turia and uraemia. The cardiac lesions probably do not cause murmurs (Eliakim & Pinchas, 1966), and where these have been heard they may have been due to anaemia or an unrelated rheumatic lesion.

HAEMATOLOGICAL DISORDERS
Anaemia

Anaemia frequently accompanies cancer, and Hyman & Harvey (1955) found that 90 per cent of a group of patients with carcinoma were anaemic and all eventually became so. The anaemia was originally attributed to bone marrow metastases, but its severity does not correlate with the presence or extent of such secondary deposits. Anaemia can sometimes be confidently attributed to factors such as blood loss, inadequate iron intake, surgery or cytotoxic drugs.

Normocytic anaemia

The majority of cancer patients with anaemia have a normochromic normocytic anaemia without any clinically apparent cause. Although an increased plasma volume is present in cancer (Kelly, Bierman & Shimkin, 1952) haemodilution is probably not an important factor. The two factors which are probably responsible are increased destruction and reduced production of red cells.

In patients with tumours haemolysis is not evident from the results of serum bilirubin, the Coombs' test, reticulocyte count, or faecal and urinary urobilinogen levels. There is, however, an accelerated rate of destruction of transfused normal red cells (Hyman, 1954). In lung cancer a modified Coombs' test using low dilutions of serum showed a positive reaction in 47 per cent of 343 patients (Green, Wakefield & Littlefield, 1957). Green et al., suggested that patients with carcinoma had incomplete cold antibodies which were possibly produced by the malignant cells. Normal tissues are known to contain haemolytic soaps and lysolecithins, and these haemolysins are also present in malignant cells but may be structurally different (Gross, 1948). Adelsberger & Zimmerman (1959) took rabbit tumour antiserum absorbed with lung sediment from normal and cancer-bearing human lungs. When added to blood the supernatant from the tumour caused clumping of red cells not seen with the supernatant from normal lung. It has been suggested that antibodies may bind to red cells without causing agglutination or haemolysis but resulting in an increased rate and altered site of destruction (Jandl & Kaplan, 1960). These authors studied a patient with hypogamma-globulinaemia who was passively immunised with anti-B serum and was then given group B red cells. With small doses of antibody there was slow splenic trapping of red cells, with larger doses rapid hepatic trapping, and with even bigger doses rapid intravascular haemolysis. The haemolytic element of normocytic paramalignant anaemia may be due to tumour haemolysins or to incomplete antibodies which cause either an increased rate or an altered site of red cell destruction.

Decreased red cell production may seem at first sight to be an unlikely cause of the normocytic anaemia of cancer since the bone marrow is usually normal or hyperactive. In carcinoma there is usually a normal or increased rate of radioactive iron turnover suggesting that marrow activity is, if any-thing, increased. Erythropoiesis may, however, be ineffective for there is often a discrepancy between the red cell mass in the peripheral circulation and total marrow red cell production, even in the absence of blood loss or haemolysis (Giblett, Coleman, Pirzio-Biroli, Donohue, Motulsky & Finch, 1956). In ineffective erythropoiesis there is a raised faecal urobilinogen, plasma iron turnover and *erythroid/myeloid* ratio. This is not accompanied by a reticulocytosis or increased red cell radioactive iron clearance which measure effective erythropoiesis. The ineffective erythropoiesis of malignancy may be due to coating of red cell precursors with antibodies (Betts, Rigby, Friedell & Emeson, 1962).

In malignancy, although total erythropoiesis is increased much of the activity is ineffective so that the marrow cannot keep pace with the increased haemolysis.

Other less common anaemias

Autoimmune haemolytic anaemia with a positive Coombs' test is usually associated with leukaemias and reticuloses although it is sometimes present in carcinomatosis. The anaemia may appear many years before the under-lying disorder becomes evident. It usually responds well to treatment with corticosteroids. It now seems probable that malignancy may be a compli-cation of autoimmune disease.

Pure red cell aplasia is a rare cause of anaemia and about half of the cases described have occurred with thymomas. The anaemia sometimes responds to tumour removal. There is a severe normochromic normocytic anaemia with a decrease or absence of reticulocytes. In the bone barrow, nucleated red cell precursors are absent or hypoplastic. In a case recorded by Entwhistle, Fentem & Jacobs (1964) the serum contained a factor which inhibited erythropoiesis in the rabbit. This factor disappeared when the tumour was irradiated, possibly indicating it was produced by the malignant cells. In 9 cases of pure red cell aplasia and thymoma, antinuclear factor was present in the serum and in all of 4 patients where it was sought the serum contained an immunoglobulin which retarded growth of bone marrow cells in culture (Barnes, 1966).

Sideroblastic anaemia and megaloblastic anaemia due to utilisation of folate by malignant cells are rare causes of cancer anaemia, except in leukaemia.

Erythrocytosis

Erythrocytosis has been related to benign and malignant renal disease, uterine myomata and cerebellar haemangioblastoma. It is also found in hepatomas and malignant tumours of the adrenal glands and ovary. In many instances assays of the tumour and plasma have claimed to demonstrate elevated levels of erythropoeitin. A critical review claimed that of 200 reports of erythrocytosis associated with tumours erythropoeitin assays had been performed in 21. In only one instance had tumour activity been satis-factorily related to a standard erythropoeitin (Malpas, Blandford, White & Wrigley, 1967). Malpas *et al.* found normal or reduced serum erythropoeitin levels in leukaemic patients. A more complex mechanism for paramalignant erythrocytosis was suggested by Gordon, Zanjani & Zalusky (1970). They found no erythropoeitic stimulating activity in tumour extract from a patient with erythrocytosis and a tumour. When tumour homogenate was incubated with renal erythropoeitic factor from hypoxic rats an erythropoeitic stimulating factor was detected. It was suggested that in tumour tissue there was increased production or availability of substrate for renal erythropoeitic factor with resultant formation of erythropoeitic stimulating factor leading to erythrocytosis. Removal of the tumour in erythrocytosis leads to a prompt return of the red cell count to normal.

Syndrome of Disseminated Intravascular Coagulation

The syndrome of disseminated intravascular coagulation consists of a bleeding tendency with shock and renal failure due to widespread blood coagulation in small vessels, resultant consumption of clotting elements leading to the bleeding tendency. It is associated with a variety of diseases and also occurs in transfusion reactions and severe trauma. In malignant disease it is especially seen in carcinomas of the pancreas and prostate. In cancer there is activation of both the coagulation and fibrinolytic systems (Miller, Sanchez-Avalos, Stefanski & Zuckerman, 1967; Soong & Miller, 1970). In most patients the opposing systems balance each other but the control mechanism is set at a higher level, and minor stimuli such as venous stasis or operation may cause either local or disseminated intravascular coagulation. It seems possible that if clotting occurs in the heart it causes thrombotic non-bacterial endocarditis, in the veins thrombophlebitis migrans and in the capillaries disseminated intravascular coagulation.

RENAL DISEASE

Renal disease in malignancy may be a complication of extrarenal paramalignant disorders such as gout, amyloid and damage due to hypercalcaemia. There is now evidence that the nephrotic syndrome may sometimes be paramalignant. In 101 cases of this syndrome 11 had malignant disease against an expected incidence of one. (Lee, Yamauchi & Hopper, 1966.) The lesion in 9 was membranous glomerulonephritis, with lobular glomerulonephritis and lipoid nephrosis each in a single case. The authors postulated that tumour antibodies resulted in soluble antigen–antibody complexes which were deposited in glomerular basement membrane. Three further cases with a review of the literature were reported by Loughridge & Lewis (1971). In one case focal changes progressed to membranous glomerulonephritis over a three-year period and the other 2 had membranous glomerulonephritis. In one case immunofluorescence was used to demonstrate the presence of IgG on the basement membrane and the nephrotic syndrome was attributed to deposition of antigen–antibody complexes in this region.

STEATORRHOEA

In view of the marked cachexia so often seen in malignancy, several studies of the small bowel have been made in cancer patients. Jejunal biopsies were reported by Deller, Murrell & Blowes (1967) in 45 patients with various malignant conditions. Normal villus structure was seen in only 38 per cent, and the remainder had combinations of simple atrophy, partial atrophy and subtotal atrophy. Steatorrhoea was present in 15 cases. Similar biopsy results were obtained in another series of 16 cases and half the patients had an abnormal xylose excretion (Dymock, Mackay, Miller, Thompson, Gray,

Kennedy & Adams, 1967). Klipstein & Smarth (1969) obtained rather different results in 24 patients with non-gastrointestinal tumours. Of 18 biopsies 15 were normal and 3 showed minor abnormalities which were regarded as probably insignificant. They pointed out that Deller *et al.* had not defined their understanding of the terms simple and partial villus atrophy and many patients had received abdominal radiotherapy which may have caused villus changes leading to steatorrhoea. Klipstein & Smarth found a dubiously abnormal faecal fat excretion in only one of 20 subjects and although xylose excretion was often reduced the peak blood xylose level was normal so the reduced xylose excretion was difficult to explain.

It seems probable that villus atrophy and malabsorption in cancer are rarer than was originally believed. Possibly, when villus atrophy is present it is due to folate deficiency from to excessive folate utilisation by tumour tissue, since folate deficiency would be likely to become manifest in gastrointestinal epithelium which has a high rate of cell turnover. (Somayaji, 1970.)

UNCLASSIFIED DISORDERS

Cachexia

Cachexia is one of the most striking effects of malignant disease and is probably the most common single cause of death in cancer patients. In general it accompanies advanced malignancy, but sometimes patients may have only small tumours yet considerable cachexia. Weight loss is most marked in the subcutaneous fat and voluntary muscles but involves all organs except the liver and brain. Cachexia is accompanied by anorexia but in spite of the reduced food intake the basal metabolic rate is inappropriately raised and may fall when the tumour is removed. (Heindl & Trauner, 1927.) Most of the experimental work in cancer cachexia has involved the Waller 256 tumour in rats. This bears little relation to human cancer since it is transplantable and may eventually form 40 per cent of the animal's weight so that great care is needed in extrapolating these results to human tumours.

Animal studies

In malignancy the tumour accumulates nitrogen while the host carcass loses nitrogen especially from the skeletal muscle. In animals during starvation tumours continue to grow and obtain nitrogen from the tissues of the host (White, 1945). This passage of amino acids is unidirectional and tumour protein is probably not available for use by the host. The tumour successfully competes with the host for the available nitrogen pool, acting as a 'nitrogen trap'. In the rat hepatoma the malignant cells have an increased power to incorporate amino acids and glucose into protein (Zamecnik, Loftfield, Stephenson & Steele, 1951). Animal tumours are associated with hyperlipaemia and in rats food fat is built into the tumour (Haven, Bloor & Randall, 1951), although unlike protein, the tumour fat can then be mobilised from the tumour for use by the host. Mider, Sherman & Morton (1949) showed that rats bearing the Waller 256 carcinoma had a greater loss of body weight and fat than control animals on the same diet. This suggested that the tumour had an action of increasing the caloric expenditure of the host by an unknown mechanism.

Human studies

In human cancer anorexia causes reduced protein intake and protein metabolism is disordered. Nitrogen balance studies have yielded conflicting results and the state of nitrogen balance may depend on the stage of tumour growth and the state of the patient's nutrition. Where overall nitrogen equilibrium is present the tumour retains nitrogen. In malignant disease there is a failure of incorporation of labelled methionine into albumen (Holland, 1970), suggesting a defect in protein synthesis, while there is also an increased level of alanine in the blood (Cahill, 1970) possibly from increased protein breakdown. Tumours may increase body energy expenditure since a negative nitrogen balance may be seen on a diet adequate for the patient without cancer (Waterhouse, Fenniger & Keutmann, 1951). Hyper-lipaemia is not found in human malignancies, but the level of free fatty acids is high and in individual patients is closely related to degree of activity of the tumour (Mueller & Watkin, 1961). These fatty acids play an important role in fat transport, and this finding may mean that they are used as an alternative energy source.

Force feeding may reverse cachexia in animal tumours, but in man this procedure is limited by anorexia. The use of tube feeding, with a high protein, high calorie diet with vitamin supplements, has been claimed to improve patients' general condition and to give a positive nitrogen balance with disappearance of anorexia and cachexia (Pareira, Conrad, Hicks & Elman, 1955). These findings were not confirmed in a careful study of 9 patients by Terapka & Watkins (1956). Although considerable weight gain took place with forced feeding this was largely due to increased intracellular water and nitrogen retention was transient.

Fever

Fever in malignancy can sometimes be attributed to intercurrent infection or tumour necrosis, but in the majority of cases neither of these factors is present and the cause of pyrexia is obscure. It is common in the presence of liver metastases (Fenster & Klatskin, 1961) and is a notable feature of renal carcinomas where it may antedate other tumour symptoms and is relieved by tumour removal. Three cases of renal carcinoma were studied by Rawlins, Luff & Cranston (1970). Two were pyrexial and injection of tumour extract from these two subjects into rabbits gave a pyrexial response with no response to extracts from the apyrexial patient. Rawlins et al. considered that in the pyrexial patients the tumour contained a pyrogen which might be a normal endogenous pyrogen from leucocytes migrating to the tumour or more probably a pyrogen released by the tumour.

Alcohol Intolerance

Alcohol induced pain is found in 17 per cent of patients with Hodgkin's disease, and where it is present the tumours tend to show more fibrosis and eosinophilia with fewer reticulum-cell mitoses (James, 1960). The pain appears within fifteen minutes of drinking and may last for several hours. It may be severe and usually occurs at the site of proliferating tissue. The pain has occasionally been described in other types of malignancy and in benign bone diseases. Brewin (1966) considered that alcohol intolerance was much more common in carcinomas than had previously been thought. He found the most common manifestation of alcohol intolerance was alcohol induced pain, but some patients experienced tumour bleeding after alcohol and others a bizarre and variable group of symptoms such as terror, vomiting and sweating. The cause of alcohol intolerance is unknown.

Finger Clubbing

Finger clubbing commonly accompanies bronchogenic carcinoma and pleural mesothelioma. It is less commonly present in pulmonary metastases and is frequently associated with a wide variety of benign disorders both within and outside the thorax. In the subungual tissues there is an increased amount of fibrous connective tissue with dilated arteries and veins and many arteriovenous anastomoses.

Precapillary bronchopulmonary anastomoses were demonstrated in patients with clubbing by Cudkowicz & Armstrong (1953), and Bashour (1961) claimed that there was an intrapulmonary left-to-right blood shunt amounting to 20 per cent of the cardiac output which might allow a vasodilator substance to by pass the lungs and result in clubbing. Barium sulphate was injected into the lungs at autopsy, via the bronchial supply in a group of patients with various chest diseases by Turner-Warwick (1963). About half the patients had clubbed fingers and in these there was a consistent bilateral increase in size of both the bronchial and pulmonary vascular bed. Turner-Warwick considered that the bronchopulmonary anastomoses previously described were due to fortuitous linking up of proliferating bronchial and pulmonary vessels while the left-to-right blood shunts could be due to passage of blood from bronchial arteries to bronchial veins and into the left atrium. This would allow 'tissue-metabolite' produced by the tumour to bypass the lungs and cause clubbing. Hall (1959) postulated that reduced ferritin was the vasodilator responsible for clubbing since it is normally oxidised in the lung. Hall measured radioactive sodium clearance in the fingers as an index of finger blood flow. A reduced clearance was found in finger clubbing presumably due to subungual arteriovenous shunts. The reduced clearance was corrected by the flavinoid rutin which is a specific antagonist to reduced ferritin suggesting that reduced ferritin was responsible for finger clubbing.

In all the diseases associated with clubbing, the affected organs are innervated by the vagus and in ulcerative colitis finger clubbing is only present if the affected part of the colon is supplied by the vagus (Young, 1966). It seems possible that clubbing arises through a reflex mechanism which, in a large variety of diseases of vagally innervated organs, results in afferent impulses to the central vagal connections. This causes pulmonary and finger vasodilatation by an unknown humoral or neural efferent reflex. This hypothesis would not require postulation of the elusive 'tissue metabolite' and would explain the presence of clubbing in so many unrelated diseases.

Hypertrophic Pulmonary Osteoarthropathy

Hypertrophic pulmonary osteoarthropathy is still sometimes regarded as an advanced variety of finger clubbing but is clinically different and is a much more specific sign of malignancy than finger clubbing. Finger clubbing may occasionally be absent. Approximately 95 per cent of patients with arthropathy have an intrathoracic tumour and it is uncommon in benign lung disease. The condition is not found in oat cell bronchogenic carcinomas (Yaccoub, 1965) and is more common in peripheral lung tumours. It may antedate the radiological appearance of the tumour by as much as five years.

The arthropathy is rapidly relieved by vagotomy (Flavell, 1956; Huckstep and Bodkin, 1958) and this seemed to incriminate a neural or neurohormonal reflex in its aetiology. Limb blood flow is increased and this increase is abolished by bilateral cervical vagotomy but not by blocking motor vagal impulses with atropine (Holling, Brodley & Boland, 1961). Holling *et al.* found no increase in blood flow in normal animals with cross circulation to dogs with hypertrophic pulmonary osteoarthropathy and their evidence suggested that it was due to a reflex mechanism with an afferent arc in the vagus while the efferent arc was unknown. This interpretation did not explain why limb blood flow fell on incision of the parietal pleura and on subperiosteal rib resection in two of the animals studied. Ginsburg & Brown (1961) claimed that urine oestrogen excretion was more than twice as high in cancer patients with arthropathy than in those without this complication. Riyami & Anderson, (unpublished observation) have been unable to confirm this and found no elevation of urinary oestrogens in 7 patients with arthropathy, 2 of whom had gynaecomastia.

The clinical manifestations are finger clubbing which is usually gross in degree, together with polyarthritis, painful bones, circulatory disturbances and sometimes gynaecomastia. The arthropathy is painful and symmetrical being most marked in the ankles, wrists and knees. The bone pain is deep seated and continuous but worse if the limbs are dependent. It is most marked in the lower thirds of the arms and legs but other bones may be involved. The limbs are hot, red and sweating, and ankle oedema is frequent. Gynaecomastia is present in about 7 per cent of patients. (Semple & McCluskie, 1955.) Thickening of the facial features is occasionally seen.

On histological examination the periosteum is infiltrated by lymphocytes, plasma cells and leucocytes. The periosteum is converted to bone forming osteoid matrix. The joint synovium is thickened and congested with areas of fibrinoid degeneration. Periosteal new bone formation can be demonstrated radiologically and gives an appearance of concentric lamellae or sometimes of candle-wax dripping down a candle. Radiographs of the joints merely show soft tissue swelling and the diagnosis may be missed if the long bones are not included in the film.

References

ADELSBERGER, L. & ZIMMERMAN, H. M. (1959). *Acta. Un. Int. Cancr.*, **15**, 480.
AMUNDSEN, M. A., SPITTELL, J. A., THOMPSON, J. H. & OWEN, C. A. (1963). *Ann. intern. Med.*, **58**, 608.
ANDREWS, J. T. (1967). *Med. J. Aust.*, **7**, 451.
AUGUST, J. T. & HIATT, H. A. (1958). *New Engl. J. Med.*, **258**, 17.

AZZOPARDI, J. G. & LEHNER, T. (1966). *J. clin. Path.*, **19**, 539.
AZZOPARDI, J. G. & WHITTAKER, R. S. (1969). *J. clin. Path.*, **22**, 718.
AZZOPARDI, J. G. & WILLIAMS, E. D. (1968). *Cancer, Philad.*, **22**, 274.
BAGSHAWE, K. D. (1960). *Lancet*, **2**, 284.
BARNES, R. D. (1966). *Lancet*, **2**, 1464.
BASHOW, F. A. (1961). *J. Lab. clin. Med.*, **58**, 613.
BECKER, K. L., COTTRELL, J., MOORE, C. F., WINNACKER, J. L., MATTHEWS, M. J.
    & KATZ, S. (1968). *J. clin. Endocr.*, **28**, 809.
BETTS, A., RIGBY, P. G., FRIEDELL, G. H. & EMESON, C. P. (1962). *Blood*, **19**, 687.
BOWER, B. F., MASON, D. M. & FORSHAM, P. H. (1964). *New Engl. J. Med.*, **27**, 934.
BRAIN, Lord & ADAMS, R. D. (1965). *In* "The Remote Effects of Cancer on the Ner-
    vous System". Ed. Lord Brain & F. Norris, p. 216. Baltimore: Grune &
    Stratton.
BRAIN, Lord, CROFT, P. B. & WILKINSON, M. (1965). *Brain*, **88**, 479.
BRAIN, Lord & WILKINSON, M. (1965). *Brain*, **88**, 465.
BREUR, R. T. & LE BAUER, J. (1967). *J. clin. Endocr.*, **27**, 695.
BREWIN, T. B. (1966). *Br. med. J.*, **2**, 437.
BRITTEN, R. J. & DAVIDSON, E. H. (1969). *Science*, **165**, 349.
BROWN, W. H. (1928). *Lancet*, **2**, 1022.
BURNET, F. M. (1965). *Lancet*, **1**, 1141.
CAHILL, K. (1970). *Cancer Res.*, **30**, 2816.
CAREY, R. W., PRETLOW, T. G., EDZINLI, E. Z. & HOLLAND, J. F. (1966). *Am. J.
    Med.*, **40**, 458.
CHRISTY, N. P. (1961). *Lancet*, **1**, 85.
COSTA, G. & HOLLAND, J. F. (1965). *In* "The Remote Effects of Cancer on the
    Nervous System". Ed. Lord Brain & F. Norris, p. 125. Baltimore: Grune &
    Stratton.
CROFT, P. B. & WILKINSON, M. (1963). *Lancet*, **1**, 184.
CUDCOWICZ, L. & ARMSTRONG, J. B. (1953). *Br. J. Tuberc.*, **47**, 227.
CURTH, H. O., HILBERG, A. W. & MACHACEK, G. F. (1962). *Cancer, Philad.*, **15**,
    364.
DELLER, D. J., NURRELL, T. G. C. & BLOWES, R. (1967). *Aust. ann. Med.*, **16**, 236.
DE MATTEIS, A. & BONUCCI, E. (1964). *J. Path. Bact.*, **88**, 597.
DOEGE, K. W. (1930). *Ann. Surg.*, **92**, 955.
DYMOCK, I. W., MACKAY, N., MILLER, V., THOMPSON, T. J., GRAY, B., KENNEDY,
    E. A. & ADAMS, J. F. (1967). *Br. J. Cancer*, **21**, 505.
EATON, L. M. & LAMBERT, E. H. (1957). *J. Am. med. Ass.*, **163**, 1117.
EDWARDS, S. (1919). *J. Indiana med. Ass.*, **12**, 296.
ELIAKIM, M. & PINCHAS, S. (1966). *Israel J. Med. Sci.*, **2**, 42.
ENTWHISTLE, C. C., FENTEM, P. H. & JACOBS, A. (1964). *Br. med. J.*, **2**, 1504.
FAIMAN, C., COLWELL, J. A., RYAN, R. J., HERSHMAR, J. M. & SHIELDS, T. W. (1967).
    New Eng. J. Med., **277**, 1395.
FENSTER, L. & KLATSKIN, G. (1961). *Am. J. Med.*, **31**, 238.
FICHMAN, M. P. & BETHUNE, J. E. (1968). *Ann. intern. Med.*, **68**, 806.
FISHER, M. M., HOCHBERG, L. A. & WILENSKY, N. D. (1951). *J. Am. med. Ass.*,
    147, 1213.
FLAVELL, G. (1956). *Lancet*, **1**, 260.
FREUND, E. (1885). *Wien med. Bl.*, **8**, 268.
FRIEDMAN, M., MARSHALL-JONES, P. & ROSS, E. J. (1967). *Q. Jl. Med.*, **35**, 193.
FUSCO, F. D. & ROSEN, S. W. (1966). *New Eng. J. Med.*, **275**, 507.
GIBLETT, E. R., COLEMAN, D. H., PIRZIO-BIROLI, G., DONOHUE, D. M., MOTULSKY,
    A. G. & FINCH, C. A. (1956). *Blood*, **11**, 291.
GINSBERG, D. M. (1964). *Adv. internal Med.*, **12**, 33.
GINSBURG, J. & BROWN, J. B. (1961). *Lancet*, **2**, 1274.

GLICKSMAN, A. S. & RAWSON, R. W. (1956). *Cancer*, **9,** 1127.

GOLDBERG, M. F., TASHJIAN, A. H., JR., ORDER, S. E. & DAMMIN, G. J. (1964). *Amer. J. Med.*, **36,** 805.

GORDON, G. A., ZANJANI, E. D. & ZALUSKY, R. (1970). *Blood*, **35,** 151.

GRACE, J. T. & DAO, T. L. (1959). *Cancer, Philad.*, **12,** 648.

GRAHAME, R. & SCOTT, I. J. (1970). *Ann. rheum. Dis.*, **29,** 461.

GREEN, W. H., WAKEFIELD, J. & LITTLEFIELD, G. (1957). *Br. med. J.*, **2,** 779.

GREENFIELD, J. G. (1934). *Brain*, **57,** 161.

GRIMES, B. J., FISHER, B., FINN, F. & DANOWSKI, T. S. (1967). *Acta endocr., Copenh.*, **56,** 510.

GROSS, L. (1948). *Proc. Soc. exp. Biol. Med.*, **70,** 656.

GUTMAN, A. B., TYSON, T. L. & GUTMAN, E. B. (1936). *Archs. intern. Med.*, **57,** 379.

HALL, G. H. (1959). *Lancet*, **1,** 750.

HATCH, H. B., SEGALOFF, A. & OCHSNER, A. (1965). *Ann. Surg.*, **161,** 645.

HAVEN, F. L., BLOOR, W. R. & RANDALL, C. (1951). *Cancer Res.*, **11,** 619.

HEINDL, A. & TRAUNER, R. (1927). *Mitt. Grenzgeb. Med. Chir.*, **40,** 416.

HENNEN, G. (1967). *J. clin. Endocr.*, **27,** 610.

HENSLEY, G. T. & GLYNN, K. P. (1969). *Cancer, Philad.*, **24,** 1051.

HENSON, R. A., HOFFMAN, H. L. & URICH, H. (1965). *Brain*, **88,** 449.

HOLLAND, J. F. (1970). *Cancer Res.*, **30,** 2816.

HOLLING, H. E., BRODLEY, R. S. & BOLAND, H. C. (1961). *Lancet*, **2,** 1269.

HOWEL-EVANS, W., MCCONNELL, R. B., CLARKE, C. A. & SHEPPARD, P. M. (1958). *Q. Jl. Med.*, **27,** 413.

HUCKSTEP, R. L. & BODKIN, P. E. (1958). *Lancet*, **2,** 343.

HYMAN, G. A. (1954). *Blood*, **9,** 911.

HYMAN, G. A. & HARVEY, J. E. (1955). *Am. J. Med.*, **19,** 350.

ISLAND, D. P., SHIMIZU, W. E., NICHOLSON, K., ABE, E., OGATA, E. & LIDDLE, G. W. (1965). *J. clin. Endocr.*, **25,** 975.

IVY, H. K. (1961). *Archs. intern. Med.*, **108,** 47.

JAMES, A. H. (1960). *Q. Jl. Med.*, **29,** 47.

JANDL, J. H. & KAPLAN, M. E. (1960). *J. clin. Invest.*, **39,** 1145.

JARRETT, L., LACY, P. E. & KIPNIS, D. M. (1964). *J. clin. Endocr. Metab.*, **24,** 543.

KAY, S. & WILLSON, M. A. (1970). *Cancer, Philad.*, **26,** 445.

KAYE, M. K. (1966). *Am. J. Med.*, **41,** 910.

KELLY, K. H., BIERMAN, H. R. & SHIMKIM, M. B. (1952). *Cancer Res.*, **12,** 814.

KLEIN, L. A., RABSON, A. S. & WORKSMAN, J. (1969). *Surg. Forum.*, **20,** 231.

KLIPSTEIN, F. A. & SMARTH, G. (1969). *Am. J. dig. Dis.*, **14,** 887.

KRITZLER, R. A. (1958). *Am. J. Med.*, **25,** 532.

LAMBERT, E. H. & ROOKE, D. E. (1965). *In* "The Remote Effects of Cancer on the Nervous System". Ed. Lord Brain & F. Norris, p. 67. Baltimore: Grune & Stratton.

LEE, J. C., YAMAUCHI, H. & HOPPER, J. (1966). *Ann. intern. Med.*, **64,** 41.

LEVIN, J. & CONLEY, C. L. (1964). *Archs. intern. Med.*, **114,** 497.

LIDDLE, G. W. (1960). *J. clin. Endocr. Metab.*, **20,** 1539.

LOUGHRIDGE, L. W. & LEWIS, M. G. (1971). *Lancet*, **1,** 256.

MCDONALD, R. A. & ROBBINS, S. L. (1957). *Ann. inter. Med.*, **46,** 255.

MALPAS, J. S., BLANDFORD, G., WHITE, R. J. & WRIGLEY, D. F. M. (1967). *Proc. R. Soc. Med.*, **61,** 463.

MANCALL, E. L. & ROSALES, R. K. (1964). *Brain*, **87,** 639.

MEADER, C. K., LIDDLE, G. W., ISLAND, D. P., NICHOLSON, W. E., LUCAS, C. P., NUCKTON, J. G. & LUETSCHER, J. A. (1962). *J. clin. Endocr.*, **22,** 693.

MIDER, G. B., SHERMAN, C. D. & MORTON, J. J. (1949). *Cancer Res.*, **9,** 222.

MILLER, D. R., BOLINGER, R. E., JAMIGAN, D., CROCKETT, J. E. & FRIESEN, S. R. (1959). *Ann. Surg.*, **150,** 624.

MILLER, S. P., SANCHEZ-AVALOS, J., STEFANSKI, T. & ZUCKERMAN, L. (1967). *Cancer, Philad.*, **20**, 1452.

MOODY, J. F. (1965). *Brain*, **88**, 1023.

MORTON, D. L., ITABASHI, H. H. & GRIMES, O. F. (1966). *J. Thorac. Cardiovasc. Surg.*, **51**, 14.

MUELLER, P. S. & WALKIN, P. M. (1961). *J. Lab. clin. Med.*, **57**, 95.

MUNSON, P. L., TASHJIAN, A. H., JR., & LEVINE, L. (1965). *Cancer Res.*, **25**, 1062.

NORRIS, F. H., JR. & ENGEL, W. K. (1965). *In* "The Remote Effects of Cancer on the Nervous System". Ed. Lord Brain & F. Norris, p. 24. Baltimore: Grune & Stratton.

ODELL, W. D., BATES, R. W., RIVLIN, R. S., LIPSETT, M. B. & HERTZ, R. (1963). *J. clin. Endocr.*, **23**, 658.

OLSON, D. R., BUCHAN, G. C. & PORTER, G. A. (1969). *Archs intern. Med.*, **124**, 741.

OMENN, G. S. (1970). *Ann. intern. Med.*, **72**, 136.

O'RIORDAN, J. L. H., BLANSHARD, G. P., MOXHAM, A. & NABARRO, J. D. N. (1967). *Q. Jl. Med.*, **35**, 137.

PAREIRA, M. D., CONRAD, E. J., HICKS, W. & ELMAN, R. (1955). *Cancer, Philad.*, **8**, 803.

PLIMPTON, C. H. & GELLHORN, A. (1956). *Am. J. Med.*, **21**, 750.

RAWLINS, M. D., LUFF, R. H. & CRANSTON, W. I. (1970). *Lancet*, **1**, 1371.

REES, J. R., ROSALKI, S. B. & MACLEAN, A. D. W. (1960). *Lancet*, **2**, 1005.

RICHARDSON, E. P., JR. (1965). *In* "The Remote Effects of Cancer on the Nervous System". Ed. Lord Brain & F. Norris, p. 6. Baltimore: Grune & Stratton.

ROHNER, R. F., PRIOR, J. T. & SIPPLE, J. H. (1966). *Cancer, Philad.*, **19**, 1805.

ROSE, A. L. & WALTON, J. N. (1966). *Brain*, **89**, 747.

ROSS, E. J. (1963). *Q. Jl. Med.*, **32**, 297.

SCHWARTZ, W. B., BENNETT, W. & CURELOP, S. (1957). *Am. J. Med.*, **23**, 529.

SEMPLE, T. & McCLUSKIE, R. A. (1955). *Br. med. J.*, **1**, 754.

SHAMES, J. M., DHURANDER, N. R. & BLACKARD, W. G. (1968). *Am. J. Med.*, **44**, 632.

SHY, G. M. & SILVERSTEIN, I. (1965). *Brain*, **88**, 515.

SIEMSEN, J. K. & MEISTER, L. (1963). *Ann. intern. Med.*, **58**, 669.

SNEDDON, I. B. (1963). *Br. med. J.*, **2**, 405.

SOMAYAJI, B. N. (1970). *Br. med. J.*, **4**, 680.

SOONG, B. C. F. & MILLER, S. P. (1970). *Cancer, Philad.*, **25**, 867.

TEREPKA, R. & WATERHOUSE, C. (1956). *Am. J. Med.*, **20**, 225.

THALASSINOS, N. & JOPLIN, J. F. (1968). *Br. med. J.*, **4**, 14.

TURNER-WARWICK, M. (1963). *Thorax*, **18**, 238.

UNGER, R. H. (1966). *Am. J. Med.*, **40**, 325.

VICTOR, M. (1965). *In* "The Remote Effects of Cancer on the Nervous System". Ed. Lord Brain & F. Norris, p. 134. Baltimore: Grune & Stratton.

VORHERR, H., MASSEY, S. G., UTIGER, R. D. & KLEEMAN, C. R. C. (1968). *J. clin. Endocr.*, **28**, 162.

WANEBO, H. J., BENUA, R. S. & RAWSON, R. W. (1966). *Cancer, Philad.*, **19**, 1523.

WATERHOUSE, C., FENNINGER, L. D. & KEUTMANN, E. H. (1951). *Cancer, Philad.*, **4**, 500.

WEISENFELD, S., HECHT, A. & GOLDNER, M. G. (1962). *Cancer, Philad.*, **15**, 18.

WHITE, F. R. (1945). *J. natn. Cancer Inst.*, **5**, 265.

WHITELAW, A. G. L. (1969). *Br. J. Cancer*, **23**, 69.

WILKINSON, P. C. (1964). *Lancet*, **1**, 1301.

WILKINSON, P. C. & ZEROMSKI, J. (1965). *Brain*, **88**, 529.

WILLIAMS, R. C., JR, (1959). *Ann. intern. Med.*, **50**, 1174.

WINKLER, A. W. & CRANKSHAW, O. F. (1938). *J. clin. Invest.*, **17**, 1.

WOODHOUSE, M. A., DAYAN, A. D., BURSTON, J., CALDWELL, I., HUME-ADAMS, J., MELCHER, D. & URICH, H. (1967). *Brain*, **90**, 863.

YACCOUB, M. H. (1965). *Thorax*, **20**, 537.

YOUNG, J. R. (1966). *Br. med. J.*, **1**, 278.

ZAMECNIK, P. C., LOFTFIELD, R. B., STEPHENSON, M. L. & STEELE, J. M. (1951). *Cancer Res.*, **11**, 592.

ZU RHEIM, G. M. & CHOU, M. (1965). *Science*, **148**, 1477.

CHAPTER 2

PERIPHERAL NEUROPATHY

PAMELA M. LE QUESNE

The use of modern tools such as the electron microscope, electronic apparatus, and radioactive isotopes has greatly increased our knowledge of peripheral nerve structure and function. Further understanding of many pathological conditions has resulted from more frequent use of diagnostic nerve biopsy and the study of experimental toxic neuropathies in animals. The contribution of these studies will be considered first, followed by a discussion of some specific disease in which important recent advances have been made.

CLASSIFICATION

Peripheral neuropathies are, at present, most conveniently classified on a pathological basis, such as suggested by Thomas (1969). This classification is based on the element primarily or predominantly affected.

1. **Disorders of neurones** (resulting in primary axonal degeneration):
    (*a*) Metabolic: uraemia, porphyria, alcoholism.
    (*b*) Toxic: organophosphates, acrylamide, *p*,bromophenyl urea, organic mercury, arsenic, isoniazid, vincristine, furadantin, thalidomide, thallium.

2. **Disorders of supporting tissues**
    Schwann cells (resulting in primary segmental demyelination):
    (*a*) Metabolic: diabetes.
    (*b*) Immunological: Guillain-Barré syndrome.
    (*c*) Toxic: lead, diphtheria.
    (*d*) Infective: leprosy.
    (*e*) Hereditary: Charcot-Marie-Tooth, sulphatide lipidosis, Krabbe's disease, hypertrophic neuropathy (Déjèrine-Sottas, Refsum's).
    Connective tissues: amyloidosis, sarcoidosis, Fabry's disease, primary biliary cirrhosis.

3. **Disorders of blood vessels.** Polyarteritis nodosa, arteriosclerosis, rheumatoid arthritis.

Vascular disorders may produce both segmental demyelination and axonal degeneration, the former change being more prominent if ischaemia is mild and the latter if more severe.

The distinction between the two types of pathological change is not absolute in the diseases listed above. For example, in uraemia, porphyria and alcoholism, although axonal degeneration is the predominant pathological change, some segmental demyelination has also been described. In chronic experimental lead poisoning segmental demyelination is the main process, but in severe acute poisoning axonal degeneration may be marked. The extent to which axons and Schwann cells are interdependent is still unknown. However, at our present state of knowledge it is still useful to classify diseases into the broad groups described above depending on the predominant change. This is helpful in diagnosis, because the electro-physiological as well as pathological findings differ in these main groups.

In the connective tissue diseases peripheral nerve biopsy is particularly likely to be helpful in diagnosis. For example amyloid deposits or sarcoid lesions can be easily recognised. The value of nerve biopsy and the problems of quantitation have been discussed in a report produced by a sub-committee of the Research Group on Neuromuscular Diseases of the World Federation of Neurology (Thomas, 1970). This report provides a useful assessment of the present diagnostic value of nerve biopsy, and stresses its usefulness in connective tissue and arteritic disorders. It also provides a basis for future development of this technique.

PATHOLOGY

Axonal degeneration

Disorders of neurones or axons result in degeneration of both axis cylinders and myelin sheaths. Trauma to nerve fibres by crush or section produces the classical pathological changes described by Waller. Most other types of axonal degeneration are indistinguishable by light microscopy from Wallerian degeneration. However, different types of degeneration may be recognised by the distribution of pathology, group of fibres predominantly affected or electron microscopic appearance of the axon or cell body.

A common pattern of degeneration is that initially the longest fibres die back from the periphery. The significance of this process has been discussed by Cavanagh (1964a). Despite the distal pathology, the most likely site of the metabolic disturbance is thought to be the cell body, the initial effects being apparent at the most remote part of the neurone. Organophosphate compounds (e.g. triorthocresyl phosphate (TOCP)), acrylamide and p-bromophenyl urea produce this type of lesion. By contrast in isonizid and organomercury neuropathy in rats, although long fibres are affected more severely than short ones, degeneration affects the proximal parts of the fibres at a much earlier stage (Cavanagh, 1967, 1969).

Different types of fibre are predominantly affected in the neuropathies produced by the substance already mentioned. In TOCP poisoned cats the main and initial damage occurs to large sensory fibres from the muscle spindle annulospinal formation (Cavanagh, 1964b). Motor and medium sized sensory fibres are mainly affected in isoniazid neuropathy, the large diameter spindle afferents being strikingly spared. In organo-mercury neuropathy damage is confined to sensory fibres. These differences presumably reflect some as yet unidentified biochemical lesion.

A further difference between different types of neuropathy is in the speed and degree of regeneration. Electrophysiological and pathological evidence of regeneration is found early after acute acrylamide intoxication. Indeed, in chronic poisoning regeneration occurs while exposure continues both in animals and man (Fullerton & Barnes, 1966; Fullerton, 1969a). On the other hand, regeneration is very poor after damage by thalidomide. Sensory disturbances persist for many years after removal from exposure in a large proportion of patients (Fullerton & O'Sullivan, 1968). These authors found a marked reduction in the number of fibres, particularly those of large diameter, in sural nerves obtained at biopsy from patients two to six years after stopping the drug. In some, an increase in the number of small fibres was taken to indicate attempted regeneration but without maturation of the regenerating fibres.

In the neuropathies already discussed, axonal changes on light microscopy are indistinguishable from those seen during typical Wallerian degeneration. Chromatolysis may be seen in the cell bodies of affected neurones, possibly associated with regenerative processes, as following nerve crush or section, but more extensive or specific changes have not been seen. Specific changes are seen in the neuropathy produced by thallium, where axonal swellings occur before fibres degenerate completely (Allsop, 1953). Another axonal neuropathy in which a characteristic change may be seen on light microscopy is that produced by the vinca alkaloids, vincristine and vinblastine. Intracellular microcrystals, although more obviously recognisable on electron microscopy, have been identified with light microscopy by Schochet, Lampert & Earle (1968).

Electron microscopy reveals characteristic early axonal changes in other neuropathies. For example, Prineas (1969b) has described an accumulation of neurofilaments in the early stages of acrylamide intoxication in cats, with prominent mitochrondrial changes occurring later. These appearances are distinct from those seen in TOCP intoxication (Prineas, 1969a), in which the earliest change is accumulation of abnormal membrane bound vesicles and tubules in the distal parts of the axons. The development of flat membrane-bound sacs in the distal axons in thiamine deficient rats (Prineas, 1970a) produces yet another different electron microscopic appearance. These changes are all different from those seen during Wallerian degeneration.

Segmental demyelination

The myelin of each internodal segment is part of the membrane of one Schwann cell (Geren, 1954; Robertson, 1955). Primary Schwann cell disorders result in patchy degeneration of myelin sheaths, the axons remaining in continuity, a process known as segmental demyelination. This process was first described in 1880 by Gombault in lead poisoned guinea pigs and has subsequently been described in many conditions, including diphtheritic neuropathy (Webster et al., 1961) and experimental allergic neuritis (Cragg & Thomas, 1964). The diseases in man in which segmental demyelination predominates have been reviewed by Gilliatt (1966) and include diabetes and the Guillain-Barré syndrome.

Light microscopic changes are essentially similar in segmental demyelination whatever its cause. The earliest change is widening of the nodes of Ranvier. Degeneration of myelin may then spread to involve either part or the whole of an internodal segment. If only a short length of myelin degenerates, repair may occur from the existing segment without the formation of a new internode. Allt (1969) has observed this process electron microscopically following the intraneural injection of diphtheria toxin in rats.

He suggests that this type of regeneration occurs if the nodal widening is less than 15 μm. If a longer length of myelin has degenerated then one or more new internodes are formed during repair. In normal nerves internodal distance increases with fibre diameter, thus large fibres have long internodes (up to 1 mm). Newly formed internodes are short (usually of the order of 200 μm). In large diameter fibres demyelination of part of a segment is repaired by formation of a single intercalated new internode. If the whole segment has degenerated several new internodes are formed. Thus, repair of segmental demyelination results in a marked variation of internodal length

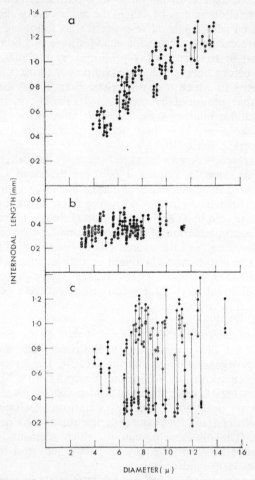

FIG. 2.1. (a) Normal guinea pig nerves.
   (b) Nerves after crush.
   (c) Nerves after segmental demyelination produced by lead or diphtheria toxin.

Closed circles indicate length of individual internodal segments. Values for different internodal segments of the same fibre are joined by a line. A single value for diameter is given for each fibre, this is the diameter of the largest internodal segment measured in the fibre concerned. (Fullerton et al., 1965).

along large diameter fibres. Previous episodes of demyelination may be recognised by measurement of single fibres as described by Fullerton et al. (1965) and shown in Fig. 2.1. The marked variation in internodal length along individual fibres following segmental demyelination in diphtheritic and lead neuropathy may be contrasted with the uniformly short internodal lengths of the large diameter fibres that have regenerated following Wallerian degeneration, a finding originally described by Vizoso & Young (1948).

Measurements of internodal distance and diameter do not distinguish between normal, regenerated or remyelinated small diameter nerve fibres, since the newly formed segments are approximately the same length as the original ones. However, distinction may be possible by electron microscopy. Ochoa (1970) was able to recognise small diameter regenerating fibres in isoniazid neuropathy by their arrangement in clusters.

From electron microscopic studies it seems that myelin may break down in more than one way. Webster et al. (1961) have described the changes in diphtheritic neuropathy. Fragmentation of myelin lamellae occurs within Schwann cells initially in the region of the nodes of Ranvier. Then loss of normal myelin compaction occurs along the internode at the axonal or Schwann cell surface and particularly near Schmidt-Lantermann incisures. Later ovoid masses of degenerating myelin are present within macrophages. Weller (1965) has suggested that the lysosomes which accumulate in the juxta-axonal Schwann cytoplasm in the early stages of diphtheritic neuropathy in the chicken are important in initiating demyelination. Cellular invasion in diphtheritic neuropathy occurs after myelin degeneration has started.

On the other hand, invasion of the nerve fibres by mononuclear cells appear to be the initiating factor in demyelination in experimental allergic neuritis (EAN) and the Guillain-Barré syndrome (Lampert, 1969; Wisniewski et al., 1969). Lampert (1969) has described focal lysis of myelin adjacent to invading mononuclear cells in EAN. Outer myelin lamallae are then split by processes of the invading cells. Schwann cells do not multiply and act as macrophages in this, in contrast to other types of segmental demyelination.

Hypertrophic neuropathy

The appearance of 'onion bulbs' in transverse sections of peripheral nerves examined by light microscopy was for long considered a specific diagnostic feature of the hypertrophic polyneuropathy of Déjèrine and Sottas. Later, similar histological appearances were recognised to occur in Refsum's disease. In 1956 Austin questioned the specificity of the 'onion bulb' appearance and more recent work has supported Austin's view. For example, Thomas & Lascelles (1966) described the appearance of 'onion bulbs' in the nerves of a patient with diabetic neuropathy, and later Ballin & Thomas (1968b) studied nerves from 9 other patients with diabetic neuropathy. Hypertrophic changes were visible on electron microscopy in 5 of them. They postulated that the hypertrophy might be a reaction to frequent episodes of demyelination and remyelination. Dyck (1969) supported this view as a result of experiments whereby a tourniquet was repeatedly inflated around rat nerves.

Before hypertrophic nerves were examined electron microscopically it was impossible to be sure whether the concentric layers of cell processes were derived from Schwann cells or from fibroblasts. However, it is now known that they are predominantly or entirely derived from Schwann cells. The processes are surrounded by a basement membrane, which is characteristic of Schwann cells but not of fibroblasts (Thomas & Lascelles, 1967; Weller, 1967; Webster et al., 1967).

Segmental demyelination was found to be the predominant degenerative process in the nerves from patients with hypertrophic neuropathy by Thomas & Lascelles (1967) and by Weller (1967). On the other hand, Webster et al. (1967) found little evidence of segmental demyelination in the nerves they studied and concluded that the hypertrophic changes occurred largely around small surviving myelinated or unmyelinated fibres. It thus appears that different pathological processes may underlie hypertrophic changes.

Nerve Conduction in Pathological Conditions

With the development of modern electronic apparatus conduction in motor and sensory nerve fibres can be studied in increasing detail. Conduction velocity in fast conducting, large diameter motor fibres is easily estimated by recording the muscle response to nerve stimulation at two sites. The distance between the stimulating points divided by the difference in conduction time of the two responses gives an estimate of conduction velocity. Conduction cannot yet easily be studied in the slower conducting alpha motor nerve fibres, nor in the gamma motor fibres to the muscle spindles.

Sensory conduction may be measured by recording nerve action potentials after stimulation of sensory nerve trunks, such as the digital nerves of the fingers. The amplitude of such potentials may be very small (1–10 μV) when recorded through the skin because of attenuation in the intervening structures. Electronic averaging of many potentials is usually necessary for accurate measurement of the amplitude and latency of the potentials. The development and refinement of electronic averagers has enabled sensory conduction to be studied in some detail. Estimation of conduction velocity in the fastest conducting sensory fibres is relatively simple. Buchthal & Rosenfalk (1971) have been able to identify late components of nerve action potentials of less than 0·5 μV in amplitude and estimate conduction in more slowly conducting sensory fibres.

The first demonstration of abnormal nerve conduction in man was by Hodes, Larabee & German in 1948, who found a marked reduction of velocity in fibres regenerating following injury. A similar phenomenon had previously been demonstrated in animal experiments by Berry, Grundfest & Hinsey (1944) and Sanders & Whitteridge (1946). A gross reduction in conduction velocity in some types of chronic neuropathy in man was demonstrated by Henriksen (1956), Lambert (1956) and Gilliatt & Sears (1958). Since these early studies technical advances have been made and an electrophysiological study of nerve conduction is now a routine and important part of the investigation of any patient with peripheral neuropathy.

Understanding of the structural changes responsible for abnormal conduction is far from complete but progress has been made by correlating conduction studies with pathological changes found in nerves obtained by biopsy in man and even more, from studies of experimental neuropathies in animals.

In diphtheritic neuropathy Kaeser & Lambert (1962) and McDonald (1963) found that marked reduction in conduction velocity occurred in association with segmental demyelination. A similar association occurs in experimental allergic neuritis (Cragg & Thomas, 1964) and lead neuropathy (Fullerton, 1966). By contrast only a slight reduction in velocity has been found in the axonal types of neuropathy, e.g. thallium neuropathy in guinea pigs (Kaeser, 1962) and acrylamide neuropathy in rats (Fullerton & Barnes, 1966). Thus, as a rough generalisation Gilliatt (1966) suggested that if in peripheral neuropathy conduction velocity was reduced by more than 40 per cent the pathological process was likely to be segmental demyelination.

Various views have been expressed about the mechanism responsible for the reduction of velocity in segmental demyelination. Kaeser & Lambert (1962) suggested that decreased current density at the widened nodes of Ranvier might lead to an increased excitation time and thus reduction of velocity. Cragg & Thomas (1964) investigated the slowing of conduction in experimental allergic neuritis. They postulated that at the acute stage, when there are many completely demyelinated segments, conduction along the damaged regions may be continuous as in non-myelinated fibres and at a similar slow rate. Conduction in normal myelinated fibres is saltatory, excitation occurring only at the nodes of Ranvier.

Following an electron microscopic study of myelin changes in experimental allergic neuritis, Ballin & Thomas (1969) suggested that the partially compacted myelin present in some fibres in the early stages of remyelination is likely to affect the electrical properties of the sheath enough to produce abnormal conduction. Morgan-Hughes (1968) measured conduction velocity serially in guinea pigs recovering from an attack of diphtheritic neuropathy. Conduction velocity remained slow but gradually increased over many months. The time course of recovery of velocity was similar to that of the increase in myelin sheath thickness of the remyelinating segments. Thus, during the later stages of recovery, conduction velocity may depend on fibre diameter as in normal nerve fibres. It is possible that all these factors may produce slowing of conduction, their relative importance varying at different stages of the disease. At some stage during segmental demyelination conduction may be blocked completely. It is obvious that this must be so since a severe clinical deficit may occur in purely demyelinating neuropathies. Also action potential size recorded from nerve or muscle following nerve stimulation may be markedly reduced (McDonald, 1963; Morgan-Hughes, 1968). At present the factors that determine whether or not conduction is blocked completely are unknown. An interesting and valuable technique has been developed by Rasminsky & Sears (1971) for recording along lengths of normal and demyelinated single nerve fibres in the rat. This opens the way for the direct demonstration of the mechanism of abnormal conduction and testing the various hypotheses discussed above.

The cause of the slight reduction in conduction velocity in axonal neuropathies is also in dispute. Kaeser (1962) and Fullerton & Barnes (1966) recorded muscle action potentials following stimulation of nerve trunks and thus measured maximal motor velocity. In both instances it was suggested that a reduction of maximal velocity of about 20 per cent was probably due to failure of conduction in the largest most rapidly conducting fibres, with normal conduction continuing in the slower, smaller fibres. Hopkins & Gilliatt (1971) found a greater reduction in maximal motor velocity in some baboons with acrylamide neuropathy. In the anterior tibial nerve of the most severely affected animals velocity was reduced by 49 per cent. However, they postulate that this was also probably due to failure of conduction in the largest fibres. Histologically the largest fibres were most severely affected and the greatest fall in velocity occurred in animals with the fewest surviving motor units. There was no dispersion of the muscle action potential when the nerve was stimulated at different levels, such as might be expected if there had been actual slowing of conduction in some fibres (Catton *et al.*, 1970). Although the normal range of velocity in the nerves they were studying is not known, such data from other nerves in the baboon (Eccles, Phillips & Chien-Ping, 1968) and cat (Wuerker, McPhedran & Heneman, 1965) suggest that some normal fibres might conduct at the velocity found by Hopkins & Gilliatt (1971). It is not possible to extrapolate from this data to man, because the velocity of the slowest conducting normal motor fibres in man is unknown. Whether failure of conduction in large fibres is the sole explanation for the reduction of velocity in axonal degeneration remains uncertain and is likely to remain so until further data is available about ranges of normal velocity.

Dyck & Lambert (1966, 1969) have described an interesting method of studying conduction in a wider range of fibres than has previously been possible in man. They have been able to stimulate and record the compound nerve action potential from isolated sural nerves obtained at biopsy. The potential has very similar characteristics to that recorded from animal nerve (Erlanger & Gasser, 1937). It has fast conducting A alpha and delta peaks produced by large and small diameter myelinated fibres and a slowly conducting C fibre peak produced by unmyelinated fibres. In nerves from patients with Charcot-Marie-Tooth disease and hypertrophic interstitial neuropathy maximal conduction velocity was greatly reduced, as was A wave size. C waves were within normal limits. These findings correlated reasonably well with histological changes in myelinated fibres. By contrast, in two patients with amyloidosis, A delta and C fibre potentials were reduced with relative preservation of the A alpha potential. As might be expected, loss of unmyelinated and small myelinated fibres was detected on histological examination. This technique is unlikely to be used routinely, but it raises most interesting possibilities for more detailed correlations between physiological and pathological findings in human diseases.

Axon Flow

The concept that material flows down the axons of nerve trunks has been accepted since Weiss & Hiscoe (1948) demonstrated that damming up of axoplasm occurs proximal to the site of a ligature or cuff round a peripheral nerve. Experiments designed to follow the movement of radioactive tracers down axons have confirmed a centrifugal movement. In recent years there has been considerable interest in the possible mechanism responsible for this flow and suggestions that certain pathological conditions may be due to its disorder.

Early autoradiographic studies of the movement of labelled amino acids demonstrated a flow rate of 0·8 mm/day in adult rat sciatic nerve (Koenig, 1958; Droz & Leblond, 1963), but Koenig (1958) was uncertain as to whether amino acids were transported in a free form or only after incorporation into protein. The latter now appears to be the case. McEwen & Grafstein (1968) found that when radioactive leucine was injected into the eye of a goldfish inhibition of protein synthesis in the retina prevented the normal transport of labelled leucine to the optic tectum. Inhibition of protein synthesis in the tectum had no influence on the transport process. Recent experiments have indicated that there appear to be two components in protein transport, one fast and one slow. In goldfish optic nerve, McEwen & Grafstein (1968) demonstrated a movement of at least and probably greater than 40 mm/day. Ochs & Johnson (1969) have estimated an even faster flow rate in ventral root fibres of up to 930 mm/day.

An elegant technique for studying axon flow in single nerve fibres has been devised by Lux et al. (1970). Labelled amino acids are iontophoretically injected into single neurones and the progress of the labelled material down the axon can be followed from autoradiographs. They have demonstrated that a greater amount of protein is transported down axons that have been stimulated than those in a resting state. This technique obviously has great potential for studying normal and pathological nerves.

The role of neurotubules in axon transport has been a subject of interest and experiment in the last few years. It has been suggested that they are responsible for rapid protein movement. McEwen & Grafstein (1968), for example, demonstrated that the fast moving protein that they studied in the optic nerve was associated with particulate matter. Acetyl cholinesterase, thought to be a fast moving protein, was shown to be related to neurotubules in an ultrastructural histochemical study by Kasa (1968).

Pathological changes in neurotubules have also been studied. Neurotubules have a similar structure to spindle tubules (Gonatas & Robbins, 1965) and mitotic spindle inhibitors, such as colchicine, aluminium and vinca alkaloids, produce their disintegration. Following administration of these substances there is a marked increase of intracellular neurofilaments (Wisniewski, Shelanski & Terry, 1968). It has been suggested that inter-conversion of tubules and filaments occurs.

Kreutzberg (1969) has studied the flow of various axon components following local injection of colchicine into a nerve. He crushed the nerve lower down. In a normal nerve axon components accumulate proximal to the site of a crush and he compared the amount of substances accumulating above a crush in normal nerve and following local colchicine. He found that colchicine had a much greater effect on the flow of acetyl cholinesterase, a fast moving component, than of diphosphopyridine nucleotide (DPN) diaphorase, a slow moving enzyme related to mitochondria. Since colchicine produces disintegration of neurotubules, this observation supports the suggestion that these structures are involved in rapid transport. It is perhaps surprising that most mitotic spindle inhibitors are not significantly neurotoxic. The vinca alkaloids, particularly vincristine, are an exception to this.

Pleasure, Mishner & Engel (1969) have followed the movement of labelled L-leucine in neuropathy produced by acrylamide and by TOCP. They studied slowly transported axon components. No abnormality was demonstrated in animals with TOCP neuropathy. However, movement of the labelled fraction was stopped in animals with acrylamide neuropathy. They concluded that the transport mechanism rather than protein synthesis was affected, since radioactive substances accumulated in the nerve trunks close to the cell bodies.

These observations are of great theoretical interest in considering basic pathological mechanisms. However, their relevance to clinical neuropathy in man is at present not established.

PERIPHERAL NERVE DISEASES

Intensive studies of a number of peripheral nerve disorders in man have been carried out by the techniques already described. Those on which the most fruitful results have been obtained will be discussed.

Diabetic Neuropathy

Several clinically distinct types of neuropathy occur in patients with diabetes. These are:

(a) diffuse, distal, predominantly sensory;
(b) autonomic;
(c) mononeuropathy multiplex;
(d) increased incidence of pressure palsies.

Some workers have suggested that diabetic neuropathy has a primary metabolic basis and others that changes are secondary to vascular abnormalities (Fagerberg, 1959). It now seems possible that the relative importance of these factors may vary in the different types of neuropathy.

Evidence is accumulating that some isolated nerve palsies and mononeuropathy multiplex are ischaemic in origin. A detailed pathological study of nerves from a diabetic patient with mononeuropathy multiplex was carried out by Raff, Sangalong & Asbury (1968). Multiple infarcts were demonstrated in the nerves and their frequency and distribution correlated well with the neurological disability that had been present before death. However, although there seems little doubt that these lesions were ischaemic in origin, the responsible vascular changes were less clearly defined. Only one completely occluded vessel was found and it was possible to attribute three infarctions to this lesion. Elsewhere only endothelial and perithelial proliferation of intraneural arterioles and capillaries was demonstrated. Although these authors were doubtful about their relevance, it seems that this type of diffuse small vessel lesion might have been important. Fagerberg (1959) has previously discussed in some detail the blood vessel changes in diabetes and their possible relation to neuropathy. Another detailed pathological study of nerves and vessels in a patient with an oculomotor palsy by Asbury et al. (1970) provides further evidence of the importance of small vessel pathology. A focal demyelinating lesion of presumed ischaemic aetiology was found.

There were extensive changes in arteriolar and capillary walls without complete vessel occlusion. Similar changes were not found in non-diabetic subjects.

On the other hand, it is possible that there is a metabolic basis for the distal symmetrical neuropathy. Diffuse pathological changes of segmental demyelination have been demonstrated by Thomas & Lascelles (1966) in diabetic neuropathy, with few blood vessel abnormalities. In severe cases, some axonal degeneration was also present, but focal lesions of the type described by Raff et al. (1968) in mononeuropathy multiplex were not seen. A non-ischaemic cause of this type of neuropathy seems possible.

Biochemical studies on nerves from animals made diabetic by treatment with alloxan may be relevant and have been summarised by Field (1966). These suggest that the alloxan-diabetic nerves are unable to metabolise glucose normally and in particular that there is a severe limitation of the conversion of glucose into the fatty acids from which myelin triglyceride and cholesterolesters are derived. Interestingly, nerve metabolism does not return to normal when animals are kept normoglycaemic with insulin. Gabbay, Merola & Field (1966) have raised the possibility that the conversion of glucose to fructose via sorbitol (the sorbitol pathway) may contribute to the development of neuropathy. Sorbitol, fructose and glucose are all increased in nerves from diabetic rats compared with controls. The inability of the metabolites to escape from the cells might have harmful osmotic effects and more energy might be required to maintain osmotic equilibrium and the sodium and potassium content. How these various metabolic studies relate to the development of neuropathy is not at present clear.

Diabetic nerves in men and in alloxan treated rats behave differently from healthy nerves when made ischaemic. Steiness (1959) found that when limbs were rendered ischaemic by a pneumatic cuff, appreciation of vibration sensation persisted for longer in diabetic than in healthy subjects. Seneviratne & Peiris (1968) found that in diabetic subjects, even in those without clinical evidence of neuropathy and with normal nerve conduction velocity, there was a much smaller change in nerve action potential size following submaximal shocks during a period of 30 minutes ischaemia than in healthy subjects. The same authors have extended these observations to nerves from alloxan-diabetic rats and also studied the effect of insulin on the excitability changes (Senevriatne & Peiris, 1969, 1970a). They attribute their results to changes in potassium equilibrium due to changes in permeability of diffusion barriers in diabetes. Until further studies have been carried out in other pathological conditions it is impossible to say how specific the findings are. Similar resistance of nerves to periods of ischaemia has been demonstrated in patients with motor neurone disease (Shahani & Russell, 1969), uraemia (Christensen & Orskov, 1969) and liver disease (Seneviratne & Peiris, 1970b). Whether the decreased membrane resistance demonstrated by Eliasson (1969) in nerves from alloxan-diabetic rats is in any way a specific phenomenon also requires further study.

An increased incidence of pressure palsies is known to occur in diabetic subjects (Mulder et al., 1961). Some interesting experimental work by Hopkins & Morgan-Hughes (1969) may be relevant. They have shown that pressure lesions in guinea pigs occur more easily in nerves mildly damaged by diphtheria toxin than in healthy animals. A similar situation might exist in diabetes.

Uraemic Neuropathy

Asbury, Victor & Adams first clearly described the syndrome of neuropathy associated with chronic renal failure in 1963. The initial symptom is usually burning feet followed by numbness and distal weakness affecting the legs more than the arms. The syndrome has become commoner since dialysis has enabled these patients to live longer. There have been several reports of neuropathy becoming worse in the early stages of dialysis (Hegstrom et al., 1962). However, now that many patients have been treated and followed for long periods it has become clear that the neuropathy improves with prolonged dialysis (Konotey-Ahulu et al., 1965). Tyler (1968) has found that improvement in neurological symptoms is much better and surer following transplantation than with dialysis.

Slight reduction in nerve conduction velocity has been found in patients with uraemic neuropathy (Konotey-Ahulu et al., 1965) and also in patients with renal failure without clinical evidence of neuropathy (Preswick & Jeremy, 1964). Jebsen, Tenckhoff & Honet (1967) found that a single dialysis had no effect on conduction velocity but that there was an improvement in patients who were treated for more than a year. Little improvement has been found in patients treated for shorter periods (Heron et al., 1965).

The predominant histological change found by Asbury et al. (1963) was degeneration of both axis cylinders and myelin sheaths. This suggests that the slight fall in conduction velocity might be explained by loss of rapidly conducting fibres. However, Nielsen (1967) recorded sensory potentials in uraemic patients and concluded that there was a disturbance in the conducting mechanism because action potential amplitude was well preserved in the presence of reduced velocity. Recently teased fibre studies of biopsy specimens from patients with uraemia by Dinn & Crane (1970) have suggested that segmental demyelination may occur in addition to axonal degeneration. The contribution of this type of pathological change to slowing of conduction in uraemia has not been fully evaluated.

It has been suggested that uraemic neuropathy might be due to deficiency of one of the B vitamins or to a disorder of carbohydrate metabolism producing a type of diabetic state. However, supplementary vitamins do not prevent or influence the course of the neuropathy and there is little evidence for the diabetic theory (Asbury et al., 1963; Tyler, 1968). In view of the greater improvement following transplantation than after dialysis it has been suggested that some unknown essential substance may be lost in the dialysis fluid but again there is no evidence to support this (Tyler, 1968). The cause of neuropathy appears to be some metabolic disturbance as yet undefined.

Rheumatoid Neuropathy

Peripheral neuropathy was described in a small proportion of patients with rheumatoid arthritis by Hart, Golding & Mackenzie in 1957. Neuropathy may be difficult to diagnose in these patients because of the pain and disuse atrophy of muscles produced by the joint disease. However, it is now recognised that nerve involvement may take one of three forms; pressure lesions secondary to joint deformity, a mild distal neuropathy which is entirely or predominantly sensory and a fulminating sensory-motor disorder (Pallis & Scott, 1965; Chamberlain & Bruckner, 1970). The mild form does not progress to the severe type, which is acute in onset. The prognosis of the mild neuropathy is good. Its course fluctuates but tends to improve. The severe form, however, has a bad prognosis since it is a manifestation of a widespread vasculitis. Death often occurs from mesenteric or coronary vessel occlusion and most patients described by the authors mentioned above died within a year of the onset of symptoms of vasculitis. Steroids are not helpful in treatment.

Chamberlain & Bruckner (1970) have carried out nerve conduction studies on 32 patients with the mild or severe type of neuropathy and Weller, Bruckner & Chamberlain (1970) have examined sural nerve biopsy specimens from five of the same patients. In some, marked slowing of conduction was found, such as is associated with segmental demyelination and this type of pathology was demonstrated in the nerves. Axonal degeneration was, however, also prominent and was particularly marked in those with severe neuropathy. There is good evidence from clinical and pathological studies that vasculitis is responsible for the severe neuropathy. The role of ischaemia when neuropathy is mild is less sure, but may be important (Weller *et al.*, 1970).

Guillain-Barré Syndrome and Experimental Allergic Neuritis

The Guillain-Barré syndrome and experimental allergic neuritis (EAN) have many features in common. Interpretation of changes in the former condition in modern immunological terms and by analogy with EAN has helped our understanding of the disease.

EAN was first produced by Waksman & Adams (1955) by immunising animals with peripheral nerve and Freund's adjuvant. After a latent interval there is cellular infiltration of the peripheral nerves, before any clinical signs are evident. At the time the animals become paralysed, myelin breakdown, predominantly of the segmental demyelinating type, is seen in the nerves. Aström, Webster & Arnason (1968) have studied the early stages of the lesion and described the passage of mononuclear cells through the cytoplasm of the vascular endotholial cells to lie amongst the nerve fibres. These cells are thought to be 'activated' lymphocytes. Lampert (1969) has recently described the electron microscopic appearances of the demyelinating process itself. The mononuclear cells penetrate the neurolemma, push aside the Schwann cell cytoplasm and destroy the myelin sheath. There is focal lysis of myelin lamallae where the mononuclear cells are in contact with them and then myelin layers are peeled off by processes of the invading cells. Vesicular degeneration of the myelin may also occur (Ballin & Thomas, 1968a).

In the classical description of histological changes in the Guillain-Barré syndrome by Haymaker & Kernohan (1949) oedema of the nerve roots was described as the first change. Myelin breakdown was thought to occur later, followed by cellular infiltration. However, the sequence of events is now thought to be similar to that in EAN. Asbury, Arnason & Adams (1969) studied nerves from 19 patients dying of this disease. They found no significant oedema. In most patients the nerves were affected diffusely and pathological changes were not confined to root level. The ultrastructural features of myelin breakdown in nerves from a patient who died of the Guillain-Barré syndrome described by Wisniewski et al. (1969) are also very similar to those shown by Ballin & Thomas (1968a) and Lampert (1969) in EAN.

Both the Guillain-Barré syndrome and EAN are thought to be cell-mediated immune diseases of the delayed hypersensitivity type. EAN has been passively transferred via lymphocytes (Aström & Waksman, 1962). Lymph node cells and peripheral blood buffy coat cells from animals with EAN and patients with the Guillain-Barré syndrome will demyelinate nerves in tissue culture (Winkler, 1965; Arnason, Winkler & Hadler, 1969). Antinerve antibodies have been detected in the serum of some animals with EAN and some patients with the Guillain-Barré syndrome. Mellnick (1963) found complement fixing antibodies to nervous tissue in 50 per cent of 38 patients with the Guillain-Barré syndrome. However, the presence of these antibodies bears an unpredictable relationship to the time of onset and severity of the disease (Caspery & Field, 1965; Waksman & Adams, 1955; Arnason et al., 1969). Asbury et al. (1969) have stressed that it is not uncommon for lymphocytes from rats with EAN to produce demyelination in tissue culture whereas serum from the same animals will not and they emphasise the primary importance of the lymphocyte in both EAN and the Guillain-Barré syndrome.

Recent extensive reviews of the clinical features of the Guillain-Barré syndrome are those by Weiderholt, Mulder & Lambert (1964), Ravn (1967) and Prineas (1970b). The typical Guillain-Barré syndrome has an acute onset with maximum involvement in less than two months. The relation of more chronic and relapsing neuropathies to the Guillain-Barré syndrome will be discussed later. That the syndrome is a specific entity is supported by the uniform pathological findings in the fatal cases examined by Asbury et al. (1969), in all of which the diagnosis had been made clinically. In the various series mentioned above, a preceding illness, most often an upper respiratory tract infarction, had occurred in between one third and three-quarters of the patients, with a mean latent interval in Ravn's series of 9 days.

The role of steroid therapy in treatment of acute polyneuropathy is still doubtful. Assessment is obviously difficult in a disease from which complete spontaneous recovery is usual. Recently there have been several reports of patients with a recurrent or relapsing polyneuropathy thought to be similar to the Guillain-Barré syndrome, in some of whom there was good evidence that steroids did play an important part in treatment (Thomas et al., 1969; De Vivo & Engel, 1970; Matthews, Howell & Hughes, 1970).

A patient described by Austin (1958) had 20 episodes of paralysis in 5 years, approximately half developing when the steroid dose was reduced and half were clearly improved by steroid treatment. The autopsy findings in one patient described by Thomas et al. (1969) support the suggestion that this syndrome is related to the acute Guillain-Barré syndrome. She had a chronic neuropathy with a relapsing course and histological findings similar to those of Asbury et al. (1969) in patients with the typical acute syndrome. It is perhaps surprising that relapses do not occur more commonly. Asbury et al. (1969) found persistent cellular infiltration of the nerves of two patients who had recovered completely from an acute neuropathy several years previously.

Lipid Disorders
Peripheral neuropathy may occur in the lipidoses and lipoprotein deficiency diseases discussed below. Signs of peripheral neuropathy often form only a minor part of the clinical picture, but sometimes may be the presenting feature. These rare conditions should therefore be considered when investigating a patient with peripheral neuropathy. It is possible that other at present unexplained neuropathies may eventually be found to be due to a primary lipid disorder.

Another important aspect of the peripheral nerve involvement in these conditions is that histological and chemical analysis of sural nerve biopsy specimens may enable an exact diagnosis to be made, and avoid the more dangerous procedures of cerebral or rectal biopsy. If reduction of peripheral nerve conduction velocity is found in a patient with a degenerative neurological disease, even if clinically there is only scanty evidence of peripheral neuropathy, then diagnostic sural nerve biopsy is likely to be rewarding.

Refsum's disease (heredopathia atactica polyneuritiformis)
This disorder was first described as a distinct condition by Refsum in 1946 and the pathology has been described and reviewed by Cammermeyer (1956). The main clinical features consist of peripheral neuropathy, cerebellar ataxia, retinitis pigmentosa and nerve deafness. Cardiomyopathy may develop and is an important cause of sudden death, which is a frequent ending to the disease. The clinical course of the neuropathy is frequently one of relapses and remissions. A characteristic pathological feature is hypertrophic changes in the peripheral nerve fibres producing an 'onion bulb' appearance indistinguishable from Déjèrine-Sottas disease. The possibility that the condition might be a form of lipidosis was raised because of the marked fatty infiltration that occurs in the liver. This has now been shown to be the case. In 1963 Klenck and Kahlke demonstrated the presence of high concentrations of an unusual fatty acid in urinary and organ extracts and this substance was identified as 3,7,11,15-tetramethyl hexadecanoic acid (phytanic acid) (Kahle & Richterick, 1965). In contrast to other lipidoses, the fatty acid stored is an abnormal one, being present only at extremely low concentrations in normal individuals.

From studies of the fate of labelled substances in patients with the disease, it has been established that the phytanic acid does not arise as a result of biosynthesis but most likely accumulates because of a failure to metabolise dietary phytanic acid and phytol (Steinberg et al., 1966; Steinberg et al., 1967). The obvious corollary was to study the effect on patients with the disease of a diet which excluded these substances as far as possible. Steinberg et al. (1966) have reported the results of such an attempt on two patients. After one year the serum phytanic acid levels had fallen to a quarter of their initial values and conduction velocity had increased from 6 to 19 m/s in one patient. The clinical effects were, however, inconclusive. The disease is characteristically relapsing and remitting which makes clinical evaluation particularly difficult, especially in small numbers of patients observed over a relatively short time. Evaluation of dietary treatment must therefore await further long term studies.

Sulphatide lipidosis (metachromatic leukodystrophy)

This familial disorder is due to a deficiency of sulphatase which results in the accumulation of sulphatide in nervous tissue, giving the characteristic metachromatic staining material after which the disease was originally named (Austin *et al.*, 1963). The dominant clinical features are usually due to degenerative cerebral changes affecting particularly the brain stem. However, from the original clinical descriptions of the disease it seemed possible that peripheral nerves might be involved. Brain & Greenfield (1950) commented on early loss of reflexes as an unusual feature for a cerebral disorder. More rarely evidence of peripheral neuropathy may dominate the clinical picture in the early stages (Yudell *et al.*, 1967).

Norman, Urich & Tingey (1960) demonstrated metachromatic granules in sciatic nerve fibres and studies of sural nerve biopsy specimens have shown clear evidence of peripheral neuropathy, with accumulation of metachromatic granules in Schwann cells and segmental demyelination of nerve fibres (Webster, 1962). As might be expected in a segmental demyelinating type of neuropathy, marked slowing of nerve conduction may occur. Fullerton (1964) found greatly reduced motor nerve conduction velocity in 6 of 7 children with this disease.

Globoid cell leukodystrophy (Krabbe's disease)

The primary metabolic disorder in this familial degenerative disease of childhood is a deficiency of cerebroside sulphotransferase, an enzyme responsible for synthesis of sulphatide (Bachhawat, Austin & Armstrong, 1967). Neutral cerebrosides accumulate in white matter. Like sulphatide lipidosis, the characteristic clinical features of globoid cell leukodystrophy are of a progressive cerebral disorder and clinically at least in the early stages, the only evidence of peripheral neuropathy may be depressed or absent reflexes.

Peripheral nerve involvement in the disease has been demonstrated histologically by Allen & de Veyra (1967) and by Sourander & Olsson (1968). The latter workers found marked axonal as well as myelin destruction. However, Dunn *et al.* (1969) demonstrated prominent segmental demyelination associated with marked slowing of nerve conduction velocity. Thus, conduction studies and nerve biopsy may be diagnostically useful. There is some doubt about the specificity of the light microscopic findings and globoid cells are not present in peripheral nerves. Bischoff & Ulrich (1969) consider that the ultrastructural features are, however, characteristic and different from other types of degeneration. Dilatation of the vesicular and tubular elements of the endoplasmic reticulum are prominent in Schwann cells and histiocytes.

Fabry's disease (angiokeratoma corporis diffusum)

This familial disorder of lipid metabolism is due to a deficiency of ceramide trihexosidase (Brady *et al.*, 1967) resulting in the deposition of unmetabolised ceremide trihexoside. The lipid accumulates and affects particularly small blood vessels. Pain in the extremities is prominent but sensory loss is rare and only recently has peripheral nerve involvement been recognised histologically. Lipid deposits in endoneurial cells, capillary pericytes and perineural connective tissue were found in the sural nerve of a patient with this disease by Bischoff *et al.* (1968). There was degeneration of unmyelinated fibres which the authors consider responsible for the sudomotor insufficiency and pain. Lipid deposits and loss of nerve fibres were also demonstrated in a sural nerve biopsy specimen by Kocen & Thomas (1970). Their patients had no sensory loss, nor electro-physiologically demonstrable abnormality, but the authors raise the possibility that the pain may be related to the nerve abnormality.

Primary biliary cirrhosis

Patients with cutaneous xanthomatosis associated with primary biliary cirrhosis may develop pain in the extremities with tenderness rather similar to patients with Fabry's disease. This has usually been thought to be due to the xanthomata. Thomas & Walker (1965), however, described three patients with primary biliary cirrhosis who had these symptoms and mild distal sensory impairment. The only electrophysiological changes were abolition of lateral popliteal nerve action potentials in 2 of the 3 patients. Xanthomatous deposits were demonstrated in the nerves obtained at biopsy and thought probably responsible for the neuropathy.

Lipoprotein deficiencies

Neuropathy may occur in the familial lipoprotein deficiencies, Tangier disease (α-lipoprotein deficiency) (Kocen *et al.*, 1967; Engel *et al.*, 1967) and the Bassen-Kornzweig syndrome (β-lipoprotein deficiency) (Sobrevilla, Goodman & Karne, 1964). Two sisters described by Engel *et al.* (1967) with Tangier disease each had frequent episodes of neuropathy starting in child-hood and a patient described by Kocen *et al.* (1967) had a chronic neuropathy with dissociated pain and temperature sensory loss. In the Bassen-Kornzweig syndrome the other features—steattorhoea, retinitis pigmentosa and central nervous system involvement, particularly of the cerebellum and long tracts, may overshadow the signs of peripheral neuropathy.

Toxic Neuropathies

Several aspects of toxic neuropathies, particularly those produced experimentally in animals, have already been considered in the introductory section. An exhaustive account of all known toxic peripheral nerve disorders will not be given, but only the commonest toxic substances will be considered. There are many others which are occasionally toxic under certain circumstances but are of little practical or theoretical importance.

Drug induced neuropathies

Drugs in common use today which have frequently caused peripheral neuropathy are isoniazid, furadantin and vincristine. Other substances which have been used as drugs in the past or which produce neuropathy only very rarely include arsenicals, chloramphenical, disulphiram, gold, some sulphonamides, thalidomide and thallium (Le Quesne, 1970). Isoniazid and furadantin are rare causes of neuropathy now, because the circumstances in which they produce neuropathy are better understood and can therefore largely be avoided. Vincristine is still a common cause of neuropathy because its value as a chemotherapeutic agent overrides the disadvantages of the side effects it produces.

Isoniazid. This drug was recognised as a cause of neuropathy very soon after it was introduced for the treatment of tuberculosis in 1952; many patients developed toxic effects when taking the high doses that were used at that time (Biehl & Skavlem, 1953; Jones & Jones, 1953; Gammon, Burge & King, 1953). The neuropathy is initially and predominantly distal and sensory.

Biochemical studies showed that isoniazid produces a pyridoxine deficiency state by inactivating pyridoxine and increasing its excretion as a hydrazone (Biehl & Vilter, 1954). Neuropathy can be prevented by giving pyridoxine without interfering with the antituberculous effect (Biehl & Nimitz, 1954). However, this is unnecessary as a routine measure because neuropathy is rare with the drug doses currently in common use. Further interesting studies revealed that the rate of acetylation, the first stage in isoniazid metabolism, may vary and patients may be divided into slow and rapid inactivators. Slow inactivators are much more likely to develop neuropathy, presumably because they have higher blood levels of the active substance for a longer time (Hughes *et al.*, 1954). The rate of acetylation is now known to be a genetically determined characteristic, slow inactivation being inherited as a recessive trait (Evans, Manley & McKussick, 1960).

The histological changes in experimental isoniazid neuropathy have already been described. Detailed histological studies of sural nerve biopsy specimens from nine patients have been described by Ochoa (1970) who found evidence of degeneration and regeneration of unmyelinated as well as myelinated fibres.

Nitrofurantoin (furadantin). This drug was first recognised as a cause of neuropathy in 1956 (Olivarius, 1956) and there have been a number of similar reports since that time (Rubinstein, 1964). The neuropathy is initially sensory, but distal weakness may develop shortly after the onset of symptoms and may progress rapidly (Willett, 1963). Complete recovery only occurs if the drug is stopped before the weakness has become severe (Rubinstein, 1964).

Nitrofurantoin rarely causes neuropathy in the absence of renal failure. Ellis (1962) found a correlation between the degree of renal impairment and the incidence of neuropathy and Loughridge (1962) found that higher blood levels of the drug developed in the presence of defective renal function. Evidence such as the relation of neuropathy to the duration of treatment and the recovery, at least partial, after drug withdrawal indicates that nitrofurantoin, and not only the renal failure itself, can cause neuropathy. This is further supported by experimental studies by Klinghardt (1965) who produced nitrofurantoin neuropathy in rats.

Vincristine. The interesting experimental studies of the effect of the vinca alkaloids on neurotubules have been discussed earlier. Vinblastine has a much greater effect on neurotubules than vincristine, whereas vincristine is much more neurotoxic than vinblastine when given to both man and animals. These differences are at present not understood.

In rats and guinea pigs vincristine produces predominantly a myopathic lesion (Anderson, Song & Slotwiner, 1967; Morgan-Hughes, Gajeree &

Le Quesne, 1972) and only a few degenerating nerve fibres are seen after prolonged dosing (Bradley, 1970). By contrast the predominant lesion in man is peripheral neuropathy (Warot, Goudemand & Habay, 1965; Bradley *et al.*, 1970; Casey, Jelliffe, Le Quesne & Millett 1972). The reasons for this difference are unexplained but may be related to the size of the dose given and the speed of development of neurotoxic symptoms. Thus, the acute lesion in animals given a high dose is a myopathy and neuropathy only develops after prolonged treatment with doses more comparable to those used in man.

The clinical features of the neuropathy in man have been described in detail by Bradley *et al.* (1970) and by Casey *et al.* (1972). The following account is based largely on the latter study of 13 patients, some of whom were treated for up to two years. Paraesthesiae are most commonly the first symptoms, but are rarely troublesome and actual sensory loss occurs later. Weakness is more troublesome and may at times progress rapidly to severe disability. When less severe the weakness affects the distal leg muscles. In the arms there is often a striking localisation of weakness to the wrist and finger extensor muscles. Thus motor and not sensory involvement is an indication for reducing the dose. Although few patients recover completely all improve when the dose is reduced or the drug stopped. Weakness and paraesthesiae improve considerably, but sensory loss may persist, although without being disabling.

Digital sensory nerve action potentials were recorded serially in the patients studied by Casey *et al.* (1972). There was a remarkably uniform decrease in amplitude in relation to dose in different patients. This observation, as well as the clinical studies indicates that the drug is toxic to all who are exposed to it.

Electrophysiological study of motor nerves showed evidence of denervation in the foot muscles and a great decrease in the number of active motor units. However, motor nerve conduction velocity was little affected, suggesting that the lesion is probably of the axonal type. This is supported by histological studies of biopsy specimens by McLeod & Penny (1969). Thus, clinical, electrophysiological and histological studies have confirmed the neuropathic nature of the lesion in man. Bradley *et al.* (1970) have, however, shown that electron microscopic changes in painful proximal muscles may be much more extensive than suspected on light microscopic examination.

Thalidomide. This substance, which was introduced as a sedative in 1955, was recognised as a cause of neuropathy in 1960 (Florence, 1960; Scheid *et al.*, 1961; Fullerton & Kremer, 1961). Thereafter, further reports of its neurotoxicity appeared and it became a common cause of neuropathy before being withdrawn at the end of 1961 on account of its teratogenic effects (Lenz, 1962). The incidence of toxic effects is difficult to estimate; the drug was extremely widely used and many patients took it irregularly.

Paraesthesiae with sensory loss and nocturnal cramps were the initial symptoms. Motor involvement was rarely severe, but was unusual in that proximal muscles were affected more than distal ones (Fullerton & Kremer, 1961). The distribution of weakness is thus different from that seen in vincristine neuropathy.

The most distressing feature of thalidomide neuropathy is that recovery is poor. This is in contrast to the toxic neuropathies already discussed. It has been claimed that recovery occurred if the drug was stopped within six weeks of the onset of symptoms (Burley, 1961); but in most reported series symptoms were present for longer before their cause was recognised. Fullerton & O'Sullivan (1968) studied 22 patients with thalidomide neuropathy four to six years after stopping the drug. One half were unchanged, a quarter improved and only a quarter had recovered. Sural nerve biopsies were taken from 6 patients between two and six years after stopping the drug. There was a marked loss of large diameter fibres. An increase in numbers of small fibres in some indicated that fibres had attempted to regenerate but failed to mature. The reasons for this are unknown.

Environmental causes of neuropathy

The important causes of neuropathy produced by substances to which people are exposed during the course of their work are lead, carbon disulphide (Vigliani, 1954) and the recently recognised hazard, acrylamide. Many accidental cases of poisoning by fluids contaminated with organo-phosphates (Cavanagh, 1964a), and by arsenic (Heyman et al., 1956) and methyl mercury used as insecticides or fungicides have been reported. Following accidents with the latter substances the cause of neuropathy is usually obvious because some specific incident has occurred shortly before the onset of symptoms. More general environmental hazards are currently attracting much attention and those which might cause neuropathy are organic mercurials in fish and lead in water or from lead-glazed pottery.

Some of the toxic substances mentioned, for example, carbon disulphide and methyl mercury, have prominent effects on the central nervous system as well as on the peripheral nerves and the neurotoxic effects of lead under certain circumstances may be confined to the central nervous system. For a more general discussion of environmental causes of peripheral neuropathy, including the substances already mentioned and others of less importance see Fullerton (1969b).

Lead. Lead palsy was once very common. Poor factory conditions and the widespread use of lead paints were largely responsible for this. It is a well-known clinical observation that the most exercised muscles are most severely affected; thus wrist drop used to occur in manual workers and painters, but foot drop was described in professional dancers who were exposed to lead (Hunter, 1969). This disorder is usually confined to the motor system and there have been only occasional descriptions of sensory involvement in lead poisoning (Goodwin, 1934).

It was suggested at one time that weakness might be due to a primary muscle rather than neural lesion (Reznikoff & Aub, 1927) but the evidence for this was not strong. Early pathological observations (Laslett & Warrington, 1898) and recent experimental and clinical studies (Fullerton, 1966; Simpson, Seaton & Adams, 1964) have shown definite neuronal involvement and no evidence of a primary muscle lesion.

Although lead poisoning remains the commonest notifiable industrial disease in Great Britain today (Department of Employment and Productivity, 1968), clinical neurological involvement is rare. However, Catton et al. (1970) carried out nerve conduction studies on 19 men working in a factory manufacturing accumulators (a common source of poisoning) and found minor differences compared with a group of control subjects. None of the workers had any abnormal neurological symptoms or signs, but 13 had raised blood lead levels and 7 had haemoglobin levels below 12g/100 ml.

Lead glazes are still used on pottery in many peasant communities throughout the world. In such circumstances severe lead poisoning is still common (Beritíc & Stahulzak, 1961). Neuropathy occurs and may present as a rapidly progressive quadriplegia usually associated with abdominal pain and anaemia (Le Quesne, personal observation).

The type of pathological change in lead neuropathy may vary in different species. Gombault's (1880) original description of segmental demyelination was in lead poisoned guinea pigs. Fullerton (1966) has confirmed that this type of lesion occurs in guinea pigs and produces a marked reduction in conduction velocity. Axonal degeneration also occurs and is more prominent in acute than chronic poisoning. In rabbits axonal degeneration seems to be the primary lesion (Shimazono, 1914). In man, slowing of conduction of the type expected with segmental demyelination is not seen (Delwaide & Chan-traine, 1965; Simpson et al., 1964), but detailed histological studies have not been carried out.

Acrylamide. This substance, although relatively new to industry, is now widely used, particularly to stabilise soil and as a flocculator. Its neuro-toxicity to animals was recognised before any cases of poisoning in exposed workers were reported (Kuperman, 1958; McCollister, Oyen & Rowe, 1964). Fullerton & Barnes (1966) demonstrated a dying back type of axonal neuropathy in rats. There have now been several reports of neurotoxic effects in man (Fujita et al., 1960; Auld & Bedwell, 1967; Garland & Patterson, 1967). Sensory symptoms occur first followed by weakness. Ataxia appears to be out of proportion to sensory loss and suggests an additional central effect. Excessive sweating is also a feature of acute poison-ing. Good recovery occurs after removal from exposure. In mild cases this is complete but there are persistent symptoms and signs in more severely affected patients at least up to eight months later (Fullerton, 1969a).

The exact structure of the acrylamide molecule is important in relation to its toxic effects. Acrylamide polymer is not toxic. Barnes (1970) investi-gated a number of related compounds and found that only N-methyl acrylamide and N-hydroxymethylacrylamide were slightly toxic, and this may have been partly because they were contaminated with acrylamide. Any other alteration to the molecule removes the neurotoxicity.

Organic mercury compounds. The main effects of these substances are on the cerebellum and occipital cortex producing ataxia and blindness, but a sensory peripheral neuropathy also occurs (Hunter, Bomford & Russell, 1940). The characteristics of methyl mercury poisoning have become well known since the cause of Minamata disease was established. Eighty-three people developed the neurological symptoms described above when fish from Minamata Bay in Japan became contaminated with mercury effluent from a factory (Kurland, Farc & Siedler, 1960). The effluent from the factory was almost entirely inorganic mercury and for some time it was not clear how this related to the much more toxic organic mercury compounds which caused the disease. However, it is now known that biological methy-lation of mercury occurs in bottom sediment and rotten fish (Jensen &

Jernelov, 1969). Recent analyses have indicated that all fish contain some organic mercury, but there is no evidence that this is harmful, except when unusual contamination occurs as in Minamata Bay.

In rats methyl mercury produces degeneration of the whole length of the sensory fibre at an early stage, rather than a slow dying back from the periphery (Cavanagh, 1969). Motor fibres are unaffected. Electrophysiological measurement of sensory nerve action potential amplitude should thus be a particularly sensitive indicator of toxic effects. Such measurements will be valuable in the investigation of possible cases of poisoning in future.

Acknowledgement

I would like to thank the Editors of the *Journal of Physiology* for permission to reproduce Fig. 2.1.

References

ALLEN, N. & DE VEYRA, E. (1967). *J. Neuropath. exp. Neurol.*, **26**, 456.

ALLSOP, J. L. (1953). *Australasian Ann. Med.*, **2**, 144.

ALLT, G. (1969). *Brain*, **92**, 639.

ANDERSON, P. J., SONG, S. K. & SLOTWINER, P. (1967). *J. Neuropath. exp. Neurol.*, **26**, 15.

ARNASON, B. G. W., WINKLER, G. F. & HADLER, N. M. (1969). *Lab. Invest.*, **21**, 1.

ASBURY, A. K., ALDREDGE, H., HERSHBERG, R. & MILLER FISHER, C. (1970). *Brain*, **93**, 555.

ASBURY, A. K., ARNASON, B. G. & ADAMS, R. D. (1969). *Medicine*, **48**, 173.

ASBURY, A. K., VICTOR, M. & ADAMS, R. D. (1963). *Archs Neurol., Chicago*, **8**, 413.

ASTRÖM, K.-E. & WAKSMAN, B. H. (1962). *J. Path. Bact.*, **83**, 89.

ASTRÖM, K.-E., WEBSTER, H. DE F. & ARNASON, B. G. (1968). *J. exp. Med.*, **128**, 469.

AULD, R. B. & BEDWELL, S. F. (1967). *Canad. med. Ass. J.*, **96**, 652.

AUSTIN, J. H. (1956). *Medicine*, **35**, 187.

AUSTIN, J. H. (1958). *Brain*, **81**, 157.

AUSTIN, J. H., BALASUBRAMANIAN, A. S., PATTABIRAMAN, T. N., SARASWATHI, S., BASU, D. K. & BACHHAWAT, B. K. (1963). *J. Neurochem.*, **10**, 805.

BACHHAWAT, B. K., AUSTIN, J. & ARMSTRONG, D. (1967). *Biochem. J.*, **104**, 15c.

BALLIN, R. H. M. & THOMAS, P. K. (1968a). *J. neurol. Sci.*, **8**, 1.

BALLIN, R. H. M. & THOMAS, P. K. (1968b). *Acta neuropath.*, **11**, 93.

BALLIN, R. H. M. & THOMAS, P. K. (1969). *J. neurol. Sci.*, **8**, 225.

BARNES, J. M. (1970). *Br. J. industr. Med.*, **27**, 147.

BERITÍC, T. & STAHULZAK, D. (1961). *Lancet*, **1**, 669.

BERRY, C. M., GRUNDFAST, H. & HINSEY, J. C. (1944). *J. Neurophysiol.*, **7**, 103.

BIEHL, J. P. & NIMITZ, H. J. (1954). *Amer. Rev. Tuberc.*, **70**, 430.

BIEHL, J. P. & SKAVLEM, J. H. (1953). *Am. Rev. Tuberc. pulm. Dis.*, **68**, 296.

BIEHL, J. P. & VILTER, R. W. (1954). *J. Amer. med. Ass.*, **156**, 1549.

BISCHOFF, A., FIERZ, U., REGLI, F. & ULRICH, J. (1968). *Klin. Wschr.*, **46**, 666.

BISCHOFF, A. & ULRICH, J. (1969). *Brain*, **92**, 861.

BRADLEY, W. G. (1970). *J. neurol. Sci.*, **10**, 133.

BRADLEY, W. G., LASSMAN, L. P., PEARCE, G. W. & WALTON, J. N. (1970). *J. neurol. Sci.*, **10**, 107.

BRADY, R. O., GAL, A. E., BRADLEY, R. M., MARTENSSON, E., WARSHAW, A. L. & LASTER, L. (1967). *New Engl. J. Med.*, **276**, 1163.

BRAIN, W. R. & GREENFIELD, J. G. (1950). *Brain*, **73**, 291.

BUCHTHAL, F. & ROSENFALK, A. (1971). *Brain*, **94**, 241.

BURLEY, D. (1961). *Br. med. J.*, **2**, 1286.

CAMMERMEYER, J. (1956). *J. Neuropath. exp. Neurol.*, **15**, 340.

CASEY, E. B., JELLIFFE, A. M., LE QUESNE, P. M. & Millett, Y.L. Brain. In press.

CASPARY, E. A. & FIELD, E. J. (1965). *J. Neurol. Neurosurg. Psychiat.*, **28**, 179.

CATTON, M. J., HARRISON, M. J. G., FULLERTON, P. M. & KAZANTZIS, G. (1970). *Br. med. J.*, **2**, 80.

CAVANAGH, J. B. (1964a). *Int. Rev. exp. Path.*, **3**, 219.

CAVANAGH, J. B. (1964b). *J. Path. Bact.*, **87**, 365.

CAVANAGH, J. B. (1967). *J. Neurol. Neurosurg. Psychiat.*, **30**, 26.

CAVANAGH, J. B. (1969). *Br. med. Bull.*, **25**, 268.

CHAMBERLAIN, M. A. & BRUCKNER, F. E. (1970). *Ann. rheum. Dis.*, **29**, 609.

CHRISTENSEN, N. J. & ØRSKOV, H. (1969). *J. Neurol. Neurosurg. Psychiat.*, **32**, 519.

CRAGG, B. G. & THOMAS, P. K. (1964). *J. Neurol. Neurosurg. Psychiat.*, **27**, 106.

DELWAIDE, P. J. & CHANTRAINE, A. (1965). In "Proceedings of 6th International Congress of Electroencephalography and Clinical Neurophysiology". p. 643. Vienna, Wiener Medizinische Akademie für ärzliche Fortbildung.

DEPARTMENT OF EMPLOYMENT AND PRODUCTIVITY. (1968). Ann. Rep. of H.M. Chief Inspector of Factories 1967 (Cmnd. 3745). London: HMSO.

DEVIVO, D. C. & ENGEL, W. K. (1970). *J. Neurol. Neurosurg. Psychiat.*, **33**, 62.

DINN, J. J. & CRANE, D. L. (1970). *J. Neurol. Neurosurg. Psychiat.*, **33**, 605.

DROZ, B. & LEBLOND, C. P. (1963). *J. comp. Neurol.*, **121**, 325.

DUNN, H. G., LAKE, B. D., DOLMAN, C. L. & WILSON, J. (1969). *Brain*, **92**, 329.

DYCK, P. J. (1969). *Archs Neurol., Chicago*, **21**, 73.

DYCK, P. J. & LAMBERT, E. H. (1966). *Trans. Am. Neurol. Ass.*, **91**, 214.

DYCK, P. J. & LAMBERT, E. H. (1969). *Archs Neurol., Chicago*, **20**, 490.

ECCLES, R. M., PHILLIPS, C. G. & CHIEN-PING, W. (1968). *J. Physiol.*, **198**, 179.

ELIASSON, S. G. (1969). *J. Neurol. Neurosurg. Psychiat.*, **32**, 525.

ELLIS, F. G. (1962). *Lancet*, **2**, 1136.

ENGEL, W. K., DORMAN, J. D., LEVY, R. I. & FREDRICKSON, D. S. (1967). *Archs Neurol., Chicago*, **17**, 1.

ERLANGER, J. & GASSER, H. S. (1937). "Electrical Signs of Nervous Activity." Philadelphia: University of Pennsylvania Press.

EVANS, D. A. P., MANLEY, K. A. & MCKUSICK, V. A. (1960). *Br. med. J.*, **2**, 485.

FAGERBERG, S. E. (1959). *Acta med. scand. Suppl.*, **345**.

FIELD, R. A. (1966). *Diabetes*, **15**, 696.

FLORENCE, A. L. (1960). *Br. med. J.*, **2**, 1954.

FUJITA, A., SHIBATA, M., KATO, H., AMOMI, Y., ITOMI, K., SUJUKI, K., NAKAJAWA, T. & TAKAHASHI, T. (1960). *Nippon Iji Shinpo*, **1869**, 37.

FULLERTON, P. M. (1964). *J. Neurol. Neurosurg. Psychiat.*, **27**, 100.

FULLERTON, P. M. (1966). *J. Neuropath. exp. neurol.*, **25**, 214.

FULLERTON, P. M. (1969a). *J. Neurol. Neurosurg. Psychiat.*, **32**, 186.

FULLERTON, P. M. (1969b). *Proc. R. Soc. Med.*, **62**, 201.

FULLERTON, P. M. & BARNES, J. M. (1966). *Br. J. industr. Med.*, **23**, 210.

FULLERTON, P. M., GILLIATT, R. W., LASCELLES, R. G. & MORGAN-HUGHES, J. A. (1965). *J. Physiol.*, **178**, 26.

FULLERTON, P. M. & KREMER, M. (1961). *Br. med. J.*, **2**, 855.

FULLERTON, P. M. & O'SULLIVAN, D. J. (1968). *J. Neurol. Neurosurg. Psychiat.*, **31**, 543.

GABBAY, K. H., MEROLA, L. O. & FIELD, R. A. (1966). *Science, N.Y.*, **151**, 209.

GAMMON, G. D., BURGE, F. W. & KING, G. (1953). *Archs Neurol. Psychiat., Chicago*, **70**, 64.

GARLAND, T. O. & PATTERSON, M. W. H. (1967). *Br. med. J.*, **4**, 134.

GEREN, B. B. (1954). *Expl Cell Res.*, **7**, 558.

GILLIATT, R. W. (1966). *Proc. R. Soc. med.*, **59**, 989.

GILLIATT, R. W. & SEARS, T. A. (1958). *J. Neurol. Neurosurg. Psychiat.*, **21**, 109.
GOMBAULT, M. L. (1880). *Archs Neurol., Paris*, **1**, 11.
GONATAS, N. K. & ROBBINS, E. (1965). *Protoplasma*, **59**, 377.
GOODWIN, T. C. (1934). *Johns Hopkins Hosp. Bull.*, **55**, 347.
HART, F. D., GOLDING, J. R. & MACKENZIE, D. H. (1957). *Ann. rheum. Dis.*, **16**, 471.
HAYMAKER, W. & KERNOHAN, J. (1949). *Medicine*, **28**, 59.
HEGSTROM, R. M., MURRAY, J. S., PENDRAS, J. P., BURNELL, J. M. & SCRIBNER, N. H. (1962). *Trans. Am. Soc. artif. intern. Organs*, **8**, 266.
HENRIKSEN, J. D. (1956). M.S. (Phys. med.) Thesis. University of Minnesota.
HERON, J. R., KONOTEY-AHULU, F. I. D., SHALDON, S. & THOMAS, P. K. (1965). *Excerpta med. Int. Congress Series*, **103**, 138.
HEYMAN, A., PFEIFFER, J. B., WILLETT, R. W. & TAYLOR, H. M. (1956). *New Engl. J. Med.*, **254**, 401.
HODES, R., LARREBEE, M. C. & GERMAN, W. (1948). *Archs Neurol. Psychiat., Chicago*, **60**, 340.
HOPKINS, A. P. & GILLIATT, R. W. (1971). *J. Neurol. Neurosurg. Psychiat*, in press.
HOPKINS, A. P. & MORGAN-HUGHES, J. A. (1969). *J. Neurol. Neurosurg. Psychiat.*, **32**, 614.
HUGHES, H. B., BIEHL, J. P., JONES, A. P. & SCHMIDT, L. H. (1954). *Am. Rev. Tuberc. pulm. Dis.*, **70**, 266.
HUNTER, D. (1969). "The Diseases of Occupations." 4th edn. London: English Universities Press.
HUNTER, D., BOMFORD, R. R. & RUSSELL, D. S. (1940). *Q. Jl. Med.*, **9**, 193.
JEBSEN, R. H., TENCKLOFF, H. & HONET, J. C. (1967). *New Engl. J. Med.*, **277**, 327.
JENSEN, J. & JERNELOV, A. (1969). *Nature, Lond.*, **223**, 753.
JONES, W. A. & JONES, G. P. (1953). *Lancet*, **1**, 1073.
KAESER, H. E. (1962). *Dt. Z. Nervenheilk.*, **183**, 268.
KAESER, H. E. & LAMBERT, E. H. (1962). *Electroen. Neurophysiol. Suppl.*, **22**, 29.
KAHLKE, W. & RICHTERICH, R. (1965). *Am. J. Med.*, **39**, 237.
KASA, P. (1968). *Nature, Lond.*, **218**, 1265.
KLENK, E. & KAHLKE, W. (1963). *Hoppe-Seyler's Z. physiol. Chem.*, **333**, 133.
KLINGHARDT, G. W. (1965). *Mitt. Max-Planck Ges.*, **3**, 142.
KOCEN, R. S., LLOYD, J. K., LASCELLES, P. T., FOSBROOKE, A. S. & WILLIAMS, D. (1967). *Lancet*, **1**, 1341.
KOCEN, R. S. & THOMAS, P. K. (1970). *Archs Neurol., Chicago*, **22**, 81.
KOENIG, H. (1958). *Trans. Am. neurol. Ass.*, p. 162.
KONOTEY-AHULU, F. I. D., BAILLOD, R., COMTY, C. M., HERON, J. R., SHALDON, S. & THOMAS, P. K. (1965). *Br. med. J.*, **2**, 1212.
KREUTZBERG, G. W. (1969). *Proc. natn. Acad. Sci., U.S.A.*, **62**, 722.
KRÜCKE, W. (1959). *Dt. Z. Nervenhilk*, **180**, 1.
KUPERMAN, A. S. (1958). *J. Pharmac. exp. Ther.*, **123**, 180.
KURLAND, L. T., FARO, S. N. & SIEDLER, H. (1960). *World Neurol.*, **1**, 370.
LAMBERT, E. H. (1956). "Clinical Examinations in Neurology". p. 287. Philadelphia: Saunders.
LAMPERT, P. W. (1969). *Lab. Invest.*, **20**, 127.
LASLETT, E. E. & WARRINGTON, W. B. (1898). *Brain*, **21**, 224.
LENZ, W. (1962). *Lancet*, **1**, 45.
LE QUESNE, P. M. (1970). *In* "Handbook of Clinical Neurology". Vol. 7. Ed. P. J. Vinken & G. W. Bruyn. p. 527. Amsterdam: North-Holland Publ. Co.
LOUGHRIDGE, L. W. (1962). *Lancet*, **2**, 1133.
LUX, H. D., SCHUBERT, P., KREUTZBERG, G. W. & GLOBUS, A. (1970). *Expl. Brain. Res.*, **10**, 197.
MCCOLLISTER, D. D., OYEN, F. & ROWE, V. K. (1964). *Toxic. appl. Pharmac.*, **6**, 172.
MCDONALD, W. I. (1963). *Brain*, **86**, 481.

McEwen, B. S. & Grafstein, B. (1968). *J. cell Biol.*, **30**, 494.

McLeod, J. G. & Penny, R. (1969). *J. Neurol. Neurosurg. Psychiat.*, **32**, 297.

Matthews, W. B., Howell, D. A. & Hughes, R. C. (1970). *J. Neurol. Neurosurg. Psychiat.*, **33**, 330.

Melnick, S. C. (1963). *Br. med. J.*, **1**, 368.

Morgan-Hughes, J. A. (1968). *J. neurol. Sci.*, **7**, 157.

Morgan-Hughes, J. A., Gajeree, T. & Le Quesne, P. M. To be published.

Mulder, D. W., Lambert, E. H., Bastron, J. A. & Sprague, R. G. (1961). *Neurology, Minneap.*, **11**, 275.

Nielsen, V. K. (1967). *Excerpta Med. Int. Congress Series. No.*, **155**, 279.

Norman, R. M., Urich, H. & Tingey, A. B. (1960). *Brain*, **83**, 369.

Ochoa, J. (1970). *Brain*, **93**, 831.

Ochs, S. & Johnson, J. (1969). *J. Neurochem.*, **16**, 845.

Olivarius, B. de F. (1956). *Ugesk Laeger*, **118**, 753.

Pallis, C. A. & Scott, J. T. (1965). *Br. med. J.*, **1**, 1141.

Pleasure, D. E., Mishner, K. C. & Engel, W. K. (1969). *Science, N.Y.*, **166**, 524.

Preswick, G. & Jeremy, D. (1964). *Lancet*, **2**, 731.

Prineas, J. (1969a). *J. Neuropath. exp. Neurol.*, **28**, 571.

Prineas, J. (1969b). *J. Neuropath. exp. Neurol.*, **28**, 598.

Prineas, J. (1970a). *Archs Neurol., Chicago*, **23**, 541.

Prineas, J. (1970b). *Acta neurol. scand.*, **46**, Suppl. 44.

Raff, M. C., Sangalang, V. & Asbury, A. K. (1968). *Archs Neurol., Chicago*, **18**, 487.

Rasminsky, M. & Sears, T. A. (1971). *4th Int. Congress of Electromyography.* p. 121. Brussels.

Ravn, H. (1967). *Acta neurol. scand.*, **43**, Suppl. 30.

Refsum, S. (1946). *Acta psychiat. neurol. scand.*, Suppl. No. 38.

Reznikoff, P. & Aub, J. C. (1927). *Archs Neurol. Psychiat., Chicago*, **17**, 444.

Robertson, J. D. (1955). *J. biophys. biochem. Cytol.*, **1**, 271.

Rubinstein, C. J. (1964). *J. Am. med. Ass.*, **187**, 647.

Sanders, F. K. & Whitteridge, D. (1946). *J. Physiol.*, **105**, 152.

Scheid, W., Wieck, H. H., Stammler, A., Kladetsky, A. & Gibbels, E. (1961). *Dt. med. Wschr.*, **86**, 938.

Schochet, S. S., Lampert, P. W. & Earle, K. M. (1968). *J. Neuropath. exp. Neurol.*, **27**, 645.

Seneviratne, K. N. & Peiris, O. A. (1968). *J. Neurol. Neurosurg. Psychiat.*, **31**, 348.

Seneviratne, K. N. & Peiris, O. A. (1969). *J. Neurol. Neurosurg. Psychiat.*, **32**, 462.

Seneviratne, K. N. & Peiris, O. A. (1970a). *J. Neurol. Neurosurg. Psychiat.*, **33**, 310.

Seneviratne, K. N. & Peiris, O. A. (1970b). *J. Neurol. Neurosurg. Psychiat.*, **33**, 609.

Shahani, B. & Russell, R. W. (1969). *J. Neurol. Neurosurg. Psychiat.*, **32**, 1.

Shimazono, J. (1914). *Archs Psychiat. Nervenkr.*, **53**, 972.

Simpson, J. A., Seaton, D. A. & Adams, S. F. (1964). *J. Neurol. Neurosurg. Psychiat.*, **27**, 536.

Sobrevilla, L. A., Goodman, M. L. & Kane, C. A. (1964). *Am. J. Med.*, **37**, 821.

Sourander, P. & Olsson, Y. (1968). *Acta neuropath.*, **11**, 69.

Steinberg, D., Mize, C., Avigan, J., Fales, H. M., Eldjarn, L. E., Try, K., Stokke, O. & Refsum, S. (1966). *Trans. Am. Neurol. Ass.*, **91**, 168.

Steinberg, D., Vroom, F. Q., Engel, W. K., Cammermeyer, J., Mize, C. E. & Avian, J. (1967). *Ann. intern. Med.*, **66**, 365.

Steiness, I. B. (1959). *Acta med. scand.*, **163**, 195.

Thomas, P. K. (1969). *In* "Fifth Symposium on Advanced Medicine". Ed. R. Williams. p. 323. London: Pitman.

THOMAS, P. K. (1970). *J. neurol. Sci.*, **11**, 285.

THOMAS, P. K. & LASCELLES, R. G. (1966). *Q. Jl. Med.*, **35**, 489.

THOMAS, P. K. & LASCELLES, R. G. (1967). *Q. Jl. Med.*, **36**, 223.

THOMAS, P. K., LASCELLES, J. F., HALLPIKE, J. F. & HEWER, R. L. (1969). *Brain*, **92**, 589.

THOMAS, P. K. & WALKER, J. G. (1965). *Brain*, **88**, 1079.

TYLER, H. R. (1968). *Am. J. Med.*, **44**, 734.

VIGLIANI, E. C. (1954). *Br. J. indust. Med.*, **11**, 235.

VIZOSO, A. D. & YOUNG, J. Z. (1948). *J. Anat.*, **82**, 110.

WAKSMAN, B. H. & ADAMS, R. D. (1955). *J. exp. Med.*, **102**, 213.

WAROTT, P., GOUDEMAND, M. & HABAY, D. (1965). *Rev. neurol.*, **113**, 464.

WEBSTER, H. DE F. (1962). *J. Neuropath. exp. Neurol.*, **21**, 534.

WEBSTER, H. DE F., SCHRÖDER, J. M., ASBURY, A. K. & ADAMS, R. D. (1967). *J. Neuropath. exp. Neurol.*, **26**, 276.

WEBSTER, H. DE F., SPIRO, D., WAKSMAN, B. H. & ADAMS, R. D. (1961). *J. Neuropath. exp. Neurol.*, **20**, 5.

WEISS, P. & HISCOE, H. B. (1948). *J. exp. Neurol.*, **107**, 315.

WELLER, R. O. (1965). *J. Path. Bact.*, **89**, 591.

WELLER, R. O. (1967). *J. Neurol. Neurosurg. Psychiat.*, **30**, 111.

WELLER, R. O., BRUCKNER, F. E. & CHAMBERLAIN, M. A. (1970). *J. Neurol. Neurosurg. Psychiat.*, **33**, 592.

WIEDERHOLT, W. C., MULDER, D. W. & LAMBERT, E. H. (1964). *Mayo Clin. Proc.*, **39**, 427.

WILLETT, R. W. (1963). *Neurology, Minneap.*, **13**, 344.

WINKLER, G. F. (1965). *Ann N.Y. Acad. Sci.*, **122**, 287.

WISNIEWSKI, H., SHELANSKI, M. L. & TERRY, R. D. (1968). *J. cell Biol.*, **38**, 224.

WISNIEWSKI, H., TERRY, R. D., WHITAKER, J. N., COOK, S. D. & DOWLING, P. C. (1969). *Archs Neurol., Chicago*, **21**, 269.

WUERKER, R. B., McPHEDRAN, A. M. & HENNEMAN, E. (1965). *J. Neurophysiol.*, **28**, 85.

YUDELL, A., GOMEZ, M. R., LAMBERT, E. H. & DOCKERTY, M. B. (1967). *Neurology Minneap.*, **17**, 103.

CHAPTER 3

CALCIUM HOMEOSTASIS IN HEALTH AND DISEASE

M. R. WILLS

The control mechanisms involved in calcium homeostasis can be divided, essentially, into physico-chemical and hormonal. In most, if not all, situations where physico-chemical factors cause alterations in calcium homeostasis these induce regulatory hormone changes and in the overall control of calcium homeostasis the hormonal mechanisms are dominant.

PHYSICO-CHEMICAL FACTORS IN CALCIUM HOMEOSTASIS

The skeleton represents an almost inexhaustible reserve of calcium, and simple exchange of ions undoubtedly takes place between bone crystal surfaces and the extracellular fluid compartment. The rate of this exchange is almost certainly influenced by physico-chemical variations in the constitution of the extracellular fluid, and by alterations in the physical factors which control skeletal homeostasis.

Physical Factors

In the maintenance of a normal skeleton and the mineralisation of bone matrix the physical factors of mechanical stress from muscular activity and gravitational weight bearing are of considerable importance. The loss of these stimulatory physical factors can cause disturbances not only in skeletal homeostasis but also in calcium homeostasis and are mainly reflected by changes in urine calcium excretion.

Acid-base Effects

It has been established that dissolution of bone salt occurs both in disease states causing a metabolic acidosis, and in response to experimental acid loading (Bernstein, Wachman & Hattner, 1970). It is probable that the dissolution of bone salt which occurs in acidotic states is due to an increase in ion exchange between the bone crystal surfaces and the extracellular fluid, as a direct consequence of the increased hydrogen ion concentration in the latter compartment. In addition to acting as a reservoir for calcium the skeleton also provides an enormous reserve of phosphate. The importance of the buffering role of the phosphate ions liberated by the dissolution of bone salt in acidotic states is, however, controversial. It has been proposed that the cellular mechanisms involved in bone formation and resorption may be responsive to alterations in acid-base status such that bone is formed or liberated during periods of alkalosis or acidosis respectively (Barzel & Jowsey, 1969). The role of metabolic acidosis in the aetiology of bone disease in conditions associated with disturbances in hydrogen ion excretion, such as chronic renal failure, is, however, controversial (Wills, 1971a). The current evidence would support the concept that in disease states associated with metabolic acidosis the latter probably does play a role in the production of bone disease although the precise extent of that role and its relationship with hormone control factors remains to be clarified. It has been proposed that the liberation of bone salt is a possible mechanism involved in the buffering of the fixed acid load imposed by the ingestion of an 'acid-ash' diet in man and this is an aetiological factor in so-called 'idiopathic' osteoporosis (Wachman & Bernstein, 1968). This interesting hypothesis awaits further clarification.

HORMONAL CONTROL OF CALCIUM HOMEOSTASIS

In normal human subjects, under standardised conditions of calcium intake, the plasma calcium concentration is maintained within remarkably narrow limits (Wills, 1970a). This is currently considered to depend on the interaction of two hormones, parathyroid hormone and calcitonin, acting primarily either on bone (Copp, 1969) or on the renal tubular handling of calcium (Nordin & Peacock, 1969). In either case the dominant role is attributed to parathyroid hormone. There is now a considerable amount of evidence that cholecalciferol (Vitamin D_3) plays an important role in the transport of calcium across cells and in any consideration of the hormone control of calcium homeostasis cholecalciferol must also be included.

The hormones involved in calcium homeostasis exert their control in an integrated manner through three main processes: (i) the balance between the rates of deposition and mobilisation of calcium in bone; (ii) the urine excretion of calcium; and (iii) the absorption of calcium from the gastro-intestinal tract. Calcium is also lost from the body in the faeces. The total faecal calcium content represents the sum of the dietary calcium intake less the amount which has been absorbed plus the endogenous faecal calcium. The endogenous faecal calcium represents the calcium content of the various intestinal secretions and as such is a passive, rather than an active, route of calcium loss from the body. The importance and extent of endogenous intestinal calcium turnover is not clearly defined.

Parathyroid Hormone

Parathyroid hormone is a single-chain polypeptide that exerts its regulatory role in calcium homeostasis through its actions on bone, the kidney, and the gastro-intestinal tract.

Action on bone

The actions of parathyroid hormone on bone are complex and apparently involve all of the osteogenic cells—the osteoclast, the osteoblast, and the osteocyte. The osteoclast is the osteogenic cell which is responsible for bone resorption, that is the removal of both the organic and inorganic phases of bone. The osteoblast is the cell responsible for the laying down of bone matrix and probably through the liberation of alkaline phosphatase plays a role in the initiation of mineralisation. The precise role of the osteo-cyte is not clearly defined although under certain conditions it is capable of removing bone by changes induced in the organic matrix. Parathyroid hormone is considered to have at least three direct effects upon bone: (i) it promotes resorption by the osteoclasts; (ii) it both inhibits and stimulates osteoblast activity; and (iii) it promotes osteolysis by the osteocytes.

Osteoclasts and osteoblasts. It has been demonstrated that following the administration of parathyroid extract there is a marked increase in osteoclast activity with after a time-interval an increase in the total number of osteoclasts (Bingham, Brazell & Owen, 1969). Bingham and her colleagues considered that the increase in total numbers of osteoclasts was a secondary effect and followed as the result of increased metabolic activity of the osteoclasts present at the time of commencement of hormone action. In this concept the resorption of bone from increased osteoclast activity accounts for the increase in plasma calcium concentration, and which precedes the increase in total number of osteoclasts. Bingham and her colleagues also reported that the changes in plasma calcium concentration, induced by osteoclastic bone resorption, were augmented by an inhibition of osteoblast activity due to a simultaneous action of parathyroid hormone on these cells. However, it was demonstrated in their studies that the initial decrease in osteoblast activity was followed by a late transient increase.

Osteocytes. In addition to the effects of parathyroid hormone on both the osteclast and the osteoblast there is also a considerable amount of evidence that parathyroid hormone acts on the osteocyte to induce osteolysis and that this cell plays a fundamental role in the action of the hormone on bone. Rasmussen & Tenenhouse (1967) considered that the osteocyte may be the cell primarily involved in the regulation of calcium concentration; whereas the osteoclasts and the surface resorption of bone were primarily of importance in skeletal homeostasis and only became involved in calcium regulation when a disturbance was either severe or prolonged. In this concept the osteocytes are considered to act as a finely controlled mechanism which is the primary 'buffer' to counteract any changes in the calcium concentration of the extracellular fluid compartment. It would seem probable that the osteocytes could fulfil such a role because these cells, and their cellular extensions the canaliculi, do form an extensive network with a large surface area throughout the entire cortical and trabecular bone which gives them ready access to the surfaces of bone crystals.

Action on kidney

The actions of parathyroid hormone on the kidney are complex, and involve not only the renal tubular reabsorption of calcium and phosphate but also the tubular reabsorption of sodium, hydrogen ion and water.

Calcium and sodium. Widrow & Levinsky (1962), using stop-flow studies in dogs, demonstrated that parathyroid extract directly increased the tubular reabsorption of calcium and that this effect was exerted, at least in part, at a distal tubular site. The mechanisms involved in the renal tubular handling of calcium are, at present, not clearly defined. Clearance studies in animals have shown that procedures which increase the urine excretion of sodium usually increase the excretion of calcium; conversely those which increase the excretion of calcium usually increase the excretion of sodium. An effect of one ion, calcium or sodium, on the tubular reabsorption of the other (Walser, 1961) with perhaps a shared transport process for the two ions

(Gutman & Gottschalk, 1966) has been proposed to explain this inter-relationship. However, in studies on the interrelationships between the urine excretion of these two ions over long periods in subjects on fixed metabolic regimens no consistent relationship was observed between the absolute mean values for urine calcium and those for urine sodium either during the control periods or during various regimens that affected the urine excretion of one or other of these ions (Wills, Gill & Bartter, 1969). Wills and his colleagues suggested that the regimens produced their effects through alteration of tubular function rather than through an effect of one ion, calcium or sodium, on the tubular reabsorption of the other. The previously reported inter-relationship of the urine excretion of these two ions, when considered in conjunction with the findings of Wills and his colleagues (1969), might represent competition within the tubular cells for a common energy source, such as ATP, and are otherwise distinct, rather than invoking a common regulatory mechanism for their renal excretion.

Phosphate. It is now generally agreed that parathyroid hormone increases urine phosphate excretion by its action on the renal tubules to decrease phosphate reabsorption and may possibly increase or start tubular secretion. Fourman & Royer (1968) considered that although parathyroid hormone is regulatory it is not part of a homoestatic mechanism for regulating plasma phosphate concentration. These views are supported by their own and other observations that the body can excrete phosphate loads in the absence of the parathyroid glands.

Hydrogen ions and water. In addition to its actions on the renal tubular handling of calcium and phosphate it has been demonstrated that the injection of parathyroid extract, or of purified parathyroid hormone, causes the urine to become more alkaline (Hellman, Au & Bartter, 1965). An inability of the renal tubules to acidify the urine normally after the administration of ammonium chloride has been demonstrated in a proportion of hyperparathyroid patients, particularly those with renal stones (Fourman, McConkey & Smith, 1960). Fourman and his co-workers concluded that defect in urine acidification in these patients which was associated with a failure to reabsorb water normally, was not simply due to the high circulating concentration of either parathyroid hormone or calcium as the defect did not disappear after removal of a parathyroid adenoma. They postulated that these changes could be the result of renal deposition of calcium. The evidence, however, suggests that the administration of parathyroid extract affects the ability of the renal tubules both to acidify urine (Hellman, Au & Bartter, 1965) and to reabsorb water (Charbon, Brummer & Reneman, 1968) independently of renal tubular cell damage or changes in either serum calcium concentration or its urine excretion. The importance of the action of parathyroid hormone on the maintenance of a hydrogen ion gradient between the body fluids and the tubular urine is not clearly defined. It is, however, possible that this action is of fundamental importance in any consideration of the evolutionary role of parathyroid hormone (Wills, 1970b; 1971b).

Action on gastro-intestinal tract

Reports of the effect of parathyroid hormone on the absorption of calcium from the gastro-intestinal tract in man have, in the main, been based on indirect evidence derived from clinical studies in patients with either hyper-parathyroidism or hypoparathyroidism. Recently, Wills *et al.* (1970) have reported evidence that parathyroid hormone plays a small but significant role in enhancing the intestinal absorption of calcium in man. Previous workers had reported that the administration of parathyroid extract had no effect on intestinal calcium absorption in normal human subjects as assessed by faecal calcium excretion (Aub, Tibbetts & McLean, 1937) or by calcium transport measured by unidirectional flux rates (Wensel *et al.*, 1969). In those studies based on faecal calcium excretion it is probable that the calcium content of faeces does not give a true estimate of intestinal calcium absorption in a situation where the plasma calcium concentration is changing, as the latter does following the administration of parathyroid extract. In such a situation the increase in plasma calcium concentration could induce an increase in endogenous faecal calcium. If the extra calcium is secreted into the intestinal tract at a point lower than the absorption site any changes in absorption would be masked. In those experiments where calcium transport was measured by the unidirectional flux rate of calcium from the intestinal lumen to the blood no significant effect upon calcium transport was demonstrated after the intravenous injection of parathyroid extract. However, the effects were only measured for 90 to 150 minutes after the injection of extract and the lack of effect in these experiments was presumably due to the relatively short follow-up time, after the injection, when compared with the long-term studies of Wills and his colleagues (1970).

Mode of action: cyclic 3′,5′-AMP

There is now a considerable amount of evidence that parathyroid hormone exerts both its renal and skeletal actions through cyclic 3′,5′-adenosine monophosphate (cyclic 3′,5′-AMP), (Chase, Fedak & Aurbach, 1969). Cyclic 3′,5′-AMP has been implicated in a wide variety of hormone-dependent biological actions as the second messenger (Hardman, Robison & Sutherland, 1971). In this concept hormones are considered to act by a two messenger system. The first messenger, the hormone itself, acts on the cells of its target tissues to cause an alteration in the intra-cellular concentration of the second messenger which initiates the cellular activity, or activities, characteristic of that hormone. As cyclic 3′,5′-AMP is a fundamental substance found in almost all cells the way in which any one cell type responds to the changes in cyclic 3′,5′-AMP would appear to depend upon the biochemical constitution of the cell, which varies between cell types.

The majority of studies that have been undertaken on the cellular mode of action of parathyroid hormone have been with respect to its action on bone, where it causes dissolution of both the organic and inorganic phases. It is generally agreed that the dissolution of the mineral phase of bone is caused by a local increase in hydrogen ion concentration while dissolution of the organic phase is the result of enzymatic degradation. In the process of bone resorption it has been demonstrated that the lysosomes and their enzymes are involved. In osteoclastic bone resorption it has been proposed that the acid hydrolases of the lysosomes are excreted in bulk, through exocytosis, into a sealed resorption zone beneath the osteoclast where they act on the organic components of bone matrix (Vaes, 1969). In his hypothesis Vaes also suggested that the simultaneous excretion of organic acids into the resorption zone would solubilise the mineral component of bone. He proposed that these two simultaneous events, which would augment each other in their actions, would be initiated through the stimulation by intracytoplasmic messengers of the synthesis and release of lysosomal enzymes, and an increased output of organic acids. In this concept the release of the intracytoplasmic messengers by the cell membrane receptors would be the consequence of the action, on those receptors, of parathyroid hormone. Vaes considered that the intracytoplasmic messengers could include cyclic 3',5'-AMP.

It is known that for cyclic 3',5'-AMP to exert some of its actions there is a requirement for calcium in the external medium for the appropriate hormone stimulus to be effective. The critical nature of this requirement for parathyroid hormone has been demonstrated by Nagata & Rasmussen (1970), who reported that although the hormone effected an increase in cyclic 3',5'-AMP in isolated rat renal tubules it did not enhance the rate of gluconeogenesis in the absence of calcium. It has been postulated that an essential step in the physiological action of parathyroid hormone is an alteration in calcium distribution between the extra-cellular and intra-cellular compartments (Tenenhouse, Rasmussen & Nagata, 1970): they proposed that the redistribution of calcium occurred subsequent to, and was perhaps the direct result of, the accumulation of cyclic 3',5'-AMP within the cell. Although the mechanism whereby cyclic 3',5'-AMP effects this redistribution remains to be clarified it is presumably accounted for by the known effects of cyclic 3',5'-AMP on cell membrane permeability. They also attributed a direct intracellular action to the increased calcium ion concentration, and proposed that as the calcium ion is known to inhibit isocitrate dehydrogenase, and thus citric acid cycle activity, there would be a consequent accumulation of citrate which would presumably act in solubilisation of the mineral phase of bone and augment the actions of cyclic 3',5'-AMP on acid production. The cellular mechanisms of action of parathyroid hormone is intimately linked with the mode of action of cholecalciferol and this will be discussed later.

Cholecalciferol (Vitamin D_3)

Although the main role of cholecalciferol in calcium homeostasis is usually considered with respect to the intestinal absorption of calcium there is evidence that it also has a direct action on bone metabolism and the renal tubular handling of both calcium and phosphate. At these sites of action cholecalciferol has effects comparable to those of parathyroid hormone, although it is not dependent on the presence of the parathyroid glands to exert its effects.

Action on bone

There is now a considerable amount of evidence that cholecalciferol has a direct effect on bone metabolism. When cholecalciferol is administered in small doses it promotes mineralisation of bone; however, when it is administered in large doses over a long period of time there is an increase in plasma calcium concentration which is associated with bone resorption. The mechanism by which cholecalciferol induces bone resorption is not clearly defined although it is undoubtedly different to the mode of action of parathyroid hormone. This view is supported by the observations that although cholecalciferol affects the bone mobilisation of calcium in contrast to parathyroid hormone it does not mobilise bone collagen or increase urine hydroxyproline excretion (Ney, Kelly & Bartter, 1968).

Action on kidney

On the kidney cholecalciferol has actions comparable to those of parathyroid hormone in that it increases the tubular reabsorption of calcium (Gran, 1960) and decreases the tubular reabsorption of phosphate (Bartter & Ney, 1967).

Action on gastro-intestinal tract

Cholecalciferol is undoubtedly the dominant factor in the absorption of calcium from the intestinal tract. There is also evidence that the absorption of phosphate is under the influence of cholecalciferol. It has been proposed that phosphate transport is mediated through two routes one of which is independent of calcium and mediated by diffusion, and the other depending on an active transport mechanism linked to calcium (Fourman & Morgan, 1969).

Mode of action

It is now generally accepted that a metabolite or metabolites of cholecalciferol act by stimulating the transport of calcium across cells in bone, intestine and kidney. In homogenates of intestinal mucosal cells the presence of a specific calcium-binding protein has been demonstrated as part of the cholecalciferol-induced transport mechanism (Wasserman, 1968). That cholecalciferol played a role in protein synthesis was demonstrated by Eisenstein & Passavoy (1964) who reported that the administration of actinomycin D blocked the cholecalciferol-mediated stimulation of intestinal calcium transport. There was some doubt initially as to whether cholecalciferol induced protein synthesis direct, via RNA, or indirectly by altering the permeability of the nuclear membrane to calcium. The evidence, however, now supports the concept that cholecalciferol metabolites act directly, via RNA, in the induction of the specific transport protein, although it is possible that alterations in intracellular calcium concentration do have a subsidiary 'triggering' role.

It is known that mitochondria are involved in calcium ion transport and bind calcium according to three different processes (Lehninger, 1970). One of these processes has been described as 'high-affinity' binding and is considered to be both reversible and mediated through a specific carrier substance (Reynafarje & Lehninger, 1969). It could be postulated that the effects of cholecalciferol on the cellular transport of calcium are effected at the mitochondrial level possibly through an action on the 'high-affinity' calcium binding site. It is known that isolated rat kidney mitochondria bind calcium by a process that is dependent upon the presence of magnesium ions, ATP and an oxidizable substrate, such as succinate, but does not require the presence of either cholecalciferol or parathyroid hormone. The subsequent release of calcium from these mitochondria is, however, stimulated by both cholecalciferol and parathyroid hormone, although the latter requires the presence of cholecalciferol to exert its effect (DeLuca, Engstrom & Rasmussen, 1962). Alterations in intracellular calcium concentration could play a role at this level in the induction of protein synthesis by cholecalciferol metabolites.

The nature of the biologically active metabolites of cholecalciferol have been intensively investigated in recent years. DeLuca (1969) reported evidence from which he proposed that the biologically active metabolite of cholecalciferol was probably 25-hydroxycholecalciferol. It has been proposed that the probable site of conversion of cholecalciferol to 25-hydroxy-cholecalciferol is the liver (Ponchon & DeLuca, 1969) and there is some evidence that the conversion rate is product-regulated (Horsting & DeLuca, 1969). Subsequently, however, it has been suggested that 25-hydroxychole-calciferol represents the circulating form of cholecalciferol in plasma and a more polar metabolite accumulates in the target tissues which accounts for the characteristic action of cholecalciferol on intestinal and other cells (Myrtle & Norman, 1971). Recently Lawson et al. (1971) have reported that the more polar metabolite in intestinal mucosal cells is 1,25-dihydroxy-cholecalciferol and its formation involves a further hydroxylation step which takes place in the kidney. Other cholecalciferol metabolites have been isolated in plasma and amongst these is 21,25-dihydroxycholecalciferol which appears to be preferentially active in the mobilisation of bone mineral (Suda et al., 1970). The further clarification of the individual metabolites of cholecalciferol and their precise role in calcium homeostasis remains to be defined. The importance of this role is stressed by the recent report that the in vivo synthesis of the dihydroxy metabolites of 25-hydroxycholecalciferol is regulated by the circulating calcium concentration (Boyle, Gray & DeLuca, 1971). Such a regulatory role for circulating calcium concentration would support the concept of cholecalciferol as a hormone under feed-back control.

Interrelationship between cholecalciferol and parathyroid hormone

Although it is now undisputed that both cholecalciferol and parathyroid hormone are involved in calcium homeostasis there is controversy over the interrelationship between these two substances. Cholecalciferol can exert its actions in the absence of parathyroid hormone while parathyroid hormone appears to be dependent on the presence of cholecalciferol to exert most, if not all, of its actions. In clinical studies it has been reported that there were negligible changes in plasma calcium concentration and urine phosphate excretion after either acute intravenous (Evanson, 1966), or repeated intra-muscular administration (Freer & Wills, 1970) of parathyroid extract to hypocalcaemic patients with chronic renal failure and acquired chole-calciferol resistance.

It has been proposed that the lack of response to parathyroid hormone in cholecalciferol-deficient or resistant states is due to a local critical lack of calcium at the site of hormone action (Raisz & Niemann, 1969). In this concept it would seem possible that the acquired resistance to parathyroid hormone in patients with hypocalcaemia due to cholecalciferol deficient or resistant states could be attributed to a critical lack of calcium to mediate some of the actions of cyclic $3',5'$-AMP. However, the administration of parathyroid extract to hypocalcaemic hypoparathyroid patients produces all of the known metabolic effects of parathyroid hormone and the results are comparable to the administration of the extract to normal subjects. It would seem unlikely, therefore, that a lack of calcium ion to mediate the actions of cyclic 3′,5′-AMP accounts for the interrelationship between parathyroid hormone and cholecalciferol.

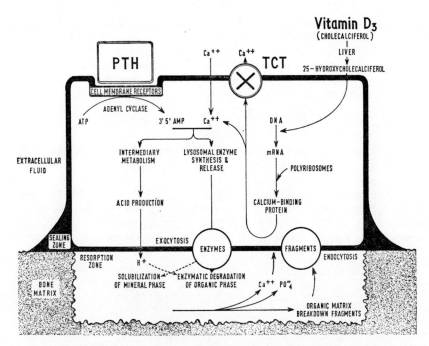

FIG. 3.1. Model of an osteoclast to indicate probable modes of action and interrelationship between parathyroid hormone and cholecalciferol.

Parathyroid hormone (PTH) acts on cell membrane receptors activating adenyl cyclase and formation of cyclic 3′,5′-AMP. The intracellular accumulation of cyclic 3′,5′-AMP is associated with the passive entry of calcium ions into the cell from the extracellular fluid compartment, probably through increased cell membrane permeability; within the cell cyclic 3′,5′-AMP acting as 'second messenger' causes an increase in H^+ ion production and stimulates both the synthesis and release of lysosomal enzymes. The release of H^+ ions and lysosomal enzymes into the sealed resorption zone beneath the cell accounts for the dissolution of both the organic and inorganic phases of bone. The intracellular events that 'trigger' the synthesis of the specific calcium-binding transport protein by 25-hydroxycholecalciferol or by the dihydroxy metabolites of cholecalciferol are unknown. It is possible, however, that transport protein synthesis and the direction of transport is initiated in some way by the increased calcium ion concentration in the resorption zone, and also changes in intracellular nuclear calcium-binding protein. Calcium ion extrusion from the cell is an active process which involves a pump mechanism and probably sodium for calcium ion exchange. It is also the probable site of the inhibitory action of calcitonin (TCT). In this model the rate limiting step is the intracellular synthesis of the specific calcium-binding transport protein, a function of 25-hydroxycholecalciferol or of the dihydroxy metabolites of cholecalciferol.

It is now generally accepted that actions of parathyroid hormone are mediated by cyclic 3',5'-AMP and that the action of cholecalciferol is to induce the synthesis of a specific transport protein. A model of an osteoclast which shows the probable relationship between these mechanisms of action of parathyroid hormone and cholecalciferol are shown in Fig. 3.1. The relationships shown in this model are consistent with the view of DeLuca (1970) who proposed that in the cholecalciferol-deficient state the intra-cellular synthesis of the specific calcium-binding transport protein is the rate limiting step such that any changes in calcium ion distribution induced by parathyroid hormone activity are ineffective. The dependence of parathyroid hormone on cholecalciferol is consistent with the late evolutionary develop-ment of the parathyroid glands and the apparent earlier evolutionary develop-ment of cholecalciferol (Wills, 1970b).

Calcitonin

In 1962 Copp *et al.* reported evidence for the existence of a hormone which was capable of lowering the plasma calcium concentration. They named the hormone calcitonin because they considered that it was involved in the regulation of the normal concentration or 'tone' of calcium in the body fluids. The existence of this polypeptide hormone which is secreted by the parafollicular or 'C' cells of the thyroid in man is now well established. However, the precise physiological role of calcitonin remains to be clarified (Copp, 1969).

Action on bone

Calcitonin rapidly inhibits the release of calcium from resorbing bone *in vitro* and *in vivo* with a time course which is similar to that for its action *in vivo* in lowering the plasma calcium concentration (Reynolds & Dingle, 1970). Reynolds & Dingle also reported that calcitonin prevented the forma-tion of new osteoclasts and inhibited the bone mineral mobilising action of existing osteoclasts. These effects of calcitonin on the osteoclast are associated with a reduction in the bone collagen resorption rate, although the hormone has no effect on collagen synthesis or deposition (Flanagan & Nichols, 1969).

Action on kidney

There is evidence that calcitonin causes a decrease in the tubular reab-sorption of both calcium and phosphate (Cochran *et al.*, 1970). However, it was demonstrated in these studies that although calcitonin has a phosphaturic action similar to that of parathyroid hormone it did not affect the renal excretion of hydrogen ions in a reproducible manner.

Action on gastro-intestinal tract

It has been reported that calcitonin has no effect on the absorption of either calcium or phosphate from the intestinal tract (Robinson, Matthews & MacIntyre, 1969).

Mode of action

The mode of action of calcitonin at the cellular level is not clearly defined. There is evidence that calcitonin inhibits the extrusion of calcium from the cell and thereby increases the intracellular calcium concentration (Borle, 1969). It has been demonstrated that the calcaemic effect of the administration of parathyroid extract is inhibited by the simultaneous injection of calcitonin (Evanson et al., 1967). These observations would suggest some 'final common pathway' in the modes of action of both parathyroid hormone and calcitonin. In his hypothesis for the mode of action of calcitonin MacIntyre (1970) proposed that the hormone acted on a membrane pump to influence the rate of extrusion of calcium from the cell. This hypothesis is consistent with the observations that the hypocalcaemic action of exogenous calcitonin is only marked in those situations where bone resorption is the dominant factor controlling the plasma calcium concentration.

HYPERCALCAEMIA

There is a risk of irreversible renal damage in all patients with hypercalcaemia, if it is allowed to continue. The accurate differential diagnosis of hypercalcaemia is therefore important if rational treatment is to be instituted for the underlying condition. The differential diagnosis of hypercalcaemia is essentially based on clinical evaluation and biochemical criteria, as the symptoms of hypercalcaemia are the same irrespective of the aetiological mechanism. The symptoms, all of which are vague and non-specific, include fatigue, muscular weakness, lassitude, headache, loss of appetite, vomiting, chronic constipation, mental disturbances, thirst and polyuria.

Conditions Giving Rise to Hypercalcaemia

The diseases in which hypercalcaemia may occur are described in an order which corresponds to the general frequency of the condition. In many patients a diagnosis can either be made or excluded by the clinical history, physical and radiological examination of the patient. Frequently, however, the history may be inadequate with ill-defined physical and radiological findings and the problem of differential diagnosis has to be undertaken. Of particular importance is the recognition of primary hyperparathyroidism.

Carcinoma

The commonest cause of hypercalcaemia is carcinoma, in which it is most frequently due to the presence of osteolytic bone metatases. The commonest source of osteolytic bone metastases are from primary neoplasms of breast, bronchus, kidney, or thyroid, and in these patients the dissolution of bone salt, by the metastatic tumour process, causes a rise in both the plasma calcium and phosphate concentrations.

In recent years an increasing number of carcinoma patients with hypercalcaemia have been reported in whom there were no demonstrable metastatic bone lesions either on radiological bone survey during life or on careful histological examination of the bones at autopsy. In these patients three possible mechanisms must be considered to account for the hypercalcaemia. These three mechanisms invoke the secretion by the primary tumour of (1) a parathyroid hormone-like polypeptide; (2) an osteolytic sterol; and (3) a substance or substances that stimulate the parathyroid glands. Of these possible mechanisms the first two are established, and the third is unestablished but is a theoretical possibility.

(1) Parathyroid hormone-like polypeptide. The secretion by a primary tumour of a polypeptide which has actions similar to those of a naturally occurring hormone allows that tumour to be classified as a non-endocrine hormone-secreting tumour. In this particular situation the primary tumours synthesize a parathyroid hormone-like polypeptide which causes hypercalcaemia and hypophosphataemia, and the syndrome has been termed 'pseudohyperparathyroidism' (Fry, 1962). The diagnostic criteria for establishing a case as one of pseudohyperparathyroidism include the following: (*a*) hypercalcaemia and hypophosphataemia, although the latter may be normal with concomitant renal damage, (*b*) tumour of non-parathyroid origin, with if possible demonstration of normal or hypoplastic parathyroid glands at either surgical exploration or autopsy, (*c*) no demonstrable osseous metastases on either radiological survey or at autopsy, (*b*) conversion of abnormal biochemical findings to normal values after either surgical resection or other treatment of the primary tumour, (*e*) demonstration in either tumour extracts or plasma of a parathyroid hormone-like polypeptide. It has been established that both tumour extracts and the plasma from patients with pseudohyperparathyroidism contain a polypeptide which is immunologically similar to the naturally occurring hormone (Omenn, Roth & Baker, 1969). Pseudohyperparathyroidism is the commonest of the endocrine syndromes associated with bronchial carcinoma and occurs most frequently with tumours of squamous-cell origin (Azzopardi, Freeman & Poole, 1970).

The differentiation of patients with pseudohyperparathyroidism from those with primary hyperparathyroidism is of importance, particularly as in the former group there may be a small relatively symptomless primary neoplasm. However, the biochemical findings in patients with pseudohyperparathyroidism differ from those with primary hyperparathyroidism and an excess of the naturally occurring hormone. In pseudohyperparathyroidism there is invariably a hypochloraemic metabolic alkalosis in contrast to the hyperchloraemic metabolic acidosis which is usually present in patients with primary hyperparathyroidism (Wills, 1971c). These observations suggest that parathyroid hormone and the parathyroid hormone-like polypeptide produced by non-endocrine secreting tumours are not identical.

(2) Osteolytic sterol. In patients with non-metastatic breast carcinoma and hypercalcaemia, associated with either a normal or slightly raised plasma phosphate concentration, an osteolytic sterol (resembling 7-dehydrocholesterol) has been isolated from the breast tumour (Gordan *et al.*, 1966). 7-dehydrocholesterol is the precursor of cholecalciferol and it is possible that an excess of the precursor could lead to a state of cholecalciferol excess.

(3) Parathyrotrophic substance. The existence of an unknown parathyrotrophic substance, or substances, that causes parathyroid hormone secretion, with consequent hypercalcaemia and hypophosphataemia in patients with non-metastatic carcinoma, would seem most unlikely. In the majority of reported cases classified as pseudohyperparathyroidism information is lacking on the state, at autopsy, of the parathyroid glands. In some reports the glands are described as normal and in a very few either atrophic or hyperplastic (Grimes *et al.*, 1967). In a recent autopsy study of hypercalcaemia in patients with bronchial carcinoma, Azzopardi & Whittaker (1969) reported that the parathyroids were usually atrophic. They considered that 'the relationship between the genuine but very rare case of parathyroid hyperplasia with hypercalcaemia and accompanying malignant disease is obscure'.

Primary hyperparathyroidism

Although not the commonest cause of hypercalcaemia, primary hyperparathyroidism is probably the best known, and its most frequent clinical presentation is associated with symptoms of either renal stones or metabolic bone disease. In a statistical review of 138 cases of primary hyperparathyroidism Lloyd (1968) reported that the mean plasma calcium concentration and mean tumour weights were significantly lower in patients with renal stones than in those with osteitis fibrosa. He proposed that there are two main types of parathyroid tumour, one rapidly growing and highly active that causes overt bone disease, and the other slowly growing and of low activity that causes kidney stones. It is also recognised that hyperparathyroidism may present in association with a wide variety of other diseases or may even be an 'accidental' finding (Dent, 1962). In this latter respect the use of routine biochemical screening, of all patients admitted to hospital, has accounted for a marked increase in diagnosis (Haff, Black & Ballinger, 1970). These latter studies support the view that primary hyperparathyroidism is by no means a rare disease.

Classically the diagnosis of primary hyperparathyroidism has been based upon the demonstration of high plasma calcium and low plasma phosphate concentrations. The finding of hypercalcaemia is undoubtedly the best index in the diagnosis of primary hyperparathyroidism. In recent years, however, it has become established that normocalcaemia may occasionally occur in patients with primary hyperparathyroidism (Wills, 1971d). It is particularly among patients with renal stones and hypercalciuria that normocalcaemic primary hyperparathyroidism may occur.

Myelomatosis

Hypercalcaemia is relatively common in patients with myelomatosis although the mechanism is not clearly defined. However, it is recognised that the hypercalcaemia is not entirely related to the degree of hyperproteinaemia or to the extent of the bone lesions.

Vitamin D intoxication

Vitamin D intoxication may occur as a complication in patients either taking the vitamin as part of a therapeutic medical regimen or self-administered for 'tonic' purposes. In either situation the vitamin acts as a cumulative toxic compound. The hypercalcaemia is due to an increase in gastro-intestinal calcium absorption and calcium release from bone, with the former predominant.

Sarcoidosis

Hypercalcaemia is a complication of sarcoidosis, and is apparently caused by an undue sensitivity to all of the actions of cholecalciferol (Dent, 1970).

Paget's disease

Hypercalcaemia is a very rare complication of patients with Paget's disease and only occurs when the patients are immobilised and confined to bed. Hypercalcaemia in this disease is related to the abnormal bone turnover rate and the disturbance in the normal balance between bone resorption and deposition as the result of immobilisation.

Thyrotoxicosis

Hypercalcaemia may occur, as a rare complication, in hyperthyroidism either as a manifestation of associated primary hyperparathyroidism or a direct complication of thyrotoxicosis (Parfitt & Dent, 1970). It is recognised that there is an association between hyperthyroidism and primary hyperparathyroidism. Parfitt & Dent (1970) who reported two cases of their own and reviewed others in the literature concluded that although the association is genuine it is not a variant of the syndrome of multiple endocrine hyperplasia. The mechanism of the hypercalcaemia which occurs as a direct complication of hyperthyroidism is not clear. There is evidence that thyroid hormones have a direct action on bone cells and in hyperthyroidism there is an increase in both bone destruction and formation. However, hypercalcaemia is a rare complication of thyrotoxicosis and in those cases where it has been reported it can usually be accounted for by some other concomitant mechanism such as immobilisation or renal failure.

TABLE 3.1

FINDINGS IN PRIMARY, SECONDARY AND TERTIARY HYPERPARATHYROIDISM

(Based on Seifert & Seemann, 1967)

			Plasma Calcium	Plasma Phosphate
PRIMARY	Adenoma (84%)	Chief cell Water-clear cell Oxyphil cell		
	Hyperplasia (12%)	Water-clear cell Chief cell	↑	↓
	Carcinoma (4%)	Chief cell		
SECONDARY	Hyperplasia	Chief cell Water-clear cell	↓	renal ↑ intestinal ↓
TERTIARY	Adenoma and/or Hyperplasia	Chief cell Water-clear cell	↑	↑ ↓

Tertiary hyperparathyroidism

Primary hyperparathyroidism (v.s.) is most commonly due to an adenoma and is only rarely due to hyperplasia or carcinoma (Table 3.1). Secondary hyperparathyroidism is due to hyperplasia of all four parathyroid glands as the direct result of continued hypocalcaemic stimulation. The development of an autonomous adenoma in one of the four hyperplastic glands of secondary hyperparathyroidism or hypercalcaemia in association with autonomous hyperplastic glands has been termed 'tertiary hyperparathyroidism' (Davies, Dent & Watson, 1968). The associated changes in the plasma phosphate concentration are related to the disease process which caused the hypo-calcaemia and 'triggered' the secondary parathyroid hyperplasia.

Milk drinker's syndrome (or milk-alkali syndrome)

This syndrome occurs in patients with peptic ulcers who have an excessive intake of milk together with an absorbable alkali, and usually also have evidence of previous renal disease. The mechanism of the hypercalcaemia would appear to be the combination of increased intestinal calcium absorp-tion together with a diminution in urine calcium excretion as a result of decreased glomerular ultrafiltration due to the renal disease. The ingestion of absorbable alkali of itself can damage the kidneys.

Acromegaly

The occurrence of hypercalcaemia with hyperplasia or adenoma of the parathyroid glands is a recognised, but rare, occurrence in patients with pituitary adenomas. The relationship between these two glands, and the occasional associated finding of pancreatic islet cell adenomas, is not clearly defined. The generally held view is that the relationship between acromegaly and hyperparathyroidism is a manifestation of the syndrome of 'multiple endocrine adenomas' or 'polyendocrine adenomatosis'. This syndrome is inherited as an autosomal dominant with a high degree of penetrance and presents with manifestations of hyperactivity of multiple endocrine organs. A common association is the Zollinger–Ellison syndrome, of pancreatic islet cell adenomas and intractable duodenal ulcers, with hyperparathyroidism.

Idiopathic hypercalcaemia of infancy

Hypercalcaemia in infancy occurs in both a mild and in a severe form, these being two different disease processes. The mild form has been attributed to an abnormal sensitivity to cholecalciferol or to an excessive dietary intake of that substance. The severe form is rare and constitutes a syndrome characterised by 'elfin-like' facies, mental retardation, osteosclerosis, hyper-calcaemia, hypercalciuria, nephrocalcinosis and uraemia. The mechanism of the hypercalcaemia in the severe form is unknown; alterations in chole-calciferol and steroid metabolism have been postulated.

Hodgkin's disease

Hypercalcaemia occurs very rarely in patients with either Hodgkin's disease or leukaemia. In both of these diseases the hypercalcaemia is usually associated with skeletal rarefaction, as a result of bone dissolution, and this presumably accounts for the increase in the plasma calcium concentration.

Addison's disease

Hypercalcaemia is an extremely rare complication of Addison's disease. The mechanism of the hypercalcaemia is not clearly defined but it is presumably related in some way to the known antagonism between cholecalciferol and cortisol. It is possible that in the absence of cortisol, or at low circulating plasma cortisol concentrations, there is some enhancement of the action of cholecalciferol on gastro-intestinal calcium absorption.

Immobilisation

Hypercalcaemia in patients who are immobilised is extremely rare. When it occurs it can be accounted for by the disruption in the normal balance between bone formation and destruction as a consequence of the loss of both weight-bearing and muscular activity, and this disturbance is accentuated by the presence of pre-existing renal disease which causes a reduction in urine calcium excretion. Immobilisation hypercalcaemia can occur in patients with osteoporosis and/or multiple fractures, especially if these are associated with paresis due to associated neurological damage or it can occur in extensive paresis alone.

Investigations for the Differential Diagnosis of Hypercalcaemia and Hyperparathyroidism

These are based on the two principal physiological actions of parathyroid hormone on the bones and the kidneys in the regulation of calcium and phosphate homeostasis. The many diagnostic tests available can be arbitrarily classified into either the specific, or direct, tests and the non-specific, or indirect, tests depending on their relationship to the actions of parathyroid hormone.

Specific tests

Plasma calcium (total). In the collection of blood for plasma calcium estimation it has been well established that venous stasis can cause a significant increase in the result. Ideally the patient should be fasting prior to collection of blood for calcium estimations, but this is not essential as increments in plasma calcium concentration of the order of only, at the most, 0·5 to 0·8 mg per 100 ml occur during a normal working day, after the intake of normal meals or large oral calcium loads (Wills, 1970a). The use of a protein correction factor as proposed by Dent (1962) is of value in the interpretation of plasma calcium values if 'artificially' high values due to venous stasis are to be excluded. The use of such a factor is also of importance in comparing the calcium values in any one patient over a period of time when alterations in total plasma protein concentration may occur.

Plasma calcium (fractions). Calcium present in blood plasma is divisible into a non-diffusible and a diffusible portion depending on its ability to pass across a semi-permeable membrane. The non-diffusible, or protein-bound, fraction constitutes approximately 40 per cent of the total plasma calcium concentration and is in the main bound to albumin (approximately 0·7 mg per g of albumin), with only a small portion attached to the globulins. The diffusible (or ultrafiltrable) fraction is further sub-divided into the ionized and complexed fractions, the major part of which is the ionized portion (approximately 51 per cent of the total). The complexed fraction consists of calcium which is held in loose complex formation with mainly bicarbonate, citrate and phosphate. The ionized fraction is considered to be the physiologically active portion which is both the controlled and controlling mechanism in the secretion of parathyroid hormone. In this now classical concept of the state and control of calcium fractions in plasma, one would expect the measurement of the concentrations of these fractions to be of value in the differential diagnosis of hypercalcaemia with particular reference to parathyroid gland overactivity. Many workers, using varying techniques, have estimated plasma calcium fractions in disease states with conflicting results (see Wills & Lewin, 1971). In recent years considerable advances have taken place in the development of calcium ion-specific electrodes for the measurement of ionized calcium concentration in plasma. However, at the present time there is a considerable variation in the reported values for the concentration of ionized calcium in normal subjects using ion-specific electrodes (Li & Piechocki, 1971). Until these discrepancies are resolved it would appear that the estimation of the concentrations of ionized and ultrafiltrable plasma calcium fractions and the calcium-binding ability of the plasma proteins are of little value in the differential diagnosis of hypercalcaemia.

Urine calcium. In the differential diagnosis of hypercalcaemia the measurement of total 24 hour urine calcium excretion is, of itself, of little value. Urine calcium excretion represents the end result of the processes of glomerular ultrafiltration and tubular reabsorption of the diffusible plasma calcium fraction; thus in any patient with hypercalcaemia there will be an increased filtered calcium load which will be reflected as an increased urine calcium excretion. It is known that parathyroid hormone increases the tubular reabsorption of calcium (v.s.). In studies on normal subjects and patients with primary hyperparathyroidism using oral calcium loading Peacock, Robertson & Nordin (1969) reported that at any given plasma calcium concentration the hyperparathyroid patients excreted less calcium in their urine than did the normal subjects. The measurement of the tubular reabsorption of calcium appears to be of value in the differential diagnosis of patients with hypercalcaemia, with increased values in primary hyperparathyroidism and decreased values in patients with hypercalcaemia due to other causes (Transbøl et al., 1970).

Plasma phosphate. Because of the action of parathyroid hormone in blocking the net tubular reabsorption of phosphate, hypophosphataemia has been, in the past, considered to be an important distinguishing feature of patients with hypercalcaemia due to primary hyperparathyroidism when compared with patients with hypercalcaemia due to other causes. In primary hyperparathyroidism, however, consistently low values for plasma phosphate concentration are usually the exception rather than the rule, even in the presence of normal renal function. It is recognised that there is a marked overlap between the plasma phosphate concentrations in patients with primary hyperparathyroidism when compared with patients with hypercalcaemia due to various other causes (Fig. 3.2). One factor which contributes to a normal or raised plasma phosphate concentration in patients with primary hyperparathyroidism is associated renal damage. A consistently low plasma phosphate concentration is highly suggestive of primary hyperparathyroidism, but the diagnosis is not excluded in the presence of a normal or high concentration. Hypophosphataemia is also a feature of patients with pseudohyperparathyroidism (v.s.).

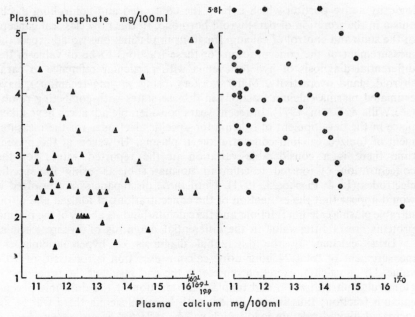

FIG. 3.2. Plasma phosphate concentrations plotted against plasma calcium concentrations for 44 patients with primary hyperparathyroidism (▲) and 44
patients with hypercalcaemia due to various other causes (●). Of the patients
in latter group the hypercalcaemia was due to carcinomatosis in 16, (primary
in breast 8, bronchus 5, prostate 1, kidney 1 and stomach 1), sarcoidosis in
10, myelomatosis in 8, vitamin D overdose in 8, Paget's disease in 1 and
Hodgkin's disease in 1.

Phosphate excretion tests. These tests are all based on the action of
parathyroid hormone at the renal tubular level in blocking net phosphate
reabsorption. They were devised in an attempt to improve both the diagnostic
accuracy in patients with borderline primary hyperparathyroidism and to
differentiate patients with hypercalcaemia due to primary hyperparathyroidism from patients with hypercalcaemia due to other causes. The tests
(Table 3.2) have been expressed in a variety of clearance equations and can be
divided into simple and more complex procedures. If the patients are on
controlled phosphate intake, have normal or nearly normal renal function

TABLE 3.2

PHOSPHATE EXCRETION TESTS

Simple procedures

Phosphate/creatinine clearance ratio (C_p/C_{cr})
Tubular reabsorption of phosphate (T.R.P.)
Phosphate excretion index (P.E.I.)
Phosphate clearance (C_p)

Complex procedures

Theoretical renal phosphate threshold (R.P.Thr.)
Maximum tubular reabsorption of phosphate (Tm_p)

and they do not have glycosuria these tests may be useful in the diagnosis of border-line cases of primary hyperparathyroidism. Abnormalities in the renal handling of phosphate do, however, also occur in a variety of other conditions which may themselves cause hypercalcaemia. Because of the technical difficulties in performing these tests, some of which require constant infusion, and the need for a rigidly controlled dietary phosphate intake, these tests are of limited differential diagnostic value.

Calcium tolerance test. The secretion of parathyroid hormone is controlled by the circulating ionized calcium concentration. The calcium tolerance tests were designed to suppress the endogenous production of parathyroid hormone in normal glands, which would not occur if the glands were autonomous, and therefore differentiate hypercalcaemia of parathyroid origin from hypercalcaemia due to other causes. The changes measured following calcium infusions are usually based on alterations in urine phosphate excretion as an index of parathyroid suppression. The value of these tests in the differential diagnosis of hypercalcaemia has, however, been questioned since hyperparathyroid-type responses have been observed in other hypercalcaemics and negative results have been obtained in patients with proven primary hyperparathyroidism (Strott and Nugent, 1968). These tests which are time-consuming and require metabolic ward facilities are thus of limited value.

Parathyroid arteriography and scan. Various radiological techniques have been used in attempts to localise functional parathyroid adenomas and foremost amongst these have been studies using selective arteriography. The main disadvantage of this technique, which requires specialised facilities, is that focal thyroid pathology can mimic most of the changes attributed to parathyroid adenomas (Newton and Eisenberg, 1966).

Methionine is a precursor for parathyroid hormone synthesis. Potchen, Watts & Awwad (1967) reported that the parathyroid gland in a hyperactive state was selectively labelled with [^{75}Se] selenomethionine, after pre-treatment with tri-iodothyronine to suppress thyroidal uptake of the selenomethionine. In their studies Potchen and his colleagues reported an excellent correlation between the parathyroid scan and surgical findings in patients later proven to have primary hyperparathyroidism. In our own experience (Wills—unpublished data), which is confirmed by that of others (McGeown et al., 1968) the scan findings do not correspond well with the position of parathyroid adenomas at subsequent surgical exploration. It is now apparent that the most important factor contributing to the visualization of parathyroid adenomas, on the scan, is the size of the tumour, and only adenomas of more than 2 g are consistently visualized by this technique (DiGiulio & Morales, 1969). The main indication at the present time for the use of the parathyroid scan would appear to be for the attempted localisation of parathyroid adenomas in patients proven or highly suspected, on other grounds, to have primary hyperparathyroidism and who have had a previous surgical exploration of the neck. The parathyroid scan would appear to have no role in the differential diagnosis of hypercalcaemia in view of the failure, with this technique, to demonstrate small functional parathyroid adenomas.

Parathyroid hormone assay. In recent years with the development of radio-immunoassay techniques for the estimation of parathyroid hormone it has become possible to establish a diagnosis in some patients with primary hyperparathyroidism who have an increased concentration of hormone in the peripheral blood. In the absence of any disorder of parathyroid hormone secretion it would be anticipated that circulating parathyroid hormone concentration would be depressed in patients with hypercalcaemia due to all other causes. There are, however, some conflicting observations that remain, as yet, unresolved. Some workers have reported that there is an overlap between the concentration of hormone circulating in normal subjects and that in patients with primary hyperparathyroidism (Deftos & Potts, 1969); while others have claimed that a clear distinction can be made (Reiss & Canterbury, 1969). Reiss & Canterbury also reported that there was an increase in plasma parathyroid hormone concentration, in patients with an adenoma, during massage of the left or right side of the neck which corresponded with the subsequent surgical findings. In the patients with parathyroid hyperplasia there was no demonstrable asymmetric rise in parathyroid hormone concentration following neck massage and in normal subjects there was no change in plasma hormone concentration during this procedure.

As well as being estimated in peripheral blood, the concentration of hormone has also been estimated in blood obtained at neck vein catheterisation in attempts to localise an adenoma prior to surgical exploration (Reitz et al., 1969). In their study of six patients with primary hyperparathyroidism, all of whom were hypercalcaemic and had elevated parathyroid hormone concentrations in peripheral venous blood, Reitz and his colleagues (1969) reported localised increases in parathyroid hormone concentration in blood samples obtained by selective catheterisation of the major veins draining the neck and the thorax. In all of the patients the location of the tumours, as assessed by blood hormone concentration, was in agreement with the findings at subsequent surgical exploration. In five of the patients there was a parathyroid adenoma in the neck and in the sixth the adenoma was located in the mediastinum. At the present time the radioimmunoassay of parathyroid hormone is not widely available as it is still a research, rather than a routine, procedure. However, it is to be hoped that this estimation will eventually become the definitive test for the diagnosis of primary hyperparathyroidism and the differential diagnosis of hypercalcaemia.

Non-specific tests

Alkaline phosphatase. In these disorders, in the absence of hepatobiliary disease, the plasma alkaline phosphatase concentration is a direct reflection of osteoblastic activity and therefore of bone remodelling. The estimation of plasma alkaline phosphatase activity is therefore of itself of little value in differential diagnosis of hypercalcaemia. In patients with primary hyperparathyroidism the plasma alkaline phosphatase concentration is correlated with the clinical presentation. In their study of seventy patients with primary hyperparathyroidism Dent & Harper (1962) divided the patients into two distinct groups on the basis of their plasma alkaline phosphatase concentration. The group of patients with raised alkaline phosphatase concentrations were those with specific radiological signs of hyperparathyroidism.

Urine hydroxyproline. Hydroxyproline is a non-essential amino acid that occurs almost exclusively in collagen, where it accounts for some 14 per cent of the total amino acids. In patients with primary hyperparathyroidism, or following the administration of parathyroid extract to normal human subjects, the urine excretion of hydroxyproline is increased. This is attributed to the accelerated bone turnover and collagen degradation. In patients with primary hyperparathyroidism the increase in urine hydroxyproline excretion appears to be a more sensitive index of bone involvement than the plasma alkaline phosphatase concentration (Smith, 1967). As urine hydroxyproline excretion is of itself directly correlated with the rate of bone destruction its estimation is of no value in the differential diagnosis of patients with hypercalcaemia where bone destruction due to a variety of causes may account for the hypercalcaemia.

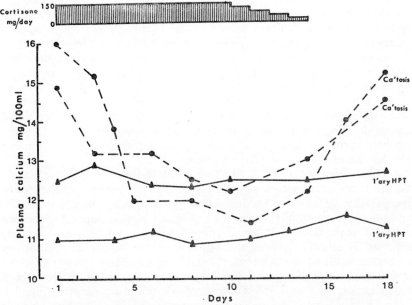

Fig. 3.3. Cortisone suppression test results in four hypercalcaemic patients. Hypercalcaemia was due to primary hyperparathyroidism in two of the patients (▲) and osteolytic bone metastases in carcinomatosis from primary breast tumours in the other two (●).

Serum proteins. The main value of serum protein electrophoresis in the differential diagnosis of hypercalcaemia is to exclude those patients with sarcoidosis and myelomatosis.

Cortisone suppression test. The test as originally described (Dent, 1956) involved the oral administration of a standard 10-day load of cortisone that was given orally in a dose of 50 mg three times a day, and recently cortisol (40 mg three times a day) has been used instead (Dent & Watson, 1968). Early observation with this test showed that unlike the hypercalcaemia of sarcoidosis, myelomatosis, thyrotoxicosis, vitamin D intoxication and malignant disease, the hypercalcaemia associated with primary hyperparathyroidism was unresponsive to the administration of cortisone. Since the original description of this test there have been many reports of patients with proven primary hyperparathyroidism who have shown suppression of their hypercalcaemia and there also have been reports of patients with hyper-calcaemia due to various other causes who have failed to show suppression. In the majority of these conflicting reports the workers have not used the method as originally described and have used other, various, steroid substitutes. Even when correctly performed it is recognised that this test is not completely reliable as both suppression of the hypercalcaemia of primary hyperparathyroidism and non-suppression of that due to other causes has been reported (Dent, 1962; Pyrah, Hodgkinson & Anderson, 1966).

The mechanism by which cortisone or cortisol lowers the plasma calcium concentration in patients with hypercalcaemia due to causes other than primary hyperparathyroidism is unexplained. In our own experience the use of cortisone or cortisol has been found to be a valuable test in the differential diagnosis of patients with hypercalcaemia due to carcinoma from those with primary hyperparathyroidism. The results from four *selected* hypercalcaemic patients are shown in Fig. 3.3. In two of the patients the hypercalcaemia was due to primary hyperparathyroidism and in the other two was associated with carcinomatosis from primary carcinomas in the breast. It is important to stress that it is unwise to suddenly stop the administration of the steroid at the end of the test period because of the potential risk of adrenocortical suppression. The steroid should be tailed off slowly over a week at least. Also parathyroid gland exploration should not be undertaken immediately after the test unless steriod cover is given.

Acid-base changes. Wills & McGowan (1964) reported that the plasma chloride concentration was significantly higher in patients with primary hyperparathyroidism when compared with patients with hypercalcaemia due to all other causes and that there was almost complete separation of the two groups of patients on this basis. These findings have been subsequently confirmed by others and found to be of value in the differential diagnosis of hypercalcaemia (Dolman & Barzel, 1971). The plasma chloride concentrations for the two groups of hypercalcaemic patients shown in Fig. 3.2 have been plotted against the plasma calcium concentrations and are shown in Fig. 3.4. It can be seen from Fig. 3.4 that the separation based on plasma chloride concentration is much better than that based on phosphate concentration. The changes in plasma chloride concentration represent a fundamental difference between patients with primary hyperparathyroidism who have a tendency towards a metabolic acidosis and those with hypercalcaemia due to all other causes who have a metabolic alkalosis (Wills, 1971c).

In order to account for changes in acid-base status and plasma chloride concentration which range in the latter case from normal to high values in the hyperparathyroid group and from normal to low values in the other group it is necessary to invoke at least two separate factors, one causing a rise and the other causing a fall in plasma chloride concentration. There are several factors which cause changes in plasma chloride concentration with a reciprocal change in bicarbonate concentration and acid-base status. From a consideration of these factors Wills (1971c) proposed that the most likely explanation for the findings in patients with primary hyperparathyroidism is that they are due to the action of parathyroid hormone on the renal tubular cells producing a hyperchloraemic metabolic acidosis in the extra-cellular fluid compartment. This explanation is supported by the known effects of

Plasma   chloride   mEq/l

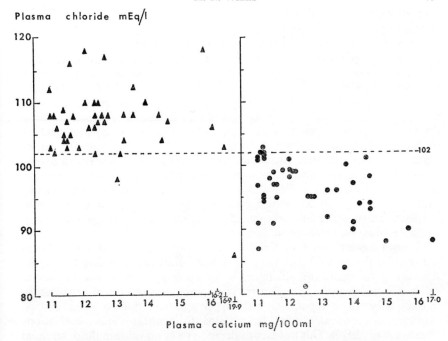

Plasma   calcium   mg/100ml

FIG. 3.4. Plasma chloride concentration plotted against plasma calcium concentration for patients with primary hyperparathyroidism (▲) and patients with hypercalcaemia due to various other causes (●). The two groups of patients are the same as shown in Fig. 3.2.

parathyroid hormone on the renal tubules and the maintenance of a hydrogen ion gradient between the body fluids and the tubular urine (v.s.). The most likely explanation for the low plasma chloride concentration and alteration in acid-base status in the patients with hypercalcaemia due to causes other than primary hyperparathyroidism is renal tubular alkalosis. It has been shown that the acute intravenous infusion of calcium, either as chloride or gluconate, causes an increase in urine hydrogen ion excretion in both animals (Verbanck, 1965) and man (Richet *et al.*, 1963). Such a factor operating over a long period would presumably cause a metabolic alkalosis of renal tubular origin. It is also possible that in the aetiology of the metabolic alkalosis found in patients with non-parathyroid hypercalcaemia suppression of endogenous parathyroid hormone secretion, by the high circulating calcium concentration, plays a role. This view is based on the demonstration of a metabolic alkalosis in patients with hypocalcaemia due to hypoparathyroidism (Barzel, 1969).

Sodium chloride infusion. Axelrod (1966) reported that the infusion of hypertonic sodium chloride produced a marked increase in urine calcium excretion in patients with primary hyperparathyroidism. However, Shane, Flink & Jones (1969) in studies using this technique in patients with primary hyperparathyroidism, idiopathic urolithiasis with and without hypercalciuria, and normal volunteers have reported that there was no significant difference in the mean increment of calcium excretion for each group following saline infusion. These findings would suggest that sodium chloride induced calciuria is of no value in the differential diagnosis of hypercalcaemia or diagnosis of primary hyperparathyroidism.

Tubular reabsorption of glucose. It has been reported that in patients with primary hyperparathyroidism the tubular maximal reabsorptive capacity for glucose and the reabsorptive capacity in relation to the glomerular filtration rate (Tm_G/G.F.R.) was elevated and following parathyroidectomy there was a pronounced decrease (Halver, 1968). It was proposed that this technique might be of value in the differential diagnosis of hypercalcaemia due to parathyroid disease as distinct from other causes. Using a modification of Halver's technique, Heath & Knapp (1969) have confirmed the earlier reports and reported that low values were obtained in patients with hypercalcaemia due to various other causes. The studies using this technique are at the present moment limited and as the test is time consuming with some overlap occurring between patient groups (Heath—personal communication) its place in the differential diagnosis of hypercalcaemia is uncertain until further evaluation has been undertaken.

Venous compression test. Krull *et al.* (1969) reported that venous compression of the arm (100 mmHg) with rhythmical fist-clenching for fifteen minutes in hyperparathyroid patients caused a substantial rise in plasma calcium concentration, in that arm, when compared with arm-occlusion in normal subjects and patients with hypercalcaemia due to other causes. However, subsequent studies have failed to confirm these observations (Buxton *et al.*, 1970). This test is considered to be of no value in the differential diagnosis of hypercalcaemia or diagnosis of primary hyperparathyroidism.

Conclusion

It is apparent that the differential diagnosis of hypercalcaemia and in particular the diagnosis of primary hyperparathyroidism is by no means a simple task. Of the tests widely available that may be performed without any specialised facilities the cortisone suppression or cortisol suppression tests appear to be of value if performed as detailed by their original proponents. Also of value is the estimation of plasma chloride concentration together with an assessment of acid-base status by independent measurements of pH, P_{CO_2} and bicarbonate concentrations. It is hoped that, when routinely available, the estimation of circulating parathyroid hormone concentration will become the definitive test in the diagnosis of hyperparathyroidism and its differentiation from other causes of hypercalcaemia.

Treatment of Hypercalcaemia

The treatment of hypercalcaemia is essentially the treatment of the causative primary disease state. There are, however, situations in which the primary disease is not amenable to therapy and in these situations treatment of the hypercalcaemia is indicated. This may be undertaken on an acute or on a long-term basis, either to provide relief from symptoms directly attributable to the increase in the plasma calcium concentration or to prevent the complications known to be associated with hypercalcaemia.

Acute treatment

In hypercalcaemia, from any cause, if there is a marked increase in the plasma calcium concentration there may be progression to a hypercalcaemic

TABLE 5.5

METHODS FOR THE ACUTE TREATMENT OF HYPERCALCAEMIA
(Based on Suki *et al.*, 1970)

Therapy	Dosage	Route of Administration	Complications (Potential)	Limitations to Use
Sodium phosphate	0·75–1 mmol sodium phosphate/kg of body weight over 8–12 h	Intravenous	Hypomagnesaemia; hyperphosphataemia; hypotension and shock; extraskeletal calcification.	Renal insufficiency
Sodium sulphate	3 litres of isotonic sodium sulphate over 9 h	Intravenous	Hypomagnesaemia; calcium depletion; hypernatraemia; sodium overload.	Hypertension; congestive heart failure; renal insufficiency
Sodium chloride	3 litres of 1·45% (0·25 mol/l) sodium chloride over 9 h	Intravenous	Sodium overload; hypernatraemia	Hypertension; congestive heart failure; renal insufficiency
Ethylenediamine-tetra-acetate	50 mg/kg of body weight over 4–6 h	Intravenous	Renal failure; hypotension	Nephrotoxicity
Mithramycin	25 μg/kg of body weight	Intravenous	Bleeding disorder; hepatic dysfunction; renal insufficiency	Hospitalised patients with cancer
Corticosteroids	150 mg of cortisone or its equivalent per day	Oral or parenteral	Hypercortisolism	Delayed effect; may not be effective in hyperparathyroidism
Frusemide	100 mg/h	Intravenous	Hypomagnesaemia; volume depletion; calcium depletion; hypokalaemia	Renal failure with oliguria not responsive to frusemide and saline

crisis. This syndrome presents with vomiting, dehydration, shock, coma, renal failure and cardiac arrhythmias, and unless treated as an emergency has a high mortality.

A number of methods have been proposed for the acute treatment of hypercalcaemia (Table 3.3) and of these the most commonly used methods are the infusion of the sodium salts of phosphate and sulphate. All of the methods listed may be associated with deleterious side effects as part of the calcium-lowering procedure. Intravenous *phosphate* lowers the plasma calcium concentration without increasing urine calcium excretion by exceeding the solubility product of $CaHPO_4$ and is associated with the extraskeletal deposition of that salt in body tissues. The extraskeletal deposition of calcium may cause, among other complications, acute renal damage with failure. Intravenous *sodium sulphate* and *sodium chloride* lower the plasma calcium concentrations by increasing urine calcium excretion. These two methods both require the administration of large volumes of fluid and in the absence of good renal and cardiac function may be hazardous. *Sodium ethylenedia-mine-tetra-acetate* (sodium edetate) infusion lowers the plasma calcium concentration by chelation and its effect is transient: also if given in repeated doses it is nephrotoxic. *Mithramycin*, an antibiotic produced by *Streptomyces plicatus*, is a highly toxic anti-neoplastic drug used in the treatment of testicular malignancy which has also been used in the treatment of symptomatic hypercalcaemia in far advanced malignancy (Perlia *et al.*, 1970). The mode of action of mithramycin in lowering the plasma calcium concentration is unknown; but it may act by blocking the peripheral effect of parathyroid hormone either by a direct action or by inducing a state of cholecalciferol resistance. *Corticosteroids* have been regarded in the past as the method of choice in the long-term treatment of the hypercalcaemia of malignant disease where treatment of the primary tumour, or the metastases, is either excluded or is unsuccessful (v.i.). The mechanism by which corticosteroids lower the plasma calcium concentration in hypercalcaemic states is unknown. The main disadvantage of the use of corticosteroids in the emergency treatment of symptomatic hypercalcaemia in malignancy and other hypercalcaemic states is the delayed response to treatment and the non-response of the hypercalcaemia due to hyperparathyroidism. The use of *frusemide*, a potent natriuretic agent which apparently increases urine calcium excretion in proportion to sodium excretion, has recently been proposed for the acute treatment of hypercalcaemia by Suki *et al.* (1970). In this therapy it is essential that there is a simultaneous water and electrolyte replacement programme which balances carefully the volume and cation (sodium, potassium and magnesium) losses associated with the frusemide-induced diuresis. Suki and colleagues using this technique reported that it was a safe method of treatment in patients with diminished cardiac reserve and effective even in patients with moderate renal insufficiency. Although more commonly used in the long-term treatment of hypercalcaemia, Buckle, Mason & Middleton (1969) have reported the successful use of *calcitonin* in the emergency treatment of a patient with thyrotoxic hypercalcaemia.

Long-term treatment

The long-term treatment of hypercalcaemia, *per se*, is only undertaken for symptomatic relief when, for various reasons, the condition which is causing the hypercalcaemia is not amenable to treatment. One of the main aims in any therapeutic regimen, for the long-term treatment of hyper-calcaemia, is to reduce gastro-intestinal calcium absorption. This can be achieved either by a low calcium diet or by rendering dietary calcium un-available for absorption by the oral administration of *sodium phytate, sulphate* or *phosphate*. In patients with hypercalcaemia in malignant disease the administration of oral sodium phosphate produces a prompt fall in the plasma calcium concentration and this is associated with marked symptomatic clinical improvement (Thalassinos & Joplin, 1968). A disadvantage of the administration of these various sodium salts are the associated gastro-intestinal tract symptoms; comprising epigastric pain, nausea and diarrhoea which are most marked in patients receiving sodium phytate. Dudley & Blackburn (1970) reported the development of extraskeletal calcification in seven out of nine patients receiving oral neutral phosphate daily over periods ranging from 9 to 87 months. In two of their hypercalcaemic patients the extraskeletal calcification was associated with progressive renal impairment which they considered to be related to nephrocalcinosis. This view is consistent with the observations of Spaulding & Walser (1970) who reported that in hypercalcaemic rats the administration of oral phosphates, and consequent lowering of plasma calcium, was associated with a significant increase in the calcium concentration of renal and cardiac tissues. The daily dose of oral neutral phosphate used in the studies of Dudley & Blackburn (1970) was larger than that used by many others. The studies do, however, stress the need for the careful monitoring of patients on long-term oral phosphate therapy for evidence of extraskeletal calcification.

Corticosteroids have, in the past, been widely used in the long-term treat-ment of hypercalcaemia in malignant disease and are considered to be effective. Recently, however, Thalassinos & Joplin (1970) reported that in twelve of thirteen unselected patients with different types of advanced malig-nant disease corticosteroids failed to lower the plasma calcium concentration. They considered that their findings 'should prompt a re-evaluation of this treatment in the hypercalcaemia of malignant disease'. All of their patients were in an advanced stage of neoplastic disease and it is possible that the corticosteroid response of the hypercalcaemia in malignancy is variable and is more responsive in the initial stages. *Mithramycin*, which has already been discussed in the acute treatment of hypercalcaemia, also has a role in the long-term treatment of hypercalcaemic patients with far advanced malignancy. *Calcitonin*, which lowers the plasma calcium concentration by inhibition of osteoclastic bone resorption, has been used successfully in the treatment of the hypercalcaemia associated with malignant disease, hyperthyroidism, and Paget's disease of bone (Foster *et al.*, 1966; Pak *et al.*, 1968; Kammerman & Canfield, 1970).

Although the basic disorder in Paget's disease of bone (osteitis deformans) is obscure, it is accepted that there is marked increase in bone turnover rate and osteoclastic activity. Because of its action in inhibiting osteoclastic activity it is to be expected that the administration of calcitonin would be of particular therapeutic value in Paget's disease of bone even in the absence of hyper-calcaemia. Recently Haddad, Birge & Avioli (1970) reported a study of the effects of the long-term administration of calcitonin to three patients with severe osteitis deformans. In all three subjects the treatment was accompanied by a marked reduction in plasma alkaline phosphatase activity and in two of them there was a reduction in total urine hydroxyproline excretion. Haddad and his colleagues considered that the well tolerated suppressive effects of calcitonin administration to patients with Paget's disease of bone suggest a role of calcitonin in the treatment of this condition. The importance and value of such treatment undoubtedly requires further evaluation as others have suggested that the inhibition by calcitonin of bone resorption is followed by an inhibition of bone formation (Bijvoet *et al.*, 1970). Bijvoet and his colleagues proposed that an excess of calcitonin might even result in osteoporosis.

HYPOCALCAEMIA

A reduction in the total plasma calcium concentration is associated with a variety of disease states. Because of the role of the calcium ion in neuro-muscular transmission a reduction in total plasma calcium concentration is frequently associated with the clinical presentation of tetany. Tetany in the overt form is usually manifested initially by numbness and tingling, in the extremities and around the mouth, followed by a sensation of stiffness in the hands and feet eventually progressing to spasms in the voluntary muscles. Spasms usually follow some voluntary contraction, such as the use of a pen or knife, but may occur spontaneously. Evidence of latent tetany can be elicited as carpopedal spasm in Trousseau's sign or as an increased irritability of the facial nerve in Chvostek's sign. As a diagnostic test the value of the latter is limited, as in many normal subjects a twitch of the facial muscles can be induced by tapping over the facial nerve. In many patients with hypo-calcaemia, despite a marked reduction in the plasma calcium concentration, there is no evidence of tetany. In the majority of cases this is due to a con-comittant acidosis which appears to play a 'protective' role due to a specific effect of the retained hydrogen ion on neuromuscular irritability. In clinical practice tetany is most commonly associated with a deficit of hydrogen ions due to a metabolic or respiratory alkalosis in patients who are normo-calcaemic.

Conditions Giving Rise to Hypocalcaemia

In the majority of patients the diagnosis of the aetiology of hypocalcaemia can be made from the clinical history and symptoms attributable to the disease state which is responsible for the hypocalcaemia. As with hypercalcae-mia, diagnostically the most important group are those patients with disorders of the parathyroid glands. The importance of the recognition of hypo-calcaemia following thyroidectomy, where there has been associated para-thyroid gland damage, is due in particular to the central nervous system damage that the hypocalcaemia may cause, both as the result of the reduction in ionized calcium concentration and as the consequence of foci of ectopic calcification. In addition to paraesthesiae and tetany the nervous system disturbances include apathy and depression, raised intracranial pressure and papilloedema, and calcification of the basal ganglia.

Surgery

The commonest cause of hypoparathyroidism is accidental damage to the parathyroid glands or their blood supply during the course of operations on the thyroid gland. Accidental removal of one or more of the parathyroid glands during thyroidectomy is rare while interference with parathyroid gland function is common.

The mechanism of post-operative hypocalcaemia after thyroidectomy for thyrotoxicosis is not clear and it has been postulated that vascular disturbances are responsible (Michie et al., 1965). During routine sub-total thyroidectomy it has been demonstrated that there is a significant fall in the plasma calcium concentration when compared with the changes in plasma calcium concentration in a group of patients following other non-thyroid operative procedures (John, Wills & Marcus, 1966). The most likely explanation for these findings is that they are due either to interference with the arterial blood supply to the parathyroid glands during the operation, or to obstruction of venous flow due to oedema or haemorrhage following the operative procedure. Recently it has been proposed that the hypocalcaemia after thyroidectomy for thyrotoxicosis is due to an avidity of the bones for calcium, as a consequence of pre-existent thyrotoxic osteodystrophy (Michie et al., 1971). This proposal is supported by the differences in the rates of fall in plasma calcium concentration after parathyroidectomy in patients with primary hyperparathyroidism and osteitis fibrosa when compared with patients without bone disease (Wills, 1971e). However, as it is routine practice to render patients euthyroid with antithyroid therapy for some months prior to thyroidectomy, it would seem unlikely that a significant degree of thyrotoxic osteodystrophy still exists at the time of operation, although this hypothesis warrants further investigation.

The reported incidence of hypoparathyroidism after thyroid surgery varies from 0·2 per cent (Swinton, 1937) to 13 per cent (Painter, 1960). This wide variation is probably related to differences in surgical technique and possibly to differences in criteria of assessment. It is usual to describe two forms of post-operative hypoparathyroidism, permanent and transient. In those cases with transient symptoms, of hypocalcaemia following thyroidectomy, it has been proposed that the disappearance of the symptoms meant that the remaining undamaged parathyroid tissue had hypertrophied and re-established biochemical control. However, Wade, Fourman & Deane (1965) proposed that if a patient had symptoms of parathyroid insufficiency after thyroidectomy then full recovery of parathyroid function was unusual and that such patients should be carefully investigated and followed up over a long period. This group of patients represents those who have a high incidence of partial parathyroid insufficiency or diminished parathyroid reserve.

The concept of partial parathyroid insufficiency or diminished reserve was originally proposed by Kramer (1936) who suggested that in some patients a state of partial parathyroid insufficiency might persist after thyroid surgery and cause symptoms, although not causing tetany, in the presence of total plasma calcium concentrations that were within the normal range. Jones & Fourman (1963) reported that this complication occurred in 28 per cent of an unselected group of post-thyroidectomy patients. Others, however, reported that the incidence was considerably lower (Rose, 1963) and proposed that a high incidence was related specifically to the surgical technique used for thyroidectomy (John & Wills, 1963). Fourman and his colleagues (Fourman *et al.*, 1967) considered that partial parathyroid insufficiency was important because of the many minor but disabling symptoms, particularly depression and lassitude, that it could produce and which were relieved by the administration of calcium. Although it is difficult to conceive how normo-calcaemic patients can experience symptoms of calcium deficiency this condition is of considerable importance because pregnancy, infection, or other intercurrent disease states may precipitate overt hypoparathyroidism. The diagnosis of diminished parathyroid reserve or partial insufficiency in a normocalcaemic patient can only be established by inducing hypocalcaemia, with either sodium edetate infusion or by calcium deprivation with oral phytate loading, and following the plasma calcium response.

Hypocalcaemia is a frequent occurrence after surgical removal of a parathyroid adenoma in patients with primary hyperparathyroidism, particularly those with osteitis fibrosa. The fall in plasma calcium concentration is usually accompanied by a simultaneous fall in plasma magnesium concentration. In this situation the hypocalcaemia, which is transient, is due to a state of relative hypoparathyroidism in the non-adenomatous glands as the result of pre-operative hypercalcaemic suppression. The hypocalcaemia is accentuated in those patients with osteitis fibrosa by the avidity of the bones for calcium.

Idiopathic

Idiopathic hypoparathyroidism is a rare disease presenting in childhood or middle age, twice as common among females as in males, and in some cases has a familial incidence. In a few patients 'idiopathic' hypoparathyroid-ism occurs in association with adrenal insufficiency and cutaneous moniliasis, and it is probable that this syndrome is a manifestation of auto-immune disease (Sweetnam, 1966).

Pseudohypoparathyroidism

Pseudohypoparathyroidism is a rare disorder inherited as a sex-linked recessive trait. It is characterised by the signs and symptoms of hypopara-thyroidism together with a round face, short stature, shortening of the metacarpals and metatarsals, and ectopic subcutaneous calcification. In pseudohypoparathyroidism the parathyroid glands are normal and the defect is considered to be in the target-organ, or tissue, response to para-thyroid hormone. This defect is characterised by the lack of a phosphaturic response following the administration of parathyroid extract in the Ellsworth-Howard test. Although calcitonin has been found in high concentrations in the thyroid glands of patients with pseudohypoparathyroidism there is evidence that this is not a primary factor in the aetiology of this syndrome (Lee *et al.*, 1968). The mechanism of the resistance to the actions of para-thyroid hormone in this condition is unknown. There is evidence that the lack of end-organ response both in pseudohypoparathyroidism and other conditions considered to be refractory to parathyroid hormone can be accounted for by a defect in parathyroid hormone sensitive adenyl cyclase in bone and kidney (Aurbach *et al.*, 1970). However, recently it has been proposed that the response to the administration of parathyroid extract in pseudohypoparathyroidism is dependent on the patients' cholecalciferol status (Suh, Fraser & Kooh, 1970). This proposal was based on the absence of a phosphaturic response following the administration of parathyroid extract in a patient with pseudohypoparathyroidism while hypocalcaemic, with a normal phosphaturic response after the plasma calcium had been raised by the administration of large doses of vitamin D_2. The need to use large doses of vitamin D_2 would suggest that in patients with pseudohypoparathyroidism there is a possible inherited defect in the metabolism of cholecalciferol and conversion to its active metabolites. The adenyl cyclase explanation seems more likely.

The occurrence of the brachydactyly, short stature and ectopic subcutaneous calcification of pseudohypoparathyroidism in the absence of associated hypocalcaemia has been termed pseudo-pseudohypoparathyroidism. Recently, Bronsky (1970) suggested that this system of nomenclature should be abandoned and proposed a new classification of parathyroid disease. In this classification the diagnostic term pseudo-pseudohypoparathyroidism would be abandoned and replaced by idiopathic brachydactyly, of either sporadic or familial type.

Chronic renal failure

Hypocalcaemia is a well recognised complication of chronic renal failure although the mechanisms involved are both complex and controversial. In the classical concept the hypocalcaemia is accounted for by phosphate retention. It has been established that phosphate infusions lower the plasma calcium concentration, and that the hypocalcaemic effect of phosphate is due to a variety of mechanisms (Stamp, 1971). Among these mechanisms is the physico-chemical precipitation of $CaHPO_4$ in the body tissues by exceeding the solubility product of that compound (Hebert *et al.*, 1966). However, if the changes in plasma calcium concentration in chronic renal disease were simply secondary to those in plasma phosphate one would expect the plasma calcium concentration to be low in all patients with phosphate retention. In practice the plasma calcium concentration may remain normal despite marked increases in phosphate concentration or it may be low in the presence of only small changes in phosphate concentration. Stanbury & Lumb (1966) proposed that the plasma calcium concentration in chronic renal disease was determined by factors other than the phosphate concentration and these included alterations in the sensitivity to the actions of cholecalciferol and responsiveness to the calcaemic actions of parathyroid hormone.

It has been well established that in patients with chronic renal disease there is a decrease in the absorption of calcium from the intestine, and that this is a manifestation of an acquired resistance to cholecalciferol. In hypocalcaemic patients with chronic renal failure there is also a diminished, or absent, calcaemic and phosphaturic response following the administration of parathyroid extract, both during intravenous infusions (Evanson, 1966) and during continued intramuscular injection (Freer & Wills, 1970). Because of the interrelationship between cholecalciferol and parathyroid hormone (v.s.) the most likely explanation for these findings is an acquired resistance, or insensitivity, to the actions of cholecalciferol as a direct consequence of the uraemic syndrome.

Although the kidney is involved in the formation of 1,25-dihydroxy-cholecalciferol it has recently been reported that the formation of this metabolite is independent of the uraemic state (Hill, Van Den Berg & Mawer, 1971). Gray, Boyle & DeLuca (1971) also reported that there was no

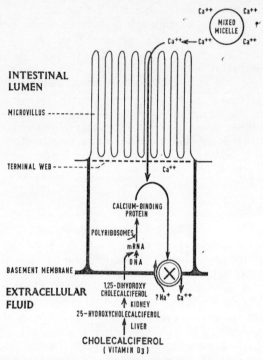

FIG. 3.5. Model of intestinal mucosal cell to indicate mode of action of cholecal-ciferol and its metabolites in intestinal calcium transport.

The mixed micelles bring the calcium in the intestinal lumen into contact with the mucosal absorption surface. The first stage in calcium transport is facilitated diffusion across the microvillar membrane, this stage involves alkaline phosphatase activity and the latter is probably initiated by 1,25-dihydroxycholecalciferol. The second stage in intestinal calcium transport involves the synthesis of a specific calcium-binding transport protein and the active extrusion of calcium from the cell at the interface with the extracellular fluid compartment. This latter stage involves an active pump mechanism and possibly sodium ion for calcium ion exchange.

defect in the entry of 1,25-dihydroxycholecalciferol into the intestinal mucosal cells. These observations would suggest that defect in intestinal calcium transport in uraemia involves the intracellular action of 1,25-dihydroxy-cholecalciferol, at the first or second stage of calcium transport across the intestinal mucosal cells (Fig. 3.5). It has been reported that the administration of cholecalciferol is associated with a marked increase in microvillar alkaline phosphate activity (Haussler, Nagode & Rasmussen, 1970). It could be postulated that the metabolic products which accumulate in the uraemic state either inhibit alkaline phosphatase activity and hence the diffusion of calcium across the microvillar membrane, or inhibit synthesis of the specific transport protein.

Dietary deficiency of cholecalciferol

In the absence of adequate endogenous cholecalciferol synthesis dietary intake becomes important and it was because of this that the steroid hormone cholecalciferol was misnamed as a vitamin. The skin content of 7-dehydro-cholesterol, the precursor of cholecalciferol, does not vary significantly between white and black skin but in the latter the melanin content acts as a protective filter (Loomis, 1967). If there is a deficiency of either endogenous or exogenous cholecalciferol there is a reduction in the absorption of calcium from the intestinal tract and consequent hypocalcaemia.

Dietary lack of cholecalciferol and nutritional osteomalacia in Britain occurs in two main groups of subjects, immigrants and elderly females. In both groups the major factor is a decrease in endogenous cholecalciferol synthesis, due either to a lack of exposure to sunlight or to the melanin content of the skin, which is not replaced by dietary intake. Among the indigenous white skinned population of Britain nutritional deficiency of cholecalciferol occurs most frequently among elderly women (Chalmers et al., 1967). But it is not confined to the elderly. One of the patients of Gough, Lloyd & Wills (1964) was a 40 year old spinster, a food faddist who seldom went out of doors because of personality defects. In their recent report Dent and Smith (1969) described seven women, aged 20 to 46 years, who had a low dietary cholecalciferol intake either because of food faddism or religious restriction.

Disorders of the gastro-intestinal tract and bile secretion

Hypocalcaemia and osteomalacia occur with a variety of disorders of the gastro-intestinal tract and bile secretion. These disorders include: (i) partial gastrectomy, (ii) obstructive jaundice, (iii) gluten-induced enteropathy, (iv) intestinal resections, (v) blind-loop syndromes, and (vi) regional ileitis. Hypocalcaemia and osteomalacia are well recognised complications of partial gastrectomy and occur most commonly after a Polya gastrectomy, but also occur after Bilroth-I gastrectomy, and vagotomy and drainage.

Morgan & Fourman (1969) used the term osteomalacia to denote only the name of that disease which is produced by cholecalciferol deficiency. They considered that 'the plasma calcium concentration in this disease may be very low but is often within the normal range, even though it may be abnormally low for that particular patient'. In their classification of the causes of osteomalacia they attributed the hypocalcaemia associated with disorders of the gastro-intestinal tract and bile secretion to cholecalciferol deficiency. In these disorders the cholecalciferol deficiency is associated with a reduction in gastro-intestinal calcium absorption.

Although it is undisputed that cholecalciferol deficiency plays an important role in the reduction in calcium absorption in this group of disorders, there is evidence that other factors are of importance. This proposal is supported by the fact that in those disorders associated with steatorrhoea it is generally agreed that the failure in fat absorption is not of itself sufficient to account for the malabsorption of both dietary cholecalciferol and calcium. It is possible that as cholecalciferol is fat soluble some is held in solution in the unabsorbed fat within the intestinal tract, but as even in severe cases of steatorrhoea fifty to eighty per cent of dietary fat is absorbed this factor is unlikely to be of major importance. This view is supported by the studies of Thompson, Lewis & Booth (1966) who reported that the absorption of [³H] vitamin D₃ was normal in two postgastrectomy patients with steatorrhoea. They also reported that osteomalacia could occur after gastrectomy even though cholecalciferol absorption was apparently normal. It is also possible that the increased intestinal fatty acid content causes a reduction in the availability of calcium for absorption by the formation of insoluble and unabsorbable calcium soaps but this too is unlikely to be of major importance. This view is supported by the lack of a consistent relationship between the degree of steatorrhoea and the absorption of calcium (Nassim *et al.*, 1959) and by the fact that hypocalcaemia and osteomalacia does not occur in patients with steatorrhoea of pancreatic origin. These observations stress the importance of normal bile secretion both in the absorption of cholecalciferol and of calcium.

The normal secretion of bile is required for the optimum absorption of dietary cholecalciferol (Schachter, Finkelstein & Kowarski, 1964). It would seem probable that the absence of bile secretion in obstructive jaundice accounts for the cholecalciferol deficiency and consequent hypocalcaemia associated with that condition. Bile probably facilitates cholecalciferol absorption by incorporating that compound into mixed micelles, bile salts and glyceride hydrolytic products. It is also recognised that bile and bile salts play a direct role in intestinal calcium absorption. Using duodenal loop preparations Olivier (1970) reported that although calcium absorption occurred in the absence of bile, the addition of bile to the loop markedly increased the percentage of calcium absorbed. He proposed that the increase in absorption of calcium was brought about by mixed micelles from bile salts and lecithin, the micelles brought the calcium into contact with the mucosal absorption surface. The facilitated diffusion of calcium across the microvillar membrane (Fig. 3.5) involves alkaline phosphatase and the presence of an active cholecalciferol metabolite. As well as playing a role in mucosal calcium transport there is some evidence that cholecalciferol metabolites play a role in the maintenance of the normal structure of the microvillar membranes (Wong *et al.*, 1970).

Bile secretion is a major route for the secretion of calcium into the intestinal tract. Briscoe & Ragan (1965) reported evidence which suggested that the calcium secreted in bile is preferentially reabsorbed by the intestinal mucosa and did not mix significantly with the dietary calcium in the gut. In those patients with absent or diminished bile secretion an alteration in endogenous faecal calcium turnover could be of importance in the aetiology of the hypocalcaemia associated with those conditions. However, this hypothesis awaits further investigation.

Although alterations in bile secretion are of importance in the aetiology of the cholecalciferol deficiency and hypocalcaemia found in some intestinal diseases, in those patients with gluten-induced enteropathy or coelic disease other mechanisms must be invoked. In a study on a group of nine patients with adult coeliac disease, Melvin *et al.* (1970) reported that the negative calcium balance in these patients was due to an excessive excretion of endogenous faecal calcium and that the true absorption of calcium was normal in every patient. Calcium absorption probably occurs throughout the whole of the intestinal tract, at variable rates depending on the segment. There is some evidence from experimental animals that active calcium transport is maximal in the most proximal parts of the small intestine (Schachter, 1963). Melvin and his colleagues (1970) considered that in coeliac disease calcium absorption took place normally at the proximal site but that the jejunal mucosa was in a secretory phase with respect to calcium as has been shown with respect to water, sodium and potassium.

Hypoalbuminaemia

Approximately 40 per cent of the total calcium present in plasma is bound by the plasma proteins. The 'protein-bound' calcium is mainly in combination with albumin; 1 g of albumin binds approximately 0·7 mg of calcium, the exact proportion depending on pH and other factors. A reduction in the total plasma protein concentration due to a reduction in the albumin fraction is a recognised cause of hypocalcaemia. Hypocalcaemia also occurs in patients with hypoalbuminaemia with normal total plasma proteins, where the latter is usually due to an increase in the gamma-globulin fraction as in patients with cirrhosis of the liver. The hypocalcaemia in hypoalbuminaemic states is due to a reduction in the protein-bound calcium fraction; and the concentrations of the ionized calcium and of the ultrafiltrable calcium fractions remain within the normal range.

Neonatal

Hypocalcaemia is the commonest of the recognised causes of generalised convulsions in the first twenty-eight days of life. In a prospective study of 100 infants with convulsions in the neonatal period, Keen (1969) reported that hypocalcaemia alone was present in 34 and was combined with hypoglycaemia in a further 4 infants. Neonatal hypocalcaemia has two peaks of incidence, one in the first forty-eight hours of life and the second between the fourth and tenth days. These two peaks represent different aetiological mechanisms for the hypocalcaemia. The less common type of hypocalcaemia, which has a poor prognosis, occurs within the first forty-eight hours of life and is usually associated with hypoglycaemia in infants of low birth-weight delivered by Caesarian section. A variety of mechanisms have been proposed to account for this type of hypocalcaemia and these include: functional immaturity of the parathyroid glands, damage by haemorrhage into the parathyroid glands, and increased maternal cortisol production during the operative delivery.

The common form of neonatal hypocalcaemia presents between the fourth and tenth day of life. This type of hypocalcaemia occurs among full-term infants of average, or above average weight who have been artificially fed. The mechanism for the hypocalcaemia in these infants has been attributed to artificial feeding and the high phosphate content of the type of artificial feed used, which induces hyperphosphataemia (Oppé & Redstone, 1968). The phosphate content of cow's milk, from which all artificial feeds are prepared, ranges from 56 to 112 mg per 100 ml compared with 6 to 26 mg per 100 ml for breast milk (Documenta Geigy, 1962). It is also possible that the high phosphate content of the artificial feeds reduces intestinal calcium transport by rendering the calcium unavailable for absorption. This view is supported by the fact that increasing the calcium content of artificial feeds abolishes their hypocalcaemic effect (Barltrop & Oppé, 1970).

Parathyroid gland suppression and neonatal hypocalcaemia is a recognised complication of maternal hypercalcaemic primary hyperparathyroidism; tetany in the neonate may be the first indication of the maternal disease.

Acute pancreatitis

Hypocalcaemia is a rare complication of acute pancreatitis and is often associated with hypomagnesaemia (Wills, 1966). The mechanism for the hypocalcaemia in patients with acute pancreatitis is the deposition of calcium with fatty acids in the areas of fat necrosis in the peritoneal cavity (Storck & Björntorp, 1971). The nodules of fat necrosis consist of areas of fat which have been made necrotic by the lipolytic activity of the pancreatic juice liberated into the peritoneal cavity. The reduction in the plasma calcium concentration in patients with acute pancreatitis is thus directly related to the extent of pancreatic involvement in the acute disease process, the amount of lipase released into the peritoneal cavity and the total mass of calcium fixed as soaps with fatty acids.

Anticonvulsant drug therapy

Many toxic or hypersensitivity reactions are known to be associated with the long-term administration of anticonvulsant drugs. Recently, hypocalcaemia and osteomalacia have been reported among patients with major epilepsy on long-term anticonvulsant therapy (Dent et al., 1970; Richens & Rowe, 1970). The hypocalcaemia was related to high dosage of anticonvulsant drugs, to multiple drug therapy and to the use of individual anticonvulsant drugs in the following order, with decreasing order of importance: pheneturide, primidone, phenytoin, and phenobarbitone. In the patients with hypocalcaemia there was no evidence, nor any history of, dietary deficiencies. Similarly in the patients with osteomalacia there was no evidence of any dietary deficiency, intestinal malabsorption abnormality or hepatic cause for the osteomalacia. Dent and his colleagues considered that the abnormalities found in these patients were the result of cholecalciferol deficiency. The liver is the probable site of conversion of cholecalciferol to 25-hydroxycholecalciferol. Dent and his colleagues proposed that drug-mediated enzyme induction could be the mechanism responsible for their findings by producing a reduction in the biological half-life and tissue deficiency of active cholecalciferol metabolites despite the adequate dietary intake of cholecalciferol. This proposal has been supported by the report of increased urine D-glucaric acid excretion (a quantitative index of increased hepatic enzyme induction) in patients on anticonvulsant drug therapy (Hunter et al., 1971). They reported a significant inverse correlation between urine D-glucaric acid excretion and serum calcium concentration in epileptic children on anticonvulsant drug therapy.

Medullary carcinoma of the thyroid

It is generally agreed that medullary carcinoma of the thyroid is a tumour of the calcitonin producing parafollicular cells (C cells) of the thyroid (Williams, 1970). It has been demonstrated that these tumours and their metastases have a high calcitonin content and in most cases this is associated with an increased plasma calcitonin concentration (Melvin, Voelkel & Tashjian, 1970). However, in the majority of the patients reported with this tumour, the plasma calcium concentration has been normal and some were even hypercalcaemic (Tubiana *et al.*, 1968). MacIntyre (1970) proposed that in patients with medullary carcinoma of the thyroid the normal plasma calcium concentration was the result of increased parathyroid hormone secretion which abolished the effects of the increased calcitonin secretion. However, if parathyroid hormone secretion was increased in all patients with medullary carcinoma of the thyroid it could be expected that the normo-calcaemia would be associated with a marked degree of hypophosphataemia, as both calcitonin and parathyroid hormone have a phosphaturic action. However, in the cases which have been reported the plasma phosphate concentration is usually within the normal range or is only slightly reduced.

Fanconi syndrome

The Fanconi syndrome is characterised by osteomalacia or rickets in association with glycosuria, aminoaciduria, and hypophosphataemia, all of which are due to defects in renal tubular reabsorption. In some patients there is also a hyperchloraemic metabolic acidosis, and this is frequently associated with an increase in urine calcium excretion. Hypocalcaemia is a rare occurrence in patients with the Fanconi syndrome and when present it has been attributed to the hypercalciuria, although there is some evidence that it is also due to a diminution in intestinal calcium absorption (Fourman & Royer, 1968).

Investigations for the Differential Diagnosis of Hypocalcaemia

The differential diagnosis of hypocalcaemia is based essentially on the clinical history and the symptoms and signs associated with the primary disease state which is responsible for the reduction in plasma calcium concentration. The clinical history of a patient found to have hypocalcaemia, for which a cause is being sought, must include details of: adequacy of diet; exposure to sunlight, particularly if there is a history of any dietary inadequacy or food faddism; previous neck surgery; disorders of genito-urinary tract, bile secretion and gastro-intestinal tract, particularly details of previous gastric or intestinal surgery; and history of long-term anticonvulsant drug therapy.

Plasma calcium (total and fractions). The effect of venous stasis during the collection of blood for the estimation of total plasma calcium concentration has already been discussed (v.s.). In patients with hypocalcaemia ultra-filtration *in vivo*, by prolonged venous stasis during the collection of blood, can artificially elevate low plasma calcium values into the normal range. It must be stressed again that a careful technique should always be used when collecting blood for the estimation of plasma calcium concentration.

In patients with hypocalcaemia it has been reported that the percentage of both the ultrafiltrable and ionized calcium fractions showed a constant relationship to the total plasma calcium concentration unless the patients were hypoproteinaemic when the percentage of ultrafiltrable calcium was increased (Fowler, Fone & Cooke, 1961). These observations have been confirmed by Wills & Lewin (1971) who also reported that the calcium-binding affinity of the plasma proteins, as determined by K_{CaProt}, did not differ significantly between hypocalcaemic patients and normal subjects.

The absence of tetanic episodes in patients with chronic renal failure and hypocalcaemia has classically been attributed to the concomitant acidosis. The 'protective' role of acidosis has been attributed either to an increase in the concentration of the ionized calcium fraction by diminishing the protein-bound fraction or to a specific effect of the hydrogen ion on neuromuscular irritability. Walser (1962) reported that in hypocalcaemic uraemic patients the percentage of ionized calcium was no higher in those patients with severe metabolic acidosis than it was in those with mild acidosis, nor did it differ from the results obtained in normal subjects. He also reported that in these patients the calcium-binding affinity of the plasma proteins did not differ significantly from that in normal subjects. These findings have been subsequently confirmed (Wills & Lewin, 1971). It would seem therefore that the absence of tetany in acidotic uraemics with hypocalcaemia cannot be attributed to an increase in the ionized plasma calcium fraction but can be attributed to the metabolic acidosis of chronic renal failure. The acidosis in chronic renal failure apparently exerts its protective role through a specific effect of the hydrogen ion on neuromuscular irritability.

Plasma phosphate. The changes that occur in the plasma phosphate concentration in disease states associated with hypocalcaemia are variable. The raised plasma phosphate concentration in hypoparathyroidism is usually attributed to an increase in the renal tubular reabsorption of phosphate due to the absence of parathyroid hormone. However, in patients with hypoparathyroidism the plasma phosphate concentration may be within the normal range. Phosphate retention and the associated high plasma concentration in patients with chronic renal failure is attributable to the decrease in glomerular filtration rate as a consequence of the renal disease. The occasional finding of a normal phosphate concentration in uraemic patients is usually accounted for by increased parathyroid hormone secretion, a consequence of secondary hyperparathyroidism due to the hypocalcaemia. The hypophosphataemia associated with nutritional cholecalciferol deficiency, disorders of the gastrointestinal tract and bile secretion is also usually attributed to secondary hyperparathyroidism. The aetiological mechanism for the hyperphosphataemia in neonates is dependent upon the type of neonatal hypocalcaemia. In the Fanconi syndrome the hypophosphataemia is attributable mainly to the increased urinary phosphate excretion and is possibly accentuated by defective intestinal absorption.

Serum proteins. The importance of variations in serum protein fractions, particularly the albumin, has already been discussed (v.s.).

Plasma alkaline phosphatase. As in the differential diagnosis of hypercalcaemia the estimation of plasma alkaline phosphatase is, of itself, of little value. However, in hypocalcaemic patients, in the absence of hepatobiliary disease, an associated increase in plasma alkaline phosphatase is indicative of osteomalacia. In the interpretation of alkaline phosphatase values, as a screening test for metabolic bone disease, it is important that the age and sex of the patient is taken into consideration (Klaassen, 1966). In a group of sixty normal men and sixty normal women, aged 25 to 85 years, Klaassen reported that with increasing age there was a rise in the alkaline phosphatase value which differed for men and women, and that in the older age groups an alkaline phosphatase activity of 12 to 18 K.A. units per 100 ml was not *per se* abnormal.

Urine calcium. In the majority of hypocalcaemic states urine calcium excretion will be reduced, as a consequence of the reduction in the renal filtered load. The estimation of urine calcium excretion is therefore of little value in the differential diagnosis of hypocalcaemia, except to confirm the low plasma value. However, in patients with the Fanconi syndrome urine calcium excretion is increased.

Acid-base status. A metabolic alkalosis has been reported in patients with either surgical or idiopathic hypoparathyroidism which was attributed to the absence of the parathyroid glands (Barzel, 1969). These findings are consistent with the metabolic acidosis found in patients with either primary or tertiary hyperparathyroidism (v.s.) and also secondary hyperparathyroidism. In a group of patients with osteomalacia, of either dietary or intestinal origin, Muldowney, Freaney & McGeeney (1968) reported that in some of them there was a metabolic acidosis, aminoaciduria and defective excretion of an acid load. They attributed these renal tubular abnormalities to parathyroid hormone excess as a consequence of secondary hyperparathyroidism. These findings would suggest that, as in hypercalcaemic states, the determination of acid-base status is of value in differential diagnosis of patients with hypocalcaemia and in particular the diagnosis of hypoparathyroidism or parathyroid gland hypofunction.

Treatment of Hypocalcaemia

Hypocalcaemia always requires treatment; either to relieve tetanic symptoms directly attributable to the low plasma calcium concentration or in the absence of tetany to avoid the long-term neurological complications associated with hypocalcaemia.

Acute treatment

The commonest cause of hypocalcaemia tetany is surgical hypoparathyroidism following operative procedures on the neck and thyroid gland. The acute treatment of hypocalcaemic tetany is the intravenous injection of a calcium salt. The calcium salt most commonly used is calcium gluconate in a dosage of 10 to 20 ml of a 10 per cent solution given intravenously over ten minutes (10 ml contains 90 mg of calcium). Calcium chloride is occasionally used because of its higher calcium content (5 ml of a 10 per cent solution contains 180 mg of calcium). Calcium chloride, however, has the disadvantages that it causes necrosis if 'spilt' into the subcutaneous tissues and may cause venous thrombosis even after successful intravenous administration. In any patient with hypocalcaemic tetany the acute relief of symptoms should be immediately followed by the institution of treatment on a long-term basis.

Long-term treatment

The aim in the institution of long-term treatment of hypocalcaemic tetany is to increase intestinal calcium absorption by the administration of calciferol (vitamin D); occasionally in combination with oral calcium supplements. Oral calcium supplements alone have no place in the long-term treatment of hypocalcaemia from any cause. The official B.N.F. preparation of calciferol which is commonly used is 'Calciferol tablets, strong, B.P.'—each tablet containing 1·25 mg calciferol (which is equivalent to 50 000 units of anti-rachitic activity). It is usual to commence calciferol therapy with an oral loading dose of 5 mg daily for 4 to 5 days and then reduce to the expected maintenance dose of 1·25 to 2·5 mg daily. The reduction to one of these maintenance dosages is dependent on the initial response in the plasma calcium concentration. The final maintenance dosage of calciferol which is required in any one individual patient has to be determined for that patient on a 'titration' basis by frequent estimations of the plasma calcium concentration. A final maintenance dosage scheme may only require calciferol therapy on alternate days, or even twice weekly. In the early stages of establishing a maintenance dosage of calciferol the plasma calcium concentration should be estimated two or three times a week. Once a dosage regimen has been established less frequent checks of plasma calcium are necessary; initially monthly and then every two or three months. The final maintenance dose of calciferol should be sufficient to maintain the plasma calcium concentration within, or slightly below, the lower half of the normal range. Calciferol (vitamin D) has a cumulative effect and it is possible for patients on long-term surveillance to progress to hypercalcaemia, if maintained at a high normal plasma calcium concentration; whereas if maintained within or just below the normal range any increase will be into or within the normal range and the dosage of calciferol can be readjusted before hypercalcaemia supervenes. If there is no plasma calcium response to the initial loading dose of calciferol, which is very rare, the daily dose should be increased by 2·5 mg for a few days, and oral calcium supplements given, until a plasma calcium response is obtained and then the dosage of calciferol should be immediately reduced. The main disadvantage of the use of oral calcium supplements in calciferol therapy is that two variables are introduced, and regulation of maintenance dosage is thus more difficult. Occasionally 'vitamin D resistance' may develop in patients with idiopathic or surgical hypoparathyroidism on long-term treatment and in such patients the use of 25-hydroxychole-calciferol has been proposed (Pak *et al.*, 1970). This form of treatment should, however, be only undertaken with the patient under strict metabolic super-vision.

In the institution of long-term treatment for hypocalcaemia in those disease states where hypocalcaemia is secondary to some primary disease such as dietary inadequacy or after partial gastrectomy, a similar regimen to that given above, may be followed although in many conditions an adequate response can be obtained with smaller doses of calciferol. In the hypocalcaemia of gluten-induced enteropathy it is essential that treatment of the primary disease is also instituted. When following treatment in those disease states associated with osteomalacia and bone pain the effectiveness of the treatment should be assessed primarily by the loss of pain, radiological improvement in the bone lesions, and reduction in the plasma alkaline phosphatase activity. In all patients receiving calciferol therapy regular surveillance must always be maintained, and the patients should be informed of the toxic symptoms associated with hypercalcaemia. The use of calciferol in prophylactic treatment is rarely, if ever, indicated and should only be given in physiological amounts.

The indications for the administration of oral calcium supplements are (i) during lactation, and (ii) in patients with a total body calcium deficit, who are reforming bone, as an addition to calciferol therapy. The calcium content of mature breast milk ranges from 17 to 61 mg per 100 ml (Documenta Geigy, 1962) and there is a daily secretion of, at the maximum, 600 to 800 ml. Thus at maximum daily secretion a lactating mother could secrete as much as 500 mg of calcium a day. In a standard man of 70 kg, the total body calcium content is approximately 1000 g (Documenta Geigy, 1962). In patients with significant radiological demineralisation a third or more of total body calcium may be lost and this would represent a total body calcium deficit of 300 g. In order to remineralise bone, this calcium has to be replaced by increased intestinal absorption. In a normal individual, in a steady-state, on a normal diet (approximately 1·0 g of calcium per day) the amount of calcium absorbed equals the daily urine calcium excretion of 0·1 to 0·3 g per day. In the face of a total body calcium deficit of 300 g, even if a patient absorbed and retained at least 1 g of calcium a day remineralisation would take almost a year. In order to achieve a daily absorption and retention of 1·0 g of calcium an oral calcium supplement of 1 to 3 g per day must be given in addition to the normal dietary calcium intake. This supplement is essential for the enhancement of calcium absorption by calciferol therapy to be effective.

TABLE 3.4

CALCIUM CONTENT OF CALCIUM SALTS

Calcium Salt	Molecular Weight	Calcium Content (g per g of Salt)	Dose of Salt necessary to provide 1 g of Calcium
Carbonate	100	0·40	2·5
Phosphate	172	0·23	4·4
Lactate	308	0·13	7·7
Gluconate	448	0·09	11·0

A variety of oral calcium supplements are available. The most palatable oral calcium supplement is cow's milk which has a calcium content ranging from 56 to 381 mg per 100 ml (Documenta Geigy, 1962). The variation in calcium content of cow's milk is partly due to seasonal variations. When used as a calcium supplement milk should be given in divided doses through the day in order to achieve maximum absorption. Of the other oral calcium supplements available the commonly used are listed in Table 3.4. It is essential in the use of these supplements to administer a sufficient amount of salt to provide 1 to 3 g of calcium a day. Although not widely used calcium carbonate is of considerable value because of its high calcium content when compared with all other preparations. Calcium carbonate can be given as a powder sprinkled over food. In our experience this method has proved to be of value in combination with calciferol therapy in the treatment of hypocalcaemia in a patient after parathyroidectomy for hyperparathyroidism and severe osteitis fibrosa (Wills, Richardson & Paul, 1961).

References

AUB, J. C., TIBBETTS, D. M. & McLEAN, R. (1937). *J. Nutr.*, **13**, 635.

AURBACH, G. D., MARCUS, R., WINICKOFF, R. N., EPSTEIN, E. H., JR. & NIGRA, T. P. (1970). *Metabolism*, **19**, 799.

AXELROD, D. R. (1966). *J. clin. Endocr. Metab.*, **26**, 207.

AZZOPARDI, J. G., FREEMAN, E. & POOLE, G. (1970). *Br. med. J.*, **4**, 528.

AZZOPARDI, J. G. & WHITTAKER, R. S. (1969). *J. clin. Path.*, **22**, 718.

BARLTROP, D. & OPPÉ, T. E. (1970). *Lancet*, **2**, 1333.

BARTTER, F. C. & NEY, R. L. (1967). *In* "L'osteomalacie". Ed. D. J. Hioco., pp. 213. Paris: Masson.

BARZEL, U. S. (1969). *J. clin. Endocr. Metab.*, **29**, 917.

BARZEL, U. S. & JOWSEY, J. (1969). *Clin. Sci.*, **36**, 517.

BERNSTEIN, D. S., WACHMAN, A. & HATTNER, R. S. (1970). *In* "Osteoporosis". Ed. U. S. Barzel. p. 207. New York: Grune & Stratton.

BIJVOET, O. L. M., VAN DER SLUYS VEER, J., WILDIERS, J. & SMEENK, D. (1970). *In* "Calcitonin 1969, Proceedings of the Second International Symposium". Ed. S. Taylor & G. V. Foster. p. 531. London: William Heinemann Medical Books.

BINGHAM, P. J., BRAZELL, I. A. & OWEN, M. (1969). *J. Endocr.*, **45**, 387.

BORLE, A. B. (1969). *Endocrinology*, **85**, 194.

BOYLE, I. T., GRAY, R. W. & DeLUCA, H. F. (1971). *Proc. natn. Acad. Sci., U.S.A.*, **68**, 2131.

BRISCOE, A. M. & RAGAN, C. (1965). *Am. J. clin. Nutr.*, **16**, 281.

BRONSKY, D. (1970). *J. clin. Endocr. Metab.*, **31**, 271.

BUCKLE, R. M., MASON, A. M. S. & MIDDLETON, J. E. (1969). *Lancet*, **1**, 1128.

BUXTON, R. L., WEBSTER, D., JOHNSTON, I. D. A. & HALL, R. (1970). *Lancet*, **2**, 498.

CHALMERS, J., CONACHER, W. D. H., GARDNER, D. L. & SCOTT, P. J. (1967). *J. Bone Jt. Surg.*, **49B**, 403.

CHARBON, G. A., BRUMMER, F. & RENEMAN, R. S. (1968). *Archs int. Pharmocydn. Thér.*, **171**, 1.

CHASE, L. R., FEDAK, S. A. & AURBACH, G. D. (1969). *Endocrinology*, **84**, 761.

COCHRAN, M., PEACOCK, M., SACHS, G. & NORDIN, B. E. C. (1970). *Br. med. J.*, **1**, 135.

COPP, D. H. (1969). *J. Endocr.*, **43**, 137.

COPP, D. H., CAMERON, E. C., CHENEY, B. A., DAVIDSON, A. G. F. & HENZE, K. G. (1962). *Endocrinology*, **70**, 638.

DAVIES, D. R., DENT, C. E. & WATSON, L. (1968). *Br. med. J.*, **3**, 395.

DEFTOS, L. J. & POTTS, J. T., JR. (1969). *Br. J. Hosp. Med.*, **2**, 1813.

DeLUCA, H. F. (1969). *Am. J. clin. Nutr.*, **22**, 412.

DeLUCA, H. F. (1970). *In* "Calcitonin 1969, Proceedings of the Second International Symposium". Ed. S. Taylor & G. V. Foster. p. 205. London: William Heinemann Medical Books.

DeLUCA, H. F., ENGSTROM, G. W. & RASMUSSEN, H. (1962). *Proc. natn. Acad. Sci., U.S.A.*, **48**, 1604.

DENT, C. E. (1956). *Br. med. J.*, **1**, 230.

DENT, C. E. (1962). *Br. med. J.*, **2**, 1419.

DENT, C. E. (1970). *Post-grad. med. J.*, **46**, 471.

DENT, C. E. & HARPER, C. M. (1962). *Lancet*, **1**, 559.

DENT, C. E., RICHENS, A., ROWE, D. J. F. & STAMP, T. C. B. (1970). *Br. med. J.*, **4**, 69.

DENT, C. E. & SMITH, R. (1969). *Q. Jl Med.*, **38**, 195.

DENT, C. E. & WATSON, L. (1968). *Lancet*, **2**, 662.

DiGIULIO, W. & MORALES, J. O. (1969). *J. Am. med. Ass.*, **209**, 1873.

DOCUMENTA GEIGY (1962). "Scientific Tables, 6th edition." Ed. K. Diem. p. 274, p. 514. Manchester: Geigy Pharmaceutical.

DOLMAN, M. & BARZEL, U. S. (1971). *N.Y. St. J. Med.*, **71**, 1201.

DUDLEY, F. J. & BLACKBURN, C. R. B. (1970). *Lancet*, **2**, 628.

EISENSTEIN, R. & PASSAVOY, M. (1964). *Proc. Soc. exp. Biol. Med.*, **117**, 77.

EVANSON, J. M. (1966). *Clin. Sci.*, **31**, 63.

EVANSON, J. M., GARNER, A., HOLMES, A. M., LUMB, G. A. & STANBURY, S. W. (1967). *Clin. Sci.*, **32**, 271.

FLANAGAN, B. & NICHOLS, G., JR. (1969). *J. clin. Invest.*, **48**, 595.

FOSTER, G. V., JOPLIN, G. F., MACINTYRE, I., MELVIN, K. E. W. & SLACK, E. (1966). *Lancet*, **1**, 107.

FOURMAN, P., MCCONKEY, B. & SMITH, J. W. G. (1960). *Lancet*, **1**, 619.

FOURMAN, P. & MORGAN, D. B. (1969). *In* "Nutritional Aspects of the Development of Bone and Connective Tissue. Proceedings of the Seventh Symposium of the Group of European Nutritionists. Cambridge 1968". Ed. J. C. Somogyi & E. Kodicek. p. 30. Bibliotheca Nutritio et Dieta, No. 13. Basel: Karger.

FOURMAN, P., RAWNSLEY, K., DAVIS, R. H., JONES, K. H. & MORGAN, D. B. (1967). *Lancet*, **2**, 914.

FOURMAN, P. & ROYER, P. (1968). *In* "Calcium Metabolism and the Bone". 2nd edn., p. 80, p. 450. Oxford: Blackwell.

FOWLER, D. I., FONE, D. J. & COOKE, W. T. (1961). *Lancet*, **2**, 284.

FREER, S. & WILLS, M. R. (1970). *Br. J. clin. Pract.*, **24**, 343.

FRY, L. (1962). *Br. med. J.*, **1**, 301.

GORDAN, G. S., CANTINO, T. J., ERHARDT, L., HANSEN, J. & LUBICH, W. (1966). *Science, N.Y.*, **151**, 1226.

GOUGH, K. R., LLOYD, O. C. & WILLS, M. R. (1964). *Lancet*, **2**, 1261.

GRAN, F. C. (1960). *Acta physiol. scand.*, **50**, 132.

GRAY, R., BOYLE, I. & DeLUCA, H. F. (1971). *Science, N.Y.*, **172**, 1232.

GRIMES, B. J., FISHER, B., FINN, F. & DANOWSKI, T. S. (1967). *Acta endocr., Copenh.*, **56**, 510.

GUTMAN, Y. & GOTTSCHALK, C. W. (1966). *Israel J. med. Sci.*, **2**, 243.

HADDAD, J. G., Jr., BIRGE, S. J. & AVIOLI, L. V. (1970). *New Engl. J. Med.*, **283**, 549.

HAFF, R. C., BLACK, W. C. & BALLINGER, W. F. (1970). *Ann. Surg.*, **171**, 85.

HALVER, B. (1968). *Acta med. scand.*, **184**, 311.

HARDMAN, J. G., ROBISON, G. A. & SUTHERLAND, E. W. (1971). *A. Rev. Physiol.*, **33**, 311.

HAUSSLER, M. R., NAGODE, L. A. & RASMUSSEN, H. (1970). *Nature, Lond.*, **228**, 1199.

HEATH, D. A. & KNAPP, M. S. (1969). *Acta endocr., Copenh.*, **61**, Suppl. 138, 190.

HEBERT, L. A., LEMANN, JR., J., PETERSEN, J. R. & LENNON, E. J. (1966). *J. clin. Invest.*, **45**, 1886.

HELLMAN, D. E., AU, W. Y. W. & BARTTER, F. C. (1965). *Am. J. Physiol.*, **209**, 643.

HILL, L. F., VAN DEN BERG, C. J. & MAWER, E. B. (1971). *Nature, New Biol., Lond.*, **232**, 189.

HORSTING, M. & DeLUCA, H. F. (1969). *Biochem. biophys. Res. Commun.*, **36**, 251.

HUNTER, J., MAXWELL, J. D., STEWART, D. A., PARSONS, V. & WILLIAMS, R. (1971). *Br. med. J.*, **4**, 202.

JOHN, H. T. & WILLS, M. R. (1963). *Lancet*, **2**, 418.

JOHN, H. T., WILLS, M. R. & MARCUS, R. T. (1966). *Br. J. Surg.*, **53**, 685.

JONES, K. H. & FOURMAN, P. (1963). *Lancet*, **2**, 121.

KAMMERMAN, S. & CANFIELD, R. E. (1970). *J. clin. Endocr. Metab.*, **31**, 70.

KEEN, J. H. (1969). *Archs Dis. Childh.*, **44**, 356.

KLAASSEN, C. H. L. (1966). *Lancet*, **2**, 1361.

KRAMER, F. (1936). *Fortschr. Ther.*, **12**, 521.

KRULL, G. H., MULLER, H., LEIJNSE, B. & GERBRANDY, J. (1969). *Lancet*, **2**, 174.

LAWSON, D. E. M., FRASER, D. R., KODICEK, E., MORRIS, H. R. & WILLIAMS, D. H. (1971). *Nature, Lond.*, **230**, 228.

LEE, J. B., TASHJIAN, A. H., JR., STREETO, J. M. & FRANTZ, A. G. (1968). *New Engl. J. Med.*, **279**, 1179.

LEHNINGER, A. L. (1970). *Biochem. J.*, **119**, 129.

LI, T. K. & PIECHOCKI, J. T. (1971). *Clin. Chem.*, **17**, 411.

LLOYD, H. M. (1968). *Medicine, Baltimore*, **47**, 53.

LOOMIS, W. F. (1967). *Science, N.Y.*, **157**, 501.

McGEOWN, M., BELL, T. K., SOYANNWO, M. A. O., FENTON, S. S. A. & OREOPOULOS, D. (1968). *Br. J. Radiol.*, **41**, 300.

MacINTYRE, I. (1970). *In* "Calcitonin 1969, Proceedings of the Second International Symposium". Ed. S. Taylor & G. V. Foster. p. 1. London: William Heinemann Medical Books.

MELVIN, K. E. W., HEPNER, G. W., BORDIER, P., NEALE, G. & JOPLIN, G. F. (1970). *Q. Jl Med.*, **39**, 83.

MELVIN, K. E .W., VOELKEL, E. F. & TASHJIAN, A. H., JR. (1970). *In* "Calcitonin 1969, Proceedings of the Second International Symposium". Ed. S. Taylor & G. V. Foster. p. 487. London: William Heinemann Medical Books.

MICHIE, W., STOWERS, J. M., DUNCAN, T., PEGG, C. A. S., HAMER-HODGES, D. W., HEMS, G., BEWSHER, P. D. & HEDLEY, A. J. (1971). *Lancet*, **1**, 508.

MICHIE, W., STOWERS, J. M., FRAZER, S. C. & GUNN, A. (1965). *Br. J. Surg.*, **52**, 503.

MORGAN, D. B. & FOURMAN, P. (1969). *Br. J. Hosp. Med.*, **2**, 901.

MULDOWNEY, F. P., FREANEY, R. & McGEENEY, D. (1968). *Q. Jl Med.*, **37**, 517.

MYRTLE, J. F. & NORMAN, A. W. (1971). *Science, N.Y.*, **171**, 79.

NAGATA, N. & RASMUSSEN, H. (1970). *Proc. natn. Acad. Sci., U.S.A.*, **65**, 368.

NASSIM, J. R., SAVILLE, P. D., COOK, P. B. & MULLIGAN, L. (1959). *Q. Jl Med.*, **28**, 141.

NEWTON, T. H. & EISENBERG, E. (1966). *Radiology*, **86**, 843.

NEY, R. S., KELLY, G. & BARTTER, F. C. (1968). *Endocrinology*, **82**, 760.

NORDIN, B. E. C. & PEACOCK, M. (1969). *Lancet*, **2**, 1280.

OLIVIER, A. H. (1970). *Experientia*, **26**, 854.

OMENN, G. S., ROTH, S. I. & BAKER, W. H. (1969). *Cancer*, **24**, 1004.

OPPÉ, T. E. & REDSTONE, D. (1968). *Lancet*, **1**, 1045.

PAINTER, N. S. (1960). *Br. J. Surg.*, **48**, 291.

PAK, C. Y. C., DeLUCA, H. F., CHAVEZ DE LOS RIOS, J. M., SUDA, T., RUSKIN, B. & DELEA, C. S. (1970). *Archs intern. Med.*, **126**, 239.

PAK, C. Y. C., WILLS, M. R., SMITH, G. W. & BARTTER, F. C. (1968). *J. clin. Endocr. Metab.*, **28**, 1657.

PARFITT, A. M. & DENT, C. E. (1970). *Q. Jl Med.*, **39**, 171.

PEACOCK, M., ROBERTSON, W. G. & NORDIN, B. E. C. (1969). *Lancet*, **1**, 384.

PERLIA, C. P., GUBISCH, N. J., WOLTER, J., EDELBERG, D., DEDERICK, M. M. & TAYLOR, S. G. (1970). *Cancer*, **25**, 389.

PONCHON, G. & DeLUCA, H. F. (1969). *J. clin. Invest.*, **48**, 1273.

POTCHEN, E. J., WATTS, H. G. & AWWAD, H. K. (1967). *Radiology Clinics N. Am.*, **5**, 267.

PYRAH, L. N., HODGKINSON, A. & ANDERSON, C. K. (1966). *Br. J. Surg.*, **53**, 245.

RAISZ, L. G. & NIEMANN, I. (1969). *Endocrinology*, **85**, 446.

RASMUSSEN, H. & TENENHOUSE, A. (1967). *Am. J. Med.*, **43**, 711.

REISS, E. & CANTERBURY, J. M. (1969). *New Engl. J. Med.*, **280**, 1381.

REITZ, R. E., POLLARD, J. J., WANG, C. A., FLEISCHLI, D. J., COPE, O., MURRAY, T. M., DEFTOS, L. J. & POTTS, J. T., JR. (1969). *New Engl. J. Med.*, **281**, 348.

REYNAFARJE, B. & LEHNINGER, A. L. (1969). *J. biol. Chem.*, **244**, 584.

REYNOLDS, J. J. & DINGLE, J. T. (1970). *Calcif. Tissue Res.*, **4**, 339.

RICHENS, A. & ROWE, D. J. F. (1970). *Br. med. J.*, **4**, 73.

RICHET, G., ARDAILLOU, R., AMIEL, C. & LECESTRE, M. (1963). *J. Urol. Néphrol.*, **69**, 373.

ROBINSON, C. J., MATTHEWS, E. W. & MACINTYRE, I. (1969). *In* "Proceedings Fifth European Symposium on Calcified Tissues, Bordeaux, 1967". Ed. G. Milhaud. p. 279. Paris: S.E.D.E.S.

ROSE, N. (1963). *Lancet*, **2**, 116.

SCHACHTER, D. (1963). *In* "The Transfer of Calcium and Strontium Across Biological Membranes". Ed. R. H. Wasserman. p. 197. New York: Academic Press.

SCHACHTER, D., FINKELSTEIN, J. D. & KOWARSKI, S. (1964). *J. clin. Invest.*, **43**, 787.

SEIFERT, G. & SEEMANN, N. (1967). *Dt. med. Wschr.*, **92**, 1943.

SHANE, S. R., FLINK, E. B. & JONES, J. E. (1969). *J. clin. Endocr. Metab.*, **29**, 401.

SMITH, R. (1967). *Clinica chim. Acta.*, **18**, 47.

SPAULDING, S. W. & WALSER, M. (1970). *J. clin. Endocr. Metab.*, **31**, 531.

STAMP, T. C. B. (1971). *Clin. Sci.*, **40**, 55.

STANBURY, S. W. & LUMB, G. A. (1966). *Q. Jl Med.*, **35**, 1.

STORCK, G. & BJÖRNTORP, P. (1971). *Scan. J. Gastroenterology*, **6**, 225.

STROTT, C. A. & NUGENT, C. A. (1968). *Ann. intern. Med.*, **68**, 188.

SUDA, T., DELUCA, H. F., SCHNOES, H. K., PONCHON, G., TANAKA, Y. & HOLICK, M. F. (1970). *Biochemistry*, **9**, 2917.

SUH, S. M., FRASER, D. & KOOH, S. W. (1970). *J. clin. Endocr. Metab.*, **30**, 609.

SUKI, W. N., YIUM, J. J., VON MINDEN, M., SALLER-HEBERT, C., EKNOYAN, G. & MARTINEZ-MALDONADO, M. (1970). *New Engl. J. Med.*, **283**, 836.

SWEETNAM, W. P. (1966). *Lancet*, **1**, 463.

SWINTON, N. W. (1937). *New Engl. J. Med.*, **217**, 165.

TENENHOUSE, A., RASMUSSEN, H. & NAGATA, N. (1970). *In* "Calcitonin 1969, Proceedings of the Second International Symposium". Ed. S. Taylor & G. V. Foster. p. 418. London: William Heinemann Medical Books.

THALASSINOS, N. C. & JOPLIN, G. F. (1968). *Br. med. J.*, **4**, 14.

THALASSINOS, N. C. & JOPLIN, G. F. (1970). *Lancet*, **2**, 537.

THOMPSON, G. R., LEWIS, B. & BOOTH, C. C. (1966). *Lancet*, **1**, 457.

TRANSBØL, I., HORNUM, I., HAHNEMANN, S., HASNER, E., ØHLENSCHLAGER, H., DIEMER, H. & LOCKWOOD, K. (1970). *Acta med. scand.*, **188**, 505.

TUBIANA, M., MILHAUD, G., COUTRIS, G., LACOUR, J., PARMENTIER, C. & BOK, B. (1968). *Br. med. J.*, **4**, 87.

VAES, G. (1969). *In* "Lysosomes in Biology and Pathology". Vol. 1. Ed. J. T. Dingle & H. Fell. p. 217. Amsterdam: North-Holland.

VERBANCK, M. (1965). *Acta clin. Belg.*, **20**, Suppl. 1, 1.

WACHMAN, A. & BERNSTEIN, D. S. (1968). *Lancet*, **1**, 958.

WADE, J. S. H., FOURMAN, P. & DEANE, L. (1965). *Br. J. Surg.*, **52**, 493.

WALSER, M. (1961). *Am. J. Physiol.*, **200**, 1099.

WALSER, M. (1962). *J. clin. Invest.*, **41**, 1454.

WASSERMAN, R. H. (1968). *Calcif. Tissue Res.*, **2**, 301.

WENSEL, R. H., RICH, C., BROWN, A. C. & VOLWILER, W. (1969). *J. clin. Invest.*, **48**, 1768.

WIDROW, S. H. & LEVINSKY, N. G. (1962). *J. clin. Invest.*, **41**, 2151.

WILLIAMS, E. D. (1970). *In* "Calcitonin 1969, Proceedings of the Second International Symposium". Ed. S. Taylor & G. V. Foster. p. 483. London: William Heinemann Medical Books.

WILLS, M. R. (1966). *Br. J. Surg.*, **53,** 174.

WILLS, M. R. (1970a). *J. clin. Path.*, **23,** 772.

WILLS, M. R. (1970b). *Lancet*, **2,** 802.

WILLS, M. R. (1971a). *In* "Biochemical Consequences of Chronic Renal Failure". p. 51. Aylesbury: Harvey Miller & Medcalf.

WILLS, M. R. (1971b). *Lancet*, **1,** 142.

WILLS, M. R. (1971c). *J. clin. Path.*, **24,** 219.

WILLS, M. R. (1971d). *Lancet*, **1,** 849.

WILLS, M. R. (1971e). *Lancet*, **1,** 797.

WILLS, M. R., GILL, J. R., JR., & BARTTER, F. C. (1969). *Clin. Sci.*, **37,** 621.

WILLS, M. R. & LEWIN, M. R. (1971). *J. clin. Path*, **24,** 856.

WILLS, M. R. & McGOWAN, G. K. (1964). *Br. med. J.*, **1,** 1153.

WILLS, M. R., RICHARDSON, R. E. & PAUL, R. G. (1961). *Br. med. J.*, **1,** 252.

WILLS, M. R., WORTSMAN, J., PAK, C. Y. C. & BARTTER, F. C. (1970). *Clin. Sci.*, **39.** 89.

WONG, R. G., ADAMS, T. H., ROBERTS, P. A. & NORMAN, A. W. (1970). *Biochim, biophys. Acta.*, **219,** 61.

CHAPTER 4

RADIOISOTOPE SCANNING

H. S. WILLIAMS

Radioisotope scanning is a comparatively recent addition to available diagnostic techniques but its remarkable rate of development has already extended its applications into most branches of medicine.

Basically the technique maps the distribution of radioactive material in the body: if a particular organ accumulates radioactive material selectively it may be possible, by using the radiation emitted, to produce an image which shows its position, size and shape. Furthermore the degree to which the organ concentrates the material may supply valuable information about its function. Lesions within an organ may have a concentration of radioactive material different from that in the rest of the organ and scanning is commonly used to detect such lesions.

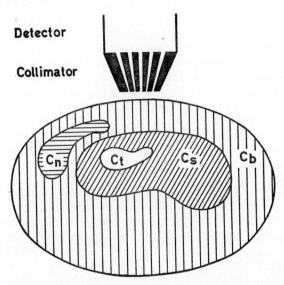

FIG. 4.1. The volume of interest (concentration of radioactivity, C_t) is embedded in an organ (C_s) situated in the body (C_b): other organs (C_n) may also be present. (By courtesy of J. R. Mallard.)

Mallard (1966) has admirably reviewed the physical aspects of the technique. Fig. 4.1 illustrates the general problem.

The aim is to visualize an organ which has a concentration of radioactivity, C_s, and, within it, an abnormality with a concentration C_t. The organ is situated within the body which has a general background concentration, C_b. Other organs with yet different concentrations, C_n, may lie close to, or even overlap, the organ of interest.

The pattern of radiation flux emerging from the body must then be translated into an image representing the distribution of radioactive material within the body. Obviously scanning can only be performed with isotopes emitting radiation sufficiently penetrating to escape from the body and reach a detector and, in practice, this means X or γ radiation of energy greater than about 50 keV. Lower energy X and γ rays and β rays are mostly absorbed in the body and are therefore unsuitable for scanning. Furthermore, it is important that only radiation travelling in a straight line from its source to the detector should be detected and the equipment should be designed and programmed to respond only to this primary (unscattered) radiation flux.

The contrast and resolution of the scan image depend on the type of scanning equipment and on the properties of the radioactively labelled substance—or 'radiopharmaceutical'—administered to the patient. Important and interdependent factors in the design of equipment and choice of radiopharmaceutical are spatial resolution (determining the size of the lesion which can be detected), the sensitivity of the equipment, the radiation dose to the patient, the time to perform the test, and cost. For example, a suitable radiopharmaceutical is one which results in C_t differing considerably from C_s, and C_b being low. But, in practice, the difference between C_t and C_s is often small and the contrast between them may be masked by statistical fluctuations in the radiation emitted from them. The decay of a radioactive isotope is a random process with a Poisson probability distribution and, therefore, even from a constant activity source, the number of γ ray photons emitted per second fluctuates. The effect on the scan image of these variations decreases as the total number of counts making up the image increases. This calls for high administered doses of radioactivity, long imaging times and high sensitivity apparatus. In their turn, however, high doses may involve unacceptable radiation hazards to the patients and high sensitivity can often only be achieved by sacrificing the ability to visualize small lesions. It is clear that compromises have to be made in the choice of radiopharmaceutical and the design of the apparatus.

INSTRUMENTATION

Instruments for observing the pattern of γ ray flux and converting it into a visible image fall into two broad classes—moving detector instruments, often called rectilinear scanners, and stationary detector instruments, the so-called gamma cameras.

Moving Detector Instruments

The detector used in all scanners is a NaI(Tl) scintillation crystal which is usually 7·5 or 12·5 cm in diameter and 5 cm thick and has a high detection efficiency. When used with a pulse height analyser, the lower energy scatter component of the radiation flux, which would have the effect of degrading the quality of the scan, can be rejected.

The region of the patient from which radiation is detected is defined by a collimating device which almost invariably consists of a tungsten block with multiple conical holes focussed at a point a few inches from the end of the collimator. By this device a large area of detector is exposed to radiation, resulting in high sensitivity. The extent to which fine detail may be detected is governed by the diameter of the holes. The greater the diameter of the holes, the greater the flux reaching the crystal but the poorer the spatial resolution. The thickness of the septa required between the holes depends on the energy of the radiation to be detected. High energy radiation requires thicker septa to absorb radiation travelling from points outside the area 'seen' by the holes. In rectilinear scanners the display system is usually linked mechanically to the detector which moves to and fro across the patient in a series of parallel lines with a preset spacing between them.

In many scanners the image is produced by a stylus which makes a mark on paper each time a preset number of pulses, called the dot factor, has been accumulated. Small differences in count rate may be made more easily detectable by recording ranges of count rate in different colours (Mallard & Peachey, 1959). Another common method of display is by photographic recording (photoscan) in which the intensity of a light source, moving across a film synchronously with the detector, is controlled by the count rate. The logarithmic response of a film enables higher contrast to be achieved than with the dot recording. Controls which vary contrast and suppress background are usually incorporated in scanning instruments. In effect, the eye detects differences in the distribution of radioisotope in the patient as differences in concentration of dots on paper, as different colours or as different densities of blackening of a film. There is no general agreement on the best method.

A disadvantage of moving detector scanners is that, at any moment, radiation from only a small volume of tissue is detected. To scan a large area therefore is a lengthy procedure and it is necessary that the distribution of radioactivity should remain constant during the period of scanning.

Specialised equipment

A useful collimator for rapid screening purposes is a slit which 'sees' a thin coronal section of the patient. By scanning at constant speed along the body axis a profile scan can be plotted on a chart recorder. Such a system is sensitive and can detect areas of abnormal uptake which can then be studied in more detail with other instruments.

Special scanners for the detection of positron emitters make use of the emission in opposite directions of the two photons of annihilation radiation which accompany positron emission. Two parallel opposed detectors with single hole collimation, on opposite sides of the patient, count only photons arriving in coincidence at the two detectors. Thus only radiation originating in a cylinder of tissue between the two detectors is counted and resolution depends on the size of the detectors. Positron scanners are used only in very few centres due to their high cost and the small number of useful positron emitting isotopes.

Stationary Detector Instruments

This type of imaging device, in which the whole field of interest is viewed at the same time, is a more recent development than rectilinear scanners but has now become well established in clinical practice.

The collimator, which may be a pinhole in a block of heavy alloy or an array of parallel holes, causes a pattern of radiation flux, corresponding to the distribution of radioactivity in the patient, to fall on to a sensitive layer. In the great majority of gamma cameras the detector is a NaI(Tl) crystal 28 cm in diameter and 1·2 cm thick, which is viewed at the back by an array of 19 photomultiplier tubes. The distribution amongst the tubes, of light produced in the crystal by the absorption of a photon of radiation, depends on the point at which absorption takes place. The outputs of the tubes are used to produce a flash of light on the screen of a cathode ray oscilloscope, at a point corresponding to the point of absorption of the γ ray on the detector. In a short period a complete picture is made up of a great number of flashes, perhaps half a million, on the screen and photographed by a Polaroid camera. The final image, therefore, is usually small but methods are available for producing a life-size image.

In the autofluoroscope (Bender & Blau, 1963) the single large detector is replaced by a mosaic of crystals, one to each hole of the collimator. The crystal in which a photon has been absorbed is identified electronically and the display system is activated at a corresponding point. Other detector systems which have been developed include spark chambers and image intensifiers. Cameras for positron emitters have also been developed and some have the ability to visualize different planes in the body, producing a type of tomographic picture.

The advantage of a gamma camera is its high sensitivity compared to that of a rectilinear scanner, allowing images to be obtained in a matter of minutes or even seconds. In practice this often means that multiple scans may be performed, and more diagnostic information obtained, in a time tolerable to the patient.

Data analysis

In adjusting the controls of the instrument before performing a scan the result of the scan must be prejudged to some degree. At the end it may be clear that the settings chosen were not optimal and the scan therefore not as useful as it might have been. However by that time information has been irretrievably lost and to repeat the scan may be too time consuming. A current trend in scanning, therefore, is to record, on magnetic tape or paper tape, all the data obtained during the test. During play back and display of the data later, adjustments can be made to levels of background subtraction and contrast enhancement so that the most informative display can be produced.

Much interest is now being shown in computer processing of scan data and there is no doubt that the diagnostic accuracy of scanning techniques will be increased by this means.

Dynamic studies

Benefits which accrue from high count rates have been mentioned. The high count rates obtained using the high sensitivity of the gamma camera and the administration of large amounts of short-lived isotopes open up new fields of dynamic studies which have great potential. For example, simultaneous studies of renal function and structure may be carred out by taking rapid sequential pictures of the kidneys with a gamma camera, following injection of [^{131}I] hippuran. By data storage and processing, graphs of the uptake and excretion of the hippuran in each kidney can be obtained, as well as displays of the distribution of hippuran within the kidneys.

RADIOPHARMACEUTICALS

The suitability of a radiopharmaceutical for scanning purposes depends on its biological and physical properties. The first essential is that it should be taken up selectively in the organ or structure of interest. In most cases the radioactive material is accumulated in normally functioning tissue and lesions are detected by absent or reduced uptake. In other cases the lesion accumulates the radioactive material to a higher concentration than normal tissue. An important requirement is that the specific activity, i.e. the fraction of the material which is radioactive, should be high in order to avoid physiological or toxic effects.

Important physical properties which determine the suitability of an isotope are its rate of decay, usually specified in terms of half life, and the type of radiation emitted. If a radiopharmaceutical is to be kept in stock, an isotope with a long half life is desirable. From the point of view of radiation dose to the patient, however, a half life just long enough to allow for the preparation and sterilisation of the pharmaceutical and the performance of the test is ideal and permits large amounts of radioactivity to be administered with minimal radiation hazard to the patient. In this context, biological half life is equally important since a short biological half life may compensate for a long physical half life.

Radioisotopes decay by various modes including the emission of negative and positive β particles. These particles have a short range in tissue and play no part in radioisotope imaging. In many cases, β^- emission is accompanied by a γ ray photon, the energy of which is characteristic of the isotope, and in some cases there is an appreciable time interval between the β^- emission and the subsequent γ emission. The emission of a β^+ particle (positron) is followed by the emission of two 0·51 MeV γ rays (annihilation radiation) travelling in opposite directions. In the use of isotopes decaying by either of these modes, it is usually β radiation which accounts for the bulk of the radiation dose to the patient. Yet another mode of decay is by the nucleus capturing an orbital electron with the consequent emission of characteristic X rays, free from undesirable β emission. ^{125}I is an example of an isotope which decays in this manner.

The energy of the γ or X radiation is of major importance. With low energy radiation only a small proportion may escape from the body, especially from organs situated deeply, but the radiation which does emerge is easily collimated and efficiently detected. With high energy radiation a greater proportion will penetrate tissue and form an emergent pattern but collimation is more difficult and absorption in the detector less efficient. The optimum energy for most scanning is about 150 keV.

Short-lived isotopes

During the last five years radioisotope imaging has been revolutionised by the introduction of short-lived isotopes which are obtained as daughter products of radioactive parents contained in generators or 'cows' (see Table 4.1).

TABLE 4.1

PHYSICAL PROPERTIES AND SCANNING APPLICATIONS OF
SHORT-LIVED RADIOISOTOPES OBTAINED FROM GENERATORS

Daughter Radioisotope	Half life	γ-ray energy keV	Parent Radioisotope	Half life	Applications of the Daughter Radioisotope
$^{99}Tc^m$	6 h	140	^{99}Mo	67 h	Brain, thyroid, lungs, liver, kidneys, placenta
$^{113}In^m$	1·7 h	392	^{113}Sn	118 d	Brain, lungs, liver, kidneys, placenta
$^{87}Sr^m$	2·8 h	388	^{87}Y	80 h	Bone
^{68}Ga	68 min	$510(+\beta^+)$	^{68}Ge	280 d	Brain, bone, lung, liver, kidney

Metastable isotopes, especially $^{99}Tc^m$ and $^{113}In^m$, which are produced as a result of β^- decay and themselves emit only γ rays, are particularly useful in scanning. The lack of β emission combined with short half life permits large amounts of radioactivity to be administered thereby shortening scanning time and improving the quality of the image as well as delivering very small radiation doses to the patient.

Technetium. $^{99}Tc^m$ is the radioactive daughter of the radioactive isotope ^{99}Mo. In the generator the ^{99}Mo is adsorbed on aluminium oxide contained in a glass cylinder with a porous disc at the bottom. When an eluant, saline in this case, is passed through the column the $^{99}Tc^m$ which has accumulated as the decay product of ^{99}Mo, is washed out, leaving the ^{99}Mo on the column. The accumulation of $^{99}Tc^m$ then recommences and the column can again be eluted after a few hours. $^{99}Tc^m$, with a half life of six hours and emitting 140 keV γ rays with no accompanying β radiation, approaches most nearly the specifications of an 'ideal' isotope. It is now very widely used, particularly for scanning the liver and brain. The useful life of a generator is determined by the half life of the parent and a $^{99}Tc^m$ generator has a useful life of only a week or ten days.

Indium. In contrast, $^{113}In^m$ generators have a much longer life. A single generator will ensure an adequate supply of $^{113}In^m$ for several months. The rather high γ ray energy, however, results in poorer resolution than with $^{99}Tc^m$. The half life of 100 min is also perhaps too short for applications involving long scanning times.

Strontium. $^{87}Sr^m$ is a suitable agent for bone scanning but its parent is produced in a cyclotron and is therefore expensive.

Gallium. ^{68}Ga is the only suitable positron emitter obtainable from a generator. Its parent is also cyclotron-produced and expensive but has a long half life. ^{68}Ga has been used for scanning several organs but so far it has not gained wide acceptance.

Developments will probably take place in the use of isotopes with even shorter half lives. If isotopes with half lives of the order of seconds were used, perhaps involving eluting generator columns directly into the patient, it would be possible to attain much higher resolutions than at present and visualize structures such as blood vessels.

One further point should be made in connection with the use of short-lived isotopes. Because of their rapid decay, radiopharmaceuticals incorporating these isotopes cannot be obtained commercially and must be prepared immediately before use, thereby precluding sterility and pyrogen testing before injection. The user must therefore assume the burden of preparation and the responsibility for the quality control of the pharmaceuticals he uses.

SPECIFIC ORGANS AND SYSTEMS

Brain

Selective uptake of radioactive material in a brain tumour was first observed using [^{131}I]diiodofluorescein and a hand-held Geiger counter as long ago as 1948 (Moore, 1948), but it is only in the last 10 years that brain scanning has become a routine procedure and it is now the most common of all scanning tests.

In the brain, in contrast to most other organs, lesions exhibit a higher concentration of radioactivity than normal brain tissue. The mechanisms whereby this difference is achieved are obscure and are currently the subject of a great deal of research. The radiopharmaceuticals which have been used for brain scanning are concentrated in many other organs of the body at least as much as in brain lesions and, in fact, it is the very low uptake of radiopharmaceuticals by the normal brain rather than specific uptake by the lesion which makes brain scanning possible.

The ability of normal brain tissue to exclude substances is due to what is termed the 'blood-brain barrier' and the uptake of radiopharmaceuticals in brain tumours and other lesions is due mainly to the breakdown of this barrier. Other factors contribute to tumour radioactivity. The vascularity of many lesions is greater than that of normal brain and increased blood content of the lesion may therefore be important, especially shortly after injection when blood activity is still high. This phase may then be followed by slower cellular uptake, which probably does not contribute much to lesion radioactivity until a considerable time after injection.

Radiopharmaceuticals

It is generally agreed that no substance has yet been found which concentrates specifically in brain tumours though Sodee (1964a) claims that chlormerodrin, a pharmaceutical used in brain scanning, accumulates selectively in all malignant tumours.

A large number of isotopes in several chemical forms have been used for brain scanning (DiChiro, Ashburn & Grove, 1968). Positron emitters—e.g. ^{74}As (Brownell & Sweet, 1953), ^{18}F (Entzian et al., 1964)—have been used successfully as scanning agents but the special equipment required for coincidence detection of annihilation radiation is expensive and confined to a few centres. [^{203}Hg]chlormerodrin, [^{197}Hg]chlormerodrin and ^{131}I-serum albumin are still widely used but [^{99}Tc^m]pertechnetate has become the agent of choice in many centres. ^{113}In^m-DTPA is a more recent addition to the range of brain scanning agents and first reports state that it gives excellent results (O'Mara et al., 1969). The ability to visualize a lesion in certain regions of the brain is affected by the radioactivity of blood and muscle—for example, suprasellar and pontine tumours are relatively difficult to diagnose due to the proximity of radioactivity in the sinuses. Therefore, the levels of blood and muscle radioactivity at the time of scanning are important and affect the choice of scanning agent.

^{131}I-serum albumin diffuses slowly and the ratio of concentration of activity in tumour to that in normal brain rises over a period of days. Scanning is usually performed 24 h after injection though blood radioactivity is still comparatively high at that time. Chlormerodrin is cleared rapidly from the blood and excreted by the kidneys, and high tumour/brain ratios with low blood and muscle activities are achieved within an hour of injection. Using [^{99}Tc^m]pertechnetate, blood activity is high at the time of scanning but the advantages to be gained, in terms of speed of scanning and improved quality of the image, by the administration of the large amounts of radioactivity permitted with this isotope, have led to the present popularity of [^{99}Tc^m] pertechnetate. Using ^{113}In^m, blood clearance is rapid and tumour/brain ratios are high. ^{131}I-albumin is not as widely used as chlormerodrin or pertechnetate because of the long time interval between injection and scanning and because of radiation dose considerations. Tumour/brain ratios of activity are between 10 and 20 for all these compounds except ^{113}In^m-DTPA where the ratio is higher.

Brain scanning has also been performed following the injection of ^{131}I-macroaggregated albumin into the carotid artery (Rosenthall, Aguayo & Stratford, 1966). The particles are filtered out by the capillary beds and both tumours and vascular lesions appear as cold areas on the scan. This is not a simple procedure however as it involves a direct puncture of the internal carotid artery and its diagnostic value remains to be proved.

Technique

Preparation of the patient depends on the isotope being used. Before administration of technetium, 200 mg of potassium perchlorate is usually given in order to minimise accumulation of technetium in the choroid plexus which otherwise may make interpretation of the scan difficult. Atropine is also commonly given to reduce uptake in the salivary glands and in the nasal and oral mucosa. When using [^{203}Hg]chlormerodrin, it is advisable to give a blocking dose of stable mercury, which causes a three-fold reduction in the radiation dose to the kidneys in most patients (Blau & Bender, 1962). Using [^{197}Hg]chlormerodrin the dose to the kidneys is so low that no precautions are necessary.

Although time-consuming when using a rectilinear scanner, it is nevertheless desirable to perform antero-posterior, postero-anterior and two lateral scans. It is sometimes helpful, in addition, to obtain a vertex view (Overton et al., 1965) and a reverse Townes view (Witcofski & Roper, 1965). Using a gamma camera four or five views should routinely be performed. Landmarks such as the external auditory meatus, nasion, and outer canthus are usually transferred to the scan as reference points. In interpreting the scan it is helpful to view it and a skull radiograph side by side. A more refined method of relating the scan image to the patient's anatomy, described by Marryat & Bull (1964), involves superimposing an underexposed X-ray image on the photoscan, using an X-ray tube attached to the scanner.

Normal scan

The appearances of normal scans using various isotopes have often been described, e.g. ^{131}I-albumin scans by McAfee & Taxdal (1961), chlormerodrin scans by Rhoton, Carlsson & Ter Pogossian (1964) and technetium scans by Webber (1965), but considerable experience is required in order to be able to recognise the detailed appearances of the normal scan (Fig. 4.2). Structures below the level of the base of the brain are shown as areas of high activity. High activity in the venous sinuses is a feature of technetium scans but blood activity is much lower using chlormerodrin.

Abnormal scan

Areas of increased uptake are not necessarily due to tumours. (Figs. 4.3, 4.4). Abnormal appearances may also be produced by cerebral infarcts, A–V malformations, subdural and intracerebral haematomas, abscesses, trauma, Paget's disease and cerebro-vascular accidents (Fig. 4.5). Burr holes and craniotomies often result in increased uptake. Epidermoid cysts do not accumulate isotopes and are not demonstrable by scanning.

Scanning using a bone seeking isotope may be useful in distinguishing lesions of the skull from brain tumours in some cases where the interpretation of a positive brain scan is doubtful (Tow & Wagner, 1967).

Tumours. The ability to visualize a tumour depends on its position and size and its concentration of radioactivity relative to the normal brain. Uptake by a tumour varies with histological type—meningiomas and glioblastomas have relatively high uptakes and astrocytomas low uptakes. Pituitary and supra-sellar lesions may be hidden by pools of circulating activity and the visualization of infratentorial tumours may be difficult because of activity in the sagittal and transverse sinuses. Chlormerodrin, giving a low blood background, is therefore superior to technetium for demonstrating posterior fossa lesions. Most reports agree that few tumours less than 2·0 cm in diameter can be visualized especially when situated near the midline.

The accuracy of brain scanning in terms of the ability to detect abnormalities is high. There have been many reports quoting success rates in detecting tumours but, in most of them, the numbers have been small especially when subdivided according to histological type. Since some types are more easily detected than others, reported variations in accuracy may be partly due to differences in the relative numbers of different tumours in the series.

Ojemann & Sweet (1969), using the positron emitter, [74]As, localised 98 per cent of proven meningiomas, 95 per cent of proven glioblastomas and 60–68 per cent of slower-growing gliomas. Bender & Williams (1966) summarised 13 previous reports in which the diagnostic rate varied between

65 per cent and 93 per cent. They found an overall rate of 78 per cent in the 473 proven tumours, all scanned using [^{197}Hg], or [^{203}Hg], chlormerodrin. Using ^{131}I-serum albumin, Budabin (1965) reported 86 per cent success and Bender & Blau (1962) 88 per cent. Similar figures have been reported using [^{99}Tc^{m}]pertechnetate—Schmukler & Workman (1966) 83 per cent and Filson & Rodriguez-Antunez (1968) 90 per cent. Positive scans in over 90 per cent of glioblastomas and meningiomas are reported by most authors. Many reports have stated that infratentorial tumours are relatively difficult to visualize. However, Bender & Williams (1966) in their figures collected from the literature, found that if acoustic neuromas were excluded, the diagnostic rate for posterior fossa tumours was 82 per cent. Acoustic neuromas are probably small at the time of scanning and only 44 per cent were correctly visualized. These results are comparable to those obtained by cerebral angiography and pneumoencephalography, which demonstrate the tumour indirectly by the displacement of vascular structures and air filled spaces.

It has been claimed that by studying the exact position and shape of the area of increased uptake on the scan it is possible to predict the pathological nature of the tumour. Takahashi, Nofal & Beierwaltes (1966) observed that meningiomas are usually spherical with a sharp outline and a high differential uptake ratio, gliomas have irregular margins with high uptake, while metastases are usually spherical with irregular margins. Bull & Marryat (1965) stress the importance of the anatomic location in relation to the convexity of the dura, the falx cerebri, the tentorium and corpus callosum. Thus if a mass crosses the midline at the frontal pole it is likely to be a meningioma whereas if it crosses in the region of the corpus callosum it is likely to be an astrocytoma. Planiol (1966, 1969) uses an entirely different technique in which the rate of uptake of a radiopharmaceutical is measured over a period of 48 h by detectors at fixed points on the skull. Radioactivity is taken up much more rapidly by meningiomas than by astrocytomas, for example. With this method, sometimes combined with scanning, a specific diagnosis may be made in a very high proportion of cases.

Non-neoplastic disease. Increasing attention is being given to the differential diagnosis of neoplastic and non-neoplastic disease by brain scanning. It has already been stated that positive brain scans are obtained in a multitude of non-malignant conditions. However, from the location, size, shape and sharpness of the images on the scan, and using serial scanning, non-neoplastic lesions can be distinguished from tumours, and their nature diagnosed, in a considerable proportion of cases (Leslie, Alker & Bakay, 1969). For example, subdural haematomas, en plaque meningiomas, Paget's disease, middle cerebral infarcts and scalp lesions may all show crescent-shaped images on the A.P. scan. However, on the lateral scan a subdural haematoma produces a typically diffuse image, in contrast to the well defined image typical of the other conditions. Strong evidence of infarction may be obtained from the position and shape of the uptake in relation to the areas supplied by the arteries, and from the results of serial scanning. Negative scans are usually obtained in the first few days after infarction and then become increasingly positive for a period. Nevertheless, angiography is often superior in differentiating between tumour, infarct, intracerebral clot and arteriovenous malformations (Overton, Haynie & Snodgrass, 1965).

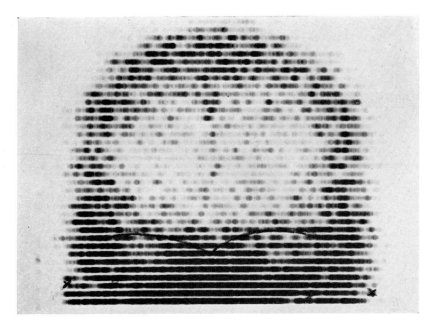

(a)

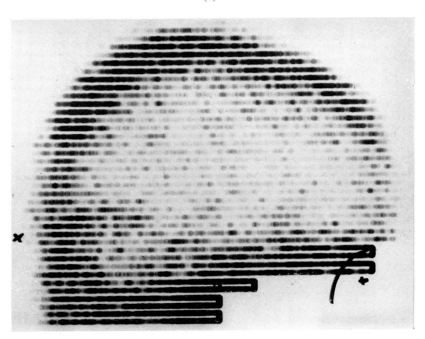

(b)

FIG. 4.2. Photoscan of normal brain using [^{99}Tc ^{m}] pertechnetate.

(a) Anterior view. The peripheral band represents circulating radioactivity in the scalp, bone and vessels on the brain surface. The superior sagittal sinus is seen extending downwards from the vertex. There is high uptake in the vascular structures below the base of the brain and the orbital fossae are visible as areas of reduced uptake.

(b) Right lateral view. The vascular rim increases in thickness towards the posterior. The lateral sinus is also visible, defining the cerebellar fossa.

[*To face p.* 112.

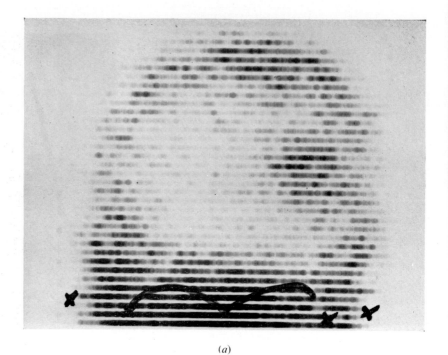

(a)

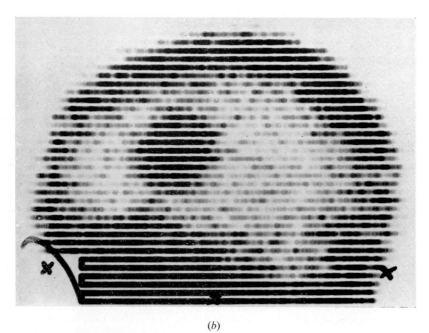

(b)

Fig. 4.3. Brain scan showing glioma in the left fronto temporal region: (a) anterior view; (b) left lateral view.

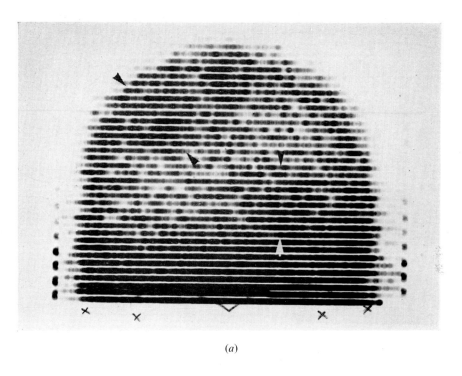

(a)

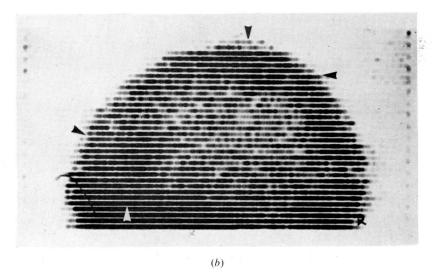

(b)

FIG. 4.4. Brain scan showing metastases from carcinoma of the bronchus. Arrows indicate the positions of the lesions: (a) anterior view; (b) left lateral view.

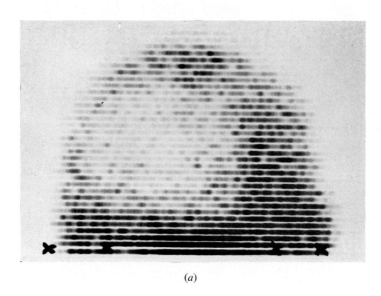

(a)

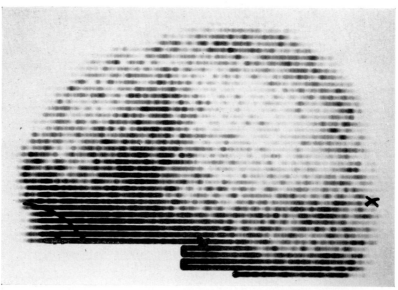

(b)

FIG. 4.5. Brain scan demonstrating a cerebrovascular lesion: (a) anterior view;
(b) left lateral view.

Summary

Brain scanning is a most important technique in the investigation of brain lesions and its accuracy compares favourably with that of other methods. It has the advantage that it is simple, does not involve any discomfort to the patient and visualizes the lesion directly. A positive scan always denotes a lesion but a negative scan in the face of positive clinical evidence should always be followed by further investigations. Scanning, therefore, should be performed before more difficult or hazardous examinations are undertaken. Scanning and angiography are complementary procedures and provide different information.

^{99}Tc^m appears to be the most suitable isotope for routine use but in some cases repeat scans with [^{203}Hg], or [^{197}Hg], chlormerodrin may be helpful. Future advances in brain scanning may well be in the field of data processing and display.

Subarachnoid Space

Cerebrospinal fluid dynamics may be assessed by serial scanning following the injection of radioactive materials into the subarachnoid space. For long term studies, perhaps up to 72 h after injection, ^{131}I-human serum albumin, which diffuses only slowly out of the C.S.F. space, is commonly used. ^{99}Tc^m-serum albumin has been used for short term studies.

C.S.F. scanning—cisternography—is used to differentiate between the communicating and non-communicating forms of hydrocephalus by showing whether or not radioactivity reaches the ventricles. Normal-pressure hydrocephalus, in which there is obstruction of flow through the subarachnoid space, can be successfully treated by surgical shunting and scanning as an aid to diagnosis is potentially valuable, though still seldom used (Patten & Benson, 1968; James et al., 1970).

Thyroid

Radiopharmaceuticals

Its shape, position and avidity for iodine make the thyroid gland very easy to scan. Three isotopes are used for thyroid scanning, namely ^{131}I, ^{125}I and ^{99}Tc^m, of which ^{131}I is still by far the most popular. In terms of the quality of scan produced, there is little to choose between the two isotopes of iodine. ^{125}I, emitting 27 and 35 keV photons and with a half life of 60, is perhaps marginally better for demonstrating superficial abnormalities but ^{131}I, because of its higher energy γ rays (364 keV), is superior in scanning deeper lesions and retrosternal goitres. Because of the high radiation dose delivered to the thyroid by these isotopes—20 microcuries of ^{131}I in a normal sized thyroid delivers about 40 rads—many workers now use ^{99}Tc^m as pertechnetate, which also concentrates in the thyroid gland but is not organically bound. Only about 4 per cent of administered ^{99}Tc^m localises in the thyroid gland but low uptake is offset by the fact that many millicuries may be given and by the efficient detection of the 140 keV radiation. Count rates therefore may be 10–20 times as high as when using a permissible amount of ^{131}I and, because of the rapid uptake, a scan may be performed one hour after administration, with settings adjusted to suppress background counts due to remaining circulating activity. Nevertheless, in spite of the advantages of $^{99}Tc^m$, ^{131}I remains the isotope of choice in most centres, if only because thyroid scanning is usually carried out in conjunction with thyroid uptake tests and ^{131}I has been the only isotope suitable for both purposes. Methods are being developed for using $^{99}Tc^m$ in thyroid function tests but have not yet reached the stage of general acceptance.

Clinical applications

Spencer & Waldman (1965) have described the appearance and dimensions of the normal thyroid scan using ^{131}I and Atkins & Fleay (1968), using $^{99}Tc^m$, were in close agreement with them.

Scanning is valuable in showing the extent of a diffusely enlarged thyroid, especially to demonstrate retrosternal extension. The size of the thyroid gland is an important factor in the calculation of doses of ^{131}I for the treatment of thyrotoxicosis and cannot be estimated accurately by physical examination. Myhill, Reeve & Figgis (1965) found good correlation between surface area measured on an A.P. scan and the frontal view of the thyroid removed at operation but concluded that the thyroid mass could be predicted only very approximately by scanning.

Evaluation of nodules. Many patients are referred for scanning because of the clinical finding of a nodule in or near the thyroid. If scanning shows a nodule to be functioning, its nature can be evaluated by repeat scanning, following either stimulation or suppression of thyroid function. For example, in some cases a hyperfunctioning nodule is seen as a 'hot' area while the rest of the surrounding thyroid tissue has very low uptake. In this case it may be useful to perform a repeat scan after a course of thyroid stimulating hormone (TSH). If the second scan shows that the extranodular tissue has been stimulated to take up iodine the nodule is 'autonomous' and the relative count rates over the nodule and normal thyroid tissue on the first scan reflect the degree of suppression of the normal thyroid by thyroxine secreted by the nodule. If however the course of TSH does not stimulate the extranodular tissue the relative count rates do reflect relative functional capacity. When a thyroid scan shows a count rate over the nodule only slightly greater than over the rest of the gland, evaluation of the nature of the nodule can be made by repeat scanning following a course of liothyronine. This will suppress function of the extranodular thyroid but not of the nodule if it is autonomous (Miller & Hamburger, 1965). The incidence of carcinoma in hyperfunctioning nodules is very low (Shimoaka & Sokal, 1964).

'Cold' areas may be due to adenomas, cysts, haemorrhagic areas, or carcinoma, and a definite diagnosis cannot be made on the scan appearances alone (Fig. 4.6). It is unusual for a carcinoma to take up iodine if any normal thyroid remains, although exceptions have been reported. (Pochin *et al.*, 1952; Bonte, 1965). Some workers have used TSH to test whether a cold nodule can be stimulated to function, the suggestion being that nodules which show an increase in function are less likely to be malignant and that nodules which are not stimulated by TSH should be removed (Gibbs *et al.*, 1965).

Carcinoma. When the normal thyroid has been removed surgically or destroyed by massive doses of ^{131}I, a remaining carcinoma and any metastases will, in a few cases, begin to take up iodine. The chances of this are greatest with well differentiated tumours and least with undifferentiated and anaplastic tumours. The sites of uptake may then be detected by scanning, using a dose of ^{131}I larger than would normally be used, in order to facilitate detection of small metastatic lesions. The value of TSH in stimulating metastatic deposits seems to be uncertain (Robinson & Hochman, 1962; Bonte, 1965). The value of thiouracil in increasing uptake in metastases has also been reported (Dobyns & Maloof, 1951; Rose & Kelsey, 1963).

If a primary thyroid carcinoma and its metastatic deposits can be stimulated to take up a significant amount of iodine, treatment with massive doses of ^{131}I may be given and the results followed by serial scanning.

Summary

Scanning is useful in the evaluation of thyroid nodules but a definite diagnosis cannot be made on the evidence of the scan alone. It is valuable in showing substernal extension of the thyroid, in locating residual thyroid tissue after thyroidectomy and in searching for functioning thyroid metastases in the management of carcinoma. An approximate thyroid mass can be estimated from the scan for the purpose of calculating therapy doses of ^{131}I.

Parathyroid

The demonstration of the parathyroid glands during surgery is often difficult because of their small size and the fact that their location is variable. The ability to demonstrate preoperatively the position of hyperactive parathyroids by scanning would therefore be valuable.

The technique involves suppression of the thyroid by giving tri-iodothyronine for a few days before the intravenous injection of 200–250 microcuries of [^{75}Se]selenomethionine. Serial scans are then performed. Hyperactive tissue such as an adenoma initially takes up a relatively large amount of the agent and Garrow & Smith (1968) showed that the most favourable time for detecting small adenomata is about 40 min after injection when the concentration of radioactivity in the gland is maximal and blood activity minimal. These workers also found that in two patients with parathyroid carcinoma the location of the tumours was shown but in only one of 10 patients with adenoma did the scan provide an accurate and useful diagnosis.

Di Guilio & Morales (1969) investigated 42 patients with a clinical diagnosis of hyperparathyroidism and correctly localised the abnormal gland in 13 out of 23 patients with parathyroid adenomas but found scanning unhelpful in 7 patients with hyperplastic glands. Centi Colella & Pigorini (1970) obtained 8 positive scans in 13 surgically proved cases, the sizes of the glands being 0·3–23 g and the relative activities in the parathyroid and thyroid in the range 1·3–5·5:1.

At present parathyroid scanning is not a routine technique but if methods of enhancing the relative uptake of [^{75}Se]selenomethionine in the parathyroids were evolved, it would become more useful.

Lung

Two procedures are currently used in lung scanning. Pulmonary arterial blood perfusion can be visualized by scanning following an intravenous injection of radioactive macroaggregates or a solution of a radioactive gas. Ventilation and diffusion patterns are shown by scanning after the inhalation of radioactive aerosols or gases. The great majority of reports of lung scanning have been concerned with blood perfusion studies using macroaggregates and it is only recently that reports of ventilation studies have appeared.

Perfusion scanning

Particles of a suitable size injected intravenously become trapped in the pulmonary capillary bed. Having been trapped the particles are broken down mechanically, pass through the capillaries and are removed from the circulation by the reticulo-endothelial system. The half life of the aggregates in the lungs is between 2 and 8 h and therefore they remain in the capillaries long enough for a scan to be performed. The number of capillary segments is about $2\cdot8 \times 10^8$ (Weibel, 1963) and since less than 10^6 particles are injected only a small proportion of the capillaries are blocked. Collateral circulation takes place and there is no physiological effect.

Radiopharmaceuticals

^{131}I-macroaggregated albumin (MAA), first introduced by Taplin et al., (1964) is still the most widely used agent for lung scanning. Count rates are rather low from the radioactivity which may be given—usually limited to 300 microcuries which delivers a radiation dose of about 2 rads to the lungs— and, as a result, scanning times are long, a serious matter in patients who are very ill. The thyroid should also be blocked to prevent uptake of the ^{131}I eventually liberated. These disadvantages have led to the introduction of agents labelled with short-lived isotopes—^{99}Tc^m-macroaggregated albumin, ^{99}Tc^m-albumin microspheres, ^{99}Tc^m-iron hydroxide aggregates and ^{113}In^m-iron hydroxide aggregates, all of which produce excellent scans. Several millicuries of these isotopes may be given without exceeding the radiation dose which would be received during a chest radiograph. However, ^{131}I-MAA, with particle sizes in the range 20–50 μm is the only commercially available preparation and for this reason will probably continue to be the agent of choice in many hospitals.

All macroaggregates contain a range of particle sizes, which ideally should be between 20 and 40 μm and most preparations, whether produced commercially or in hospitals according to published recipes, lie at least within the range 10–100 μm. If particles less than 5 μm are present in appreciable numbers they will pass through the capillaries and be taken up in the liver and spleen making interpretation of the lung scan more difficult. Also, if a considerable proportion of the particles go to sites other than the lung the quality of the scan will suffer due to low radioactivity in the lungs.

Attention has been drawn to a potential hazard in the use of macroaggregates in patients who have right to left shunts in the heart since then particles will bypass the lungs and some will be trapped in the cerebral circulation. However, in animal experiments no side effects resulted when particles reached the cerebral circulation in much larger number than could do so in lung scanning (Kennady & Taplin, 1965) and no ill effects have been reported in patients. There have been reports of lung scans showing a single 'hot' spot (Moser & Miale, 1968; Quinn, 1969) most probably due to blood clots forming in the syringe and taking up most of the radioactive material, as blood is mixed with the macroaggregates before injection. However, no untoward symptoms have occurred in the cases reported.

Technique

Most lung perfusion scanning has been performed using radioactive macroaggregates and rectilinear scanners. With a gamma camera it is not necessary to use agents which are trapped in the capillaries for a considerable time. Perfusion scans may be obtained with short exposures following the intravenous injection of 2–5 mCi of ^{133}Xe in saline solution (Loken & Westgate, 1968).

The distribution of pulmonary blood flow is affected by gravity and if the injection of macroaggregates is made with the patient erect the greatest concentration appears in the bases of the lungs. Therefore, in order to achieve good distribution, injection is usually made with the patient supine. Anterior and posterior views are normally taken. Lateral views, to show the anterior and posterior profiles of the lungs may be helpful and can be obtained more easily with gamma cameras than with most rectilinear scanners. If they are to be taken, using macroaggregates, it is best to inject half the material with the patient prone and the other half with the patient supine in order to ensure even distribution between the anterior and posterior regions of the lungs.

Ventilation scanning. The second technique demonstrates ventilation of the lung by scanning following inhalation of either a radioactive aerosol or a radioactive gas (Taplin & Poe, 1965; Quinn & Head, 1966; Loken & Westgate, 1968; De Nardo *et al.*, 1970). ^{131}I-albumin, ^{99}Tc^m-albumin, ^{198}Au colloid and ^{99}Tc^m-sulphur colloid have been used as aerosols which on inhalation are deposited in the air passages down to alveoli. The aerosol is inhaled for 10–15 min and the scan carried out 1–2 h later. Alternatively, using a gamma camera, a ventilation scan may be performed while the breath is held, following inspiration of 10–25 mCi of ^{133}Xe gas (De Nardo *et al.*, 1970).

Combined perfusion and ventilation scanning. Both ventilation and perfusion patterns may be visualized by taking serial gamma camera pictures during inhalation of ^{133}Xe and then, when the patient stops breathing xenon and returns to breathing air, as the dissolved xenon is cleared from the lung by the blood flow (Loken & Westgate, 1968).

Normal scan

The normal perfusion and ventilation scans show a relatively uniform distribution of radioactivity with smooth convex borders. On the anterior view, the heart is seen as an area of absent radioactivity; on the posterior view it is not so prominent and the lung images are more symmetrical.

In pulmonary arterial hypertension there is increased blood flow to the upper lobes of the lungs and even if the injection is made with the patient erect the radioactivity in the upper lobes may be higher than in the lower, in marked contrast to the situation in normal subjects. The ratio of counts in the upper lobe to counts in the lower lobe can show whether pulmonary venous pressure is also raised in patients with pulmonary arterial hypertension (Friedman & Braunwald, 1966).

Clinical applications

The major application of lung perfusion scanning is in the diagnosis of pulmonary embolism. Scanning has shown that pulmonary emboli are much more common than was previously thought and that many emboli produce no symptoms and resolve spontaneously. A pulmonary embolus results in diminished perfusion of a section of the lung which then appears on the scan as an area of low radioactivity. It should be emphasised that scanning does not show the embolus itself but reduced perfusion of that part of the lung normally supplied by the occluded artery. In many cases of pulmonary embolism the perfusion scan is abnormal well before any defect is visible on a plain X-ray film. In fact, it has been reported that X-ray findings are positive in only about 20 per cent of cases of severe embolism (Wagner, 1968). Angiography is the most specific test for demonstrating the site of an embolus since it visualizes the arteries themselves and scanning and angiography should be considered as complementary tests. Scanning should normally be performed first since it is a simple test and may itself provide enough information to make angiography unnecessary.

Many diseases other than pulmonary embolism result in reduced pulmonary blood perfusion and therefore the appearances of an abnormal lung scan are not diagnostic of a specific pathology. Nevertheless the perfusion scan, when considered together with the clinical signs and the results of other tests is a most useful screening test for pulmonary embolism.

A positive scan, especially if it shows multiple areas of diminished perfusion or concave bites out of the lateral border of the scan is very suggestive of pulmonary embolism particularly if the chest radiograph is normal, since some other diseases which cause abnormal perfusion are usually seen on the radiograph (Fig. 4.7). If both the scan and X-ray findings are negative, pulmonary embolism is unlikely though it must be remembered that small areas of reduced activity may not be detected. Symptoms such as tachycardia, tachypnoea and systemic hypotension can be caused only by large lesions and therefore if the scan is normal in a patient with these symptoms, the presence of pulmonary embolism as a cause of the symptoms is virtually ruled out. Nevertheless difficult diagnostic problems remain. In the case of scan defects corresponding to X-ray abnormalities the diagnosis is often doubtful. For example, cysts and emphysematous bullae and pulmonary emboli may give similar appearances on both perfusion scans and X-rays and the diagnosis of pulmonary embolism co-existing with other pulmonary diseases can be difficult. In these cases, serial scanning and, especially, ventilation scanning can be helpful.

Because of its safety and simplicity scanning may be performed repeatedly and serial scanning may be helpful in distinguishing pulmonary embolism, in which scan appearances change as the embolus spontaneously resolves, from other, chronic, lung diseases where the scan tends to remain unchanged. Serial scanning is also useful in evaluating the results of anticoagulant or fibrinolytic treatment.

Ventilation scanning maps the distribution of aerated lung. In combination with perfusion scanning it is useful in distinguishing pulmonary embolism, where ischaemic areas are usually well ventilated, from chronic obstructive diseases, where ventilation is impaired.

In emphysema patchy areas of reduced activity correspond to areas of poor ventilation and capillary destruction. In a study of 62 patients with emphysema, 95 per cent of the scans showed areas of diminished perfusion (Lopez-Majano, Tow & Wagner, 1966). Mishkin & Wagner (1967) found areas of reduced perfusion during acute attacks of asthma but normal scans between attacks. Taplin et al. (1969) using combined perfusion and ventilation scans reported that, in acute asthma, lung perfusion scans showed multiple areas of ischaemia similar to those seen in pulmonary embolism and that inhalation scans were characteristic of obstructive bronchopulmonary disease, showing aerosol deposition in the main bronchi and diminished activity in the peripheral areas of normally perfused lung. In bronchiectasis, tuberculosis and pneumonia, perfusion scanning shows areas of reduced activity which are often larger than would be expected from X-ray appearances (Lopez-Majano et al., 1965).

Combined perfusion/ventilation scans may be helpful in the diagnosis of bronchogenic carcinoma. A tumour can compromise pulmonary arterial flow either directly by compression of a pulmonary artery or indirectly through impaired ventilation. It may also produce an abnormal ventilation scan by causing obstruction of an airway. Regional defects on the perfusion scan are often much larger than would be expected from radiographic findings.

In reporting studies on almost 4000 patients, many of whom had both types of scan, Taplin et al. (1969) stress the value of the combined procedure in distinguishing pulmonary embolism from other lung disorders. Pircher (1969) studied 500 patients, two-thirds of whom had both perfusion and ventilation scans. He found ventilation scanning useful in the assessment of bronchial obstruction in patients with asthma and bronchitis but only occasionally helpful in detecting carcinoma of the bronchus. Combined scanning was useful in distinguishing between emphysematous and purely obstructive changes and in the recognition of pulmonary embolism in the presence of emphysema.

Summary

Perfusion scanning is a safe and simple procedure and has proved valuable in the diagnosis and management of pulmonary embolism. Developments in combined perfusion and ventilation scanning promise to extend the usefulness of the technique in the diagnosis of pulmonary embolism and other lung diseases. Scanning and pulmonary angiography are complementary procedures and scanning should be performed first as a screening test before the more major procedure of angiography.

Liver

Radiopharmaceuticals

The liver may be scanned using radioactive colloids which are rapidly taken up by reticulo-endothelial cells, chiefly in the liver. Since liver scanning was first performed in 1953, denatured ^{131}I-albumin, ^{198}Au colloid, ^{99}Tc^m-

aggregated albumin, $^{99}Tc^m$ sulphur colloid, $^{113}In^m$ colloid and $^{113}In^m$-iron complex have all been used but ^{198}Au colloid and $^{99}Tc^m$ sulphur colloid have proved the most popular. Uptake of these materials by reticulo-endothelial tissue other than in the liver is variable, and in certain conditions this variability may provide useful diagnostic information. Colloids, apart from denatured ^{131}I-albumin, which is rapidly degraded and released from the liver, are retained in the liver and result in a stable count rate during the time required to perform a scan with a rectilinear scanner.

Alternatively, radiopharmaceuticals taken up by the parenchymal cells may be employed, of which [^{131}I]Rose Bengal is the most commonly used though ^{99}Mo and ^{131}I-BSP (bromsulphthalein) have also been tried. Using Rose Bengal, measurements of the rates of clearance from the blood, of uptake by the liver and of entry into the intestine have been useful in distinguishing cirrhosis from hepatitis and intra-hepatic from extra-hepatic cholestases (Lum et al., 1959). In scanning, however, the rapid excretion of Rose Bengal into the bile means that the radioactivity in the liver may change by 30–50 per cent during the period of scanning, producing an uneven image. Using a gamma camera a change in activity does not, of course, matter. Radioactivity in the biliary tree and small bowel may make interpretation of the Rose Bengal scan difficult but, on the other hand, may be useful in the differential diagnosis of jaundice.

Using $^{99}Tc^m$, the greater amounts which may be administered and the almost ideal radiation energy result in scans superior in quality to those using ^{198}Au colloid or [^{131}I]Rose Bengal.

Antero-posterior and right lateral scans are usually taken and an oblique view is sometimes useful. The positions of the costal margin and, if it is palpable, the lower edge of the liver should be marked on the scan as landmarks.

Normal scan

On the A.P. view of a normal liver the count rate is highest over the right lobe and uniform over the left lobe. Interpretation of liver scans is complicated by the great variation in size and shape of normal livers. According to McAfee, Ause & Wagner (1965) about 65 per cent have a triangular shape on the A.P. scan, of which 15 per cent have an indentation on the inferior border. Other variations include a Riedel's lobe, high right lobe due to a high diaphragm, indentation due to pressure of the rib cage, and indentation by the right kidney. The scan accurately visualizes the position, size and shape of the liver and, when filling defects are shown, may provide a valuable guide to suitable sites for hepatic biopsy.

Abnormal scan

Hepatomegaly. As might be expected, many scans show an enlarged liver, since patients are often referred for scanning in the first instance on the clinical discovery of enlargement of the liver. However, the fact that the liver is palpable well below the costal margin does not necessarily mean that it is enlarged, and vice versa. The surface area on the A.P. scan is a reliable index of liver size (Naftalus & Leevy, 1963) but does not correlate with body weight, height or surface area in normal subjects (McAfee et al., 1965). There

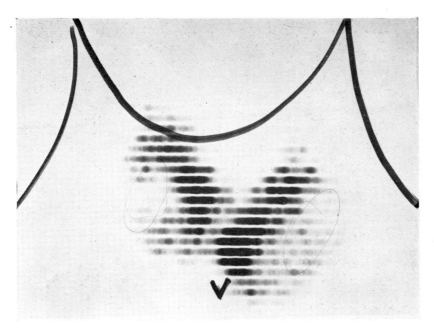

Fig. 4.6. Scan of nodular colloid goitre demonstrating 'cold' nodules. Outlines indicate neck and chin.

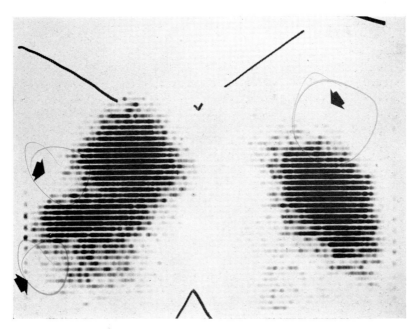

Fig. 4.7. Lung perfusion scan, using ^{131}I-MAA, of patient with multiple pulmonary emboli. Arrows indicate areas of diminished perfusion, including 'bites' out of the border of the scan.

[To face p. 120.

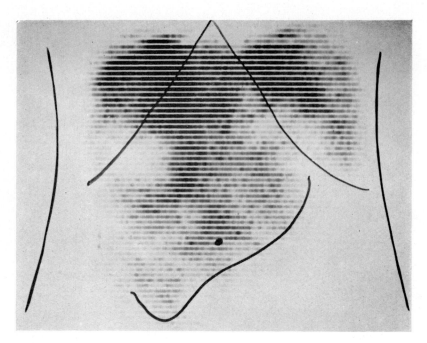

FIG. 4.8. Liver scan, using $^{113}In^m$ colloid, showing hepatomegaly and several metastatic deposits. Lines represent the costal margin and palpable lower edge of the liver.

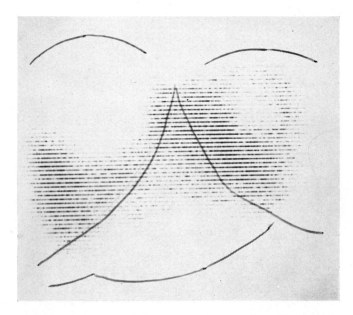

FIG. 4.9. Liver scan with hydatid cysts appearing as well defined filling defects. The costal margin and the boundaries of the liver are shown as landmarks.

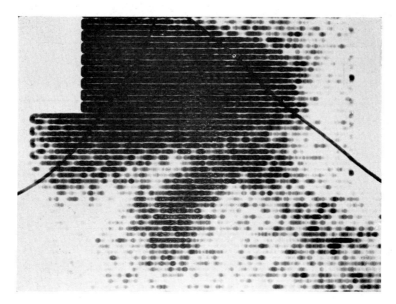

FIG. 4.10. Scan of normal pancreas. In this case the pancreas is not overlapped by the liver which also concentrates the [^{75}Se]selenomethionine.

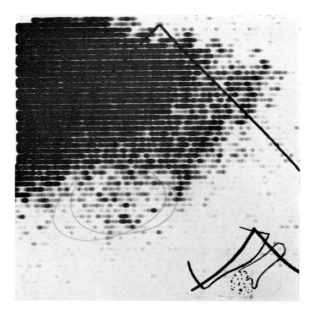

FIG. 4.11. Pancreas scan of a patient with carcinoma of the head of the pancreas which is visualized by its failure to concentrate the [^{75}Se]selenomethionine.

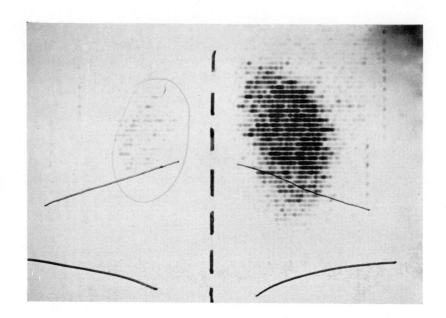

FIG. 4.12. Renal scan. Unilateral hydronephrosis showing almost total absence of radioactivity in the diseased left kidney.

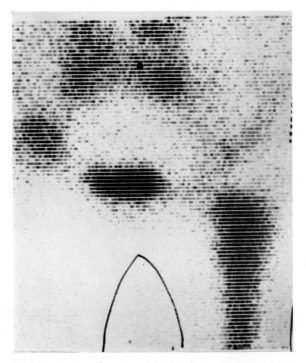

FIG. 4.13. Bone scan using ^{18}F. Several areas of increased uptake in metastatic lesions are shown.

are many causes of hepatomegaly—diffuse diseases of the parenchyma usually cause generalised enlargement, while enlargement of a single lobe may be due to cirrhosis or to an expanding lesion. In livers with hydatid cysts the uninvolved lobe is sometimes enlarged (Caroli & Bonneville, 1962).

Liver scanning is particularly helpful in the differential diagnosis of upper abdominal masses, showing whether such masses comprise functioning liver tissue. The liver can move under pressure and scanning will provide information about its displacement by ascites or subphrenic abscess, for example.

Space-occupying lesions. All space-occupying lesions, whether cyst, abscess, haematoma, hepatoma or metastatic tumour, will show as filling defects on the scan, whether radioactive colloid or Rose Bengal is used as the scanning agent (Fig. 4.8). The bulk and shape of the liver determine the size of defect which can be detected. A single defect 4 cm in diameter situated deep in the right lobe and overlaid by several cm of functioning liver might easily be missed on an A.P. scan but it should be possible to detect a defect 2 cm in diameter lying superficially in the left lobe. For this reason it is an advantage to obtain scans from several directions, thereby increasing the chance of visualizing the defect, wherever it is situated. Ozarda & Pickren (1962) reported that in 31 per cent of patients the maximum diameter of metastatic nodules measured at autopsy was less than 2 cm and therefore probably undetectable by scanning. It must be remembered therefore that a normal scan does not exclude the presence of disease.

Unfortunately the appearances of the scan are not specific—hepatomas, hydatid cysts, and pseudomasses in advanced cirrhosis can produce identical scan images showing large focal defects (Fig. 4.9). The patchy scans sometimes obtained with multiple metastatic deposits are similar to those seen in diffuse liver disease. Nevertheless, liver scanning is valuable in providing suggestive information to be considered together with clinical findings and he results of other tests such as coeliac angiography. For example, if the scan shows multiple filling defects in a patient with a known primary neoplasm it is highly likely that metastases are present in the liver. In the case of a solitary defect shown on the scan the diagnosis may be less obvious and other investigations such as biopsy or angiography indicated. Serial scanning can be helpful both in the diagnosis, and in assessing the results of chemotherapy, of abscesses and neoplasms.

It is difficult to make briefly a meaningful comparison of published reports on the success rate in liver scanning since it is noticeable that presentations of results and even definitions of the terms 'false positive' and 'false negative' are not consistent.

McAfee et al. (1965) used [198]Au colloid for liver scanning in 112 patients with proven hepatic metastases and found positive scans in 101. In 22 patients with proven hepatomas 20 scans were positive. Gollin, Sims & Cameron (1964), using [198]Au colloid in almost all cases, scanned 101 patients with proven localised disease and visualized 74 on the scans. In 28 proven normals there were 3 false positive scans. Nagler, Bender & Blau (1963) investigated 548 patients whose liver status was proved by laparotomy, biopsy or postmortem examination. Of 351 patients with hepatic cancer 333 had positive, and 18 negative, scans. In 197 normal livers the scan was positive in 69 and negative in 128. Smith & Williams (1968) found that of 120 patients whose liver scans were normal, 13 were later proved to have space occupying lesions in the liver, and 3 diffuse liver disease. Of 95 patients whose scans were reported as showing diffuse liver disease 10 were proved to be normal and 5 to have space occupying lesions. In 81 patients whose scans were reported as showing discrete lesions 17 were normal, 13 had diffuse disease and in the remaining 51 the scan report was correct.

Conn & Elkington (1968) reviewed five reports which dealt with the accuracy of liver scanning and which claimed that liver scans were positive in 72–90 per cent of patients in whom liver cancer was proved by biopsy, laparotomy or autopsy, and negative in 88–100 per cent of patients with normal livers. They point out that these quoted figures are open to criticism in view of the non-random way in which data was collected, the time interval between scanning and obtaining proof of the diagnosis, and the fact that failure to demonstrate cancer during surgery cannot be regarded as proof of its absence. According to Ozarda & Pickren (1962), in more than 10 per cent of patients with liver cancer, the tumour is not demonstrable on the surface of the liver.

Diffuse parenchymal disease. Scanning using colloids is helpful in the diagnosis of cirrhosis, where the scan usually shows poor uptake of isotope in the liver due to diminished effective hepatic perfusion and to cellular malfunction. The consequent statistical variations in the low count rate result in the scan having a patchy appearance. At the same time, probably due to shunting of blood in the liver, there is marked uptake of colloid in the spleen, sometimes exceeding that in the liver, and some uptake in the bone marrow. According to Castell & Johnson (1966) splenic uptake correlates well with the degree of collateral shunting as measured by the ammonia tolerance test, but Whang, Fish & Pollycove (1965) found little correlation between the scan appearance and the results of liver function tests. High splenic uptake helps to distinguish cirrhosis from multiple small metastases but similar scan appearances can be obtained in other diseases such as bilharzia (Mustafa et al., 1966) and sarcoidosis (McAfee et al., 1965). In some cases of cirrhosis the liver is enlarged and in others reduced in size. A focal defect may be present in advanced cirrhosis and on the scan can easily be mistaken for a malignant tumour (Rozental, Miller & Kaplan, 1966; Johnson & Sweeney, 1967).

Budd-Chiari syndrome. In the Budd-Chiari syndrome the liver scan shows very reduced uptake of colloid by the whole liver except for the caudate lobe situated near the mid line, presumably due to the venous drainage of the caudate lobe being retained while that from the rest of the liver is occluded. The caudate lobe is sometimes enlarged and there is increased uptake in the spleen also.

Jaundice. As already mentioned, when using [^{131}I]Rose Bengal, activity normally appears in the intestine soon after administration of the compound. The Rose Bengal scan may therefore be used in the differential diagnosis of jaundice, failure to detect radioactivity in the intestine being consistent with obstructive jaundice. In severe hepatitis also the dye may not be excreted (Eyler et al., 1965). Rose Bengal may also be excreted via the kidneys and renal uptake may easily be mistaken for intestinal activity, leading to an erroneous diagnosis of the cause of jaundice. However, by serial scanning and taking extra views, renal and non-renal activity can be distinguished (Freeman, Kay & Derman, 1968).

Summary

Liver scanning is well established and is useful in the differential diagnosis of upper abdominal masses, as a guide to sites for biopsy, and in helping to establish the diagnosis of cirrhosis and the Budd-Chiari syndrome. Its main application is the detection of focal lesions and, although filling defects shown on scanning are not specific for a particular pathology, scanning is an extremely valuable adjunct to clinical examination and liver function tests.

Spleen

Radiopharmaceuticals

Spleen scanning is usually performed using labelled red blood cells which have been treated in such a way that they localise in the spleen. The two isotopes most commonly used are ^{51}Cr and ^{197}Hg.

In the case of ^{51}Cr labelled red cells, treatment consists of heating the labelled cells at 49·5°C for 20 min (Marsh, Lewis & Szur, 1966). Peak activity in the spleen is reached about 4 h after injection of the damaged cells, and there is also always appreciable uptake of the damaged cells in the liver. In the preparation of heat denatured red cells the temperature and duration of heating are critical—for example, if heating is prolonged, an increasing proportion of the cells are sequestered by the liver. ^{99}Tc^{m} has also been used as a red cell label, with similar denaturation by heating (Burdine & Legeay, 1968).

Denaturation by chemical means is quicker and simpler. BMHP (1–bromomercuri–2–hydroxypropane), labelled with ^{197}Hg, when mixed with the patient's blood both labels and denatures the red cells, over 90 per cent of the BMHP combining with the red cell membrane (Wagner et al., 1964). Peak activity in the spleen is attained 1–2 h after re-injection of the labelled cells and considerable radioactivity also appears in the kidneys from which it is slow to clear so that the kidneys receive a higher dose of radiation than the spleen. The retention of activity in the kidneys is so prolonged, in fact, that a renal scan can be performed at 24 h.

Labelling of red cells with ^{81}Rb, followed by denaturation using BMHP, has been described (Friedmann et al., 1968) and also the denaturation of ^{51}Cr labelled red cells by means of excess acid-citrate-dextrose solution (Sharma et al., 1970). ^{99}Tc^{m} and ^{113}In^{m} colloids used for liver scanning may also be taken up by the spleen in sufficient quantity to make scanning of that organ possible (Nelp & Kuhn, 1966).

Normal scan

With a rectilinear scanner, two views of the spleen are usually taken—a left lateral and either an anterior or a posterior view. With a gamma camera, more views may be taken in less total time. The rectilinear scan image is more accurate in obtaining a measurement of spleen size, which is often an important requirement. The greatest area of spleen is shown on the lateral view and lies within a fairly narrow range, 70–90 cm^2 (Holzbach et al., 1962; Fischer &

Wolf, 1964). The volume of the spleen (V) may be calculated from the area (F) measured on the lateral scan, using the formula $V = 0 \cdot 3\ F^{1 \cdot 5}$ (Fischer, Leon & Wolf, 1969).

Abnormal scan

Splenomegaly has diagnostic significance and may be present without the spleen being palpable. McCready, Gwyther & Stringer (1969) found that only 34 spleens were palpable in 76 patients with Hodgkin's disease though 43 had areas over 100 cm² on the lateral view. According to Fischer *et al.* (1969) only 26 per cent of cases of splenomegaly can be detected clinically. Scanning is therefore useful in cases where the size of the spleen affects the treatment policy. Splenomegaly is associated with portal hypertension in cirrhosis and the response to treatment may be assessed by repeat scans. It is sometimes impossible to distinguish clinically between splenomegaly and a non-splenic abdominal mass and the scan will show whether or not a mass is splenic in nature.

Space occupying lesions in the spleen result in filling defects, but lesions less than $2 \cdot 5$–3 cm in diameter are not detectable. Tumours of the spleen, apart from lymphomas, are rare and very few have been reported. However, the scan appearances of haemangiomas, abscesses and cysts have been described. Diffuse disease shows as a non-uniform distribution of radio-activity caused by masses too small to be resolved individually. Infarction results in an area of absent uptake on the scan, usually extending to the periphery (Nelp & Kuhn, 1966), but clinical findings may be expected to distinguish between an infarct and an intra-splenic mass. If the infarct is resolved, the appearance of the scan reverts to normal.

Summary

Spleen scanning is valuable in the estimation of spleen size, in the differential diagnosis of upper abdominal masses and in the detection of intrasplenic masses and infarcts, and provides information which cannot readily be obtained by other means. Serial scans are useful in assessing the results of treatment.

Pancreas

Radiopharmaceuticals

Despite a continuing search for radioactive tracers which will concentrate selectively in the pancreas, the only one which has proved of value is [75Se]sele-nomethionine. The high rate of enzyme synthesis by the pancreas requires a high uptake of the sulphur-containing amino acid, methionine. Methionine contains no atom for which a suitable gamma emitting isotope is available but sulphur and selenium have similar chemical properties and by substituting selenium-75 for sulphur, [75Se]selenomethionine is produced, having the same biological properties as methionine and being secreted in the pancreatic juice. 75Se has a half life of 120 d and emits several γ rays, the principal one having an energy of 270 keV.

Studies in dogs have shown that about 6 per cent of a dose of [75Se]selenomethionine is present in the pancreas 1–2 h after administration and that the uptake per gram in the pancreas is 8 or 9 times that in the liver (Blau & Manske, 1961).

Technique

Various procedures designed to increase the uptake in the pancreas have been tried but the consensus of opinion is that none of these regimes, except perhaps a high protein meal before the test, results in a better scan and most workers consider that a reasonably complete diet for a few days and a large breakfast on the morning of the test is adequate preparation.

The usual dose of [^{75}Se]selenomethionine is either 3 μCi/kg body weight or 200–250 μCi, and the time of commencement of scanning varies from a few minutes to one hour, after injection. This amount of radioactivity delivers a whole-body radiation dose of about 1·3 rads. The positions of the costal margin, umbilicus and, if palpable, the liver edge are marked on the scan. A scan takes about 40 min to complete and during this period the isotope remains well distributed throughout the normal parenchyma. Scans performed later than 2–3 h after injection are less satisfactory since the distribution of isotope in the gland becomes less uniform (Melmed, Agnew & Bouchier, 1968).

Visualization of the pancreas is made difficult by the uptake of [^{75}Se]selenomethionine in the liver, which lies close to the pancreas and often overlaps it on an antero-posterior view. The concentration of isotope is far lower in the liver than in the pancreas but the liver, because of its size, accumulates a greater amount of the amino acid homologue. Attempts at displacing the liver edge away from the pancreas by tilting the patient have not been successful (Centi Colella & Pigorini, 1967). A lead shield placed on the patient to mask the radioactivity in the liver, previously located precisely using a radioactive colloid scan, does not improve the quality of the scan and makes interpretation more difficult (Sodee, 1964b). A better method of achieving good visualization of the pancreas is to perform a separate liver scan in conjunction with the pancreas scan, and to subtract one from the other, either visually or by electronic techniques. A dual-channel scanning machine described by Kaplan *et al.* (1966) either subtracts liver from liver-plus-pancreas and prints out an image of the pancreas or, alternatively, displays liver and pancreas in different colours. Eaton *et al.* (1967) described a similar subtraction technique. Scanner settings to produce the subtraction image are critical because of the necessity of carefully balancing the signals from the two isotopes in order to eliminate the liver image and because the counting statistics of the subtraction output, which is obtained as the difference between two fluctuating signals, are inevitably poor, leading to a patchy scan appearance which may make interpretation difficult.

Subtraction scanning is undoubtedly sometimes valuable and even essential but, in most cases, it is easier to make a diagnosis using the unsubtracted scans because of their superior statistics. Although it is not necessary to perform a scan of the whole liver as part of the investigation of the pancreas, nevertheless a complete liver scan is often worthwhile in order to detect possible hepatic or bile duct lesions.

Normal scan

The position and shape of the normal pancreas as seen on the scan has been described by many workers. Generally it lies obliquely and its shape is usually straight or sigmoid. Some have included a 'horse-shoe' shaped pancreas in the normal group (King *et al.*, 1966) but others believe that this appearance is due to uptake of isotope in the jejunum (Saldino & Mishkin, 1968; Melmed *et al.*, 1968). There is often an area of reduced uptake in the body of the pancreas, probably due to compression by blood vessels. A filling defect is sometimes seen on the duodenal margin of the head presumably caused by the termination of the pancreatic and common bile ducts (Fig. 4.10).

Abnormal scan

Cold areas on the scan reflect reduced enzyme synthesis and may be caused by carcinomas, cysts, penetrating ulcers, stones or pancreatitis. The smallest focal defect which can be detected by scanning is 2·5–3 cm in diameter.

A carcinoma may result in a diffuse failure of uptake or a discrete filling defect (Fig. 4.11). Pseudocysts have usually been reported as showing reduced uptake (Centi Colella & Pigorini, 1967; Kaplan & Ben Porath, 1969). Uptake is also often reduced in patients with diabetes mellitus and in cirrhotics (Lahdevirta, 1967; Melmed *et al.*, 1968; McCarthy *et al.*, 1972).

Chronic pancreatitis results in reduced or totally absent uptake of [75Se]selenomethionine by the pancreas (Sodee, 1964b; Burdine & Haynie, 1965; Centi Colella & Pigorini, 1967; Melmed *et al.*, 1968). Patients with acute pancreatitis show no uptake at the time of attack, but scans performed more than two weeks after an attack are frequently normal (Leger, Roucayrol & Lenriot, 1971).

It is clear, then, that the scan appearance is relatively non-specific. Only very occasionally is it characteristic of a specific pathology—for example, a localised filling defect, particularly if it has a concave rounded edge, strongly suggests a neoplasm. Otherwise the chief value of scanning is simply in differentiating between normal and abnormal without being able to suggest the cause of an abnormality.

Many reports agree that a proportion of pancreatic scans are not interpretable, the number depending on the scanning technique used. Sodee (1966) found that in 251 patients only 18 scans were unsatisfactory. More recently, McCarthy *et al.* (1972) reported 6 scans to be uninterpretable in a series of 393 scans. Inevitably, however, a larger proportion of scans can only be reported on with limited confidence. This particularly applies to scans where the pancreatic image is overlapped by that of the liver.

Brown *et al.* (1968) routinely scanned the liver, using 99Tcm sulphur colloid, as part of the test. They found 8.1 per cent false negatives in 37 scans reported as normal and 15.4 per cent false positives in 39 abnormal scans. Melmed *et al.* (1968) reported 200 pancreas scans all of which were combined with liver scans using 198Au colloid. In 36 of the 67 normal cases there was a degree of overlap of the pancreas by the liver but the scans were still readable. Six scans were uninterpretable and there was diffuse reduction of uptake in 4 patients—all over 65 years of age—in these 67 normal cases. Thirteen patients had proven primary carcinoma and in 10 the scan was abnormal, 3 having a localised filling defect and 7 a diffuse reduced activity. Liewendahl & Kvist (1970) reported 4 per cent false negative results in 53 patients with scans interpreted as abnormal. The majority of these false positive scans were found in patients with liver, biliary or gastrointestinal disease.

The incidence of false negative reports in cases of pancreatic carcinoma is low—the proportion of normal scans found in such patients is generally less than 6 per cent (Sodee, 1966; Hatchette, Shuler & Murison, 1972; McCarthy et al., 1972).

Many workers have stressed the value of the normal pancreas scan in excluding the presence of significant pancreatic disease. The high incidence of false positive reports reflects the fact that many non-pancreatic diseases can affect pancreatic uptake of selenomethionine.

Several reports have compared the usefulness of scanning and radiological tests in the diagnosis of pancreatic disease and have suggested appropriate combinations of tests whereby diagnostic accuracy may be improved (Eaton et al. 1968; McCarthy et al. 1969).

Summary

Pancreas scanning is a lengthy and expensive examination and interpretation requires considerable expertise. Only a few centres may have the time or the experience in interpretation to carry out this investigation. The radiation dose is higher than in the scanning of most other organs and the long half life of [^{75}Se]selenomethionine means that it may interfere with subsequent isotope tests. However, the test is painless and well tolerated by the patient.

Although an abnormal scan is not diagnostic of a particular disorder, the test often provides useful information in cases of difficulty. A completely normal scan is strong evidence of the absence of pancreatic disease.

Kidney

Radiopharmaceuticals

The first compounds used for renal scanning were ^{131}I labelled contrast media but these proved to be excreted from the kidneys too rapidly for a scan to be obtainable. In 1956 Borghgraef & Pitts labelled chlormerodrin (3–chlormercuric–2 methyl propylurea) with ^{203}Hg in order to study the pharmacology of mercurial diuretics and found a high concentration in the renal cortex. In fact, chlormerodrin was shown to have the highest selective concentration of all the mercurial diuretics (Kessler, Lozano & Pitts, 1957) and, labelled with either ^{203}Hg or ^{197}Hg, it has been used for most renal scanning. ^{203}Hg emits penetrating (280 keV) gamma rays which are suitable for scanning the deeply situated kidneys in a large patient, but its long half life (47 d) results in a high radiation dose to the kidneys, variously estimated as between 10–30 rads/100 μCi. ^{197}Hg, emitting 77 keV gamma rays and with half a life of 65 h is a preferable label, the radiation dose to the kidneys‘ including that due to contamination by ^{203}Hg, being less than 1 rad/100 μCi.

Other renal scanning agents which also concentrate in the cortex are the chelates, ^{197}Hg-EDTA (Krasznai, Pal & Foldes, 1965) and ^{99}Tc^{m}-iron complex (Harper et al., 1965; Aquino & Cunningham, 1969). The ability of the gamma camera to produce images in a very short time has enabled compounds with a short transit time through the kidneys, such as $^{113}In^m$-DTPA (Reba, Hosain & Wagner, 1968) and [^{131}I]hippuran, to be used for scanning. In patients with renal insufficiency the passage of hippuran through the kidney may be so prolonged that a rectilinear scan can be performed (Freeman *et al.*, 1969). The radiation doses using the latter compounds are extremely small and serial pictures taken during uptake and excretion by the kidneys have the advantage of providing additional information on kidney function (Hayes, Swanson & Taplin, 1968).

However, because of its ready commercial availability, [^{197}Hg]chlormerodrin remains the most commonly used scanning agent. Scanning is generally performed 1–2 h after injection of 100–150 μCi and, at this time, approximately 60 per cent of the dose is present in the renal cortex. Excretion is slow and, though most of the chlormerodrin is excreted in the urine in 24 h, about 10 per cent remains permanently in the renal tubules.

Normal scan

A renal scan using chlormerodrin visualizes the distribution of functioning cortex. On a normal scan the count rates from the two kidneys are usually similar though a 15 per cent difference has been reported (Morris *et al.*, 1967). Sometimes a small uptake in the liver is observed in normal subjects and increased hepatic uptake reflects impairment of renal function (Gottschalk, 1967; Chisholm, Aye & Evans, 1967). The scan demonstrates renal position and shape satisfactorily but it is difficult to determine size accurately because of blurring of the edges of the scan caused by movement. The length of the image on the scan is 1–3 cm less than on a radiograph and the width is the same on both (Chisholm *et al.*, 1967). Nevertheless, a scan may be useful as a guide to renal biopsy and in localising the kidney for radiotherapy although it does not visualize renal size and contour as accurately as do X-ray techniques.

Abnormal scan

Congenital abnormalities such as horseshoe kidney in which the lower poles are joined but the upper poles are separate, and renal ectopia, are readily demonstrated by scanning. Visualization of a displaced kidney may prevent an erroneous diagnosis of aplasia.

When renal function is impaired as, for example, in pyelonephritis, the uptake of chlormerodrin is correspondingly reduced (Fig. 4.12).

In renal failure the kidneys may occasionally be shown by scanning when pyelography has failed but the uptake of chlormerodrin by the liver often masks the upper pole of the right kidney (Chisholm *et al.*, 1967). Scanning is also useful in renal trauma in evaluating the extent of damage to a kidney and ascertaining whether the contra-lateral kidney is normal (Freeman, Kay & Meng, 1966; Kazmin, Swanson & Cockett, 1967).

Space-occupying lesions. Lesions affecting the parenchyma, such as tumours and cysts, show as filling defects on the scan. Peripheral lesions as small as 1 cm in diameter may be detected (Quinn & Maynard, 1965) but central lesions of 2–3 cm diameter which are covered by normal cortex are very difficult to detect by scanning and X-ray techniques are more satisfactory. The multiple filling defects caused by polycystic disease are characteristic

(Quinn & Maynard, 1965) and scanning will also demonstrate areas of impaired function caused by stones or staghorn calculi.

Generally, however, it is impossible on a chlormerodrin scan to distinguish between tumours and cysts. The fact that most malignant tumours are vascular while cysts are avascular has been used to distinguish between them by taking gamma camera pictures following the injection of a vascular scanning agent such as [^{99}Tc^m]pertechnetate (Rosenthall, 1967). If the filling defect demonstrated on the chlormerodrin scan shows uptake of pertechnetate it is considered to be due to a neoplasm and if the two scans are similar it is considered to be a cyst. Nevertheless, renal angiography has a far higher resolution and also distinguishes between tumours and cysts by their vascular patterns. In the investigation of renal masses, therefore, angiography is a superior technique.

Renovascular disease. The problem of diagnosing renovascular hypertension is a difficult one. Opinions on the value of scanning as a screening test for selecting patients for more intensive investigation vary. Most workers consider scanning alone to be unreliable as a test for unilateral renal ischaemia (Gyftaki et al., 1966; Graham et al., 1967; Wagner, 1968). Wagner (1968) considered that the measurement of the rate of accumulation of chlormerodrin by each kidney, followed by scanning, constituted a reliable screening procedure for hypertension, though even the combined test is not specific in indicating aetiology. Computer analysis of serial gamma camera images following injection of ^{131}I-inulin has given more specific results (zum Winkel, 1968).

Uptake of chlormerodrin in a functioning kidney depends on blood flow. Schlegel, Varela & Stanton (1966) proved that the amounts of radioactivity in the two kidneys 48 h after injection of radioactive chlormerodrin are proportional to the relative plasma flows through the two kidneys. Knowing total plasma flow, which may be measured by para-amino hippurate, or [^{131}I]sodium iodohippurate, clearances, the plasma flow in each of the kidneys may be obtained without catheterisation. A difference between relative amounts of radioactivity in the kidneys at 48 h and relative renal sizes indicates ischaemia which should be investigated further (Schlegel, Merlin & Varela, 1967).

Evaluation of transplants

Recently, scanning has been used to supplement renography for the evaluation of function of renal transplants. According to Hor, Pabst & Hanbold (1969), rejection episodes do not alter the size of the scan image and filling defects are the most important criteria in recognising rejection. In a study of 13 patients who had received renal transplants and who had clinical evidence of rejection, complete lack of uptake was never found. This is in contrast to the findings of Figueroa et al. (1965). Lubin et al. (1969) also found renal scanning a helpful complement to renography in differentiating between prerenal, intrarenal and postrenal causes of anuria.

By performing sequential scanning, using [^{131}I]hippuran, zum Winkel et al. (1969) combined the dynamic studies usually obtained by renography with images showing the distribution of isotope in the kidney. The most frequent signs of transplant rejection were abnormally slow uptake and delayed intrarenal transport of the hippuran. In acute tubular necrosis there was some uptake of radioactivity in the transplant but in renal artery thrombosis no uptake was detected. Infarction could be detected by reduced uptake in segments of the kidney.

Weiss *et al.* (1970) also performed serial studies with a gamma camera. They visualized transplant vascular perfusion with [^{99}Tc^m]pertechnetate and showed that changes in perfusion were associated with early symptoms and signs of rejection. Using [^{131}I]hippuran, delayed appearance in the kidney parenchyma and the bladder, and abnormally slow clearance from the blood, were characteristic of transplant rejection.

Summary

Renal scanning is complementary to other established tests—urography, arteriography and isotope renography—and is useful in demonstrating calculi, polycystic disease and the effects of trauma, and in evaluating transplants. The role of scanning is very limited in the investigation of renal masses because of the superior results obtainable by arteriography, both in resolution and in distinguishing between tumours and cysts.

Scanning alone is unreliable in the assessment of renovascular disease but is useful if combined with dynamic studies using the gamma camera.

Placenta

Localisation of the placenta is important in distinguishing placenta praevia from other causes of bleeding in the later stages of pregnancy. Scanning involves demonstrating the placental blood pool after radioisotope labelling of the maternal blood. Browne & Veall (1950) carried out point-to-point counting over the abdomen using a poorly collimated hand held counter, following the intravenous injection of ^{24}Na. Subsequently many other workers have performed manual counting using ^{51}Cr labelled red cells and serum albumin labelled with ^{131}I, ^{51}Cr or ^{99}Tc^m. The introduction of ^{99}Tc^m-serum albumin (McAfee *et al.*, 1964), however, enabled automatic scanning to be used, giving better visualization of the placenta than can be obtained by manual scanning. In order to avoid having to perform a labelling procedure the use of ^{99}Tc^m as pertechnetate ion has been proposed (Fish *et al.*, 1967) but because of the rapid clearance from the blood the short imaging time of a gamma camera is required. More recently ^{113}In^m has become the isotope of choice (Stern *et al.*, 1967). When given intravenously at a suitable pH it binds to β globulin and is thereby prevented from crossing the placenta. Finally, placenta localisation following blood labelling by inhalation of [^{11}C]carbon monoxide has been described (Glass *et al.*, 1968). ^{11}C is a positron emitter with a half life of 20 min and for its use, therefore, a cyclotron is required near at hand.

The radiation hazard is an important factor in the choice of isotope in this application but there is no doubt that all isotope methods result in much smaller radiation doses than that received from a plain abdominal X-ray.

Johnson, Bragg & Sciarra (1966), using manual counting with either 5 μCi ^{131}I-albumin or 35 μCi ^{51}Cr-albumin correctly demonstrated the position of the placenta in 96·5 per cent of 86 verified cases. Hibbard (1969) using a similar method and 200 μCi or ^{99}Tc^m-albumin made only 9 errors in

301 diagnoses. Using a rectilinear scanner Wright (1970), using 250–500 μCi ^{113}In^m, made only one major error in 200 cases but, contrary to the experience of Huddlestun et al. (1969), found failure of the ^{113}In^m to bind to the plasma proteins at pH 4 a problem and in 3 cases obtained a pyelogram but saw no placenta. Reduction of the pH to 1·6 resulted in better binding of the indium. Mishkin, Carter & Reese (1970) employed scanner and gamma camera and, using 4 mCi of ^{113}In^m, predicted the position of the placenta correctly in 71 cases out of 75 but stressed the importance of the lateral view in cases where the placenta lies on the posterior wall of the uterus. Glass et al. (1968) obtained gamma camera pictures and scans in 50 cases using ^{11}CO and all placentas were successfully visualized. The life size image obtained with a scanner was found to be an advantage in accurately identifying the placental position.

Placental scanning therefore, is a simple test with a very low radiation hazard and with an accuracy of localisation approaching 100 per cent.

Bone

Radiopharmaceuticals

Since Treadwell et al. (1942) showed by autoradiography using ^{89}Sr that strontium is deposited in regions of osteogenesis, radioisotopes have been used in the study of bone disease. Much later ^{85}Sr was found to be useful in detecting metastatic bone tumours (Sklaroff & Charkes, 1963) and, as for some time it was the only suitable isotope available, ^{85}Sr has had wide application in bone scanning. ^{85}Sr emits 0·513 MeV γ rays and has a half life of 65 d. These properties, together with a long biological half life, limit the amount of ^{85}Sr which may be given to patients to 100 μCi, because of radiation dose considerations. Assuming uniform distribution in the skeleton this amount of radioactivity delivers a dose of about 4·5 rads to bone (Fleming, McIlraith & King, 1961). It should be remembered however, that distribution is, in fact, markedly non-uniform; local doses must be much higher than this figure and, therefore, the use of ^{85}Sr is permitted only in patients with malignant disease. On the other hand the long shelf life of ^{85}Sr is convenient and, in spite of the restrictions on its use, ^{85}Sr is still the most widely used isotope in bone scanning.

However, short lived isotopes have become increasingly popular in recent years, since better quality scans can be obtained in a shorter time with less radiation hazard, using the larger quantities of radioactivity which may be given. Myers (1960) introduced the use of ^{87}Sr^m which has a half life of 2·8 h and emits 0·388 MeV γ rays with no associated particle emission. ^{87}Sr^m is obtained from a ^{87}Y generator having a half-life of 80 h which unfortunately is rather short and makes the use of this isotope costly since the generator has to be replaced frequently. ^{18}F, produced by either a reactor or cyclotron, has a half life of 1·8 h and is a positron emitter, leading to the emission of 0·51 MeV γ radiation, which is not quite as suitable for scanning as the less energetic radiation from ^{87}Sr^m. The average radiation dose to the bone is 0·36 rads from 2 mCi of ^{18}F, which is the radioactivity commonly administered (Blau, Nagler & Bender, 1962). Recently ^{68}Ga citrate has been used successfully as a bone scanning agent (Hayes, Carlton & Byrd, 1965). The latest introduction, ^{99}Tc^m-polyphosphate, gives excellent scans (Bell *et al.*, 1972) and may well become the agent of choice for bone scanning. The abnormally high vascularity of bone tumours has also enabled positive scans to be obtained using [$^{99}Tc^m$]pertechnetate (Whitley *et al.*, 1966) and ^{131}I-serum albumin (Bone *et al.*, 1967). Other isotopes not yet tried but which are potentially useful are ^{139}Ba and ^{132}Cs.

The main mechanism of uptake of bone seeking isotopes is by ion exchange with exposed bone crystal. Strontium ions exchange with calcium ions and fluoride ions with hydroxyl or bicarbonate ions, in the hydroxyapatite crystals of bone. Following intravenous injection a proportion of the isotope is rapidly taken up into the skeleton and the remainder excreted at various rates, depending upon the isotope used.

A detailed comparative study of the uptake of bone seeking isotopes into normal bone, bone lesions and soft tissue has been made by Weber *et al.* (1969) and a comparison of ^{18}F and ^{85}Sr by French & McCready (1967). These studies showed that at present ^{18}F is the best isotope available for bone scanning. It is taken up very rapidly by bone, has the highest ratio for lesion to normal bone uptake, and the most rapid clearance of the remaining isotope from the blood. This last property results in a low soft tissue background activity very soon after injection and the scan is usually performed after $1-1\frac{1}{2}$ h, though precautions must be taken to avoid confusion in interpretation due to radioactivity in the bladder. Strontium clears from the blood more slowly and, therefore, using ^{85}Sr, the best scans are obtained 24 h, or even longer, after injection. Because of faecal excretion of strontium the bowel must be washed out before the test. The short half life of $^{87}Sr^m$ precludes waiting for the optimum period and scans are usually performed within 2 or 3 h of injection. Charkes (1969) has pointed out that, using ^{87}Sr, the high level of circulating activity at the time of scanning may make interpretation difficult and that lesions may be missed which longer accumulation of ^{85}Sr might have made demonstrable. On the other hand, it is, of course, a practical advantage to be able to scan the patient soon after giving the isotope.

A major disadvantage of bone scanning is the length of time required to carry out a scan of the complete skeleton if this is called for. Many patients are in considerable pain and find it difficult to keep still for long periods. The projections used depend on circumstances but sometimes both anterior and posterior views are justified. A saving of time can be achieved by first performing a rapid profile scan of the complete length of the patient. Suspicious areas can then be investigated in more detail. The higher scanning speeds which are possible with the short lived isotopes are a great advantage in this situation and help to make the test more viable as a screening procedure.

Bone seeking isotopes are deposited mainly in areas where new bone is being formed and so, in normal subjects, there is increased radioactivity at the ends of the long bones, around the acetabula and sacroiliac joints and in the vertebrae, carpal and tarsal bones. The increased uptake in these sites is more marked in children than in adults. On a typical scan it is not usually possible to distinguish individual vertebrae (Rosenthall, 1965). In interpreting scans, differences in uptake in symmetrical areas of the skeleton should be particularly looked for and it is most important that the scan should be compared to a radiograph taken with minimum distortion in order to localise accurately the isotope deposition.

Clinical applications

Bone scanning is used to visualize primary bone tumours, bone metastases from various malignant tumours, lymphomas involving bone, osteomyelitis, fractures and metabolic bone diseases such as Gaucher's disease and Paget's disease. The uptake of isotope is a function of the rate of metabolism and lesions with the greatest metabolic activity have the highest uptake. When mineralisation of an active lesion is complete the radioisotope is not taken up though radiographic findings at that time will probably be positive. A negative scan is therefore obtained in the case of a bone island or anaplastic tumour which has little metabolic activity.

Scanning visualizes isotope uptake which depends on a change currently taking place whereas radiology detects the results of a change which has already taken place. Metabolic processes, which may be osteolytic or osteoblastic, may be active for a long time before producing the 30–50 per cent change in mineral content of the bone which is said to be required before detection is possible on a radiograph. Malignancy is characterised by both sclerosis and lysis taking place at the same time. Scanning is useful therefore in localising active bone lesions before they can be seen by X-ray examination. In prostate cancer, for example, the majority of patients have either occult or detectable bone involvement at the time of first diagnosis (Fig. 4.13) and knowledge of their presence may affect the treatment policy (Rubin, 1969). Several reports have quoted the proportion of cases studied in which scanning has demonstrated a lesion before radiography. In 50 patients with various bone disorders De Nardo & Volpe (1966), using ^{85}Sr, found 14 cases where the scan was positive and X-rays negative and also considered the test useful in the early detection of osteomyelitis. Charkes & Sklaroff (1966), using ^{85}Sr, found that bone metastases were detectable by scanning before being detectable by radiography in 28 out of 118 patients. Positive bone scans and normal X-ray appearances were found in 25 per cent of 20 patients with prostate cancer by Williams & Blahd (1967) and in 56 per cent of 32 similar patients by Faber et al. (1967). Both groups used ^{85}Sr. Blau, Laor & Bender (1969), using ^{18}F, reported that in more than 10 per cent of their patients it was possible to demonstrate bone metastases on the scan before X-ray changes appeared. These figures are only a rough guide to the usefulness of scanning in this context since in some cases patients were referred for scanning because of pain and negative X-ray findings. However, it might be expected that about 20 per cent of lesions detected by scanning would be missed by X-ray examination alone. Nevertheless, bone scanning should not be considered as a substitute for radiography but as a useful complementary test.

Finally scanning is a useful guide to the field size required in radiotherapy since it often shows a greater region of involvement than is shown by radiography (Spencer et al., 1967).

Summary

Bone scanning demonstrates new bone formation and positive scans are therefore obtained in many bone disorders. The chief value of the technique is its ability to detect metastases in the bone before they are demonstrable by radiography. A disadvantage is the time involved in performing a complete skeletal survey even with the short lived isotopes though whole body profile scanning, which is not yet widely performed, may resolve this.

Bone Marrow

The distribution of bone marrow may be visualized using either radioactive iron, preferably ^{52}Fe, which concentrates in sites of erythropoeisis, or radioactive colloids, preferably ^{99}Tc^m sulphur or ^{113}In^m colloids, which are taken up by the reticuloendothelial cells. It has been shown that the two types of agent are similarly distributed in the marrow (Nelp, Larson & Lewis, 1967). Only a small fraction of a colloid is taken up by the marrow, the bulk going to the liver and spleen.

Expansion or contraction of the amount of marrow in the central areas—particularly the lumbar spine and pelvis—can be demonstrated and also extension of marrow into the long bones in response to an increased demand for erythropoeisis. The results are extremely inconsistent however, and the applications of bone marrow scanning are very limited at present (Kniseley *et al.*, 1966; Rosenthall & Chartrand, 1969).

Lymph Nodes

Scanning of lymph nodes is not a widely used test. The technique involves injecting subcutaneously a small volume of radioactive colloid, which is carried along the lymphatic channels to be phagocytosed in the lymph nodes. The injection is made into the first interdigital space of the foot for visualizing the inguinal, iliac and para-aortic chains, into the hand for the axillary chain, beneath the liver capsule or intra-peritoneally for the mediastinal chain and into the buccal mucosa for the jugular chain. The scan is usually performed 24 h after an injection of about 100 μCi of ^{198}Au colloid by which time 40–50 per cent will have been cleared from the injection site in the foot, for example. The slow clearance means that the injection site may receive a high dose of radiation. This can be reduced by using ^{99}Tc^m labelled macroaggregates of albumin (Kazem, Galinsky & Schenck, 1967) or ^{99}Tc^m sulphur colloid (Hauser, Atkins & Richards, 1969).

Uptake of the colloid reflects the phagocytic activity of the lymphatic tissue. In normal subjects the scan shows the individual nodes but often activity is demonstrated as a more or less continuous band, especially in the inguinal and iliac regions where there are large numbers of lymph glands and where, following injection into the foot, the radioactivity is highest since they are the first sites to trap the colloid. Small areas of absent uptake may well be due to normal anatomical variations. In Hodgkin's disease, enlargement of the lymphatic chain may be demonstrated. Failure to take up the colloid may be due to infection or to metastatic involvement and the test has limited value in the detection of metastases in the lymph nodes. The limited resolution of the instrument does not permit small defects in individual nodes to be detected.

Seaman & Powers (1955) using ^{198}Au colloid found that, of 63 nodes with known metastatic involvement, only 43 showed no uptake. zum Winkel & Muller (1965) carried out both isotope scanning and lymphangiography on 133 patients and found reasonably good correlation between the two, though the X-ray examination, because of its superior resolution, gave more definite morphological information. They agreed with other authors (Kazem *et al.*, 1968; Herting *et al.*, 1970) that the technique is sufficiently accurate to be useful as a screening test.

In summary, lymph node scanning may be useful in planning treatment, in demonstrating enlarged nodes as found in Hodgkin's disease and as a screening test. It gives less morphological information than lymphangiography but has the virtue of simplicity.

Blood Pool

Scanning of the heart blood pool was introduced by Rejali, MacIntyre & Friedell (1958) using ^{131}I-serum albumin but this agent has been superseded by [^{99}Tc^m]pertechnetate, ^{99}Tc^m-serum albumin and ^{113}In^m, all of which give better images. Rectilinear scanners have been used for most cardiac scanning but, when using [^{99}Tc^m]pertechnetate, a gamma camera is preferable because of the rapid diffusion of the isotope.

The main application of the test is in the demonstration of pericardial effusion, based upon observing a discrepancy between the size of the scan image and the size of an X-ray image of the heart. An increased separation of heart and liver blood pools is also characteristic of pericardial effusion. Effusions less than 150 ml cannot be demonstrated by scanning (Bonte & Curry, 1966).

By rapid sequential imaging with a gamma camera following the injection of several millicuries of [^{99}Tc^m]pertechnetate intravenously or directly into the chambers of the heart during cardiac catheterisation, the heart and great vessels have been visualized in a variety of congenital and acquired diseases. Aneurysms and stenosis of the aorta have been detected (Mason *et al.*, 1969; Tori, Marabini & Fattovich, 1970) as well as obstruction of the superior vena cava (Maxfield & Meckstroth, 1969).

Myocardium

Myocardial scanning for the detection of infarction has been performed using ^{86}RbCl (Carr *et al.*, 1962), ^{131}CsCl (Carr *et al.*, 1964) and ^{131}I-oleic acid (Gunton *et al.*, 1965). Normal myocardium takes up these agents whereas ischaemic areas do not and are shown as 'cold' areas on the scan.

Myocardial perfusion has also been successfully visualized by scanning after the injection of ^{99}Tc^m-macroaggregates into the left coronary artery at the time of coronary angiography (Ashburn *et al.*, 1970).

Salivary Glands

[^{99}Tc^m]pertechnetate concentrates in the salivary glands and although uptake in each salivary gland is less than in the thyroid, it is adequate for successful scanning (Harden *et al.*, 1967). Decreased uptake by the salivary glands has been demonstrated with benign and malignant tumours (Sorsdahl, Williams & Bruno, 1969).

Stomach

^{131}I, given intravenously, is taken up by the gastric mucosa to a sufficient degree to permit gastric scanning. The technique has been applied to detect cancer of the stomach but with limited success (Clode *et al.*, 1964). ^{99}Tc^m

also accumulates in the stomach wall and scanning may be performed a few minutes after the administration of about 2 mCi of [^{99}Tc^m]pertechnetate. The ability to concentrate ^{99}Tc^m is lost by a stomach wall invaded by neoplasm but is not affected by inflammatory changes. Scanning may therefore be useful in differentiating between these two conditions (Fridrich, 1969).

GENERAL CONCLUSIONS

The technique of radioisotope visualization or scanning, has grown at a tremendous rate during the last decade and is now firmly established in clinical practice. In this chapter it has been possible to cover the subject only in broad terms and many interesting aspects have had to be omitted. The literature on the subject is vast and only a fraction has been quoted here.

Developments in the fields of radiopharmaceuticals and instrumentation go hand in hand. New radiopharmaceuticals with shorter lives and more suitable gamma ray energies are required. Scanning is commonly used to demonstrate malignant tumours and for this purpose many radioactive agents are used. Much effort is devoted to the search for a single agent concentrated by all tumours but with only limited success so far. In the field of equipment, sensitivity and resolution are continually being improved as new types of scanner, camera and hybrid instruments are evolved. Data storage and processing, still in its early stages, is already improving diagnostic efficiency and widening the whole field of application of imaging techniques.

References

AQUINO, J. A. & CUNNINGHAM, R. M. (1969). *Medical Radioisotope Scintigraphy*, 1968, vol. 2, p. 255. I.A.E.A., Vienna.

ASHBURN, W. L., BRAUNWALD, E., SIMON, A. L. & GAULT, J. H. (1970). *J. nucl. Med.*, 11, 618.

ATKINS, H. L. & FLEAY, R. F. (1968). *J. nucl. Med.*, 9, 66.

BELL, E. G., BLAIR, R. J., SUBRAMANIAN, G. & McAFEE, J. G. (1972). *J. nucl. Med.*, 13, 413.

BENDER, M. A. & BLAU, M. (1962). *In* "Progress in Medical Radioisotope Scanning". Ed. R. M. Knisely, G. A. Andrews & C. C. Harris. p. 388. Oak Ridge, Tennessee: Oak Ridge Institute of Nuclear Studies.

BENDER, M. A. & BLAU, M. (1963). *Nucleonics*, 21, 52.

BENDER, M. A. & WILLIAMS, C. M. (1966). *Am. J. Roentg.*, 96, 698.

BLAU, M. & BENDER, M. A. (1962). *J. nucl. Med.*, 3, 83.

BLAU, M., LAOR, Y. & BENDER, M. A. (1969). *Medical Radioisotope Scintigraphy*, 1968, vol. 2, p. 341. I.A.E.A., Vienna.

BLAU, M. & MANSKE, R. F. (1961). *J. nucl. Med.*, 2, 102.

BLAU, M., NAGLER, W. & BENDER, M. A. (1962). *J. nucl. Med.*, 3, 332.

BONTE, F. J. (1965). *Am. J. Roentg.*, 95, 1.

BONTE, F. J. & CURRY, T. S. (1966). *Am. J. Roentg.*, 96, 690.

BONTE, F. J., CURRY, T. S., OELZE, R. G. & GREENBERG, A. J. (1967). *Am. J. Roentg.*, 100, 801.

BORGHGRAEF, R. R. M. & PITTS, R. F. (1956). *J. clin. Invest.*, 35, 31.

BROWN, P. W., SIRCUS, W., SMITH, A. N., DONALDSON, A. A., DYMOCK, I. W., FALCONER, C. W. A. & SMALL, W. P. (1968). *Lancet*, 1, 160.

BROWNE, J. C. M. & VEALL, N. (1950). *J. Obstet. Gynaec., Br. Commonw.*, 57, 566.

BROWNELL, G. L. & SWEET, W. H. (1953). *Nucleonics*, 11, 40.

BUDABIN, M. (1965). *J. Mt Sinai Hosp.*, **32**, 527.

BULL, J. W. D. & MARRYAT, J. (1965). *Br. med. J.*, **1**, 474.

BURDINE, J. A. & HAYŃIE, T. P. (1965). *J. Am. med. Ass.*, **194**, 979.

BURDINE, J. A. & LEGEAY, R. (1968). *Radiology*, **91**, 162.

CAROLI, J. & BONNEVILLE, B. (1962). *Archs Mal. Appar. dig.*, **51**, 55.

CARR, E. A., BEIERWALTES, W. H., WEGST, A. V. & BARTLETT, J. D. (1962). *J. nucl. Med.*, **3**, 76.

CARR, E. A., GLEASON, G., SHAW, J. & KRONTZ, B. (1964). *Am. Heart J.*, **68**, 627.

CASTELL, D. O. & JOHNSON, R. B. (1966). *New Engl. J. Med.*, **275**, 188.

CENTI COLELLA, A. & PIGORINI, F. (1967). *Br. J. Radiol.*, **40**, 662.

CENTI COLELLA, A. & PIGORINI, F. (1970). *Am. J. Roentg.*, **109**, 714.

CHARKES, N. D. (1969). *J. nucl. Med.*, **10**, 491.

CHARKES, N. D. & SKLAROFF, D. M. (1966). *Radiol. Clin. N. Am.*, **3**, 499.

CHISHOLM, G. D., AYE, M. M. & EVANS, K. (1967). *Br. J. Urol.*, **39**, 38.

CLODE, W. H., RODRIGUES, M. S., FERNANDEZ, M. A. P., MURTEIRA, M. A. & BAPTISTA, A. M. (1964). *Medical Radioisotope Scanning*, 1964, vol. **2**, p. 175, I.A.E.A., Vienna.

CONN, H. O. & ELKINGTON, S. G. (1968). *Gastroenterology*, **54**, 135.

DE NARDO, G. L., GOODWIN, D. A., RAVASINI, R. & DIETRICH, P. A. (1970). *New Engl. J. Med.*, **282**, 1334.

DE NARDO, G. L. & VOLPE, J. A. (1966). *J. nucl. Med.*, **7**, 219.

DI CHIRO, G., ASHBURN, W. L. & GROVE, A. S. (1968). *Neurology, Minneap.*, **18**, 225.

DI GUILIO, W. & MORALES, J. (1969). *J. Am. med. Ass.*, **209**, 1873.

DOBYNS, B. M. & MALOOF, F. (1951). *J. clin. Endocr.*, **11**, 1323.

EATON, S. B., FLEISCHLI, D. J., POLLARD, J. J., NEBESAR, R. A. & POTSAID, M. S. (1968). *New Engl. J. Med.*, **279**, 389.

EATON, S. B., POTSAID, M. S., LO, H. H. & BEAULIEU, E. (1967). *Radiology*, **89**, 1033.

ENTZIAN, W., ARONOW, S., SOLOWAY, A. H. & SWEET, W. M. (1964). *Medical Radioisotope Scanning*, 1964, vol. **2**, p. 109. I.A.E.A., Vienna.

EYLER, W. R., SCHUMAN, B. M., DU SAULT, L. A. & HINSON, R. E. (1965). *Radiology*, **84**, 469.

FABER, D. D., WAHMAN, G. E., BAILEY, T. A., FLOCKS, R. H., CULP, D. A. & MORRISON, R. T. (1967). *J. Urol.*, **97**, 526.

FIGUEROA, J. E., RODRIGUEZ-ANTUNEZ, A., NAKAMOTO, S. & KOLFF, W. J. (1965). *New Engl. J. Med.*, **273**, 1406.

FILSON, E. J. & RODRIGUEZ-ANTUNEZ, A. (1968). *Acta radiol.*, **7**, 380.

FISCHER, J., LEON, A. & WOLF, R. (1969). *Medical Radioisotope Scintigraphy*, 1968, vol. **2**. p. 381. I.A.E.A., Vienna.

FISCHER, J. & WOLF, R. (1964). *German med. Mon.*, **8**, 89.

FISH, M. D., LAVINE, D., POLLYCOVE, M. & KHENTIGAN, A. (1967). *J. nucl. Med.*, **8**, 350.

FLEMING, W. H., MCILRAITH, J. D. & KING, E. R. (1961). *Radiology*, **77**, 635.

FREEMAN, L. M., GOLDMAN, S. M., SHAW, R. K. & BLAUFOX, M. D. (1969). *J. nucl. Med.*, **10**, 545.

FREEMAN, L. M., KAY, C. J. & DERMAN, A. (1968). *J. nucl. Med.*, **9**, 227.

FREEMAN, L. M., KAY, C. J. & MENG, C. H. (1966). *Radiology*, **86**, 1021.

FRENCH, R. J. & MCCREADY, V. R. (1967). *Br. J. Radiol.*, **40**, 655.

FRIDRICH, R. (1969). *Germ. med. Mon.*, **14**, 621.

FRIEDMAN, W. F. & BRAUNWALD, E. (1966). *Circulation*, **34**, 363.

FRIEDMANN, B., LEWIS, S. M., GLASS, H. I., SZUR, L. & WATSON, I. A. (1968). *Br. J. Radiol.*, **41**, 815.

GARROW, J. S. & SMITH, R. (1968). *Br. J. Radiol.*, **41**, 307.

GIBBS, J. C., HALLIGAN, E. J., GRIECO, R. V. & McKEOWN, J. E. (1965). *Archs Surg., Chicago*, **90**, 323.

GLASS, H. I., JACOBY, J., WESTERMAN, B., CLARK, J. C., ARNOT, R. N. & DIXON, H. G. (1968). *J. nucl. Med.*, **9**, 468.

GOLLIN, F. F., SIMS, J. L. & CAMERON, J. R. (1964). *J. Am. med. Ass.*, **187**, 111.

GOTTSCHALK, A. (1967). *J. Am. med. Ass.*, **202**, 221.

GRAHAM, A. G., SCOTT, J. S., KENNEDY, I. & MACK, W. S. (1967). *Br. J. Urol.*, **39**, 718.

GUNTON, R. W., EVANS, J. R., BAKER, R. G., SPEARS, J. C. & BEANLANDS, D. S. (1965). *Am. J. Cardiol.*, **16**, 482.

GYFTAKI, E., BINOPOULOS, D., RIGAS, A. & ALEVIZOI, V. (1966). *Nuclear-Medezin*, **5**, 397.

HARDEN, R. M., HILDITCH, T. E., KENNEDY, I., MASON, D. K., PAPADOPOULOS, S. & ALEXANDER, W. D. (1967). *Clin. Sci.*, **32**, 49.

HARPER, P. V., LATHROP, K. A., JIMINEZ, F., FINK, R. & GOTTSCHALK, A. (1965). *Radiology*, **85**, 101.

HATCHETTE, J. B., SHULER, S. E. & MURISON, P. J. (1972). *J. nucl. Med.*, **13**, 51.

HAUSER, W., ATKINS, H. L. & RICHARDS, P. (1969). *Radiology*, **92**, 1369.

HAYES, M., SWANSON, L. A. & TAPLIN, G. V. (1968). *Radiology*, **91**, 984.

HAYES, R. L., CARLTON, J. E. & BYRD, B. L. (1965). *J. nucl. Med.*, **6**, 605.

HERTING, S. E., FREDERIKSEN, P. B., JAGT, T. & JEPPESEN, P. (1970). *Acta. radiol.*, **10**, 359.

HIBBARD, B. M. (1969). *Br. med. J.*, **3**, 85.

HOLZBACH, R. T., CLARK, R. E., SHIPLEY, R. A. & LINDSAY, G. E. (1962). *J. Lab. clin. Med.*, **60**, 902.

HOR, G., PABST, H. W. & HANBOLD, U. (1968). *Medical Radioisotope Scintigraphy*, 1968, **vol. 2**, p. 209. I.A.E.A., Vienna.

HUDDLESTUN, J. E., MISHKIN, F. S., CARTER, J. E., DUBOIS, P. D. & REESE, I. C. (1969). *Radiology*, **92**, 587.

JAMES, A. E., DeLAND, F. H., HODGES, F. J. & WAGNER, H. N. (1970). *Am. J. Roentg.*, **110**, 74.

JOHNSON, P. M., BRAGG, D. G. & SCIARRA, J. J. (1966). *Am. J. Roentg.*, **96**, 681.

JOHNSON, P. M. & SWEENEY, W. (1967). *J. nucl. Med.*, **8**, 451.

KAPLAN, E. & BEN PORATH, M. (1969). *Med. Clin., N. Amer.*, **53**, 189.

KAPLAN, E., BEN PORATH, M., FINK, S., CLAYTON, G. D. & JACOBSON, B. (1966). *J. nucl. Med.*, **7**, 807.

KAZEM, I., ANTONIADES, J., BRADY, L. W., FAUST, D. S., CROLL, M. N. & LIGHTFOOT, D. (1968). *Radiology*, **90**, 905.

KAZEM, I., GALINSKY, P. & SCHENCK, P. (1967). *Br. J. Radiol.*, **40**, 292.

KAZMIN, M. A., SWANSON, L. E. & COCKETT, A T. K. (1967). *J. Urol.*, **97**, 189.

KENNADY, J. C. & TAPLIN, G. V. (1965). *J. nucl. Med.*, **6**, 566.

KESSLER, R. H., LOZANO, R. & PITTS, R. F. (1957). *J. clin. Invest.*, **36**, 656.

KING, E. R., SHARPE, A., GRUBB, W., BROCK, J. S. & GREENBERG, L. (1966). *Am. J. Roentg.*, **96**, 657.

KNISELEY, R. M., ANDREWS, G. A., TANIDA, R., EDWARDS, C. L. & KYKER, G. C. (1966). *J. nucl. Med.*, **7**, 575.

KRASZNAI, I., PAL, I. & FOLDES, J. (1965). *Nuclear–Medizin*, **5**, 56.

LAHDEVIRTA, J. (1967). *Acta med. scand.*, **182**, 345.

LEGER, L., ROUCAYROL, J. C. & LENRIOT, J. P. (1971). *Acta gastro-ent. belg.*, **34**, 159.

LESLIE, E. V., ALKER, G. J. & BAKAY, L. (1969). *In* "Brain Tumour Scanning with Radioisotopes". Ed. Bakay & Klein. p. 169. C. C. Thomas.

LIEWENDAHL, K. & KVIST, G. (1970). *Acta med. scand.*, **188**, 75.

LOKEN, M. K. & WESTGATE, H. D. (1968). *J. nucl. Med.*, **9**, 45.

LOPEZ-MAJANO, V., TOW, D. E. & WAGNER, H. N. (1966). *J. Am. med. Ass.*, **197**, 81.

LOPEZ-MAJANO, V., WAGNER, H. N., TOW, D. E. & CHERNICK, V. (1965). *J. Am. med. Ass.*, **194**, 1053.

LUBIN, E., LEWITUS, Z., ROSENFELD, J. & LEVI, M. (1969). *Medical Radioisotope Scintigraphy*, 1968, vol. 2, p. 219. I.A.E.A., Vienna.

LUM, C. H., MARSHALL, W. J., KOZOLL, D. D. & KEYER, K. A. (1959). *Ann. Surg.*, **149**, 353.

MCAFEE, J. G., AUSE, R. G. & WAGNER, H. N. (1965). *Archs intern. Med.*, **116**, 95.

MCAFEE, J. G., STERN, H. S., FUEGER, G. F., BAGGISH, M. S., HOLZMAN, G. B. & ZOLLE, I. (1964). *J. nucl. Med.*, **5**, 936.

MCAFEE, J. G. & TAXDAL, D. R. (1961). *Radiology*, **77**, 207.

MCCARTHY, D. M., BROWN, P., MELMED, R. N., AGNEW, J. E. & BOUCHIER, I. A. D. (1972). *Gut*, **13**, 75.

MCCARTHY, D. M., KREEL, L., AGNEW, J. E. & BOUCHIER, I. A. D. (1969). *Gut*, **10**, 665.

MCCREADY, V. R., GWYTHER, M. M. & STRINGER, A. M. (1969). *Medical Radioisotope Scintigraphy*, 1968, vol. 2, p. 419. I.A.E.A., Vienna.

MALLARD, J. R. (1966). *Int. J. appl. Radiat. Isotopes*, **17**, 205.

MALLARD, J. R. & PEACHEY, C. J. (1959). *Br. J. Radiol.*, **32**, 652.

MARRYAT, J. & BULL, J. W. D. (1964). *Br. J. Radiol.*, **37**, 711.

MARSH, G. W., LEWIS, S. M. & SZUR, L. (1966). *Br. J. Haemat.*, **12**, 161.

MASON, D. T., ASHBURN, W. L., HARBERT, J. C., COHEN, L. S. & BRAUNWALD, E. (1969). *Circulation*, **39**, 19.

MAXFIELD, W. S. & MECKSTROTH, G. R. (1969). *Radiology*, **92**, 913.

MELMED, R. N., AGNEW, J. E. & BOUCHIER, I. A. D. (1968). *Q. Jl Med.*, **37**, 607.

MILLER, J. M. & HAMBURGER, J. I. (1965). *Radiology*, **84**, 66.

MISHKIN, F. S., CARTER, J. E. & REESE, I. C. (1970). *Am. J. Roentg.*, **109**, 776.

MISHKIN, F. S. & WAGNER, H. N. (1967). *Radiology*, **88**, 142.

MOORE, G. E. (1948). *Science*, **107**, 569.

MORRIS, J. G., COOREY, G. J., DICK, R., EVANS, W. A., SMITANANDA, N., PEARSON, B. S., LOEWENTHAL, J. I., BLACKBURN, C. R. B. & MCRAE, J. (1967). *J. Urol.*, **97**, 40.

MOSER, K. M. & MIALE, A. (1968). *Am. J. Med.*, **44**, 366.

MUSTAFA, A. G., RAZZAK, M. A., MAHFOUZ, M. & GUIRGIS, B. (1966). *J. nucl. Med.*, **7**, 909.

MYERS, W. G. (1960). *J. nucl. Med.*, **1**, 125.

MYHILL, J., REEVE, T. S. & FIGGIS, P. M. (1965). *Am. J. Roentg.*, **94**, 828.

NAFTALUS, J. & LEEVY, C. M. (1963). *Am. J. dig. Dis.*, **8**, 236.

NAGLER, W., BENDER, M. A. & BLAU, M. (1963). *Gastroenterology*, **44**, 36.

NELP, W. B. & KUHN, I. N. (1966). *J. Am. med. Ass.*, **197**, 368.

NELP, W. B., LARSON, S. M. & LEWIS, R. J. (1967). *J. nucl. Med.*, **8**, 430.

OJEMANN, R. G. & SWEET, W. H. (1969). *In* "Brain Tumour Scanning with Radioisotopes". Ed. Bakay & Klein. p. 121. C. C. Thomas.

O'MARA, R. E., SUBRAMANIAN, G., MCAFEE, J. G. & BURGER, C. L. (1969). *J. nucl. Med.*, **10**, 18.

OVERTON, M. C., HAYNIE, T. P., OTTE, W. K. & COE, J. E. (1965). *J. nucl. Med.*, **6**, 705.

OVERTON, M. C., HAYNIE, T. P. & SNODGRASS, S. R. (1965). *J. Am. med. Ass.*, **191**, 431.

OZARDA, A. & PICKREN, J. (1962). *J. nucl. Med.*, **3**, 149.

PATTEN, D. H. & BENSON, D. F. (1968). *J. nucl. Med.*, **9**, 457.

PIRCHER, F. J. (1969). *Medical Radioisotope Scintigraphy*, 1968, vol. 2, p. 131. I.A.E.A., Vienna.

PLANIOL, T. (1966). *Progr. Neurol. Surg.*, **1**, 94.
PLANIOL, T. (1969). *In* "Brain Tumour Scanning with Radioisotopes". Ed. Bakay & Klein. p. 111. C. C. Thomas.
POCHIN, E. E., MYANT, N. B., HILTON, G., HONOUR, A. J. & CORBETT, B. D. (1952). *Br. med. J.*, **4794**, 1116.
QUINN, J. L. (1969). *Am. J. Roentg.*, **105**, 251.
QUINN, J. L. & HEAD, L. R. (1966). *J. nucl. Med.*, **7**, 1.
QUINN, J. L. & MAYNARD, C. D. (1965). *Radiol. Clin.*, *N. Am.*, **3**, 65.
REBA, R. C., HOSAIN, F. & WAGNER, H. N. (1968). *Radiology*, **90**, 147.
REJALI, A. M., MACINTYRE, W. J. & FRIEDELL, H. L. (1958). *Am. J. Roentg.*, **79**, 129.
RHOTON, A. L., CARLSSON, A. M. & TER POGOSSIAN, M. M. (1964). *Archs Neurol.*, **10**, 369.
ROBINSON, E. & HOCHMAN, A. (1962). *Cancer*, **15**, 1130.
ROSE, R. G. & KELSEY, M. P. (1963). *Cancer*, **16**, 896.
ROSENTHALL, L. (1965). *Radiology*, **84**, 75.
ROSENTHALL, L. (1967). *Am. J. Roentg.*, **101**, 662.
ROSENTHALL, L., AGUAYO, A. & STRATFORD, J. (1966). *Radiology*, **86**, 499.
ROSENTHALL, L. & CHARTRAND, R. (1969). *Can. med. Ass. J.*, **100**, 54.
ROZENTAL, P., MILLER, E. B. & KAPLAN, E. (1966). *J. nucl. Med.*, **7**, 868.
RUBIN, P. (1969). *J. Am. med. Ass.*, **210**, 1079.
SALDINO, R. M. & MISHKIN, F. S. (1968). *Archs Surg., Chicago*, **97**, 558.
SCHLEGEL, J. U., MERLIN, A. S. & VARELA, R. (1967). *Sth. med. J.*, **60**, 623.
SCHLEGEL, J. U., VARELA, R. & STANTON, J. J. (1966). *J. Urol.*, **96**, 20.
SCHMUKLER, M. & WORKMAN, J. B. (1966). *J. nucl. Med.*, **7**, 252.
SEAMAN, W. P. & POWERS, W. E. (1955). *Cancer*, **8**, 1044.
SHARMA, S. M., PATEL, M. C., RAMANATHAN, P., GANATRA, R. D. & BLAU, M. (1970). *J. nucl. Med.*, **11**, 228.
SHIMOAKA, K. & SOKAL, J. E. (1964). *Archs intern. Med.*, **114**, 36.
SKLAROFF, D. M. & CHARKES, N. D. (1963). *Radiology*, **80**, 270.
SMITH, L. B. & WILLIAMS, R. D. (1968). *Archs Surg.*, **96**, 693.
SODEE, D. B. (1964a). *Medical Radioisotope Scanning*, **vol. 2**, p. 147. I.A.E.A., Vienna.
SODEE, D. B. (1964b). *Medical Radioisotope Scanning*, **vol. 2**, p. 289. I.A.E.A., Vienna.
SODEE, D. B. (1966). *Radiology*, **87**, 641.
SORSDAHL, O. A., WILLIAMS, C. M. & BRUNO, F. P. (1969). *Radiology*, **92**, 1477.
SPENCER, R., HERBERT, R., RISH, M. W. & LITTLE, W. A. (1967). *Br. J. Radiol.*, **40**, 641.
SPENCER, R. P. & WALDMAN, R. (1965). *J. nucl. Med.*, **6**, 53.
STERN, H. S., GOODWIN, D. A., SCHEFFEL, U., WAGNER, H. N. & KRAMER, H. H. (1967). *Nucleonics*, **25**, 62.
TAKAHASHI, M., NOFAL, M. M. & BEIERWALTES, W. H. (1966). *J. nucl. Med.*, **7**, 32.
TAPLIN, G. V., JOHNSON, D. E., DORE, E. K. & KAPLAN, H. S. (1964). *Health Phys.*, **10**, 1219.
TAPLIN, G. V. & POE, N. D. (1965). *Radiology*, **85**, 365.
TAPLIN, G. V., POE, N. D., DORE, E. K., SWANSON, L. A., ISAWA, T. & GREENBERG, A. (1969). *Medical Radioisotope Scintigraphy*, 1968, **vol. 2**, p. 111. I.A.E.A., Vienna.
TORI, G., MARABINI, A. & FATTOVICH, G. (1970). *Br. J. Radiol.*, **43**, 344.
TOW, D. E. & WAGNER, H. N. (1967). *J. Am. med. Ass.*, **199**, 104.
TREADWELL, A. de G., LOW-BEER, B. V. A., FRIEDELL, H. L. & LAWRENCE, J. H. (1942). *Am. J. med. Sci.*, **204**, 521.

WAGNER, H. N. (1968). *In* "Principles of Nuclear Medicine". Ed. H. N. Wagner. Philadelphia: Saunders.

WAGNER, H. N. (1968). *Radiology*, **91**, 1235.

WAGNER, H. N., WEINER, I. M., MCAFEE, J. G. & MARTINEZ, J. (1964). *Archs intern. Med.*, **113**, 696.

WEBBER, M. M. (1965). *Am. J. Roentg.*, **94**, 815.

WEBER, D. A., GREENBERG, E. J., DIMICH, A., KENNY, P. J., ROTHSCHILD, E. O., MYERS, W. P. L. & LAUGHLIN, J. S. (1969). *J. nucl. Med.*, **10**, 8.

WEIBEL, E. R. (1963). *In* "Morphometry of the Human Lung". New York: Academic Press.

WEISS, E. R., BLAHD, W. H., WINSTON, M. A., HARTENBOWER, D. L., KOPPEL, M. & THOMAS, P. B. (1970). *J. nucl. Med.*, **11**, 69.

WHANG, K. S., FISH, M. B. & POLLYCOVE, M. (1965). *J. nucl. Med.* **6**, 494.

WHITLEY, J. E., WITCOFSKI, R. L., BOLLIZER, T. T. & MAYNARD, C. D. (1966). *Am. J. Roentg.*, **96**, 706.

WILLIAMS, D. F. & BLAHD, W. H. (1967). *J. Urol.*, **97**, 1070.

WITCOFSKI, R. L. & ROPER, T. J. (1965). *J. nucl. Med.*, **6**, 754.

WRIGHT, F. W. (1970). *Br. med. J.*, **2**, 636.

ZUM WINKEL, K. (1968). *Br. J. Radiol.*, **41**, 558.

ZUM WINKEL, K., HARBST, H., SCHENCK, P., FRANZ, H. E., RITZ, E., ROHL, L., ZIEGLER, M., AMMANN, W. & MAIER-BORST, W. (1968). *Medical Radioisotope Scintigraphy*, 1968, **vol. 2**, p. 197. I.A.E.A., Vienna.

ZUM WINKEL, K. & MULLER, H. (1965). *Radiologe*, **5**, 381.

CHAPTER 5

IMMUNOLOGY OF THE RESPIRATORY TRACT

MARGARET TURNER WARWICK

If the term 'allergy' is reinstated as suggested by Gell & Coombs (1968), in line with Von Pirquet's original concept to indicate all forms of altered immunological reactivity, then allergy involves the specific processes that are protective as well as those resulting in hypersensitivity, which may be tissue damaging.

It is perhaps unfortunate that the term 'immune response' is now also used to include specific processes that may be either protective or tissue damaging. To abandon the word 'immune' altogether would be both awkward and pedantic and so the common usage of the terms 'allergy' and 'immune' will be retained and used in context as seems sensible.

With this understanding it is recognised that virtually all lung disease has immunological implications and the present discussion should properly include all acute and chronic bacterial, viral and fungal infections, not forgetting pulmonary tuberculosis and infective chronic bronchitis; all pulmonary hypersensitivity diseases including the asthmas, pulmonary eosinophilia, the 'extrinsic allergic alveolitis' group of lung disease and connective tissue disorders. It should include an increasing number of the pneumoconioses and perhaps with the recognition of tumour antibodies, carcinoma and other malignant disease of the lung.

The anatomical and physiological arrangements of the lungs exposes them to a range of exogenous and endogenous agents capable of inducing immunological reactions. Antigens of many types may be inhaled; including actively multiplying bacteria, viruses and fungi, as well as non living organic and inorganic dusts. These antigens stimulate several different types of host immune response, depending on the nature of the antigen, the amount inhaled and the duration of exposure. The types of reaction induced are also greatly influenced by the particular immunological responsiveness of the host.

Antigens and antigen–antibody complexes may also reach the lung through the pulmonary and perhaps the bronchial circulations. The lung is the only organ of the body to be perfused by the total cardiac output and it is therefore not surprising that the lungs are involved in a number of systemic allergic reactions, such as anaphylaxis, serum sickness and drug reactions.

Different types of immune response may occur predominantly in different parts of the lung, some affecting particularly the bronchi, and others mainly damaging bronchioles, alveoli or pulmonary vessels. It would be erroneous to regard the lung as a 'passive' connective tissue target organ on to which exogenous inhaled antigen and antibody, preformed at distant sites, interact, because in the majority of diseases we shall discuss it can be shown that antibody is formed locally in the lung itself; IgE and IgA in plasma cells located in the lamina propria of the bronchi (Tomasi *et al.*, 1965) and IgG and IgM within plasma cells and lympoid collections, which develop in the course of various diseases affecting predominantly the peripheral parts of the lung.

Antigens stimulate and react with antibody or sensitized cells in several different ways, inducing a variety of distinct patterns of tissue damage. In general these patterns remain constant, irrespective of the organ in which the response occurs. Four types of tissue damaging hypersensitivity are now well recognised (Gell & Coombs, 1968) and recently a fifth type has been added.

Free antigen reacting with antibody passively sensitizing cell surfaces (Type I). An immediate response usually mediated by reaginic antibody. This reaction is typically initiated by antigen reacting with tissue cells which have been passively sensitized by IgE antibody produced elsewhere. The reaction results in an immediate release of vasoactive humoral mediators, such as histamine, bradykinin and SRS-A (slow reacting substance of anaphylaxis) which cause local vasodilation, exudation and smooth muscle contraction. The 'immediate' weal and flare response occurring within ten minutes on prick testing and bronchial asthma on inhalation challenge are common examples of this type of reaction.

Antibody reacting with an antigenic component of a cell or a hapten closely associated with a cell surface (Type II). The reaction usually involves complement. Circulating basement membrane antibody reacting with pulmonary capillary basement membrane in Goodpasture's syndrome (Beirne *et al.*, 1968) represents a Type II reaction in the lung.

Antigen reacting with potentially precipitating antibody to form antigen–antibody complexes (Type III). This type is initiated when antigen reacts in tissue spaces with potentially precipitating antibody forming antigen–antibody complexes; the antibody in this reaction is commonly IgG and complement is usually involved. Different types of histological tissue response may be seen depending on the proportion of antigen to antibody (Spector & Heesom, 1969). These workers showed that in antibody excess a typical 'Arthus' reaction was seen with polymorphonuclear accumulation together with fibrinoid necrosis of neighbouring small vessels, while injection of antigen–antibody complexes in equivalence stimulated the formation of granulomas. A Type III reaction also occurs when antigen in excess reacts in the blood with potentially precipitating antibody to form soluble circulating complexes: under certain circumstances these complexes become deposited on the endothelial lining of vessel walls causing local inflammation. There is indirect evidence that a number of hypersensitivity lung diseases, including extrinsic allergic alveolitis, and certain forms of aspergillus hypersensitivity are at least in part determined by a Type III response. It is probable that the haemorrhagic oedema found in some viraemias and in gram-negative septicemia may be further examples of immune complex disease. Some of the pulmonary lesions in patients with systemic lupus erythematosus and allied clinical syndromes may represent further examples of complex deposition in the lungs. The 'late' skin reaction occurring after 4–6 hours following an intracutaneous injection of certain antigens such as avian protein is an example of a Type III response in man.

'Delayed' tuberculin-type, cell mediated reaction (Type IV). This is initiated by specifically modified, sensitized mononuclear cells reacting with antigen deposited at local sites. The tissue damage of tuberculosis is the classic example of a Type IV reaction, homograft rejection is another example and blast transformation of lymphocytes also depends upon lymphocyte sensitization. Type IV hypersensitivity may also be important in other chronic granulomatous diseases, such as histoplasmosis and coccidioidomycosis and may also account for some particularly florid infections affecting the partially immune host. For instance the necrotising pulmonary lesions seen in severe adult chicken pox may be determined by cell mediated hypersensitivity. The delayed Type IV skin reactions occurs after an interval of 48–72 hours and is characterised on histological examination by the presence of mononuclear cells.

Reaction initiated by antibody reacting with an antigen causing stimulation rather than destruction of a cell (Type V). No examples of this type are yet known in relation to pulmonary disease and it will not therefore be discussed further.

Although in some diseases the major feature is apparently explained on the basis of one of these types of immune mechanisms, occurring alone, it must be emphasised that there are many examples where multiple immune reactions can be demonstrated, proceeding simultaneously. Indeed there is accumulating evidence that in human disease the development of more than one type of immunological reaction is the rule rather than the exception; humoral and cell mediated responses being interdependent and proceeding together (Roitt et al., 1969). For this reason, the clinical and histological features in human pulmonary disease are often more complicated than is seen in animal experiments where single responses have been induced selectively.

ASTHMA

There is now increasing evidence that the narrowing of airways which is recognised as bronchial asthma can be triggered by many different agents, stimulating several different reactions, only some of which are immunologically determined (summarized by Turner Warwick, 1971).

Type I. Immediate IgE Mediated Reactions in the Lung
Causing Asthma
Antigens

Inhalation of certain common vegetable and animal protein contaminants of the atmosphere, especially domestic dust, pollens and certain moulds stimulate, especially in susceptible subjects, the production of IgE reaginic antibody.

A number of different factors determine whether an antigen stimulates IgE or IgG formation. The nature of the antigen is important; some pollens for instance, are much more allergenic than others, but the explanation for this is not at present fully known. Recent work on the antigenic structure of grass pollen has shown that a number of different fractions may be separated by electrophoresis, some of which stimulate reaginic antibody formation while others do not (Augustin, 1959).

TABLE 5.1

EXAMPLES OF DIFFERENT MODES OF INDUCTION
OF THE ASTHMATIC RESPONSE

| External Antigens | Allergic Response | |
	Antibody	Reaction
Common allergens, e.g. house dust, pollens	IgE	Type I 'Immediate' asthma
Organic dusts, e.g. avian protein, micropolyspora, proteolytic enzymes	IgG (? + IgE)	Type III 'Late' or 'intermission' asthma
Aspergillus fumigatus	IgE + IgG	Type I & Type III Dual asthma

Other External Agents	Non Allergic Response
Cotton, castor oil	Stimulate histamine release
Drugs, e.g. Propranolol	β receptor blockade
'Irritants', e.g. Halogens, acrid fumes . .	? parasympathetic stimulation
Exercise	Unknown

Unknown Agents	Unknown Mechanism
	Intrinsic Asthma

Many crude extracts of antigens are known to stimulate both reaginic and precipitating antibody. Moulds such as *Candida albicans* and *Aspergillus fumigatus*, respiratory bacteria, and foods, especially eggs and milk, are common examples. The molecular nature of the antigen not only influences the type of antibody produced but also its specificity. For instance, precipitins to some antigenic protein fractions are the more specific while polysaccharide components, certainly in the case of moulds, are frequently shared by unrelated species and so give rise to production of cross reacting antibody (Longbottom & Pepys, 1964).

Factors other than the molecular structure of antigens are also important in determining the type of antibody induced. They include the route of antigenic administration and the propensity of the part of the host to produce different types of antibodies.

Antibody

It is now known that reaginic antibody is formed in the lymphoid tissue of the upper respiratory tract and in plasma cells of the bronchial and gastro-intestinal mucosa (Ishizaka & Ishizaka, 1970). It is therefore understandable that inhalation or ingestion of antigens is especially liable to induce this type of antibody. For example, inhalation of grass pollen in atopic subjects tends to produce reagin while intracutaneous injection tends to promote IgG antibody. The latter having a higher avidity for antigen than IgE, may successfully compete for antigen and act as 'blocking' antibody, resulting in so-called 'desensitization' of the host (Stanworth, 1971).

Reaginic antibody has recently been fully characterised, following its solation in a patient with IgE multiple myeloma (Johansson, 1967). This antibody is now known to belong to a separate immunoglobulin class (Ishizaka, Ishizaka & Hornbrook, 1966; Johansson, Bennich & Wide, 1968), termed IgE (WHO, 1968). It is non-agglutinating and non-precipitating by standard laboratory procedures, does not fix complement and is present in very low amounts in serum. Hence in the past, *in vitro* tests for its measurement have been unsuccessful. Its capacity to bind to cell surfaces determines its cell sensitising properties, and thus its role in the Type I response. It must be recognised however, that this is not a unique property of IgE; other types of antibody, especially IgG, have recently been shown to mediate an immediate type of skin response (Parish, 1970). Whether IgG cell sensitising antibody is ever responsible for bronchial reactions is not yet established, but this is certainly a possibility since Parish has demonstrated a Type I skin response with IgG antibodies to milk, a well recognised allergen, especially in childhood asthma.

IgE reaginic antibody is a normal immunoglobulin in man and is found in minute amounts in the serum of healthy individuals (<500 ng/ml). It has been found increased (>700 ng/ml) in 63 per cent of a series of patients with skin test-positive asthma. It is also increased in children with 'atopic' eczema, and very high levels have been found in Nigerian children, relating to the high incidence of ascaris and other helminth infestations. Specific IgE to individual antigens can now be measured quantitatively by radio immuno assay (Wide, Bennich & Johansson, 1967) and the correlation between clinical symptoms of asthma or rhinitis, prick skin test reactivity, bronchial and nasal challenge tests and the serum level of specific IgE has been shown in the case of grass pollen and *D. pteronyssinus*, to be remarkably close (Stenius & Wide, 1969; McAllan, Assem & Maunsell, 1970; Stenius *et al.*, 1971).

Certain individuals have a propensity to produce IgE and this is at least in part genetically determined. Coca (1922) recognised the hereditary factors in clinical allergy and used the word 'atopy' to define 'a type of hypersensitivity peculiar to man subject to hereditary influence presenting the characteristic immediate type reaction, having circulating antibody reagin and manifesting peculiar clinical symptoms such as asthma and hay fever'. Pepys (1969) has shown that highly atopic individuals tend to develop asthma at an early age and that the age of onset of asthmatic symptoms is related to the number of positive skin tests, irrespective of the age at the time of testing: positive skin tests to more than three antigens were found in his series of patients in 70 per cent of those with symptoms starting before the age of five years, but in only 10 per cent of those in whom symptoms developed after the age of 30 years. In several studies it has been shown that atopic subjects with multiple skin sensitivities developing reaginic antibody and asthmatic symptoms are more readily sensitized to new antigens, than their non-atopic counterparts, when exposed for the first time in adult life. Examples of this have been seen with locust antigen (Frankland, 1953), cotton dust (Voisin *et al.*, 1966), gum arabic (Fowler, 1952; Turiaf *et al.*, 1966), and probably also proteolytic enzymes (Greenberg, Milne & Watt, 1970), although in this instance the majority of 'atopic' individuals were sensitive to a single antigen only, namely *D. farinae*.

Antigen–antibody interaction

It is the binding of IgE antibody to the surface of certain cells which determines both the immediate weal and flare response on prick testing and the immediate increase of airways resistance on bronchial challenge.

Evidence recently summarised by Ishizaka & Ishizaka (1971) shows that IgE binds through the Fc portion of the molecule to sites on the surfaces of certain cells, particularly mast cells and basophils. Allergen reacting with Fab portions of two adjacent antibody molecules activates the release of vasoactive substances from the cytoplasmic granules of these cells. This immune reaction does not destroy the mast cells, and with time, the cytoplasmic granules reform and may be stimulated to discharge again. Humoral mediators thus released, act on the bronchial wall and cause the pathological features of the asthmatic response; vasodilation with exudation of serous fluid and cells, especially eosinophils, mucosal oedema, basement membrane thickening and shedding of the epithelium, increased mucous gland secretion and smooth muscle contraction with eventual muscle hypertrophy (Dunnill, Massarella & Anderson, 1969).

The varying degree of sensitization of mast cells in the skin on the one hand, and the bronchial mucosa on the other, may account for some patients with negative skin tests but positive bronchial challenge tests, and vice versa. It should also be noted that the influence of certain drugs on the skin and bronchial Type I reactions is somewhat different. Antihistamines given locally or systemically by any route, effectively block the Type I skin reaction but have little effect on bronchial asthma and are of no practical value in the treatment of the majority of cases. However, disodium cromoglycate, although having no antihistamine or anti-inflammatory properties, injected locally into the skin inhibits the immediate skin reaction, and given by inhalation also blocks the immediate bronchial reaction (Cox, 1967). Corticosteroids have no effect on immediate skin reactions but effectively block asthma due to inhaled allergens.

Asthma Induced by Precipitating IgG Antibody

Although wheeze developing within a few minutes of challenge is the usual response to inhaled allergens in a sensitized subject, under certain circumstances asthmatic symptoms may develop after an interval of several hours from the time of antigenic exposure. This is the so called 'late' asthmatic response or perhaps better termed 'intermission' asthma.

In this chapter we shall use the word 'intermission' asthma to describe the clinical features of these patients, but when referring to experimental challenge tests we have retained the words 'late asthmatic response' because it corresponds in many cases (see below) to the late skin test reaction thought to reflect an arthus type reaction. Intermission asthma is used in preference to 'late' asthma because it is more clearly distinguished from *late onset* asthma, meaning asthma developing for the first time in later life. Late onset asthma may be induced by many different sorts of immunological and non-immunological mechanisms. In bronchial challenge tests a late fall in the forced expiratory volume is one second, often accompanied by clinical wheeze, has been observed with *Aspergillus fumigatus*, *Micropolyspora faeni*, proteolytic enzymes extracted from *B. subtilis* and avian protein antigens (Pepys, 1969). It is probable that this late fall in FEV_1 reflects an increase in airways resistance, and not a restrictive ventilatory defect, because it is immediately reversible at least in part by sympathomimetic bronchodilator drugs and a fall in FEV_1/FVC ratio is seen in some cases.

FEATURES OF INTERMISSION ASTHMA WITH AND WITHOUT OTHER LUNG DISEASE CONTRASTED WITH THOSE OF EXTRINSIC ALLERGIC ALVEOLITIS

Clinical	Pathology	Radiography	Ventilatory Defect			Precipitins	Probable Tissue Response	Antigens
			Restrictive	Obstructive				
				Immediate	Late			
I Extrinsic allergic alveolitis *without* asthma	Granuloma with giant cells, alveolar wall thickening extending to bronchioles, lymphoid tissue and germinal centres and plasma cells prominent	Widespread mottling	+	−	−	+	Type III	Micropolyspora Faeni, Avian proteins, Porcine pituitary and serum proteins, A. Clavatus, A. Fumigatus, Sitophilus Granarius, also antigens of mouldy Bagasse, mushroom compost, mouldy oakbark, Cryptostroma, etc.
II Extrinsic allergic alveolitis *with* intermission *asthma*	Granuloma, alveolar wall thickening. ? Changes in bronchial walls	Widespread mottling	+	often −	+	+	Type III (+ ? Type I)	Micropolyspora Faeni, Avian proteins
III Pulmonary Eosinophilia and intermission *asthma*	Eosinophilic pneumonia and bronchial wall damage	Transient segmental shadows	−	+	+	+	Type I + Type III	A. Fumigatus (and ? C. Albicans)
IV Intermission asthma alone	Unknown	No abnormality	−	+ (variable)	+	+*	Unknown	Proteolytic enzymes Cotton dust Canadian red cedar Platinum salts. Flux
	Unknown	No abnormality	−	−	+	−	Unknown	

* Precipitins commonly found but correlate poorly with asthma.

In some of these patients specific precipitating IgG antibody can be demonstrated and on skin testing with the appropriate antigen a late (4–6 hour) 'Arthus' Type III reaction can be demonstrated, having the same time-relationships as the late bronchial reaction after challenge. On this evidence Pepys (1967) has suggested that in some instances asthma developing after a latent interval of several hours may be mediated by IgG precipitating antibody.

In some individuals with intermission asthma relating to avian protein and aspergillus hypersensitivity, intracutaneous testing has shown an immediate Type I skin reaction in addition to the late 4 hour response, and Pepys (1969) has suggested that for the development of intermission asthma an additional Type I 'conditioning' reaction is necessary. Evidence supporting this suggestion comes from the blocking effect of disodium cromoglycate on challenge tests and from experimental studies. Disodium cromoglycate is thought to act principally upon the Type I response preventing release of histamine and yet it will effectively block both the immediate and late asthmatic components in subjects sensitized to avian protein (Pepys et al., 1968). Cochrane (1963) has provided experimental support for this suggestion by demonstrating that circulating antigen–antibody complexes were only precipitated at local sites after an independently induced anaphylactic, reagin mediated reaction.

Intermission asthma has been observed as a feature in three different clinical groups of patients; those in which alveolitis is a usual concomitant feature; those in which there is associated pulmonary eosinophilia (i.e. transient pulmonary shadows and blood eosinophilia) and those in which there is no alveolar tissue reaction (Table 5.2).

When late asthmatic reactions are being sought in challenge tests with antigens known to induce alveolitis, it is obvious that care has to be taken in the interpretation of the observed fall in vital capacity, to distinguish between the restrictive defect of alveolitis and airways obstruction.

Late asthmatic reactions associated with pulmonary eosinophilia are seen most characteristically in *Aspergillus fumigatus* hypersensitivity (see page 161) and here high levels of IgE in addition to specific IgG are found. The intradermal skin test usually shows a dual reaction (with high degrees of sensitization, dual reactions may be seen following prick tests) with an immediate and late component. Challenge tests usually show an immediate as well as late fall in FEV_1.

Intermission asthma without an alveolar component (i.e. neither alveolar nor pulmonary eosinophilia infiltrations) is found with a number of agents and although precipitating antibody has been identified in some instances, such as patients exposed to proteolytic enzymes and to cotton dust (Massoud & Taylor, 1964) the correlation with the late asthmatic symptoms is usually not close, perhaps because the appropriate antigenic fraction for identification of specific antibody has not yet been identified. In other instances intermission asthma has been observed and reproduced on challenge tests but precipitating antibody has not yet been identified. Examples include intermission asthma due to Canadian red cedar (Gandevia & Milne, 1970), flux asthma (Sterling, 1967) and platinum salts (Pickering, in press).

Cotton dust asthma

Byssinosis occurs in factory workers especially in the carding rooms after years of exposure. The symptoms are characteristic; chest tightness and wheeze with cough and dyspnoea occurring after the first day back at work after the weekend break. At first the symptoms are confined to the first day only, but with continued exposure they may persist to the second or third day, eventually persisting the whole week. Wheeze and dyspnoea are the chief clinical features and physiological assessment shows airways obstruction (McKerrow et al., 1958). The chest radiograph however remains normal.

Although the delayed onset of asthmatic symptoms suggests an allergic basis for byssinosis, clear evidence for this has not yet been obtained. Detailed skin tests observing both immediate and late responses to different cotton extracts has shown a high proportion of positive reactions in the control groups as well as the affected, and in the non-affected but exposed factory workers (Cayton, Furness & Maitland, 1952). Bouhuys, Lindell & Lundin (1960) have demonstrated the development of airways obstruction on inhalation challenge of cotton extracts in normal unexposed subjects, and on this basis, and in vitro studies on chopped lung, have suggested that cotton extracts may act as histamine liberators. However, the time relationships of 'Monday morning fever' are not readily explained on this basis.

Proteolytic enzymes and asthma

'Biological' washing powders containing certain proteolytic enzymes, especially alcalase, are prepared from cultures of B. subtilis as the enzyme source. Recent reports have demonstrated that many workers in this industry become sensitized when exposed to high concentrations, developing both skin sensitizing antibody and precipitins (Pepys et al., 1969; Gandevia, 1970). Some patients develop immediate asthmatic symptoms and others inter-mission asthma, often during the night following exposure on the previous day. The correlations between measurements of the allergic response and symptoms varies in different reports—a poor correlation being found by Mitchell and Gandevia (1971), but a reasonable correlation between positive skin tests, the presence of asthmatic symptoms and of IgG precipitating antibodies being demonstrated by Newhouse, Tagg & Pocock (1970).

Two reports (Greenburg et al., 1970; Newhouse et al., 1970) suggest that 'atopic' subjects are more liable to develop symptoms than non-atopics, but as the definitions of 'atopy' in the two studies were quite different, the point remains unsettled.

Skin and bronchial challenge tests have shown that proteolytic enzymes may induce immediate, late or dual skin responses, and bronchial reactions with similar time relationships (Pepys et al., 1969).

Whether proteolytic enzymes cause permanent damage to the lung is still unproven. Gandevia & Mitchell (1970) have described persistent fine rales in some heavily exposed workers accompanied by some decrease in lung compliance, but without radiographic changes. If this work is confirmed it suggests that a peripheral bronchiolitis, perhaps with accompanying alveolitis, may occur in occasional individuals. Sensitization of housewives using domestic preparations of biological washing powders is considered to be very unlikely, but a few cases of asthma have been reported (Belin *et al.*, 1970).

Asthma related to Canadian red cedar

Occasionally, carpenters exposed to sawdust of the Canadian red cedar develop asthma some hours after exposure. In the small number of reports so far published these subjects are not atopic, have no immediate skin or bronchial response, but develop a late bronchial reaction without alveolitis. Although precipitins to a number of other conifers have been identified, components of the Canadian red cedar have not yet been implicated in these patients (Gandevia & Milne, 1970).

Asthma in Which the Agents are Unknown

Intrinsic asthma

There remains for discussion a group of patients who develop asthma, usually in adult life, and often associated with a pronounced blood eosino-philia, in whom no external agent can be identified either from a detailed clinical history or on skin testing to a large range of common allergens. The term 'intrinsic' has been applied to this type of asthma to distinguish these patients from those in whom an extrinsic cause can be established, or seems probable (Rackemann, 1947). For clinical purposes intrinsic asthma may be *defined* as that type of asthma in which no extrinsic cause is suggested by the history and in which the skin tests are negative.

It is probable that intrinsic asthma defined in this way represents a heterogeneous group and that a number of different aetiological factors will be found important in individual cases. In some cases it is theoretically possible, although not yet demonstrated, that reaginic sensitisation of the bronchus, but not of the skin, may be important. However, in a personal series of cases, studied in collaboration with Assem, nasal and bronchial challenge to the commonest allergens, house dust and pollens, proved negative in a carefully selected group of skin test negative asthmatics. In others the explanation may depend upon the reaginic sensitisation to ubiqui-tous and unidentified allergens omitted in routine selections of skin testing agents.

Further systematic study of specific immunoglobulins directed against antigens, especially those liable to be overlooked from the history, such as bacterial, viral, or those derived from foods may prove rewarding.

Thus so far we have only fragmentary information about the immuno-logical responses in intrinsic asthma. Before this problem is fully elucidated, wide ranging possibilities will have to be considered. For instance the inter-play between normal and abnormal bronchomotor 'tone' or reactivity and immunological events has not yet been explored and it is possible that in intrinsic asthma there develops an imbalance in nervous control of bronchial smooth muscle against which very minor immunological reactions trigger an asthmatic response.

That intrinsic asthma cannot be accounted for entirely on the basis of overlooked allergens causing reaginic sensitisation, is suggested by the number of clinical differences seen when patients with intrinsic and extrinsic asthma are compared (Table 5.3).

TABLE 5.3

EXTRINSIC AND INTRINSIC ASTHMA CONTRASTED

Extrinsic	Defining Criteria	*Intrinsic*
Known external allergens	Defining	No known external allergens
Positive immediate skin responses	Criteria	Negative skin tests
IgE raised in 60% of subjects		IgE normal or low
Onset usually in childhood or early adult life		Onset usually but not invariably in older adults
Intermittent asthma		More continuous asthma
Wide range of severity of asthma in different individuals		Asthma often severe
Other allergies (hayfever and eczema) often present		Other allergies uncommon
Family history of multiple allergies (asthma, hayfever, eczema) common		Family history of multiple allergies uncommon
Aspirin sensitivity and nasal polyps less common		Aspirin sensitivity and nasal polpys more common in some reports
Complicating pulmonary eosinophilia usually due to *A. fumigatus* hypersensitivity		Pulmonary eosinophilia often unrelated to *A. fumigatus*

NOTE: Blood and sputum eosinophilia common in BOTH groups.

Of particular importance is the observation that total IgE levels are low or normal in intrinsic asthma (Johansson, 1967). This observation has been confirmed in a recent study, but although total serum IgE levels were normal, about half the cases showed evidence of increased IgE and IgG coating of their leucocytes (Assem *et al.*, 1971) in a way similar to that found in extrinsic asthmatic patients (Assem & McAllen, 1970). In another recent study, the effect of disodium cromoglycate on the blockade of exercise asthma was investigated and found to be more effective in extrinsic asthma (Silverman, 1971). Thus at the present time there is apparent conflict between certain studies suggesting indirectly that the immunological mechanisms of intrinsic and extrinsic asthma may be similar, and other evidence suggesting that there are immunological differences.

In one study, gastric and thyroid antibodies and antinuclear antibodies were found more commonly in intrinsic asthmatics than in extrinsics, matched for age and sex with non-asthmatic controls (Hall *et al.*, 1966). Smooth muscle antibody has also been found more frequently in intrinsic asthmatics (Turner Warwick & Haslam, 1970) and many patients having this type of auto-antibody also had antinuclear factor or thyroid antibodies in addition. It seems probable that this finding is a reflection of a generally heightened immunological responsiveness and that it has no specific bearing on aetiology.

PULMONARY EOSINOPHILIA

The term 'pulmonary eosinophilia' refers to those clinical conditions characterised by pulmonary infiltration of various types together with a blood eosinophilia. Asthma is associated with some types of pulmonary eosinophilia but is notably absent in others. A clinical classification is suggested in Table 5.4.

TABLE 5.4

A CLINICAL CLASSIFICATION OF PULMONARY EOSINOPHILIA

	Extrinsic Asthma (allergens)	*Intrinsic Asthma* (unknown allergens)
Pulmonary eosinophilia WITH asthma	Moulds *Aspergillus fumigatus* *Candida albicans* (rare)	

	Known Extrinsic Agents	*Unknown Agents*
Pulmonary eosinophilia WITHOUT asthma	Moulds *Aspergillus fumigatus* Helminths Ascaris Toxocara Schistosoma Drugs Nitrofurantoin Gold, PAS, etc.	

Clinical features of pulmonary eosinophilia in extrinsic asthma

This is probably the most common complication of extrinsic asthma. The patients develop a marked blood eosinophilia, often between 1000 and 2000 per mm³, accompanied by transient and rapidly clearing, ill defined, non-segmental radiographic shadows, with or without increase in their asthmatic symptoms. These shadows may be seen occurring in rapid succession or simultaneously in different areas of one or both lungs. They may recur frequently over a period of months or years and then cease to occur spontaneously. They are uncommon in children and occur especially frequently during the winter months. During such episodes, characteristic plugs of rubbery firm mucus may be expectorated, in which aspergillus mycelium may be identified with appropriate silver stains.

Mycelial plugs have been identified on bronchograms and tomograms, lodged in the proximal branches of segmental bronchi, and at this site a characteristic proximal bronchiectasis may develop leaving the more peripheral parts of the bronchial tree normal. The proximal bronchiectasis probably occurs as a result of local tissue damage caused by a Type III Arthus reaction in the bronchial wall, between localised mould antigen and precipitating antibody. The immunopathogenesis of the transient peripheral shadows is somewhat less clear. In some instances, especially those with segmental features, the shadows are due to pulmonary collapse following obstruction by mucus plugs; others showing no evidence of collapse, cannot be accounted for on such a mechanical basis, and in the very occasional biopsies that have been done on these, the alveoli are shown to be packed with eosinophils. These histological features, together with the very rapid clearing, suggests that the peripheral eosinophilic infiltration may perhaps represent a Type I reagin mediated reaction occurring in the alveoli.

While complete clearing of the peripheral lesions is usual, in some, residual scarring occurs, resulting in patchy pulmonary fibrosis. This is particularly common in the upper lobes which may become contracted and easily mistaken for healed pulmonary tuberculosis (Henderson, 1968). Residual persisting radiographic abnormalities related to bronchiectasis may also be seen (McCarthy & Simon, 1970).

Pulmonary eosinophilia due to *Aspergillus fumigatus* can usually be suppressed by corticosteroids, but is usually not effectively treated by disodium cromoglycate. Eradication of the fungus is not usually possible by inhalation of antifungal agents, such as brilliant green, Nystatin and Natamycin but newer antifungal agents, currently on trial may prove to be useful in the future. Desensitisation to *A. fumigatus* has not proved successful because repeated intracutaneous inoculation of antigen causes a progressive increase in local reaction at the inoculation site.

Pulmonary eosinophilia in intrinsic asthma

Although occasional patients with skin test negative asthma develop pulmonary eosinophilia related to infestation with *Aspergillus fumigatus*, this mould cannot be incriminated on skin testing, challenge or serological tests in the majority of intrinsic asthmatics developing pulmonary eosinophilia. While the cause of intrinsic pulmonary eosinophilia remains unknown it can be distinguished from that due to *A. fumigatus* by a number of clinical features. The patients are frequently more severely ill with fever and malaise, there is often greater respiratory distress, the blood sedimentation rate is frequently high and the eosinophilia marked. Counts of 2000 or greater are common. The radiographic shadows are often more widespread and more peripheral, and in the few cases in which bronchograms have been done these have proved normal. There have been no published reports on total IgE levels in intrinsic pulmonary eosinophilia, but in a personal series while this was high in occasional cases, in the majority they were normal, suggesting once again that while a few cases may be related to unidentified extrinsic allergens, many are not due to reaginic sensitisation.

The histological features of pulmonary eosinophilia found in skin test negative patients, fall into three groups (Carrington *et al.*, 1969). Some show an eosinophilic pneumonia without vascular involvement, and others show pulmonary vasculitis in addition. Still others have associated systemic vasculitis and may then be classified as polyarteritis nodosa.

Pulmonary eosinophilia without asthma

A number of circulating agents have been identified which cause pulmonary eosinophilia without asthma and different immunological features have been observed depending on the nature of the agent.

Helminth infestations. Lung disease induced by a variety of circulating helminth antigens displays several different immunological features. The larvae of *Ascaris lumbricoides*, circulating to the lungs, commonly cause the clinical syndrome of pulmonary eosinophilia, usually without asthma (Loeffler's syndrome). In these patients there is often a high blood eosinophilia, high circulating total IgE (Johanssen, Mellbin & Vahlquist, 1968), and an immediate skin reaction with appropriate extracts (Kent, 1960). However, IgG antibody can also be demonstrated by haemoagglutination (Oliver-Gonzales, 1954) and precipitation (Kent, 1960). It seems probable that the pulmonary lesions are due to a Type I and Type III response. The clinical picture of pulmonary disease due to Toxocara canis is rather different, with intermittent fever, widespread nodular or diffuse shadows and breathlessness, with or without asthma but associated with enlargement of the liver and hypergammaglobulinaemia (Woodruff, 1971). A blood eosinophilia is usually present and skin tests giving immediate (Woodruff, Bissera & Bowe, 1966) and delayed (Duguid, 1961) responses have been reported, presumably related to different preparations of antigen. Circulating IgG antibodies have also been detected by complement fixation and immunofluorescent methods. These findings suggest that immunopathogenesis may depend on a Type I + Type III and/or Type IV response, but the relative importance of the various types of antibody and cellular sensitisation in the production of *pulmonary* lesions in toxocara infection is not yet clearly defined. Schistosomiasis is yet another example of a helminth induced pulmonary eosinophilia where immunopathogenesis has to be worked out.

The antigen responsible for the clinical syndrome of tropical eosinophilia presenting with breathlessness, usually without asthma, but with widespread bilateral fine shadows and a high blood eosinophilia occurring especially in certain parts of Asia has not yet been identified. Microfilariae have been found in the circulation in some of these patients (Danaraj, 1958), but their causative role in pathogenesis has not been conclusively demonstrated. Indirect evidence suggests that reaginic antibody is likely to be important, but whether other immune responses are involved is unproven.

Pulmonary eosinophilia due to drugs. The immune responses induced by drugs in hypersensitivity reactions are incompletely understood.

Pulmonary and blood eosinophilia with transient radiographic shadows has been reported with a large number of drugs including PAS (Wold & Zahn, 1956), penicillin (Reichlin, Loveless & Kane, 1953), *Myocrisin* (Rodman, Fraimow & Myerson, 1958) and arsenic (see also review by Davies, 1969). Nitrofurantoin is of particular interest because pulmonary eosinophilia occurs as an acute hypersensitivity, but if the drug is continued the pulmonary changes may become irreversible since an established diffuse pulmonary fibrosis develops which is then indistinguishable from cryptogenic fibrosing alveolitis (Nicklaus & Snyder, 1968).

Intrinsic pulmonary eosinophilia without asthma

A blood eosinophilia associated with widespread pulmonary involvement, but without asthma, is also seen in patients with polyarteritis nodosa (Rose & Spencer, 1957) where the causal agent remains unknown, and until recently evidence as to the nature of the immunological disturbance has been lacking. However, Gocke *et al.* (1970) demonstrated circulating Australian antigen in 4 of 11 patients with polyarteritis, vascular deposition of immune complexes and low levels of complement during the acute stage. These four cases however, did not appear to have had pulmonary involvement, and a case of pulmonary eosinophilia and systemic polyarteritis related to Australian antigen is yet to be reported.

The association between polyarteritis nodosa and Wegener's granuloma has often been suggested (Fahey *et al.*, 1954), but again the nature of the presumed immunological disturbance is unknown.

EXTRINSIC ALLERGIC ALVEOLITIS

Inhalation of certain organic dusts, usually in non-atopic subjects, has been found to induce, in certain individuals, an acute inflammatory reaction in the peripheral parts of the lung. The classical example of this reaction is farmers' lung (Fuller, 1953; Dickie & Rankin, 1958). Farmers exposed to mouldy hay, particularly while clearing hay barns towards the end of winter, develop, after a latent period of 4–6 hours, cough and breathlessness often accompanied by fever, malaise and limb pains. All of these symptoms have been reproduced by bronchial challenge using extracts of mouldy hay or the thermophylic actimomycete, *Micropolyspora faeni* (Williams, 1963). Circulating IgG precipitating antibody to these antigens was identified in 89 per cent of 205 farmers with such symptoms (Pepys & Jenkins, 1965).

A similar clinical pattern is also seen in subjects exposed to a wide variety of other organic dusts often containing microflora, and a list of some of the best authenticated examples of these is shown on Table 5.5.

TABLE 5.5

SOME ORGANIC DUST ANTIGENS IN EXTRINSIC ALLERGIC
ALVEOLITIS

Disease	Antigen
Farmers' lung	*Micropolyspora faeni* (and other actinomycetes)
Bagassosis	Mouldy bagasse (Thermoactinomyces Sacchari).
Mushroom pickers' lung	? Thermophilic actinomycetes
Malt workers' lung	*A. fumigatus, A. clavatus*
Wheat weevil disease	*Sitophilus granarius*
Bird breeders' lung	Avian serum proteins
Pituitary snuff takers' lung	Heterologous serum protein and pituitary antigens
Suberosis	Fungal contaminants of cork dust

Well-documented examples of antigens causing extrinsic allergic alveolitis with characteristic clinical, challenge and serological features, besides farmers' lung and avian protein hypersensitivity (Reed, Sosman & Barbee, 1965; Riddle *et al.*, 1968) are *Aspergillus clavatus* in malt workers, *Sitophilus granarius* in mill workers (Lunn & Hughes, 1967), mouldy bagasse in sugar cane workers (Hargreave, Pepys & Holford Strevens, 1968), mushroom compost dust in mushroom workers (Sakula, 1967), heterologous porcine protein and pituitary antigens in pituitary snuff takers (Pepys *et al.*, 1966) and mouldy oak bark in cork workers (Avila & Villar, 1968). There is an increasing list of other antigens, especially moulds inhaled in large amounts in certain occupations, which probably cause similar reactions but in which the evidence is less complete and some of the clinical, radiographic and pathological features are atypical. The term 'extrinsic allergic alveolitis' (Pepys, 1969) has been given to this group of pulmonary diseases which have similar clinical, pathological and immunological features.

Detailed studies on avian protein hypersensitivity (bird fanciers' lung) have proved valuable in our understanding of the immunopathology of this group of diseases, and on the basis of the skin test responses, together with the results of challenge tests, Pepys and his co-workers have suggested that the intrapulmonary response is due to a Type III reaction (Hargreave et al., 1966; Pepys, 1969).

While prick tests are often negative in patients with bird fanciers' lung, intracutaneous skin tests usually show an immediate reaction followed after an interval of 4–6 hours by a large oedematous non-irritant swelling which subsides over the next few hours. Biopsies of the late reaction show perivascular collections of mainly mononuclear inflammatory cells, and immunofluorescent studies show perivascular 'granular' collections of immunoglobulin and complement, at first outside cells, but in later biopsies, contained within the cytoplasm of inflammatory cells (Pepys et al., 1968). These features suggest that complement fixing antigen–antibody complexes are formed in tissue spaces and are taken up into phagocytic cells. These findings provide supporting evidence that late skin reactions are due to an 'Arthus' Type III reaction. Polymorphs and fibrinoid necrosis were not prominent in these skin biopsies, probably because the dose of antigen was far less than is commonly given in animal experiments.

Bronchial challenge with avian protein causes systemic and focal pulmonary signs and symptoms, having the same time relationship as the late skin reaction (Hargreave et al., 1966), suggesting that the pulmonary response is also a Type III Arthus reaction. The histological features of the lesions found in bird fanciers' lung require explanation. In lung biopsies from acute cases, the characteristic lesions are small granulomata scattered through the alveolar walls and in the walls of small bronchi, and are not those characteristic of Arthus type lesions seen in experimental animals. However, Spector & Heesom (1969) have shown in animal experiments that the histological response of tissues depends on the proportion of antigen and precipitating antibody, and that when complexes form in equivalence, granulomata can indeed be demonstrated. Cellular hypersensitivity resulting in Type IV reactions may also play an important associated role in determining the granulomatous rather than the typical Arthus type of histological pattern.

Clinical features of extrinsic allergic alveolitis

Acute exposure. Patients with intermittent exposure to antigen tend to have a different clinical presentation from those with continuous low dosage exposure, such as is found in those exposed to domestic budgerigars (parakeet in the U.S.A.). Sensitised individuals subjected to occasional heavy exposure, for example, farmers exposed to mouldy hay, develop systemic symptoms of fever and malaise often accompanied by limb pains 4–6 hours after exposure; respiratory symptoms include an unproductive cough, tightness in the chest and breathlessness. A pyrexia of 100–101°F (38–39°C) is typical and in severe cases cyanosis may be seen. On examination of the chest basal crepitations may be heard but usually no rhonchi. Functionally there is a restrictive ventilatory defect *without evidence of airways obstruction*. The total lung volume is reduced, the forced vital capacity in one second may approximate to the total forced vital capacity and the peak expiratory flow remains normal.

The transfer factor (T_{LCO}) is reduced. The arterial P_{O_2} may fall while increase in ventilation maintains a normal or low P_{CO_2}.

The chest radiograph shows a widespread nodular shadowing in the acute stages often most prominent in the middle zones. The size of the nodules is variable, ranging from a 'ground glass' appearance to more discrete nodules of 2–3 mm.

If further antigenic exposure is avoided the symptoms and signs subside. While the acute and systemic respiratory symptoms abate within 24–36 hours, the abnormal auscultatory sounds and the radiographic and physiological changes resolve more gradually over a two to three week period in the majority of cases without treatment. In a minority however, changes may persist in spite of withdrawal of antigen. In these, treatment with cortico-steroids usually leads to complete resolution. Evidently further exposure to antigen should be avoided, but as practical advice to small-holding farmers this is often difficult or impossible to achieve in practice.

Chronic exposure. In patients exposed more continuously to low doses of antigen, symptoms develop insidiously and these patients frequently present

TABLE 5.6

EXTRINSIC ALLERGIC ALVEOLITIS CONTRASTED WITH
CRYPTOGENIC FIBROSING ALVEOLITIS

		Extrinsic Allergic Alveolitis	Cryptogenic Fibrosing Alveolitis
Clinical			
Symptoms	Breathlessness	Yes	Yes
Signs	Clubbing	±	+ or + + (60%)
	Crepitations	±	+ +
X-ray		Upper lobes (especially)	Lower lobes (especially)
Physiology	Restrictive defect	Yes	Yes
Pathology			
Acute	Granuloma	Yes	No
	Giant cells	Yes	No
	Inclusions	Yes	No
	Alveolar wall infiltration	Patchy	Diffuse
	Desquamative pneumonia	No	Some cases
Chronic	Wall fibrosis	Yes (patchy)	Yes
	Honeycombing	Yes	Yes
	Plasma cells	+ + +	+
	Lymphoid follicles	+ + +	+
Immunology			
Circulating antibody		Precipitins	Autoantibodies
Antibody formation in the lung		Yes	Yes
Pathogenesis		Probably Arthus Type III	Uncertain ? Immune complex in some

with advanced irreversible fibrotic changes in the lung (Pepys, 1969). Breathlessness is the commonest symptom, sometimes accompanied by cough. Signs in the chest however, may be slight, crepitations are often scanty and finger clubbing is usually absent or slight; these features contrast with those found in cryptogenic fibrosing alveolitis (Table 5.6.)

The chest radiograph shows widespread irregular shadows often more prominent in the upper zones and associated with contraction of the upper lobes (McCarthy, Simon & Hargreave, 1970). Within the shadowing, 'honeycombing' with small transradient areas 2–10 mm in diameter may be observed, correlating with destructive and fibrotic changes in the respiratory bronchioles and alveoli. Even with this clinical evidence of destruction, some improvement may be observed with corticosteroids, because acute granulomatous lesions may co-exist with old scarring, especially if antigenic exposure continues.

In the most advanced cases pulmonary hypertensive cor pulmonale may develop relating to destruction of the capillary bed and to hypoxia, and this can occur without functional evidence of airways obstruction. However, in some cases of chronic extrinsic allergic alveolitis, clinical evidence of airways obstruction is apparent, some cases being attributed to chronic bacterial infection of the distorted bronchi (Hapke *et al.*, 1968).

Combined Type I and Type III reactions in extrinsic allergic alveolitis. Over the past few years and again dependent on the interpretation of skin tests and challenge studies on patients with presumed Type III pulmonary lesions and extrinsic allergic alveolitis, it has become apparent that in occasional individuals an immediate Type I immune response co-exists. This has been noted from the clinical history in patients with farmers' lung who develop immediate wheezing as well as a typical late reaction with a restrictive defect. Challenge studies have confirmed an immediate increase in airways resistance followed by a latent period with subsequent development of a typical restrictive ventilatory defect *without* late airways obstruction.

A combination of immediate airways obstruction (Type I) and a late restrictive defect (Type III) has also been demonstrated on bronchial challenge

TABLE 5.7

THE PATTERNS OF RESPONSE OBSERVED IN SENSITIZED PATIENTS
ON CHALLENGE WITH AVIAN PROTEIN

Antigen	Skin Testing			Challenge		
	Prick	Intracutaneous		Airways Obstruction	Restriction	Airways Obstruction
Avian Protein		Immediate	Late	Immediate	Late	Late
Usual response	−	+	+	−	+	−
Occasional— especially atopics	+	+	+	+	+	−
Occasional— non-atopics	−	+	+	−	+	+

with *Aspergillus clavatus* (Riddle *et al.*, 1968) and *Sitophilus granarius* (Lunn & Hughes, 1967).

ALLERGIC RESPONSES IN THE LUNG TO
ASPERGILLUS FUMIGATUS

Aspergillus fumigatus is the commonest mould associated with human lung disease in the United Kingdom. Its spores of 2μ diameter are constant environmental contaminants in damp climates and are particularly prevalent during the autumn and winter months (McCarthy, 1970). Unlike many other moulds requiring different conditions it can grow within the human bronchial lumen, and this feature results in its persistence as a mycelium in the lung leading to continuous antigenic challenge (Pepys, 1969). Several clinical syndromes result from the different types of immune response stimulated by this fungus under different circumstances (Table 5.8).

TABLE 5.8

IMMUNE RESPONSES TO *ASPERGILLUS FUMIGATUS* IN
PULMONARY DISORDERS

Clinical	Skin Response		Precipitins
	Immediate 10 min	Late 4–8 h	
Fortuitous culture in sputum in normals or patients with any chest disease, including asthma: i.e. a harmless commensal	—	—	—
Type I asthma	+	—	—
Asthma and pulmonary eosinophilia	+	+	+ 1–3 precipitin lines
Asthma with chronic lung changes, especially contracted upper lobes	+	+	+ 1–3 precipitin lines
Mycetoma (aspergilloma)	±	±	+ usually more than 3 lines
Asthma and pulmonary eosinophilia and mycetoma (this clinical picture is uncommon)	+	+	+ more than 3 lines

A. *fumigatus* may be isolated from as many as 10 per cent of routine sputum samples and is not invariably associated with lung disease (Pepys *et al.*, 1959). Subjects from whom these incidental cultures have been obtained show no allergic response to *A. fumigatus*.

In asthmatic subjects *A. fumigatus* sensitivity is common, causing an immediate Type I skin and bronchial response. In these patients reaginic antibody can usually be demonstrated to other common allergens, but occasionally lone sensitisation to *A. fumigatus* is found, and this is more common in asthma presenting in adult life (McCarthy, 1970). In these patients with asthma only, no precipitins are found by standard laboratory methods.

In some atopic asthmatics *A. fumigatus* stimulates production of both reaginic antibody and precipitins, and this is associated with the clinical syndrome of pulmonary eosinophilia (see also page 154). In these patients a dual skin and asthmatic response is seen on bronchial challenge; the immediate fall of FEV_1/FVC is transient but after a latent interval of 4–6 hours there is a more profound and persistent increase in airways resistance which is usually only partially reversible with sympathomimetic drugs. A restrictive ventilatory defect is not observed and there is no radiographic evidence of alveolitis. Total IgE levels are high and associated IgG precipitating antibody to *A. fumigatus* is also demonstrated in over 90 per cent of patients with extrinsic asthma and pulmonary eosinophilia: although in about a quarter of these concentration of serum is necessary. Disodium cromoglycate, which is believed to block the immediate Type I bronchial component, has been shown to prevent the late asthmatic reaction in challenge tests, but is not usually helpful in preventing the transient infiltrations of pulmonary eosinophilia.

Inhalation of *A. fumigatus* has been found in association with *A. clavatus* in high concentrations in non-atopic malt workers but was thought not to contribute to the resulting typical extrinsic allergic alveolitis (Riddle *et al.*, 1968). Features of widespread chronic alveolitis have however been seen in two personal cases with asthma and *A. fumigatus* hypersensitivity.

A. fumigatus infestation is a common complication of sterile cysts or cavities in the lung, especially when they result from healed tuberculosis or infarction. The mycelial mat extends round the cavity and gradually fills it with a ball of fungus. This mode of growth is reflected in the radiograph as a thick walled cavity almost filled by a homogenous mass, except for a characteristic crescentric air space. The aspergilloma is associated with minimal tissue reaction, the fungus growing as a saprophyte on tissue debris lining the pre-existing cavity. In these cases the skin tests are usually negative, but an immediate or late reaction has been reported in about 20 per cent of patients with mycetoma (Longbottom & Pepys, 1964). Precipitating antibody, however, is a constant finding and is characterised by numerous, often 7–10, precipitin lines to crude extracts of aspergillus. There is no evidence that these precipitating antibodies are playing any tissue damaging role in aspergilloma. More probably they simply reflect the presence of persisting antigen in the lung. Precipitins clear after surgical removal of a fungus ball.

A. fumigatus may also cause an invasive infection in the lungs, especially in patients with immune deficiency or paresis from any cause, for instance, those on corticosteroid or immunosuppressant therapy, and in patients with malignant lymphomas or with leukaemia. In some of these patients precipitins have been demonstrated. In immune deficiency disorders fungus infections are particularly common in those with evidence of impairment of cellular immunity, suggesting that protective immunity to fungal infection involves both antibody and sensitized lymphocytes.

IMMUNE RESPONSES TO ORGANISMS
MULTIPLYING IN THE LUNGS

Protective mechanisms

Specific immunological protection of the lungs is directed towards overcoming the different types of invasive properties possessed by multiplying organisms. For instance, the capsular polysaccharide of *Streptococcus pneumoniae* and some strains of *Haemophilus influenzae* and capsular hyaluronic acid of *Staphylococcus pyogenes* act either as a mechanical barrier to host defences or by interference with adsorption of natural opsonins. In other instances the extracellular bacterial toxins, such as the leucocidins of *Staphylococcus pyogenes* may be directly toxic to phagocytes.

Natural *non-specific* protection is offered by the special properties of mucus, respiratory tract epithelium and by wandering phagocytic cells. Mucus helps to prevent invasion of the respiratory tract by inhaled substances in a number of ways—it traps inhaled particles; its normal viscosity, pH and quantitative secretion are essential for synchronised cilial motility, and its lysozyme content acting together with complement, enhances the bacteriolytic action of secreted antibody (Adinolfi *et al.*, 1966). Mucus with entrapped particles is constantly cleared from the lungs by ciliary action of the epithelial cells; particles penetrating the alveoli are taken up by phagocytes which migrate towards the respiratory bronchiole and hence to the cilial escalator. Phagocytosis of inhaled organisms is probably very important in the respiratory tract and many common respiratory pathogens are known to be digested rapidly by intracellular lysozomes.

Understanding of the *specific* allergic mechanisms of host resistance to bacterial organisms of the respiratory tract in human disease are still fragmentary. It is however, known that following infection by certain respiratory pathogens, such as *Streptococcus pneumoniae*, *Haemophilus influenzae*, *Staphylococcus pyogenes* and *Pseudomonas pyocyaneus* precipitating IgG antibody can usually be demonstrated (Burns & May, 1967). Although these antibodies are absent in hypogammaglobulinaemia, and severe recurrent infection by these organisms is frequent in antibody deficiency states, it cannot be assumed that these precipitating antibodies are necessarily involved in the protective immune response. Their presence in chronic bronchitis, associated with persisting infection by these organisms, suggests that the precipitins are either not successful in overcoming or preventing reinfection or that other types of antibody are more important in protective immunity. Indeed it is not yet known whether the precipitins found in infective chronic bronchitis are directly and exclusively bactericidal (acting with or without complement), whether they facilitate phagocytosis or whether in part they are directed against non-toxic antigenic components of bacteria, thus representing markers of infection rather than playing an immediate protective role.

Immune deficiencies involving *selective* deficiency of IgG, IgM and IgA have all been reported, associated with susceptibility to bacterial infection, from which it may be inferred that each may be individually important.

Following a primary bacterial infection, IgM antibodies appear first. These may be especially important for opsonising bacteria, because the active antigenic sites on the IgM molecule react especially against surface components of particulate antigens (Gordon-Smith, 1970). Later, IgG antibodies are formed; these have a higher antigenic affinity and acting in association with complement are capable of destroying antigen. IgA is related especially to protection of the mucous surfaces of the respiratory and alimentary tracts (Tomasi *et al.*, 1965), and has special importance in respiratory infections.

IgA is produced mainly, but not exclusively, in the immunologically competent plasma cells in the lamina propria of the bronchial mucosa (Keimowitz, 1964). It is actively secreted by the respiratory and gastro-intestinal epithelium where an additional peptide chain, the secretory piece, becomes attached to the immunoglobulin molecule. IgA in the secretions of the respiratory tract is of higher molecular weight (11s) and can also be distinguished from 7s serum IgA by the antigenic determinants of the secretory piece. While serum IgA rarely fixes complement, secretory A in the presence of lysosome will do so. Destruction of foreign antigens within the lumen of the bronchi by antibody and complement is thus facilitated.

Some virus neutralising antibodies have been identified as IgA; this antibody prevents intracellular invasion by virus, and it may therefore play an important role in the prevention of viral reinfection.

The role of cellular immunity in protection of the respiratory tract has not yet been worked out in detail. Its importance in protection from viruses is suggested by the frequency of these infections in immune deficiency states involving depression of cellular responses.

In general terms, as cell mediated immunity develops, responsive thymus dependent lymphocytes transform to lymphoblasts which provide cells with three distinct actions: killer cells which destroy cells carrying antigen, antigen sensitive cells which react with antigen to release factors responsible for the manifestations of delayed hypersensitivity and antigen sensitive cells of long life span, responsible for immunological memory (Roitt *et al.*, 1969).

When living organisms invade the lung, humoral and cell mediated immunological reactions develop. These may result in localisation and eradication of infection, i.e. protective immunity, but if they fail to achieve this, active fulminating or chronic slowly progressive hypersensitivity disease may result. The clinical pattern of disease thus in part depends upon the immunological state of the host. Almeida & Waterson (1969) studied antigen and antibody in serum from patients infected with human hepatitis virus and suggested some of the immunological factors determining the clinical outcome. They suggested that a 'carrier' has circulating antigen but no antibody, and no disease; the normal self limiting case of acute hepatitis had immunological responses that are efficient in amount and timing to localise the disease and eradicate the virus; fulminating necrotic disease depends upon an anaphylactic response where larger antigen–antibody complexes are formed in massive quantities during *antibody excess*, when an infection occurs in an immunologically primed individual; chronic and progressive disease is attributed to a prolonged state of *antigen excess* where antibody is formed in sufficient quantity to form immune complexes but is not adequate in amount to eradicate antigen. However, recent work has failed to confirm this attractive hypothesis.

Nevertheless this concept could account for the varying clinical responses seen in other infections, especially where the organism is confined to a single organ, and may by analogy be applicable to the lung.

IMMUNE DEFICIENCY DISEASE

There have been many excellent recent reviews on the immunological aspects of these syndromes and for detailed discussion readers are referred to some of them (Franglen, 1970; Hobbs, 1966, 1970). In this section only clinical aspects of the respiratory problems will be considered.

Broncho-pulmonary symptoms are the commonest presentation of immune deficiency of any type, accounting for 153/518 infective episodes in 82 patients reported by Squire (1962). In his series severe associated nasal sinusitis was frequent, accounting for 109 further episodes. Patients with immune deficiency commonly present with established bronchiectasis and in the past have often undergone lobectomy for this. Symptoms of chronic infected bronchitis are also common, often with persistent or recurring infection by *Haemophilus influenzae*: recurrent and often severe pneumonia due to common bacteria such as *Streptococcus pneumoniae* or *Staphylococcus pyogenes* in the absence of circulating bacterial precipitins is a characteristic presentation, especially in hypogammaglobulinaemia.

The chest radiograph reflects the heritage of these infections, showing irregular peripheral 'scar' shadows and evidence of bronchial wall thickening with or without dilatation, and sometimes pleural shadows as evidence of previous inflammatory involvement. In some patients hilar shadows are prominent reflecting lymph node enlargement. This may form part of a widespread lympho-reticular hypertrophy, perhaps due to stimulation of cellular immune responses to compensate for the deficient humoral immunity. Other evidence of this may be found in associated hepatosplenomegaly.

Rarely, cases have been described showing a widespread nodular infiltration of the lung fields occurring in association with hilar node enlargement and with evidence of widespread systemic granulomata, both in the lungs and other organs. In at least one report, a diagnosis of sarcoidosis was accepted on the basis of a positive Kveim test (Bronsky & Dunn, 1965), while other cases have been Kveim negative. It seems unlikely that the granulomatous response can be accounted for by a cellular reaction to compensate for antibody deficiencies against common respiratory infections because it occurs in only a very small minority of antibody deficient patients. Possibly these granulomas result from persisting infections in antigen excess; alternatively some other component of the immune response is deficient in patients with granulomatous lesions, such as a defect in phagocytic function, but this is unproven.

Other types of immunological disturbance of clinical importance are observed in patients with immune deficiency. Certain diseases regarded as 'auto allergic' have been reported as relatively common (Good, Rolstein & Mazzeiltto, 1957), especially rheumatoid arthritis (Gitlin, Janeway & Craig, 1959), pernicious anaemia (Twomey et al., 1969), haemolytic anaemia (Hobbs, 1968) and systemic lupus erythematosus. In each case the relevant autoantibodies are usually not detected when there is a generalised hypo-gammaglobulinaemia. In selective IgA deficiency, clinical autoimmune disease is not uncommon and was found in 16/69 cases reported by Hobbs (1968), and in these cases the relevant autoantibodies could be detected.

Diarrhoea and malabsorption are also common and may reflect a disturbance of the normal gastro-intestinal bacterial flora, due to the absence of normal protective secretory IgA. Amyloidosis is also described in hypo-gammaglobulinaemia (Teilum, 1964).

While many gross and often familial antibody deficiencies appear in infancy and are rapidly fatal, many non-familial cases present in later childhood or adult life. In these the reduction in immunoglobulin levels may be less profound and may be selective, detectable only by quantitative estimation of individual immunoglobulins. In other cases individual immuno-globulins are present in normal amounts but antigenic challenge suggests that they are qualitatively deficient.

In other cases there is evidence of impairment of cellular immunity in addition to antibody deficiency, and this combined defect is found both in primary familial deficiencies and in patients with so called primary acquired immune deficiency presenting in later life. Impairment of cellular immunity may be suspected at the bedside by the total absence of tonsils (in the absence of previous surgery), and the absence of delayed hypersensitivity responses on skin testing to antigen causing such responses, for example Tuberculin, Candida protein and mumps antigen.

In these mixed types of immune deficiency not only are common pyogenic respiratory tract infections frequent, but in addition patients appear to be susceptible to viral and some fungal infections, such as invasive infection with *Candida Albicans*. Invasive fungal infections of the lung produce very variable radiographic features, but may be suggested by confluent or patchy shadows in the absence of demonstrable bacteria. The fungi can often be identified on culture of sputum. In gross immune deficiency *Pneumocystis* pneumonia may be found. The clinical features of gradually increasing and severe dyspnoea with cyanosis are characteristic and the chest radiograph shows extending widespread shadows often with perihilar concentrations, not dissimilar to a 'batswing' shadowing familiar in pulmonary oedema. Defini-tive diagnosis usually depends on examination of lung tissue but *Pneumocystis* can occasionally be found in tracheal washings. However, this is often impossible in severely ill patients and in some, a therapeutic trial of pent-amidine may be justified when the clinical features are characteristic.

Because patients with impaired cellular immunity have difficulty in handling virus infections, vaccination with live viral or bacterial vaccines is contra-indicated, and the importance of this is emphasised by reports of generalised disseminated vaccinia infection (Keidan, McCarthy & Haworth, 1953) and of disseminated lesions following BCG vaccination (Bouten, Mainwaring & Smithells, 1963).

Repeated lung infections may also be seen in other rare types of deficiency of the immune reaction including, for example, deficiency of the normal complement system and deficiencies in normal phagocytosis, namely, chronic granulomatous disease (Holmes *et al.*, 1970).

CELL MEDIATED HYPERSENSITIVITY IN
RESPIRATORY TRACT INFECTIONS

Sensitization of lymphocytes and their transformation on subsequent antigenic challenge can be demonstrated *pari passu* with antibody formation (Roitt *et al.*, 1969) as part of the complete immune response directed towards a large number of different inhaled antigens.

In certain instances, the classic example being infection by *Myco. tuberculosis* delayed-type hypersensitivity is demonstrated by the Type IV skin reaction after injection of tuberculin, and this response has been shown to be due to thymus dependent lymphocytes derived from the paracortical areas of lymph nodes (Turk, 1967). It is generally believed that the histological lesions forming a tubercle containing epithelioid cells and lymphocytes are the result of delayed hypersensitivity.

In experimental animals resistance to *M. tuberculosis* infection develops at about the same time as delayed hypersensitivity, but is independent of it because desensitization can be achieved with purified protein derivative so that delayed hypersensitivity can no longer be demonstrated, while protection from tuberculous infection persists.

Delayed hypersensitivity reactions may account for the tissue damage due not only to certain microbial protein antigens, such as *M. tuberculosis*, but also to that due to fungal proteins as in histoplasmosis and coccidioidomycosis, blastomycosis and toxoplasmosis. In all of these a Type IV reaction can be identified on skin testing and the basic pathological lesions in the lung resemble those seen in tuberculosis.

Some of the special pulmonary features seen in certain viral infections may also depend upon cellular hypersensitivity. A possible example is the severe varicella pneumonia which occurs in adults and is commonly associated with necrotising nodular lesions which later calcify. Cellular hypersensitivity has also been incriminated in the tissue damage seen in mycoplasma pneumonia (Turk, 1969).

Evidence of lymphocyte sensitisation is now being obtained from *in vitro* studies in lung disorders where humoral antibody formation is prominent, such as pollen sensitive patients with asthma (Brostoff, Greaves & Roitt, 1969) and also in patients whose delayed hypersensitivity has been considered impaired, as in sarcoidosis (Caspary & Field, 1971).

Sarcoidosis

While the pathogenesis of sarcoidosis is not yet understood, there is evidence that patients with sarcoidosis show a number of immunological deviations from control groups.

It has been recognised for more than half a century that the delayed skin reactions to tuberculin may be negative. In published reports the proportion of tuberculin negative cases varies depending on the concentration of the antigen used. In Scadding's series (1967) 68 per cent were negative to 100 TU, but a small percentage were positive to tuberculin in quite low concentrations, 16 per cent giving positive reactions to 10 TU or less. The behaviour of the tuberculin reactivity does not appear to be closely related to the activity of the disease (Israel & Sones, 1965). Delayed skin test responses to other antigens, including mumps virus, *Candida albicans* and *Trichphyton* are reduced in patients with sarcoidosis (Friou, 1952; Citron, 1957). Observations on the effect of corticosteroids on skin sensitivity to tuberculin suggests that in spite of the negative skin response, tuberculin sensitivity is in fact still present, because 50 per cent of tuberculin negative patients gave a positive response when cortisone was added to tuberculin administered intradermally (Citron & Scadding, 1957; Citron, 1957). These results are similar to those obtained in patients with pulmonary tuberculosis who have been desensitised to tuberculin, and contrast with studies on patients with diminished delayed skin responses in various forms of reticulosis who continue to have negative skin tests after cortisone addition to intradermal PPD. In contrast to patients with sarcoidosis those with reticulosis appear to have true impairment of cell mediated immunity (Fairley & Matthias, 1960).

In vitro studies have shown that lymphocytes from patients with sarcoidosis with negative tuberculin tests are nevertheless normally sensitised (Caspary & Field, 1971). Clinical evidence also supports the suggestion that protective cellular immunity in general is not fundamentally impaired since patients with sarcoidosis are not unusually prone to fungal or viral infection.

Antibody formation is not impaired; Type I immediate reactions can be detected in patients with sarcoidosis, and challenge with pertussis or typhoid vaccines and natural responses to staphylococci have all been normal (Greenwood *et al.*, 1958).

Quantitative measurements of total immunoglobulin show that IgA and IgM are increased in some patients with sarcoidosis irrespective of the clinical stage of the disease (Goldstein, Israel & Rawnsley, 1969) suggesting that antibody responses may actually be heightened, and this is reflected in the finding of circulating antibodies to a number of distinct antigens by Caspary & Field (1971). In a series of 150 patients Doniach & Karlish found a normal incidence of thyroid and other autoantibodies, but when present the titres were higher than normal.

Several studies have now confirmed the finding that when patients with sarcoidosis are vaccinated with B.C.G. their tuberculin response remains negative in spite of an apparently normal histological lesion produced at the site of inoculation (Forgacs, McDonald & Skelton, 1957). It would be interesting to know whether the tuberculin test when combined with corticosteroids following B.C.G. is restored to normal and whether lymphocytes from patients with sarcoidosis receiving B.C.G. are apparently normally sensitised to PPD, because this would provide further evidence suggesting that cellular sensitisation in sarcoidosis is normal.

The Kveim reaction in sarcoidosis has bearing both on the aetiology of the syndrome and on the immune status of these patients. Injection of a particulate suspension from human spleen containing sarcoid lesions gives rise to a papule in 3–4 weeks with the histological appearances of a non-caseating granuloma, similar to a naturally occurring sarcoid lesion. A positive Kveim test was found in 84 per cent of biopsy confirmed cases in one series (Silzbach, 1961). The test is most frequently positive in cases with hilar gland enlargement.

The Kveim test is not only positive in cases with clinical features of sarcoidosis but has been reported positive in healthy tuberculin negative subjects failing to convert after two technically satisfactory B.C.G. vaccinations (D'Arcy Hart, Mitchell & Sutherland, 1964). Positive Kveim tests have also been shown in about 50 per cent of a group of patients with Crohn's disease (Mitchell *et al.*, 1969). Recently it has been shown by *in vitro* studies that lymphocytes from patients with sarcoidosis are sensitised to Kveim antigen, once more suggesting that cellular immunity is normal (Caspary & Field, 1971). These workers also showed similar lymphocyte sensitisation in two patients failing to convert after B.C.G. inoculation. Very recently Mitchell *et al.* (1969) have shown that mice injected with human sarcoid material will develop local granuloma and a successful first passage of this agent has now been obtained. If this work is confirmed the likelihood of a transmissible agent being involved in the pathogenesis of sarcoidosis seems to be increased, but even if a transmissible agent is established the explanation of the observed immune responses summarised here still remains to be explained.

IMMUNE RESPONSES IN THE LUNG POSSIBLY RELATED TO CIRCULATING IMMUNE COMPLEXES

Exogenous antigens

Fulminating haemorrhagic pulmonary oedema has been found especially where there are larger amounts of virus or bacteria in the presence of high levels of antibody derived from previous immunisation or infection by the same or a related organism. An example of this is severe measles pneumonia following a natural infection in children previously vaccinated with an inactivated measles virus (Fulginiti *et al.*, 1967), or infants possessing maternal antibody to respiratory syncytial virus (Kapikian *et al.*, 1969). Large amounts of virus with scanty deposits of immunoglobulin have been found by immunofluorescence in severe pneumonia due to respiratory syncytial virus and the possibility of these complexes causing Type III tissue damage has been suggested (Gardner, McQuillin & Court, 1970). Pulmonary oedema occurring in gram negative septicaemia and fulminating pneumonia in patients with viral influenza, are likely further examples of respiratory disease where high levels of antigen and antibody precipitate as immune complexes on vessel walls in the lung, resulting in widespread increase in vascular permeability.

Pulmonary oedema following institution of bactericidal antibiotic therapy, especially in septicaemias after liberation of large amounts of bacterial antigens, may depend upon a similar mechanism.

The possibility of exogenous food antigens reaching the circulation, forming intravascular complexes capable of precipitation in the lung and resulting in immune complex disease is suggested by the following observations. Food antigen may reach the circulation after absorption through the gastro-intestinal tract, either due to abnormal permeability of the mucus membrane due to atrophy as in malabsorption syndromes, or in immune deficiencies in consequence of impaired production of IgA with loss of secretory IgA and diminution of normal protective immunity. A pulmonary syndrome resembling fibrosing alveolitis and associated with a restrictive and diffusion defect has been reported in association with adult coeliac disease (Hood & Mason, 1970), and in this syndrome precipitins to egg have been identified. However, so far adequate histological studies have not been reported. A high incidence of milk antibodies has also been reported in 15 cases with selective IgA deficiency in whom a variety of auto immune disorders were also found (Ammann & Hong, 1970). Although lung disease was not observed in the cases reported by these workers, the association of auto-antibodies with fibrosing alveolitis of unknown cause (to be discussed below) suggests that a further study of food antigens in fibrosing alveolitis might be rewarding. Milk precipitins have also been reported in patients with pulmonary haemosiderosis (Luz & Todd, 1964), but their role in pathogenesis remains speculative.

Endogenous antigens

Tomasi, Fudenberg & Finby (1962) demonstrated circulating immune complexes in patients with high titre rheumatoid factor, rheumatoid arthritis and fibrosing alveolitis, and suggested that deposition of IgG/IgM complexes on the alveolar walls might be responsible for the pulmonary lesion. Evidence of IgG and IgM deposits on capillary walls in a patient with rheumatoid arthritis and fibrosing alveolitis has been reported (Turner Warwick, 1967). Circulating DNA complexes with ANA (antinuclear antibody) have been reported in systemic lupus erythematosus (Tan *et al.*, 1966), and deposition of these complexes on renal glomeruli is well established (Dixon, 1963; Freedman & Markowitz, 1962). Deposition on the alveolar capillaries as well as the glomeruli, has been reported in one case with systemic lupus erythematosus in whom there was renal involvement, chronic active hepatitis, pleural effusions and minimal fibrosing alveolitis (Turner Warwick, Haslam & Weeks, 1971). Evidence of capillary deposits of complement and immuno-globulin was also reported in five other cases of fibrosing alveolitis whose serum contained antinuclear antibodies in moderately high titres.

Pulmonary manifestations of systemic lupus erythematosus

The features of SLE affecting the lungs are commonly bilateral pleural effusions and linear opacities over the lower lobes, with elevation of the diaphragm. Breathlessness is a common symptom, but rales are uncommon and clubbing is usually absent. Physiological studies show a restrictive ventilatory and gas transfer defect (Hoffbrand & Beck, 1965). On pathological examination, alveolar wall fibrosis is very uncommon although occasionally seen (Olsen & Lever, 1970); vasculitis with or without infarction is a promi-nent feature and areas of atelectasis are also common (Hoffbrand & Beck, 1965). Whether these lesions are always due to immune complex deposition, or whether other immune processes, perhaps cell mediated, also play a part is not yet known, but *in vitro* evidence of a cell mediated response to nuclear antigens has been demonstrated in patients with various clinical syndromes associated with the presence of ANA (Brostoff, personal communication).

Immune disorders of the lung related to the presence of circulating auto-antibodies

Recent evidence suggests that a number of chronic lung diseases in which external aetiological agents cannot be established are nevertheless charac-terised by the presence of circulating tissue antibodies. In the majority of instances these antibodies are non-organ specific in nature, and while they may form various types of intravascular complexes in occasional cases, it appears probable that under many circumstances their presence is not directly related to pathogenesis. In some instances they may result from tissue damage while in others they may arise as a result of cross reactivity with ingested or even inhaled antigens, as suggested by Amman & Hong (1970). The possibility that autoantibodies may result from persisting viral infections where tissue proteins become incorporated into the molecular structure of the virus during reduplication has been suggested (Gordon-Smith, 1970) and may be relevant in pulmonary as well as other diseases.

The lungs in rheumatoid arthritis

There is growing acceptance that there are three types of intrathoracic lesion occurring especially in relation to rheumatoid arthritis (Scadding, 1968; Turner Warwick, 1969), namely pleural effusion, necrobiotic intrapulmonary nodules and fibrosing alveolitis.

Pleural effusion. Pleurisy with or without effusion is probably the most common of the albeit rare intrathoracic complications of rheumatoid arthritis (Baggenstoss & Rosenberg, 1943); 19 cases of pleural effusion were found in 516 patients with rheumatoid arthritis compared to only 2 amongst 301 with osteoarthritis (Walker & Wright, 1967). They occur more frequently in men (Emerson, 1956), and this contrasts with the higher incidence of rheumatoid arthritis without pulmonary complications in women. Lymphocytes are the usual predominant cell in the effusion, but occasionally a blood and pleural fluid eosinophilia has been reported (Portner & Gracie, 1966). A low sugar content of less than 10 mg/100 ml without obvious evidence of bacterial infection has been found in some, but by no means all, cases (Carr & Mayne, 1962). Pleural biopsy very occasionally shows characteristic necrobiotic lesions in the parietal pleura (Basten, Carmens & Schwartz, 1966). Of clinical diagnostic importance is the fact that circulating rheumatoid factor may be demonstrated in rare cases with lone pleural effusion years before the development of joint symptoms.

Intrapulmonary necrobiotic nodules. Intrapulmonary nodules ranging in size from 1–5 cm are a rare complication of rheumatoid arthritis. Their histology is similar to that of subcutaneous rheumatoid nodules showing central necrosis, palisading by histiocytes with a surrounding zone of inflammatory cells, mainly lymphocytes, plasma cells and fibroblasts, often associated with an obliterative vasculitis of small vessels.

Necrobiotic nodules may be single or multiple, occurring especially in the upper and middle zones of the lung; they may appear successively and remit spontaneously; cavitation is not uncommon (Panettiere, Chandler & Libcke, 1968). As with pleural effusion they have been reported more frequently in men. In a series of 26 cases reported by Panettiere et al. (1968), long standing joint symptoms preceded the demonstration of intrapulmonary nodules in the majority, but in 9, nodules were found where joint symptoms had been present for less than five years. In occasional cases, intrathoracic nodules with characteristic histology have preceded the development of joint symptoms. In some of these, circulating rheumatoid factor was found before the arthritis, but others have been sero-negative.

Caplan's nodules. Caplan (1953) described a particular radiographic appearance in coalminers with pneumoconiosis and rheumatoid arthritis. The characteristic picture was of multiple well-defined nodules 0·5–5·0 cm, usually in the upper and middle zones with only a slight background of simple pneumoconiosis. A similar radiographic appearance was sometimes seen in coalminers without rheumatoid arthritis, and in these about 60 per cent had circulating rheumatoid factor. Later Caplan, Payne & Withey (1962) described small nodular lesions, 0·3–1·0 cm in coalminers also associated with rheumatoid arthritis and rheumatoid factor. In this group 32 per cent had rheumatoid arthritis; and of those without joint symptoms 46 per cent had circulating rheumatoid factor. Caplan's syndrome has also been described with other inorganic dust pneumoconioses, including silicosis and asbestosis (Telleson, 1961). Immunofluorescent studies of Caplan's nodules have demonstrated deposits of immunoglobulin and complement within the lesions (Pernis, 1968) and rheumatoid factor has been reported in adjacent plasma cells (Wagner & McCormack, 1967).

While the exact immunopathogenesis of Caplan's nodules is not known it appears that the altered immune response of these individuals modifies in a characteristic way the lung responses to coal dust. Whether coal acts as an adjuvant to the underlying allergic response, or whether autoantibodies alter the macrophage handling of dust has to be clarified.

Fibrosing alveolitis and rheumatoid arthritis. The histological features of interstitial pulmonary fibrosis *alias* fibrosing alveolitis (Scadding, 1964), has been described in association with rheumatoid arthritis (Ellman & Ball, 1948), and many reports have confirmed its greater frequency in men. As has already been seen with rheumatoid pleural effusion and necrobiotic nodules, several reports have confirmed the presence of circulating rheumatoid factor in fibrosing alveolitis without joint symptoms. In a review of 109 cases of fibrosing alveolitis 34 (31 per cent) had significant titres of rheumatoid factor, but only about half of these had rheumatoid arthritis. Thus 17 per cent of the whole series had rheumatoid factor without joint symptoms (Turner Warwick, 1967). In a few of these, joint symptoms developed some years after the lung changes. While some reports have suggested that fibrosing alveolitis occurs particularly when rheumatoid factor titres are high (Tomasi *et al.*, 1962), in our series the distribution of rheumatoid factor titres in patients with fibrosing alveolitis and rheumatoid arthritis was identical to that observed in a group of patients with rheumatoid arthritis alone (Turner Warwick & Doniach, 1965).

Histological examination of the lungs of patients with fibrosing alveolitis and rheumatoid arthritis frequently show prominent collections of lymphoid tissue in the periphery of the lungs, often showing numerous germinal follicles and clusters of plasma cells. Immunofluorescent studies of individual cases have demonstrated antibody formation, both in the germinal follicles and in the plasma cells. The stimulus to rheumatoid factor production in lung disease may be due to a number of different factors; that antiglobulin production may be stimulated by the slightly altered gammaglobulin circulating concomitantly as immune complexes, associated with a variety of antigens is supported by the experiments of Abruzzo & Christian (1961). Another possibility has been suggested recently by Williams, Brostoff &

Roitt (1970): *Mycoplasma fermentans* infection may be the causative infective agent in rheumatoid arthritis and, by surface adsorption of gamma-
globulin, stimulates rheumatoid factor production.

The evidence that potential damaging immune complexes identified
around joints and in joint fluid in patients with rheumatoid arthritis (Winchester, Agnello & Kunkel, 1970) may also be deposited in the alveolar
capillaries has already been mentioned.

Cryptogenic fibrosing alveolitis. Cryptogenic fibrosing alveolitis (Scadding,
1964) is now being recognised in association with an increasing number of
other systemic diseases characterised by the presence of autoantibodies;
namely, rheumatoid arthritis as discussed above, Sjogren's syndrome
(Bunim, 1961; Tomasi *et al.*, 1962), systemic sclerosis (Hayman & Hunt,
1952), dermatomyositis (Hyun, Diggs & Toone, 1962), chronic active
hepatitis (Turner Warwick, 1967), polymyositis (Thompson & Mackay,
1970). Perhaps coeliac disease (Hood & Mason, 1970; Lancaster *et al.*, 1971)
and renal tubular acidosis (Mason & Golding, 1970) are further examples,
although histological confirmation of fibrosing alveolitis has not yet been
reported in the latter two instances. The frequency of these conditions in a
personal series of 130 cases of fibrosing alveolitis is shown on Table 5.9.

TABLE 5.9

ASSOCIATED CONDITIONS IN A SERIES OF 130 PATIENTS WITH
CRYPTOGENIC FIBROSING ALVEOLITIS

Fibrosing alveolitis	Total 130		
Rheumatoid arthritis	23	18%	} 30%
Transient polyarthritis	16	12%	
Chronic active hepatitis	9		} 11%
Hepatosplenomegaly	5		
Sjogren's syndrome	3		
Systemic sclerosis	3		} 5%
Raynaud's phenomenon	3		
Ulcerative colitis	2		
Cardiomyopathy	1		
Polymyositis	1		
Macroglobulinaemia with purpura	1		
Myelosclerosis	1		
Thyroid disease Hyperthyroidism, Hashimoto thyroiditis and myxoedema)	7		5%

In fibrosing alveolitis both with and without evidence of other systemic
disease, a range of non-organ specific autoantibodies are frequently found.
In a personal series, ANA was found in 28 per cent of lone fibrosing alveolitis
and in 24 per cent of alveolitis associated with systemic disease: rheumatoid
factor was found in 9 per cent of lone fibrosing alveolitis and in 42 per cent
when systemic disease, especially when polyarthritis (including transient and
typical rheumatoid arthritis) was present.

In lung biopsies from 33 cases of fibrosing alveolitis, evidence of capillary deposits of complement and immunoglobulin was found in 6 out of 14 with positive tests for antinuclear antibodies, but in none of 19 with negative ANA, suggesting that immune complex deposition may account for alveolar wall damage in a small number of cases of fibrosing alveolitis associated with this antibody. An additional finding of interest was fluorescence of occasional macrophage nuclei in cases with circulating ANA (Turner Warwick, Haslam & Weeks, 1971). Hughes & Rowell (1970) have recently shown that turpentine pleurisy in rats is aggravated by injected human antinuclear antibodies and in their immunofluorescence studies, showed nuclear fluorescence of macrophages in the pleural fluid. It was suggested that antinuclear antibodies might gain access to nuclei of dead inflammatory cells, forming immune complexes which in turn might accelerate local tissue damage initiated in their experimental case by turpentine. Recently similar macrophage nuclear fluorescence using conjugated anti-IgM and anti-complement has been found in the pleural fluid from a patient with rheumatoid arthritis and a strongly positive ANA (Turner Warwick, unpublished).

The presence of antinuclear antibody and rheumatoid factor in chronic lung disease has often been regarded as a consequence of any type of chronic destructive disease. That this is not the entire explanation is supported by the different incidence of ANA and rheumatoid factor in different types of fibrosing lung disorders (Turner Warwick & Haslam, 1970) and especially their absence in chronic extrinsic allergic alveolitis and fibrosing sarcoidosis.

An increased incidence of non-organ specific complement fixing antibodies has been reported in fibrosing alveolitis (Turner Warwick & Doniach, 1965), and was associated with either antinuclear antibody or rheumatoid factor in 70 per cent of these showing complement fixation with tissue extracts. Mitochondrial antibody has been detected in 15/116 (13 per cent) and smooth muscle in 7/70 (10 per cent), but the latter were found mainly in those cases associated with chronic active hepatitis.

Of recent interest is the high incidence of autoantibodies, including mitochondrial, ANA, and rheumatoid factor in renal tubular acidosis (Pasternak & Linder, 1970) because many of the reported cases have radiographic appearances and a physiological defect similar to patients with fibrosing alveolitis. Detailed histological studies are now required.

Lung reactive antibodies

Antibodies specific to lung have often been demonstrated in experimental animals, but in clinical disease they have proved much more difficult to find. Lung *reactive* antibodies directed against crude connective tissue fractions of human lung and now shown to be directed against collagen (Esber & Burrell, 1970) are cross reactive in tissue absorption studies (Burrell *et al.*, 1966). Their characteristics have been intensively studied by Burrell and his co-workers (Hagadorn, Burrell & Andrews, 1966; Hagadorn & Burrell, 1968). These antibodies, demonstrated as IgG, IgM and IgA have been identified using an antiglobulin consumption technique in a wide range of lung diseases, including pulmonary tuberculosis, pulmonary fibrosis, chronic bronchitis and coalminers' pneumoconiosis. Their correlation with other types of non-organ specific autoantibodies has not been reported by these workers. In one other study reported by Turner Warwick & Haslam (1971) only a small number of sera from patients with various fibrosing lung diseases were found positive by AGCT (perhaps due to slight differences in antigen preparation) and these correlated closely with the presence of complement fixing antibodies, again providing supporting evidence of their non-organ specific nature.

Antibody to basement membrane in the lung has been demonstrated in Goodpasture's syndrome (Beirie *et al.*, 1968), but in so far as basement membrane in the lung possesses antigenic determinants cross reactive with renal glomerular basement membrane, this antibody may be regarded as non-organ specific. Immunofluorescent studies in other lung disease especially cryptogenic fibrosing alveolitis have failed to demonstrate tissue fixed antibody to components of normal lung.

In summary, while there is good evidence of many different types of *non-organ specific* autoantibodies (including antibody reacting with denatured globulins, crude lung extracts, collagen and basement membrane) in various chronic lung diseases but especially in fibrosing alveolitis, antibodies reacting exclusively to a component of human lung (i.e. lung specific antibody), has not yet been identified in human pulmonary disease.

CONCLUSION

Throughout this chapter the emphasis has been on the range of different immunological responses which can be identified in lung disease, and which are reflected in their corresponding distinct and often characteristic clinical patterns. The specification of the conditions determining these responses are of great importance in current research.

As the frontiers of immunological knowledge expand so will our understanding of the immunopathogenesis of most recognised pulmonary diseases. Moreover this knowledge is likely to throw light on the many baffling cases seen from time to time in clinical practice of thoracic medicine, which have so far defied all attempts at classification.

References

ABRUZZO, J. L. & CHRISTIAN, C. L. (1961). *J. exp. Med.*, **144,** 791.

ADINOLFI, M., GLYNN, A. A., LINDSAY, M. & MILNE, C. M. (1966). *Immunology*, **10,** 517.

ALMEIDA, J. D. & WATERSON, A. P. (1969). *Lancet*, **2,** 983.

AMMAN, A. J. & HONG, R. (1970). *Clin. exp. Immunol.*, **7,** 833.

ASSEM, E. S. K. & McALLEN, M. K. (1970). *Br. med. J.*, **2,** 504.

AUGUSTIN, R. (1959). *Immunology*, **2,** 230.

AVILA, R. & VILLAR, T. G. (1968). *Lancet*, **1,** 620.

BAGGENSTOSS, A. H. & ROSENBERG, E. F. (1943). *Archs Path.*, **35,** 503.

BASTEN, A., CARMENS, I. & SCHWARTZ, C. J. (1966). *Aust. Ann. Med.*, **15,** 175.

BEIRNE, G. J., OCTAVIANO, G. N., KOPP, W. L. & BURNS, R. O. (1968). *Ann. intern. Med.*, **69,** 1207.

BELIN, L., FALSEN, E., HOLBORN, J. & ANDRE, J. (1970). *Lancet*, **2,** 1153.

BOUHUYS, A., LINDELL, S. E. & LUNDIN, G. (1960). *Br. med. J.*, **1,** 324.

BOUTON, J., MAINWARING, D. & SMITHELLS, R. W. (1963). *Br. med. J.*, **1,** 1512.

BRONSKY, D. & DUNN, Y. O. L. (1966). *Am. J. med. Sci.*, **250,** 11.

BROSTOFF, J. Lymphocyte sensitisation. Personal communication.

BROSTOFF, J., GREAVES, M. F. & ROITT, I. M. (1969). *Lancet*, **1**, 803.
BUNIM, J. J. (1961). *Ann. rheum. Dis.*, **20**, 1.
BURNS, M. W. & MAY, J. R. (1967). *Lancet*, **1**, 354.
BURRELL, R. G., ESBER, H. J., HAGADORN, J. E. & ANDREWS, C. E. (1966). *Am. Rev. Resp. Dis.*, **94**, 743.
CAPLAN, A. (1953). *Thorax*, **8**, 29.
CAPLAN, A., PAYNE, R. B. & WITHEY, J. L. (1962). *Thorax*, **17**, 205.
CARR, D. T. & MAYNE, J. G. (1962). *Am. Rev. Resp. Dis.*, **85**, 345.
CARRINGTON, C. B., ADDINGTON, W. W., GOFF, A. M., MADOFF, I. M., MARKS, A., SCHWABER, J. R. & GAENSLER, E. A. (1969). *New Engl. J. Med.*, **280**, 787.
CASPARY, E. A. & FIELD, E. J. (1971). *Br. med. J.*, **2**, 143.
CAYTON, H. R., FURNESS, G. & MAITLAND, H. B. (1952). *Br. J. Ind. Med.*, **9**, 186.
CITRON, K. M. (1957). *Tubercle*, **38**, 33.
CITRON, K. M. & SCADDING, J. G. (1957). *Q. Jl Med.*, **26**, 277.
COCA, A. F. (1922). *J. Immun.*, **7**, 163.
COCHRANE, C. G. (1963). *J. exp. Med.*, **118**, 503.
COLE, P., SHAW, K., ASSEM, E. S. K. & TURNER WARWICK, M. (1971). In preparation.
COX, J. S. G. (1967). *Nature*, **216**, 1328.
DANARAJ, T. J. (1958). *Q. Jl Med.*, **27**, 243.
D'ARCY HART, P., MITCHELL, D. N. & SUTHERLAND, I. (1964). *Br. med. J.*, **1**, 795.
DAVIES, P. D. (1969). *Br. J. Dis. Chest*, **63**, 59.
DICKIE, H. A. & RANKIN, J. (1958). *J. Am. med. Ass.*, **167**, 1069.
DIXON, F. J. (1963). *Harvey Lectures*, **58**, 21.
DUGUID, I. M. (1961). *Br. J. Opthal.*, **45**, 789–796.
DUNNILL, M. S., MASSARELLA, G. R. & ANDERSON, J. A. (1969). *Thorax*, **24**, 176–179.
ELLMAN, P. & BALL, R. E. (1948). *Br. med. J.*, **2**, 816.
EMERSON, P. A. (1956). *Br. med. J.*, **1**, 428.
ESBER, H. J. & BURRELL, R. G. (1970). *Arch. Environ. Health*, **21**, 502.
FAHEY, J. L., LEONARD, E., CHURG, J. & GODMAN, G. (1954). *Am. J. Med.*, **17**, 168.
FAIRLEY, G. H. & MATTHIAS, J. Q. (1960). *Br. med. J.*, **2**, 433.
FORGACS, P., McDONALD, C. K. & SKELTON, M. O. (1957). *Lancet*, **1**, 188.
FOWLER, P. B. S. (1952). *Lancet*, **2**, 755.
FRANGLEN, G. (1970). *Br. J. Hosp. Med.*, **3**, 651.
FRANKLAND, A. W. (1953). *Ann. Allergy*, **11**, 445.
FREEDMAN, P. & MARKOWITZ, A. S. (1962). *Br. med. J.*, **1**, 1175.
FRIOU, G. L. (1952). *J. clin. Invest.*, **31**, 630.
FULGINITI, V. A., ELLER, J. J., DOWNIE, A. W. & KEMPE, C. H. (1967). *J. Am. med. Ass.*, **202**, 1075.
FULLER, C. J. (1953). *Thorax*, **8**, 59.
GANDEVIA, B. (1970). *Med. J., Aust.*, **2**, 332.
GANDEVIA, B. (1970). *Med. J., Aust.*, **2**, 372.
GANDEVIA, B. & MILNE, J. (1970). *Br. J. ind. Med.*, **27**, 235.
GANDEVIA, B. & MITCHELL, C. A. (1970). *Aust. Ann. Med.*, **19**, 408.
GARDNER, P. S., McQUILLIN, J. & COURT, S. D. M. (1970). *Br. med. J.*, **1**, 327.
GELL, R. G. H. & COOMBS, R. R. A. (1968). *In* "Clinical Aspects of Immunology". Oxford: Blackwell.
GITLIN, D., JANEWAY, C. A., APT, L. & CRAIG, J. M. (1959). *In* "Agammaglobulinaemia, Cellular and Humoral Aspects of the Hypersensitivity State". London Cassell.

GOCKE, D. J., MORGAN, C., LOCKSHIN, M., HSU, K., BOMBARDIERI, S. & CHRISTIAN, C. L. (1970). *Lancet*, **2**, 1149.

GOLDSTEIN, R. A., ISRAEL, H. L. & RAWNSLEY, H. M. (1969). *J. Am. med. Ass.*, **208**, 1153.

GOOD, R. A., ROLSTEIN, J. & MAZZEILTTO, W. F. (1957). *J. Lab. clin. Med.* **49**, 343.

GORDON SMITH, C. E. (1970). *J. R. Coll. Phycns., Lond.*, **5**, 31.

GREENBERG, M., MILNE, J. F. & WATT, A. (1970). *Br. med. J.*, **2**, 629.

GREENWOOD, R., SMELLIE, H., BARR, M. & CUNLIFFE, A. C. (1958). *Br. med., J.*, **1**, 1388.

HAGADORN, J. E. & BURRELL, R. G. (1968). *Clin. exp. Immun.*, **3**, 263.

HAGADORN, J. E., BURRELL, R. G. & ANDREWS, C. E. (1966). *Am. Rev. Resp. Dis.*, **94**, 751.

HALL, R., TURNER WARWICK, M. & DONIACH, D. (1966). *Clin. exp. Immun.*, **1**, 285.

HAPKE, E. J., SEAL, R. M. E., THOMAS, C. O., HAYES, M. & MEEK, J. C. (1968). *Thorax*, **23**, 451.

HARGREAVE, F. E., PEPYS, J. & HOLFORD-STREVENS, V. (1968). *Lancet*, **1**, 619.

HARGREAVE, F. E., PEPYS, J., LONGBOTTOM, J. L. & WRAITH, D. G. (1966). *Lancet*, **1**, 445.

HAYMAN, L. D. & HUNT, R. E. (1952). *Dis. Chest*, **21**, 691.

HENDERSON, A. H. (1968). *Thorax*, **23**, 501.

HOBBS, J. R. (1966). *Scientific Basis of Medicine*, 106.

HOBBS, J. R. (1968). *Lancet*, **1**, 110.

HOBBS, J. R. (1970). *Br. J. Hosp. med.*, **3**, 669.

HOFFBRAND, B. I. & BECK, E. R. (1965). *Br. med. J.*, **1**, 1273.

HOLMES, B., PARK, B. H., MALAWISTA, S. E., QUIE, P. G., NELSON, D. L. & GOOD, R. A. (1970). *New Engl. J. Med.*, **283**, 217.

HOOD, J. & MASON, A. M. S. (1970). *Lancet*, **1**, 445.

HUGHES, P. & ROWELL, N. R. (1970). *J. Path.*, **101**, 141.

HYUN, B. H., DIGGS, C. L. & TOONE, E. C. (1962). *Dis. Chest*, **42**, 449.

ISHIZAKA, K. & ISHIZAKA, T. (1970). *Clin. exp. Immun.*, **6**, 25.

ISHIZAKA, K. & ISHIZAKA, T. (1971). *Clin. Allergy*, **1**, 9.

ISHIZAKA, K., ISHIZAKA, T. & HORNBROOK, M. M. (1966). *Immunology*, **77**, 75–85.

ISRAEL, H. L. & SONES, M. (1965). *New Engl. J. Med.*, **273**, 1003–1006.

JOHANSSON, S. G. O. (1967). *Lancet*, **2**, 951.

JOHANSSON, S. G. O., BENNICH, H. & WIDE, L. (1968). *Immunology*, **14**, 265.

JOHANSSON, S. G. O., MELLBIN, T. & VAHLQUIST, B. (1968). *Lancet*, **1**, 1118.

KAPIKIAN, A. Z., MITCHELL, R. H., CHANOCK, R. M., SHVEDOFF, R. A. & STEWART, C. E. (1969). *Am. J. Epidem.*, **89**, 405.

KEIDAN, S. E., McCARTHY, K. & HAWORTH, J. C. (1953). *Archs Dis. Childh.*, **28**, 110.

KEIMOWITZ, R. I. (1964). *J. Lab. Clin. Med.*, **63**, 54.

KENT, H. N. (1960). *Expl. Parasit.*, **10**, 313.

LANCASTER SMITH, M. J., BENSON, M. K. & STRICKLAND, I. D. (1971). *Lancet*, **1**, 473.

LONGBOTTOM, J. L. & PEPYS, J. (1964). *J. Path. Bact.*, **88**, 141.

LUNN, J. A. & HUGHES, D. T. D. (1967). *Br. J. ind. Med.*, **24**, 158.

LUZ, A. Q. & TODD, R. H. (1964). *Am. J. Dis. Child.*, **108**, 479.

McALLEN, M. K., ASSEM, E. S. K. & MAUNSELL, K. (1970). *Br. med. J.*, **2**, 501.

McCARTHY, D. S. (1970). Ph.D. Thesis (London).

McCARTHY, D. S., SIMON, G. & HARGREAVE, F. E. (1970). *Clin. Radiol.*, **21**, 366.

McKERROW, C. B., McDERMOTT, M., GILSON, J. C. & SCHILLING, R. S. F. (1958). *Br. J. ind. Med.*, **15**, 75.

MASON, A. M. & GOLDING, P. L. (1970). *Br. med. J.*, **3**, 143.

MASSOUD, A. & TAYLOR, G. (1964). *Lancet*, **2**, 607.

MITCHELL, C. A. & GANDEVIA, B. (1971). *Am. Rev. Dis. Chest*, **104**, 1.

MITCHELL, D. N., CHANNON, P., DYER, N. H., HINSON, K. F. W. & WILLOUGHBY, J. M. T. (1969). *Lancet*, **2**, 571.

NEWHOUSE, M. L., TAGG, B. & POCOCK, S. J. (1970). *Lancet*, **1**, 689.

NICKLAUS, T. M. & SNYDER, A. B. (1968). *Archs intern. Med.*, **121**, 151.

OLIVER-GONZALES, J. (1954). *J. infect. Dis.*, **95**, 86.

OLSEN, E. G. J. & LEVER, J. V. (1970). *Thorax*, **25**, 509.

PANETTIERE, F., CHANDLER, B. F. & LIBCKE, J. H. (1969). *Am. Rev. Resp. Dis.*, **97**, 89.

PARISH, W. E. (1970). *Lancet*, **2**, 591.

PASTERNACK, A. & LINDER, E. (1970). *Clin. exp. Immun.*, **7**, 115.

PERNIS, B. (1968). *In* "Silicosis". Vol. 1, p. 293. Ed. P. A. Miescher, & H. J. Muller-Eberhard, New York: Grune & Stratton.

PEPYS, J. (1967). *J. R. Coll. Phycns.*, **2**, 42.

PEPYS, J. (1969). *In* "Monographs in Allergy", Vol. 4. Ed, S. Karger, Switzerland: Basle.

PEPYS, J., HARGREAVE, F. E., CHAN, M. & MCCARTHY, D. S. (1968). *Lancet*, **2**, 134.

PEPYS, J., HARGREAVE, F. E., LONGBOTTOM, J. L. & FAUX, J. (1969). *Lancet*, **1**, 1181.

PEPYS, J. & JENKINS, P. A. (1965). *Thorax*, **20**, 21.

PEPYS, J., JENKINS, P. A., LACHMANN, P. J. & MAHON, W. E. (1966). *Clin. exp. Immun.*, **1**, 377.

PEPYS, J., RIDDELL, R. W., CITRON, K. M., CLAYTON, Y. M. & SHORT, E. I. (1959). *Am. Rev. Resp. Dis.*, **80**, 167.

PEPYS, J., TURNER WARWICK, M., DAWSON, P. L. & HINSON, K. F. W. (1968). *Excerpta med.*, **162**, 221.

PICKERING, C. A. C. (1971). *Proc. R. Soc. Med.*, in the press.

PORTNER, M. M. & GRACIE, W. A. (1966). *New Engl. J. Med.*, **275**, 697.

RACKEMANN, F. M. (1947). *Am. J. Med.*, **3**, 601.

REED, C. E., SOSMAN, A. & BARBEE, R. A. (1965). *J. Am. med. Ass.*, **193**, 261.

REICHLIN, S., LOVELESS, M. H. & KANE, E. G. (1953). *Ann. intern. Med.*, **38**, 113.

RIDDLE, H. F. V., CHANNELL, S., BLYTH, W., WEIR, D. M., LLOYD, M., AMOS, W. M. G. & GRANT, I. W. B. (1968). *Thorax*, **23**, 271.

RODMAN, T., FRAIMOW, W. & MYERSON, R. M. (1958). *Ann. intern. Med.*, **48**, 668.

ROITT, I. M., GREAVES, M. F., TORRIGIANI, G., BROSTOFF, J. & PLAYFAIR, J. H. L. (1969). *Lancet*, **2**, 367.

ROSE, G. A. & SPENCER, H. (1957). *Q. Jl Med.*, **26**, 43.

SAKULA, A. (1967). *Br. med. J.*, **3**, 708.

SCADDING, J. G. (1964). *Br. med. J.*, **2**, 686.

SCADDING, J. G. (1967). *In* 'Sarcoidosis'. London: Eyre and Spottiswoode.

SCADDING, J. G. (1969). *Proc. Roy. Soc. Med.*, **62**, 227.

SILTZBACH, L. E. (1961). *Am. Rev. Resp. Dis.*, **84**, 89.

SILVERMAN, M. (1971). Exercise Studies in Intrinsic and Extrinsic Asthma. Unpublished.

SPECTOR, W. G. & HEESOM, N. (1969). *J. Path.*, **98**, 31.

SQUIRE, J. R. (1962). *Proc. R. Soc. Med.*, **55**, 393.

STANWORTH, D. R. (1970). *Clin. Allergy*, **1**, 25.

STENIUS, B. & WIDE, L. (1969). *Lancet*, **2**, 455.

STENIUS, B., WIDE, L., SEYMOUR, W. M., HOLFORD-STREVENS, V. & PEPYS, J. (1971). *Clin. Allergy*, **1**, 37.

STERLING, G. M. (1967). *Thorax*, **22**, 533.

TAN, E. M., SCHUR, P. H., CARR, R. I. & KUNKEL, H. G. (1966). *J. clin. Invest.*, **2**, 1732.

TEILUM, G. (1964). *J. Path. Bact.*, **88**, 317.

TELLESON, W. G. (1961). *Thorax*, **16**, 372.

THOMPSON, P. L. & MACKAY, I. R. (1970). *Thorax*, **25**, 504.

TOMASI, T. B., FUDENBERG, M. D. & FINBY, N. (1962). *Am. J. Med.*, **33**, 243.

TOMASI, T. B., TAN, E. M., SOLOMAN, A. & PRENDERGAST, R. A. (1965). *J. exp. Med.*, **121**, 101.

TURIAF, J., MARLAND, P., PETIT, C. & TABART, J. (1966). *Le poumon and Le coeur*, **22**, 475.

TURK, J. L. (1967). *Br. med. Bull.*, **23**, 3.

TURK, J. L. (1969). *In* "Clinical Medicine". London: Heinemann.

TURNER WARWICK, M. (1967). *J. R. Coll. Phycns., Lond.*, **2**, 57.

TURNER WARWICK, M. (1968). *Q. Jl Med.*, **37**, 133.

TURNER WARWICK, M. (1969). *Br. J. Hosp. Med.*, **2**, 507.

TURNER WARWICK, M. (1971). *Br. J. dis. Chest*, **65**, 1.

TURNER WARWICK, M. & DONIACH, D. (1965). *Br. med. J.*, **1**, 886.

TURNER WARWICK, M. & HASLAM, P. (1970). *Clin. exp. Immun.*, **7**, 31.

TURNER WARWICK, M. & HASLAM, P. (1971). *Clin. Allergy*, **1**, 83.

TURNER WARWICK, M., HASLAM, P. & WEEKS, J. (1971). *Clin. Allergy*, **1**, 209.

TWOMEY, J. J., JORDAN, P. H., JARROLD, T., TRUBOWITZ, S., RITZ, N. D. & CONN, H. O. (1969). *Am. J. med.*, **47**, 340.

VOISIN, C., JACOB, M., FURON, D. & LEFEBURE, J. (1966). *Le poumon et le coeur*, **22**, 529.

WAGNER, J. C. & MCCORMICK, J. N. (1967). *J. R. Coll. Phycns.*, **2**, 49.

WALKER, W. C. & WRIGHT, V. (1967). *Ann. rheum. dis.*, **26**, 467.

WIDE, L., BENNICH, H. & JOHANSSON, S. G. O. (1967). *Lancet*, **2**, 1105.

WILLIAMS, J. V. (1963). *Thorax*, **18**, 182.

WILLIAMS, M. H., BROSTOFF, J. & ROITT, I. M. (1970). *Lancet*, **2**, 277.

WINCHESTER, R. J., AGNELLO, V. & KUNKEL, H. G. (1970). *Clin. exp. Immun.*, **6**, 689.

WOLD, D. E. & ZAHN, D. W. (1956). *Am. Rev. Resp. Dis.*, **74**, 445.

WOODRUFF, A. W. (1970). *Br. med. J.*, **3**, 663.

WOODRUFF, A. W., BISSERU, B. & BOWE, J. C. (1966). *Br. med. J.*, **1**, 1576.

WORLD HEALTH ORGANIZATION (1968). *Bull. Wld Hlth Org.*, **38**, 151.

CHAPTER 6

VIRUS INFECTION OF THE RESPIRATORY TRACT

R. B. HEATH

The discovery in recent years of so many of the causative organisms of respiratory virus disease must be regarded as one of the most remarkable stories in the history of infectious disease. It is perhaps regrettable that much of the knowledge of these advances has tended to remain confined to laboratory-bound specialists. This must, to some extent, be inevitable in an age of increasing specialisation, but is also due to the fact that respiratory viral disease, at least in its uncomplicated form, is rarely the concern of hospital physicians. Indeed the majority of these illnesses are so trivial and sufficiently well understood by patients, that medical advice of any kind is rarely sought. In spite of this, respiratory viral disease remains a major problem to general practitioners and medical officers responsible for the health of school children, students, factory and military personnel, etc. It has, for example, been shown by Fry (1957) that by far the highest proportion (30 per cent) of diseases that he saw in his suburban London practice were respiratory infections. Most of these involved the upper air passages and so were probably of viral origin.

The high incidence of respiratory viral diseases in the community and their effect on absenteeism amongst the working population provides adequate reason for regarding them as a major medical problem. In addition it now appears that these infections are an important predisposing cause of much of the more serious illness which fills medical wards in the winter months.

This chapter will mainly deal with the evidence upon which the above statements are based but will firstly deal with our current knowledge of the aetiology, pathology and pathogenesis of these diseases.

Nomenclature and Classification of Respiratory Viruses

Table 6.1 lists the important families of viruses which are known to cause respiratory disease. They are collectively known as the respiratory viruses, a term which simply means that they replicate and produce disease which is, for the most part, confined to the respiratory tract. Some laxity is required in the use of this term because the adenoviruses, for example, although mainly associated with respiratory virus infection, frequently spread down to infect the gastro-intestinal tract. It is unusual for adenoviruses to produce intestinal disease, although they are thought to be responsible for the rare cases of acute intussusception of infants (Ross & Potter, 1961). Again it is known that nearly all human viruses are able to infect tissues of the respiratory tract and indeed it is replication at this site which is the initiating process in such well known diseases as measles, mumps and poliomyelitis. These viruses are not, of course, regarded as respiratory viruses because characteristically they spread from this portal of entry and produce disease elsewhere in the body.

TABLE 6.1

RESPIRATORY VIRUSES

Virus Group	Date of First Isolation	Physical Characteristics and Approx. Diameter	Type of Nucleic Acid	Antigenic Types
'Myxoviruses'				
(a) Influenza	1932 (1)	Helical symmetry with envelope. 100 n.m.	RNA	Basically 3 types (A, B and C) but the type A and B strains are constantly varying (see text)
(b) Parainfluenza	1956 (2)	Helical symmetry with envelope. 120 n.m.	RNA	Types 1 to 4
(c) Respiratory syncytial virus	1957 (3)	Helical symmetry with envelope. 120 n.m.	RNA	One only
Picornaviruses				
(a) Rhinoviruses	1953 (4)	Cubical symmetry. No envelope. 25 n.m.	RNA	At least 100
(b) Enteroviruses	—	Cubical symmetry. No envelope. 25 n.m.	RNA	Only a few strains have been associated with respiratory disease, e.g. Coxsackie A7 and A21 and Echo 11 viruses
Adenoviruses	1953 (5)	Cubical symmetry. No envelope. 80 n.m.	DNA	At least 28
Coronaviruses	1965 (6)	No obvious symmetry but characteristic envelope. 100 n.m.	RNA	Not known but more than one

(1) Smith, Andrewes & Laidlaw (1933).
(2) Chanock (1956).
(3) Chanock, Roizman & Myers (1957).

(4) Andrewes et al. (1953).
(5) Rowe et al. (1953).
(6) Tyrrell & Bynoe (1965).

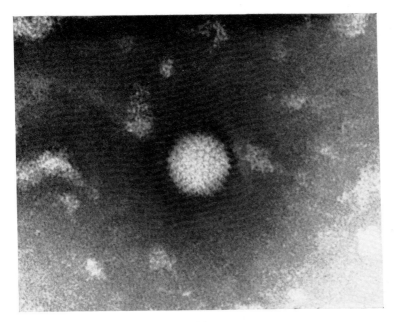

(a)

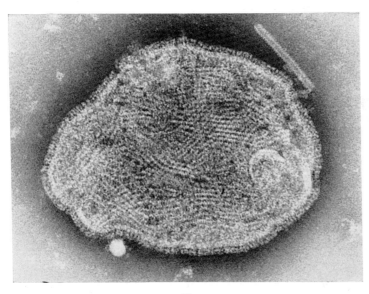

(b)

Fig. 6.1. *Electron micrographs of two common respiratory viruses.*

(a) Adenovirus, showing the cubical symmetry of the protein sub-units (× 186,500).

(b) Parainfluenza virus, showing the helical symmetry of the protein sub-units and the well defined envelope (× 128,000).

(Photomicrographs by Mr. C. Barber, Bland Sutton Institute).

[*To face p.* 182.

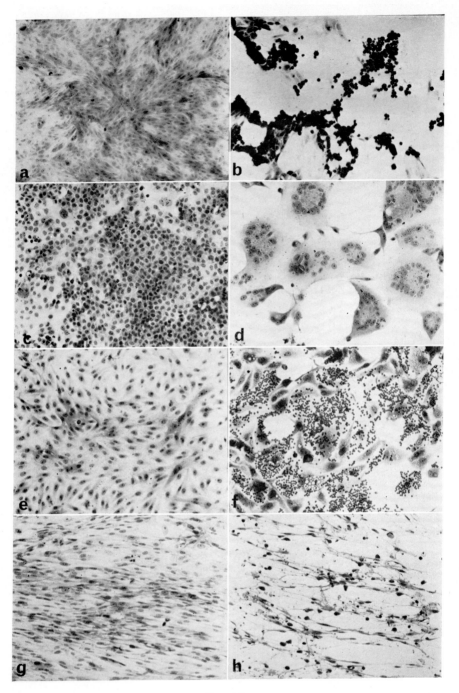

Fig. 6.2.

(a)

(b)

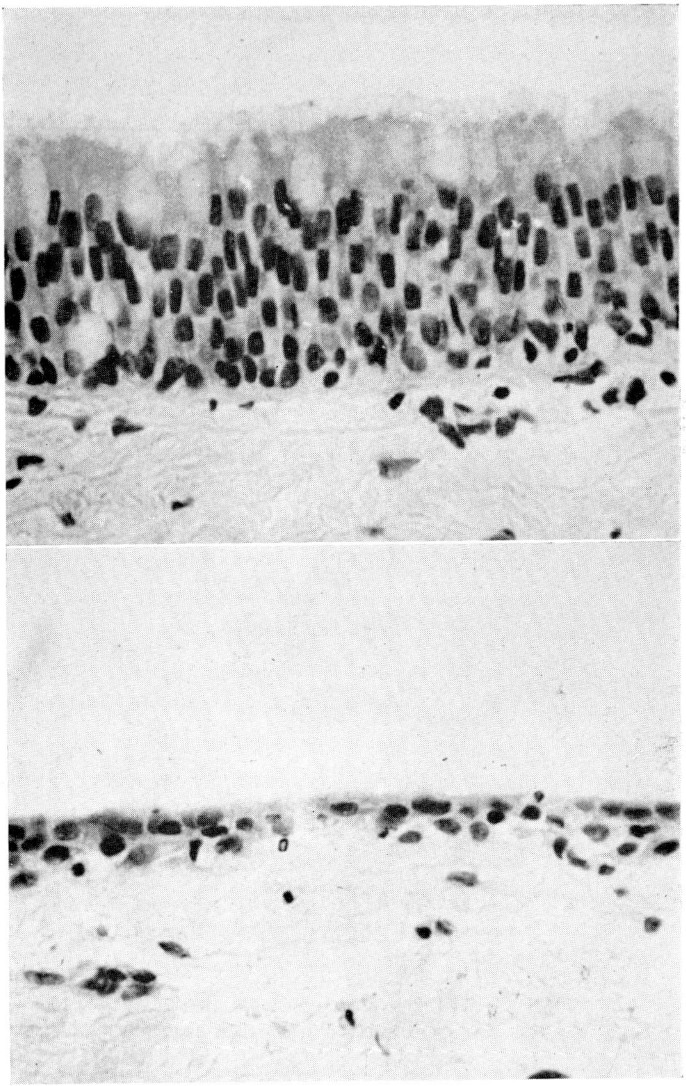

FIG. 6.3. *Organ culture of dog trachea.*
   (a) Normal.
   (b) Infected with influenza virus.

(Photomicrographs by Dr. E. A. Wickham, Pfizer Ltd.)

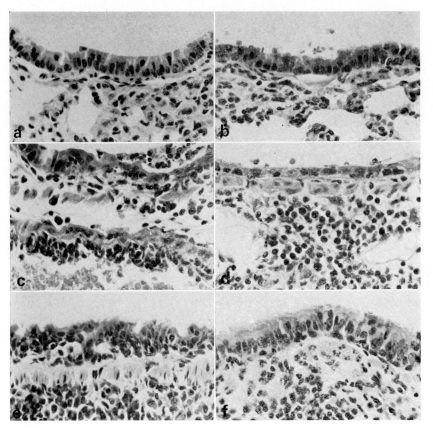

Fig. 6.4. *Sequential changes in the respiratory mucosa of mice infected with Sendai virus.*

(*a*) Day 0. Normal mucosa.

(*b*) Day 2. Early damage to the columnar epithelium.

(*c*) Day 3. More extensive epithelial damage with underlying inflammatory changes. Note the diapedesis of polymorphs from a greatly dilated blood vessel.

(*d*) Day 5. Only the basal layer of the epithelium remains. The cellular infiltration of the submucosa is now dominantly mononuclear.

(*e*) Day 13. Regenerating epithelium.

(*f*) Day. 33. Repaired epithelium. The collection of mononuclear cells in the submucosa is the sole remaining sign of the infection.

Virological terminology must inevitably cause some bewilderment to those not working in the field but must at this point be briefly described to ensure subsequent comprehension. There is unfortunately no standard procedure for naming viruses. They have either been called after the disease they cause, as with influenza, or have names which have derived from the organs or tissues from which they are commonly isolated. For example, adenoviruses are so named because they were first isolated from adenoids and in the same way the names enterovirus and rhinovirus imply that they are most commonly isolated from the intestinal tract and nose respectively. The name respiratory syncytial virus is a description of the cytopathic effect this virus produces when grown in tissue culture. The word coronavirus describes the 'crown-like' appearance of the virus when viewed with an electron microscope and picornavirus signifies the small size and kind of nucleic acid possessed by this large family of viruses.

Modern classification of viruses is primarily based upon such constant characteristics as the chemical nature of their nucleic acids and their morphological appearances. In this way, viruses are first divided into two groups depending on whether they contain RNA or DNA, since by definition a virus cannot contain both kinds of nucleic acid. Further subdivision is dependent on whether the viral protein subunits are arranged in a *cubical* pattern around the nucleic acid, as occurs with the adenoviruses (see Fig. 6.1(*a*)), in a *helical* pattern as occurs with the influenza and parainfluenza viruses (see Fig. 6.1(*b*)), or if there is *no obvious* pattern to the arrangement of these subunits. The other morphological characteristic which is taken into consideration is the presence or absence of an outer envelope. From Fig. 6.1(*b*), it can be seen that parainfluenza virus has a well-defined structure of this kind.

The above characteristics enable viruses to be arranged into well-defined groups. Further subdivision of viruses within these groups is dependent on their biological and antigenic properties. Variation in antigenic properties of different strains of the same group of viruses is an important feature of respiratory virology.

The essential characteristics of the respiratory viruses are given in Table 6.1 and also the dates when these were first isolated. From this emerges the important fact that infection of the respiratory tract can be effected by a large number of viruses which differ not only in their basic characteristics but also show wide variation in their antigenic make-up. Finally it should be noted that most of the respiratory viruses have been isolated in the years since 1945. Since respiratory viral disease is still under intensive investigation it is more

---

FIG. 6.2. *Degenerative changes (cytopathic effects) produced in tissue cultures by some common respiratory viruses.*

(*a*) Normal human kidney cultures.
(*b*) Human kidney cultures infected with an adenovirus.
(*c*) Normal Hep. 2 cells.
(*d*) Hep. 2 cells infected with respiratory syncytial virus.
(*e*) Normal monkey kidney cells.
(*f*) Monkey kidney cells showing haemadsorption produced by an influenza virus.
(*g*) Normal human embryo lung cells.
(*h*) Human embryo lung cells infected with a rhinovirus.

than likely that in the coming years many more viruses will have to be added to this list.

Laboratory Procedures in Respiratory Virology

Only a brief account of the laboratory procedures used to isolate viruses will be given which it is hoped will be sufficient for clinicians to understand the basis of laboratory diagnosis of these diseases. The specific aetiology of these diseases can be determined by two basic procedures, firstly by isolating the causal organism and secondly by demonstrating specific rises in antibody titre.

Isolation procedures

An essential requirement for the growth of any virus is a source of living cells and this in practice entails the use of laboratory animals, fertile hens' eggs or tissue cultures. Laboratory animals are nowadays practically never used for the isolation of respiratory viruses but it should be remembered that it was the use of the ferret for the isolation of influenza viruses by Smith, Andrewes & Laidlaw in 1933, which marked the beginning of respiratory virology. Laboratory animals are nevertheless still extensively used for research purposes.

The fertile hen's egg has proved most useful for the isolation of influenza viruses (Beveridge & Burnet, 1946), although it is today being replaced to some extent by tissue culture procedures. Cultivation of influenza viruses in eggs is still the only satisfactory method of bulk preparation for vaccine production. It is of interest that influenza viruses which grow well in this host rarely damage the chick embryo or its membranes and its growth can only be detected by the appearance of viral haemagglutinins in the embryonic fluids.

The advances in respiratory virology in the post-war years has been due to the introduction of tissue culture techniques. Monolayer cultures are most commonly used and for respiratory virology these must be prepared from human or other primate tissues. This type of culture has the advantage that the presence of virus can be detected by the appearance of degenerative (cytopathic) changes which can easily be visualized with a simple light microscope. Some examples of the cytopathic effects of respiratory viruses in monolayer type cultures are shown in Fig. 6.2.

Monolayer cultures have unfortunately proved to be too insensitive for the growth of the more fastidious respiratory viruses and these have only been isolated by the use of organ cultures (Hoorn & Tyrrell, 1965). For the isolation of respiratory viruses, fragments of human embryonic trachea have been used and their viability has been assessed by simply observing ciliary movement with a microscope. Addition of virus to these cultures results in cessation of the ciliary movement and this may be associated with extensive destruction of the mucosal surface of the fragments as is shown in Fig. 6.3.

Isolation of a virus by any of the above procedures must always be followed by some serological test to establish the identity of the isolate. This makes the whole process so lengthy that there must inevitably be considerable delay before a report can be submitted. To overcome this problem, serious attempts are now being made to develop more rapid methods of diagnosis employing electron microscopy and immunofluorescent staining procedures (see Gardner, 1970).

Serological procedures

It is an almost invariable rule that infection with a respiratory virus induces a good antibody response and advantage is taken of this to provide a most useful method of diagnosis. Complement fixation is the procedure most commonly used and most diagnostic laboratories are capable of testing sera for antibodies against all the viruses listed in Table 6.1 with the important exception of the rhinoviruses. In practice, however, few laboratories undertake enterovirus and coronavirus serology. In addition, virus laboratories will also test submitted sera for antibodies against the non-viral agents *Mycoplasma pneumoniae* (Eaton Agent), *Coxiella burneti* (Q fever) and psittacosis, since these agents produce illnesses which closely resemble viral respiratory disease.

The demonstration of a significant (at least four-fold) rise in antibody titre against one of the above organisms can be taken as reliable evidence of concurrent infection with that organism. It does not, of course, follow that the virus infection is always the cause of the observed illness. To obtain reliable information from serology it is essential to submit a serum which has been taken during the early days of the illness. This may be difficult when the physician first sees the patient at what must be regarded as the convalescent stage of the viral disease. Results obtained from a single serum taken at this late stage are rarely of any value because it is not possible to distinguish between recent antibodies and those acquired months or years previously. A very high level of antibody in a serum taken during the convalescent period can occasionally provide presumptive evidence of recent infection and this is particularly true of transient antibodies such as those that appear against the soluble influenza antigens. Nevertheless it must again be stressed that reliable information can only be obtained from tests carried out on paired sera taken at the correct time. Indeed there are some laboratories that refuse to perform tests on single sera.

Those requiring more information about laboratory techniques should consult the excellent monographs by Stuart-Harris (1965) and Tyrrell (1965).

Pathology of Respiratory Viral Infection

Studies of the pathology and pathogenesis of respiratory viral infection are valuable for two reasons. Firstly they demonstrate how these infections impair an important defence mechanism of the respiratory tract, leaving it particularly vulnerable to secondary bacterial infection, and they also demonstrate the remarkable effects of natural antiviral defence mechanisms which enable the host to rid itself of these organisms.

Histological changes

It will be appreciated that it has rarely been possible to study the effects of viruses on the respiratory tissues of man for the obvious reason that most of the patients with these illnesses recover and so do not become available for study in the post-mortem room. When there has been a fatal outcome to one of these illnesses, the basic histological changes have frequently been obscured by either rapid autolysis of the respiratory mucous membrane or by secondary bacterial infection. Occasionally it has been possible, especially during influenza outbreaks, to obtain suitable human material for histological studies (Walsh *et al.*, 1961), but most of our knowledge on this subject has come from studies of experimental infection of laboratory animals.

The essential feature of respiratory viral infections is necrosis and desquamation of the tall ciliated columnar epithelium which extends from the nose down to the terminal bronchi. This membrane is normally covered with a thin layer of mucus which is produced by the goblet cells. Because of the high incidence of respiratory viral infection it is apparent that this substance affords little protection against viruses, although it is known to contain inhibitors of influenza viruses (Fazekas de St. Groth, 1952). Viral infection of the respiratory tract is associated with excessive mucus production which is responsible for one of the characteristic clinical features of these illnesses. The cellular damage produced by these infections also induces marked inflammatory changes which can be seen in the submucosa. There is dilatation of the blood vessels with out-pouring into the tissues of both oedema fluid and leucocytes. In the early stages of the infection these cells are mainly polymorphonuclear leucocytes and are presumably induced by products of the damaged epithelial cells, since it is not thought that viruses have chemotactic properties. Later in the infection the cells are dominantly mononuclear and are present in large numbers; they probably represent the immune response to viral antigens. The other common clinical features of respiratory viral disease, redness of the membrane, pain and elevated temperature. result from these secondary inflammatory changes.

During the recovery phase of the illness repair of the mucous membrane occurs and the underlying inflammatory changes resolve. Small collections of the mononuclear cells persist for several weeks and are usually the last signs of the infection.

The pathological changes just described have been recognised since the earliest days of respiratory virology. Just one year after Smith and his colleagues had isolated the first human influenza virus, they were able to adapt it to the lungs of mice. In this model they noted the necrosis and desquamation of the respiratory epithelium and the leucocyte response (Andrewes, Laidlaw & Smith, 1934). Subsequent to this work there has appeared a vast literature on the pathological changes induced in mice by adapted influenza viruses. These papers will not be discussed in detail because in this model the adapted virus also infects the alveolar epithelial cells and produces pneumonitis (Hers *et al.*, 1962). This type of pathology is rarely seen in man, although it bears some resemblance to that seen in the uncommon cases of true influenza pneumonia (Hers & Holder, 1961).

A far better model of human viral respiratory disease is influenza virus infection of the ferret (Francis & Stuart-Harris, 1938 a and b; Stuart-Harris & Francis, 1938). By using strains of virus which have not been adapted to the ferret and by inoculating non-anaesthetised animals they showed that it was possible to obtain an infection which is restricted to the upper air passages. This infection is remarkably like human influenza; after a 48 hour incubation period, the ferrets become listless, refuse food and develop a high temperature. A mucoid nasal discharge and sneezing are local manifestations of the infection. The illness usually lasts 2–3 days and high levels of antibody are present some 2–4 weeks later. Necrosis and desquamation of the nasal epithelium is obvious by the second day of the infection and repair starts as early as the fourth day. At this stage of the illness there is an intense inflammatory reaction in the submucosa. During the repair phase, the denuded areas of the epithelium are first covered by a stratified squamous epithelium and then by the normal columnar epithelium.

Virtually identical changes to those just described have been noted in mice infected with a parainfluenza virus (Robinson, Cureton & Heath, 1968) and these are illustrated in Fig. 6.4. They have also been seen in ferrets and mink inoculated with respiratory syncytial virus (Coates & Chanock, 1962), in chickens inoculated with Newcastle Disease Virus (Beard & Easterday, 1967), and in natural influenza infections of man (Walsh *et al.*, 1961).

Pathogenesis

Greater understanding of respiratory viral disease can be obtained by studying the dynamics of the various pathological changes that occur in these infections. From histological studies it is apparent that many of the observed changes result from the initial damage to the epithelial cells. It is therefore of prime importance to understand how the latter is brought about.

Necrosis of respiratory epithelium

As described in an earlier section, practically all the respiratory viruses have been shown to replicate in cells in tissue culture. This process usually disrupts the normal metabolic processes of the cells to such an extent that they develop degenerative (cytopathic) changes and die. There are several experimental studies which support the view that exactly the same process occurs when respiratory epithelial cells are infected with the same viruses. For example, the presence of replicating influenza virus has been directly demonstrated in respiratory epithelial cells by procedures such as immunofluorescence (Denk & Kovak, 1965), and electron microscopy (Harford, Hamlin & Parker, 1955). It would seem, therefore, that we can regard the necrosis of the respiratory epithelium as being a simple lytic effect of the infecting virus.

It is possible that this is an oversimplified concept. In recent years there has been much speculation on the harmful effects of the immune response in viral infections. It is known that if large doses of non-replicating influenza viruses are given intranasally to sensitised animals, an allergic inflammatory reaction, with destruction of epithelial cells and a mixed polymorph and mononuclear cell response occurs (Ogasawara, Aida & Nagata (1961) and Tong and Fong (1964). It is now considered that acute bronchiolitis of infants, which is caused by respiratory syncytial virus (RSV) is a disease of this kind. The evidence for this emerged from trials of an inactivated RSV vaccine (Kapikian *et al.*, 1969; Kim *et al.*, 1969; Fulginiti *et al.*, 1969). In brief it was found that this vaccine induced good antibody responses but when the vaccinees later became naturally infected with this virus, they showed no evidence of protection and indeed developed illnesses which were more severe than those occurring in non-vaccinated individuals. It is thought that the cause of this abnormal response is the reaction on the epithelium that occurs between serum IgG antibodies induced by the vaccine and the infecting virus.

A similar reaction could be responsible for acute bronchiolitis of infancy; in these infections the IgG taking part in the reaction is passively acquired maternal antibody. The type of immunological reaction responsible for these infections is not known; it has been postulated that it might be a Type I allergic reaction or a Type III Arthus reaction (*Lancet*, 1969; Gardner, McQuillin & Court, 1970; Blandford, 1970). Interesting as these findings are, it must be appreciated that RSV is the only respiratory virus that is known to cause these allergic type reactions. They are not, for instance, produced by the structurally similar parainfluenza Type III virus, which also infects very young children and which was also used as an inactivated vaccine in the trials referred to above. The finding that the immunosuppressant compound cyclophosphamide causes deterioration rather than amelioration of a respiratory viral infection in an animal model (Robinson, Cureton & Heath, 1969) again makes it unlikely that immunological processes commonly exert harmful effects in virus infections of the respiratory tract. With the data so far available it seems wise, in most instances, to regard the initial necrosis of the epithelium to result directly from viral replication in the cells of this membrane.

Recovery from respiratory viral infection

Following the establishment of infection, virus titres rise in affected tissue for a few days and then decline; it is unusual to be able to detect any virus by the second week of the infection. Once virus eradication has started, cellular necrosis stops and repair of the tissue follows.

Termination of these infections is a complex but nevertheless very efficient process. It is brought about by a number of interdependent factors which are induced by the infection. These include the inflammatory response, interferon production and the immune response. The assessment of how much each of these factors contributes to the recovery process is particularly difficult.

The sequence of events in a typical respiratory infection are shown diagrammatically in Fig. 6.5. It can be seen from this figure, that virus titres rapidly rise in the infected tissues reaching peak levels after a few days. They then decline with equal rapidity so that virus can rarely be detected during the second week of the infection. The figure also shows the time of appearance of various substances and tissue changes which have been induced by viral replication. These will now be described individually and their possible role in the recovery process discussed.

Non-specific factors. Those thought to be involved in the recovery process are interferon and various components of the inflammatory response.

Interferon. This is an antiviral protein which is synthesised by cells in which viral replication is taking place. From Fig. 6.5 it can be seen that there is a close association between interferon production and virus growth and that as soon as peak interferon titres are reached, virus titres begin to fall. This relationship between virus growth and interferon production has been consistently found in experimental virus infections, including those which do not involve the respiratory tract (Friedman *et al.*, 1962; Sydiskis & Schultz, 1966). These findings strongly suggest that interferon is an important factor in the termination of virus infections.

Inflammatory changes. Fig. 6.5 shows that the inflammatory changes have roughly the same relationship to the virus growth curve as interferon but their antiviral effects are less clearly understood. The increased vascular and tissue permeability in the inflamed submucosa will bring various serum constituents in contact with infected cells and this may include non-specific viral inhibitors as well as antibody resulting from previous infection. The raised temperature, low oxygen tension and low pH of the inflamed tissue are thought to be antiviral (Lwoff, 1959) and this may be a result of their enhancement of interferon activity.

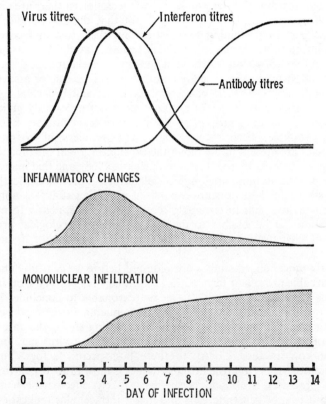

FIG. 6.5. Sequential changes in respiratory tissues infected with viruses.

Recent work has, however, shed some doubt on the importance of both interferon and the inflammatory changes as factors in the recovery process. A study of an experimental respiratory virus infection has shown that when the infected animals were given immunosuppressive agents a more serious disease with intense inflammatory changes was produced (Robinson, Cureton & Heath, 1969). Antibody production was, of course, found to be depressed but surprisingly it was found that there was an increased amount of interferon in the affected tissues. This sequence of events has also been observed in non-respiratory viral infections (Murphy & Glasgow, 1967; Nathanson & Cole, 1968).

Immune responses. The mononuclear response which develops in tissues infected with respiratory viruses (see Fig. 4(*d*)) contains large numbers of lymphocytes. plasmablasts and plasma cells known collectively as 'immuno· cytes'. They are concerned with the production of at least two classes of immunoglobulin. The most interesting of these is secretory IgA which is a dimer consisting of two IgA molecules joined together by a component made in the epithelial cells known as *secretor piece*. In respiratory viral infections secretory IgA is only found in the mucus. IgG is the other immunoglobulin made by the immunocytes and this is mainly released into the circulation although it may appear in the secretions if there are underlying inflammatory changes. There is little doubt that these antibodies play an important part in preventing re-infection but their role in recovery from primary infection has been more difficult to understand. The reason for this is shown in Fig. 6.5, where it can be seen that antibodies cannot be detected until the eradication process is virtually completed. This is true of assays carried out on both serum, extracts of respiratory tissue and bronchial secretions. This delay in the appearance of antibody does not necessarily indicate that immune processes have no part in the recovery from primary infection. It has, for example, been shown that large numbers of pyroninophilic lymphocytes are present in the mononuclear infiltration at the time that virus titres begin to fall (Robinson, Cureton & Heath, 1968), and that many of these cells are producing immunoglobulins (Blandford, Cureton & Heath. 1971). It is possible that these cells are capable of providing sufficient antibody in the micro-environment to terminate the infection. These early formed antibodies would be impossible to detect by standard serological procedures because of their fixation to excess virus that is present in the tissues at this time.

Clearly more refined studies are required before we can fully understand the remarkable process of termination of primary respiratory viral infection. From the data so far available it seems reasonable to conclude that non-specific factors such as interferon and the inflammatory response exert a moderating influence on the infection by slowing down the rate of viral replication. It is also possible that the virulence of a virus may in part be dependent on its susceptibility to these non-specific factors. The actual eradication of virus from the affected tissues is most probably carried out by immune processes. Antibody is the most likely effector mechanism, for although it cannot penetrate cells and arrest intracellular replication, it can combine with released virus and so prevent infection of the remaining susceptible cells. The progression of the infection could thus be effectively stopped and the resulting absence of infectious virus in the tissues would permit repair of damaged membranes.

Clinical Aspects of Respiratory Infection

Classification

The clinical manifestations of infections with respiratory viruses show considerable variation and there is, unfortunately, no uniformity to the terminology used to describe them.

The quasi medico-scientific method of using anatomically-rooted terms such as 'tracheitis' etc., enjoys a considerable vogue. This method merely suggests the supposed site of origin of the dominant symptom. This is clearly unsatisfactory for the obvious reason that symptoms change during the course of an illness. For example, a simple uncomplicated cold of moderate severity could successively be labelled 'pharyngitis', 'rhinitis' and 'laryngitis'.

Ideally one would prefer a classification based on aetiology but this is not possible because a single virus type can, even during one outbreak, be the

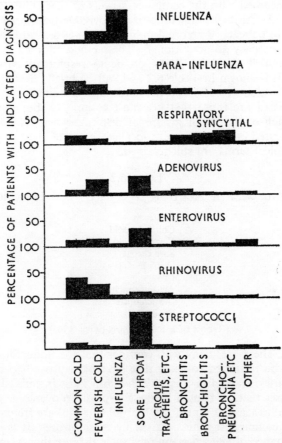

FIG. 6.6. The aetiology of various respiratory viral syndromes.
(Report of MRC working party, 1965)

cause of a wide range of clinically different illnesses. It is, however, generally true that each of the well-recognised syndromes of respiratory virus infection is most commonly caused by one group of viruses (see Fig. 6.6).

Bacterial involvement, either primary or secondary, in acute respiratory infection is another factor which confuses classification. It is not generally considered that these organisms are of much importance in infection of the upper air passages, although streptococcal sore throat and otitis media are obvious exceptions to this rule. There is, however, no doubt that there is a close association between viral and bacterial infections of the bronchi and lung parenchyma and this will be discussed in greater detail below.

In certain instances it suffices to lump together all the various syndromes under a common name such as 'acute respiratory infection'. If required a further subdivision into mild or severe could be made depending on whether the illness prevents the patient from carrying out his normal activities. Such a scheme would provide a simple but nevertheless useful terminology for those concerned with the economic aspects of these diseases.

Confronted with these difficulties it is inevitable that some sort of compromise has to be reached before deciding upon a classification which can be satisfactorily used by all practitioners. The method adopted by the Medical Research Council Working Party on acute respiratory virus infections (Report 1965) is shown in Table 6.2 and will be briefly described. It uses a terminology which consists for the most part of simple lay terms. The syndromes listed are those that are most commonly, but not exclusively, caused by each of the major groups of respiratory viruses. Since many of these viruses predominantly involve localised areas of the respiratory tract, a few anatomical terms are still retained.

TABLE 6.2

SYNDROMES OF ACUTE RESPIRATORY VIRAL INFECTION

Influenza
Common cold
Feverish cold
Sore throat
Otitis media
Croup
Acute bronchitis
Bronchiolitis
Pneumonia

(Report of MRC working party, 1965)

Influenza. There are many who consider that the unqualified use of this term should be restricted to cases that have been proved to be caused by influenza viruses. If used in this way the term must include all the various clinical illnesses that are caused by these viruses. To overcome this difficulty the terms 'influenza-like illness' or the popular 'flu' are frequently used to describe the commonest illness caused by these viruses. It is characterised by the dominance of general symptoms such as feverishness, malaise, headache and muscle pain whereas the symptoms attributable to respiratory tract involvement such as sore throat and cough are a comparatively minor cause of complaint. The illness frequently has a sudden onset and another unusual feature is marked debility which some patients experience in the convalescent stage. A detailed account of this syndrome can be found in the monograph by Stuart-Harris (1965).

Common cold. This is an illness which is as familiar to the layman as it is to the doctor because it is by far the commonest clinical manifestation of respiratory virus infection. It has a fairly well defined symtomatology which results from involvement of the nasal mucosa and hence includes sneezing, nasal discharge and nasal obstruction. Sore throat is nearly always present.

It is an afebrile illness with few if any constitutional symptoms. Although this illness is the cause of much inconvenience it is unusual for it to result in any restriction of the patients' normal activities.

Feverish cold. This syndrome has all the features of an ordinary cold which have just been described but with the addition of pyrexia and general constitutional signs such as malaise, shivering and headache. A productive cough is usually present. This condition resembles the influenza-like illnesses but is distinguished from them by the early appearance and dominant nature of the localised symptomatology. It is commonly no more than a severe rhinovirus infection but under this heading must now be included the conditions formerly known as 'febrile catarrh' (Stuart-Harris, Smith & Andrewes, 1937) and 'acute respiratory disease' or ARD (Commission, 1948) which are commonly caused by adenoviruses.

Sore throat. Practically all patients infected with respiratory viruses experience soreness of the throat. In some this is the overriding or only symptom and these illnesses should be recorded under this heading. Fever, headache and malaise are common associated symptoms. Nearly all the respiratory viruses and bacteria such as the haemolytic streptococcus can cause this illness. It is, however, impossible clinically to distinguish between the illnesses caused by viruses or bacteria.

Otitis media. Earache commonly occurs in respiratory viral infections and is thought to be due to pressure changes resulting from inflammation near the openings of the eustachian tubes. There may be infection of the aural membranes but this is difficult to demonstrate. In the majority of cases there are no physical signs. Reddened drums or perforation with a purulent discharge are usually an indication of secondary bacterial infection. These comments could equally well apply to acute sinusitis which perhaps might also be regarded as a respiratory viral syndrome.

Croup. This simple lay term is being increasingly used to replace the more cumbersome 'acute laryngo-tracheobronchitis'. In this illness, which mainly occurs in young children, the infection predominantly involves the larynx and is characterised by hoarseness, stridor and other evidence of upper airway obstruction. The severe forms of this illness are serious paediatric emergencies. Parainfluenza viruses are the commonest causative organisms.

Acute bronchitis. This illness can be regarded as an extension of a cold or influenza-like illness downwards into the chest. It begins with the symptoms of one of these upper respiratory tract infections and proceeds to the development of a cough with mucoid sputum, wheezing and dyspnoea. Bronchitis is not associated with any particular virus group.

Bronchiolitis. The probability of this condition being an immune mediated tissue reaction to respiratory syncytial virus has been discussed above. It will be recalled that it is thought to be brought about by the reaction between passively acquired maternal IgG antibody and viral antigens and is therefore mainly a disease of young babies. The typical case, with the cyanosed infant struggling to ventilate its lungs, is frightening to see. The illness is characterised by rapid wheezing respirations and retraction of the chest wall on inspiration. Rhonchi and fine rales are heard on auscultation. It is distinguished from croup by the absence of stridor and from pneumonia by the absence of radiological evidence of consolidation.

This condition is not commonly diagnosed in older children and adults although any respiratory infection which extends downwards into the chest can involve the bronchioles. In these age groups bronchiolar involvement can be caused by any of the respiratory viruses but it is difficult to distinguish from bronchitis and bronchopneumonia.

Pneumonia. The association between viral infection and pneumonia is extremely important but complex. In the discussion on pathogenesis it was pointed out that these viral infections primarily involve the ciliated columnar epithelium which extends from the nose down to the bronchioli. This membrane is structurally very different from the endothelial lining of the alveoli and it appears that the latter is very much less susceptible to virus infection. Because of this, primary viral pneumonitis is comparatively rare. It has, however, been reported following infection with influenza viruses (Hers, 1955), adenoviruses (Miller *et al.*, 1963), and even rhinoviruses (George & Mogabgab, 1969).

The term viral pneumonia is frequently used to describe lung infections caused by *Mycoplasma pneumoniae* (Eaton agent), psittacosis and *Coxiella burneti* (Q fever). This terminology is strictly incorrect as these organisms are not viruses. The condition sometimes known as 'primary atypical pneumonia' with high levels of cold red cell agglutinins and antibodies against streptococcus MG, is now known to be caused by *M. pneumoniae*.

Secondary bacterial infection is the most important cause of pneumonia associated with respiratory viral infection.

Secondary bacterial infection

It has been stressed above that the destruction of the columnar epithelium by viruses leaves the respiratory tract particularly susceptible to bacterial infection. This must in part be due to the loss, over large areas, of cilia which normally provides an efficient clearing mechanism for particulate matter. It is also possible that the inflammatory exudate and excess mucus that appears on the surface of the respiratory tract during these infections is conducive to the growth of bacteria.

Pneumococci are the organisms most frequently responsible for secondary infection, although *haemophilus influenzae*, staphylococci, streptococci and various gram negative bacilli have also been incriminated. These infections may be either exogenous or endogenous in origin.

Upper respiratory tract. Bacterial infection is thought to be an infrequent complication of viral infections which are restricted to the upper respiratory tract. This view is supported by the finding that antibiotics have little or no effect on these infections (Cecil, Plummer & Smillie, 1944; Wynn-Williams, 1961; Fraser, Hatch & Hughes, 1962).

The relationship between viral infection and both otitis media and sinusitis has been discussed above. Since virus infection can interfere with drainage from the ear and sinuses it is not surprising that they can predispose to secondary bacterial infection. Chronic infections of these cavities can also be exacerbated by virus infection.

Lower respiratory tract. In contrast to this situation in the upper air passages, there is no doubt that viral infections are an important predisposing cause of bacterial infection of the lungs and bronchi.

The association between viral infection and pneumonia is suggested by the fact that patients frequently recall symptoms of a cold or influenza at the onset of the illness. This association between viral and bacterial infection of the lung is best demonstrated during influenza outbreaks when there is a marked increase in the incidence of pneumonia. It is, for example, only at these times that one commonly sees cases of staphylococcal pneumonia (Oswald, Shooter & Curwen, 1958). The latter is the most serious complication of influenza but secondary infection with pneumococci occurs much more frequently. There is such good correlation between influenza viral infection and pneumonia that death from the latter has been found to be a reliable index of influenza epidemics. This will be discussed in greater detail below.

The association between pneumonia and viral infection other than influenza is less well established and there are several reasons for this. Influenza is the only infection of this kind which occurs in sharp widespread epidemics so that its effect on pneumonia statistics can be determined. It will be appreciated that by the time a typical case of pneumonia has been admitted to the wards, the virus infection is in its convalescent stage. It is usually impossible to isolate virus at this time and there is rarely an acute stage serum available for satisfactory serological tests. In spite of these difficulties it has been demonstrated that viruses other than influenza can predispose to pneumonia (Mufson et al., 1967; Schonell et al., 1969).

From information of this kind, it seems reasonable to assume that much of the pneumonia that occurs in previously healthy individuals is not in fact a primary bacterial infection but is secondary to viral infection of the respiratory tract. Before this assumption is established it is clearly necessary to carry out more elaborate prospective studies, particularly with rhinovirus infections.

The relationship between viral infection and chronic bronchitis is of particular interest. The chronic inflammatory state of the mucosa in this disease is generally regarded to be the result of the interaction of several factors such as air pollution as well as bacterial infection. No one seriously considers that viruses play a direct part in the maintenance of the abnormal changes of the respiratory mucosa for the reason that chronic inflammatory changes are not a feature of viral infection. It is theoretically possible that the repair processes which occur after each virus infection are impaired by pollution and this could be one of several factors that lead to the establishment of this disease.

It is, however, well known that chronic bronchitics are at special risk during influenza outbreaks and it is now well established that acute viral infections are one of the causes of acute exacerbations of this condition. This has been shown to occur after infection with influenza virus (Tyrrell, 1952), parainfluenza virus (Stark, Heath & Curwen, 1965), and rhinoviruses (Eadie, Stott & Grist, 1966).

Epidemiology of Respiratory Virus Infection

Respiratory viruses are highly infectious and apart from immunity derived from past infection, there is little to bar their spread in the community. However, each of the major groups of these viruses has a fairly distinct pattern of spread which will be briefly described.

Influenza. The three types of influenza virus, epidemiologically, behave quite differently. The type A strains are responsible for the much publicised pandemics which occur roughly every ten years. These extensive outbreaks usually originate in south-east China and spread via the trade routes to the rest of the world. In the years following a pandemic it has been found in most countries that epidemics of decreasing intensity appear about every other year. In Britain these smaller epidemics are nearly always restricted to the period just after the Christmas holidays.

The cause of this extraordinary epidemiology is now known to be due to variation in the antigenic structure of these viruses. Each pandemic is caused by a novel antigenic type of virus and since they originate in a fairly localised area of China it has been speculated that the virus originates from some animal reservoir. The epidemics that occur in the inter-pandemic years are associated with minor antigenic variation which is thought to be brought about by mutation.

The influenza B viruses show a similar but less dramatic variation in both antigenic structure and epidemiological behaviour. They never give rise to pandemics but can be responsible for extensive national outbreaks such as the one that occurred in Britain during the winter of 1961–62. Influenza C virus does not show antigenic variation and only causes sporadic illnesses of a relatively mild nature.

This variable epidemiological behaviour of influenza causes immense problems particularly in the field of prevention. Because of it, the components of influenza vaccines have to be constantly changed and advice on their use is hampered by the difficulty of predicting the intensity of the forthcoming winter's epidemic. Our recent experience with Hong Kong influenza illustrates these problems. In the summer of 1968, widespread outbreaks of influenza developed in the Far East and were shown to be due to a virus which antigenically differed considerably from previous strains. This new virus spread in the characteristic way along the trade routes and as the British population had very little immunity to the new strain, it was confidently predicted that we would experience a severe epidemic during the winter of 1968–69. It will be recalled that although cases of Hong Kong influenza occurred that winter, they were so infrequent that it cannot be said that we experienced an epidemic. It looked at that time that Britain was going to be fortunate and 'miss out' on Hong Kong influenza but hopes were dashed in the next winter (1969–70) when we endured a particularly severe outbreak. The reason for this peculiar behaviour of the Hong Kong virus in Britain is obscure, but will be discussed in greater detail in the following section.

Parainfluenza and respiratory syncytial viruses. These viruses, although physically and biologically similar to the influenza viruses, epidemiologically behave very differently. They are endemic viruses predominantly affecting young children. It has been shown that over 90 per cent of children have been infected with types 1, 2 and 3 parainfluenza viruses by the age of 10 (Stark, Heath & Peto, 1964), and over 85 per cent with respiratory syncytial virus by the age of 14 (Hambling, 1964). Re-exposure to all of these viruses in adult life can result in infection and mild upper respiratory tract disease.

Adenoviruses. These viruses are, on epidemiological grounds, divided into two groups, the so-called *endemic* and *epidemic* groups. The former, mainly types 1, 2 and 5, are common infectious agents of young children causing sporadic pyrexial illnesses sometimes with respiratory symptoms. The latter, such as the types 3, 4 and 7, are frequently associated with epidemics of fairly severe respiratory disease in semi-closed communities such as military recruit camps and boarding schools.

Rhinoviruses. To date there is insufficient information to be able to give a precise description of the epidemiology of the infections caused by these common viruses. Because of the multiplicity of antigenic types, it is obvious that the pattern will be complex. It appears that rhinovirus infections are more common in the spring and autumn. Some types produce sharp epidemics and then vanish completely whilst others reappear after a few years. Others produce a small number of infections at frequent intervals (Hamre, 1968).

Statistical Analyses of Respiratory Viral Infection

In recent years much effort has been made to obtain accurate information on this subject and the results obtained are beginning to yield useful information on the importance of these diseases. Investigators in this field have attempted to answer three basic questions:

1. How frequently do individuals experience these diseases?
2. What effect do they have on the economic competence of the individual?
3. How often are they responsible for serious illness or death?

This information is not easy to obtain particularly since respiratory viral infections are not notifiable diseases and in any case not all affected patients consult a doctor about them. Another problem is the difficulty of precise diagnosis and description. For example, cases of pneumonia and acute exacerbations of chronic bronchitis induced by viral infection will rarely be attributed to this cause. On the other hand it has been asserted that there is a sharp increase in the incidence of these illnesses in areas where mid-week football cup ties are being played!

Because of these difficulties it is obvious that the information required has often to be obtained by indirect means and must therefore be lacking in great precision.

Incidence

How frequently individuals experience acute respiratory viral infections is perhaps the most difficult but probably the least important question to answer. Difficulty is experienced with trivial symptoms such as discomfort of the throat and stuffiness of the nose which can wrongly be attributed to viral infection. Again, as has been frequently stressed, viral involvement in more serious chest disease is invariably underestimated.

The only way to obtain precise information on incidence is to carry out prospective studies of groups of all ages and from all the social strata. These should preferably be continued for a number of years to average the effect of the variable annual incidence of influenza. Few studies of this kind have been carried out but all have indicated a very high incidence of these diseases. One of the best of these studies was that carried out by Dingle and his colleagues (1953) in Cleveland, Ohio. They closely observed 61 families of high socio-economic class for 2 years. They found that on average an individual had 10 illnesses per year and that 6 of these were upper respiratory tract infections. In a similar investigation carried out in Britain it was estimated that the average number of colds per person was 7 per year and each lasted about 10 days (Hope Simpson, 1958). From the latter figures it can be calculated that a 70-year-old would have spent about 16 years of his life suffering from a cold-like illness. To many, the figures obtained from these intensive surveys seem incredibly high and one wonders if there has been some over reporting of symptoms which have no association with respiratory viral infection. Other investigators have recorded an average of 2 colds per year (Lidwell & Williams, 1961) which is the sort of figure usually given by adults on retrospective questioning. These investigations have also shown that acute respiratory disease occurs much more frequently in children than it does in adults (Fry, 1957; Lidwell & Sommerville, 1951; Brimblecombe et al., 1958), and that they occur with greater frequency in winter months (Dingle et al., 1953; Hope Simpson, 1958).

Absenteeism

Studies of work loss because of respiratory viral infection can be regarded as more important than mere assessment of incidence, because they ignore the trivial effects of these infections and instead concentrate on those aspects which are of considerable importance to the national economy. Here again one encounters difficulties. Absenteeism is not simply related to illness but is dependent to some extent on the type of work, the availability and value of sickness benefits and the attitude of the individual to sickness. It must be appreciated that relatively mild illnesses such as the acute respiratory virus infections can be an excuse for absenteeism, rather than a cause. Most of the data on this subject has been obtained from an analysis of sickness benefit claims submitted to the Ministry of Pensions. The validity of analyses of respiratory viral infection obtained from this source is dependent on the accuracy of the recorded diagnosis and must of necessity be poor. The term 'flu', for example, is often used to describe any acute pyrexial illness, and in consequence only occasionally indicates infection with an influenza virus. Again the term 'bronchitis', which is so frequently found on sickness certificates, is one which is most difficult to interpret. It is sometimes used to describe an infection by a respiratory virus which has extended down into the chest and which may or may not be associated with secondary bacterial infection. At other times it denotes sudden deterioration in a chronic bronchitic, which may be caused by a virus or by a transient increase in atmospheric pollution or some other factor. These problems should be kept in mind when examining data such as that presented in Table 6.3. This shows the number of illnesses, the number of work days lost and the cost of sickness benefit attributed to various illnesses in the year 1962–63. It can be seen that over 40 per cent of the illnesses that resulted in absence from work were those that involved the respiratory tract and that they were responsible for over a quarter of both work days lost and the amount paid out in sickness benefit. For the reasons discussed above, it is not possible to accurately determine how many of these respiratory illnesses have been caused or initiated by viruses but there can be little doubt that the proportion will be high. If one considers the syndromes

TABLE 6.3

WORK LOST THROUGH RESPIRATORY ILLNESS IN 1963–64

Recorded Illness	Spells of Illness Commencing ($\times 10^3$)	Total Work Days Lost ($\times 10^6$)	Cost of Benefits (£m)
Acute nasopharyngitis (common cold)	480·4	4·64	3
Acute pharyngitis and tonsillitis	524·0	5·07	3
Influenza	1192·7	13·88	8
Bronchitis	916·2	39·25	22
Other respiratory diseases	501·8	13·41	7
TOTAL RESPIRATORY ILLNESSES	3615·1	76·25	43
TOTAL ALL ILLNESSES	8444·5	288·86	162

(Derived from the Report of the Ministry of Pensions and National Insurance for the year 1963.)

which most likely have a viral aetiology, e.g. common cold, pharyngitis and influenza, it can be calculated that they accounted for 60 per cent of the respiratory illnesses recorded but for only 25 per cent of the work days lost. In contrast to this, the corresponding figures for bronchitis are only 30 per cent of the illnesses but 50 per cent of the work days lost. It seems probable therefore that the illnesses recorded as common cold, pharyngitis and influenza, because of their short duration, give a fairly accurate measure of uncomplicated respiratory virus infection. The more prolonged illnesses described as bronchitis must be more complicated than this. As discussed above, they may be no more than severe forms of simple respiratory viral infection or they may be exacerbations of chronic bronchitis.

Confronted with the problem of inaccurate diagnoses on the health certificates it is not surprising that some have succumbed to the temptation of ignoring the clinical data and have instead analysed *total* applications for sickness benefit irrespective of cause.

For reasons that will be discussed below, this analytical procedure can give very little information on the total effect of respiratory virus infection on absenteeism but it has been shown to provide a most useful index of influenza infection (Roden, 1963). The reason for this is that the latter occur in extensive outbreaks of such short duration that their effect on absenteeism, at these times, can be compared with estimates made at periods in the same year when influenza is not prevalent and at corresponding times in non-influenzal years.

The effect of an influenza epidemic on the weekly number of benefit claims is shown in Fig. 6.7. The years 1968 to 1970 were selected because they demonstrate the peculiar behaviour of the Hong Kong strain of influenza virus in Britain, which has been described in the section on epidemiology. It can be seen from this figure that during the winter of 1968–69, when it was confidently expected that the new Hong Kong variant would produce a severe outbreak, that the number of claims remained fairly constant at about a quarter of a million per week. Influenza due to this virus did not become epidemic until the next winter. This is reflected in the weekly number of claims that year which started a dramatic increase in mid-December and which reached a peak of just over three quarters of a million for the week ending the 6th January 1970. The unexpected dip in both curves towards the end of December is merely an artificial effect due to the Christmas holiday period

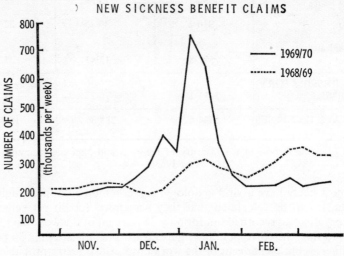

FIG. 6.7. Weekly numbers of new claims for sickness benefit submitted to the Department of Health and Social Security during the winters of 1968/69 and 1969/70.

(Data obtained from the Registrar General's weekly returns.)

and does not indicate a temporary abatement of the epidemic. The difference between the 1968–69 and 1969–70 curves provides most convincing evidence of the effect of influenza infections on absenteeism. Comparative data of this kind excludes to a large extent the individuals attitude to illness, particularly if one remembers that the 1969–70 epidemic was not preceded by near hysterical press prognostication as occurred in the previous year.

If one virus can have such a marked influence on absenteeism it is certain that the other respiratory viruses have a similar effect, even though we have no easy method of assessing this, although such a conclusion must be tempered by the fact that influenza infections are, in general, more severe than those caused by the other respiratory viruses.

Serious illness resulting from respiratory virus infection

Since respiratory virus infections occur with increased frequency in the winter months and as this is the time of greatest demand for hospital beds, it is tempting to assume that there is a causal relationship between these two events. Unfortunately, because there are so many respiratory viruses and so many difficulties to diagnosis, it is impossible to obtain precise information on their total effect on serious illness. We can, however, make a reasonable guess as to their importance by again restricting our observations to influenza epidemics. It is important to realise that with analyses of this kind we are comparing the incidence of illnesses caused by just one virus, with illness due to all other causes including those due to the remaining respiratory viruses.

It has been shown that amounts of serious illness resulting from influenza can best be estimated by consideration of the numbers requiring hospital admission at these times and the effect on mortality from the certified number of deaths attributed to influenza and also to pneumonia and bronchitis (Miller & Lee, 1969). The use of these procedures will be illustrated by again considering the strange behaviour of the Hong Kong influenza strains during the winters of 1968–69 and 1969–70.

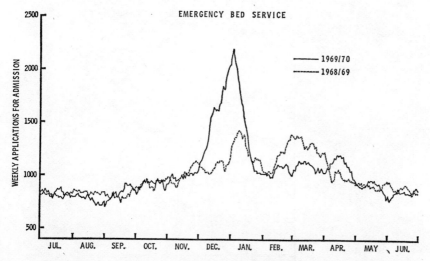

FIG. 6.8. Weekly numbers of applications for hospital admission submitted to the Emergency Bed Service during the winters of 1968–69 and 1969–70.

(From data kindly provided by the Director of the Emergency Bed Service.)

Effect of influenza on hospital admission rates. In the London area there is an independent organisation known as the Emergency Bed Service (E.B.S.) which arranges hospital admissions for general practitioners. The service is mainly used by the latter when there is difficulty in obtaining beds in the patients' local hospital. The weekly number of requests received by the E.B.S. are therefore a measure of the stress being experienced by the London hospitals during that week and are indirectly a measure of the incidence of serious illness at that time. Examination of their records shows that as winter approaches there is a steady rise in the number of requests for hospital admission. In the years when influenza is epidemic there is a marked increase in the number of these requests. Because of this the E.B.S. returns has proved to be a most valuable indicator of the onset and progress of influenza epidemics.

From Fig. 6.8 it can be seen that during the abortive epidemic of 1968–69, requests for admission did not rise above 1500 per week. The epidemic due to this new virus which developed the next winter is clearly reflected in the returns for that year which showed a dramatic increase in the number of requests for admission, which finally reached a peak of about 2300 at the beginning of January. This increased demand for hospital beds must primarily have been due to infection with influenza but the ultimate reason for admission

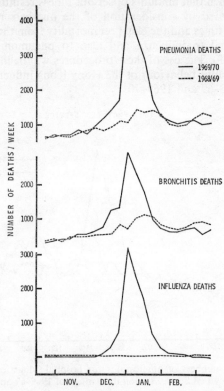

FIG. 6.9. Weekly numbers of deaths attributed to pneumonia, bronchitis and influenza in the winters of 1968–69 and 1969–70.

(Data obtained from the Registrar General's weekly returns.)

would mainly have been complications of this infection such as pneumonia, exacerbations of chronic bronchitis, sudden deterioration in the health of the aged and those with chronic disease of the heart and kidneys.

Effect of influenza on death rates. The Registrar Generals' weekly returns show the number of deaths attributed to influenza (International Classification of Diseases (ICD) Nos. 470–4) and also to pneumonia (ICD Nos. 480–6) and bronchitis (ICD Nos. 490–3). As with the E.B.S. returns the weekly number of deaths attributed to all these causes rises as winter approaches and declines again in the spring. The effect of an influenza epidemic on these statistics can be seen by again comparing the various death rates in the winter months of the non-epidemic and epidemic years of 1968–69 and 1969–70. These are shown in Fig. 6.9. It can be seen that the 1970 epidemic resulted in a dramatic increase in the number of deaths attributed to influenza, pneumonia and bronchitis. At the peak of the epidemic deaths due to these causes were at least three times higher than in the corresponding period of 1969.

One further aspect of influenza infection must be mentioned and that is that during certain epidemics *deaths from all causes* show a significant increase over those occurring at the same time in non-epidemic years (Roden, 1963).

From the information obtained from the E.B.S. returns and death rates there can be little doubt that influenza is responsible for a considerable amount of serious illness which frequently proves fatal. For reasons that have been discussed above, it is not possible to obtain comparable information on the other respiratory viruses. Infections caused by these viruses are much commoner than influenza but are probably less severe. They must nevertheless be responsible for some part of the increased morbidity and mortality which is seen in the winter months of the years when influenza is not epidemic. At present, it is not possible to distinguish between the effects of these viruses and the effects of environmental factors such as low temperature and increased air pollution.

Prevention and Treatment of Respiratory Viral Disease

The considerable success that has been achieved in understanding the aetiology, pathogenesis and prevalence of these diseases has not unfortunately been matched by comparable success in developing means for either their prevention or treatment. In line with developments in other fields of virology, most effort has been concentrated on the production of vaccines. It has been hoped that, by these means, it would be possible to simulate the successful poliomyelitis eradication programme of the last decade or the comparable campaigns currently being carried out against measles and rubella. Only with influenza vaccines has some partial success been achieved. Antiviral chemotherapy is still in its infancy and to date only one anti-respiratory viral compound is available and its efficacy is questionable.

Vaccination

The vast number of different antigenic types of respiratory viruses (see Table 6.1) makes the development of a broad spectrum vaccine incredibly difficult and perhaps even impossible. The problem can best be understood by considering the possible prevention of rhinovirus infection. There are at least one hundred different antigenic types of this virus and although inactivated rhinovirus vaccines can be made it is clearly not going to be possible to incorporate an adequate number of antigenic types into a single vaccine.

Inactivated vaccines against the parainfluenza viruses and respiratory syncytial virus have also been developed (Kapikian *et al.*, 1969) and should be capable of reducing an appreciable amount of respiratory illness in childhood. In spite of this there is little enthusiasm for the introduction of further vaccines which have to be injected into young children and the sensitisation which is produced by respiratory syncytial virus vaccines, is a further discouragement.

Influenza is obviously the first of the respiratory virus diseases to be prevented since we have only to deal with one antigenic type at any one time and we are well aware of its devastating effects. Here again there are many difficulties, such as the appearance of new antigenic variants and the constant problem of trying to predict whether the current strain is going to produce an epidemic the next winter.

Inactivated influenza vaccines have been available for a number of years and have been shown to provide between 40 and 70 per cent protection. The indications for the use of these vaccines are now well defined. At the time of an impending pandemic, as many people as possible should be vaccinated. Since supplies of vaccine containing the new strain are invariably in short supply at these times, some priority scheme has to be worked out. Special consideration should be given to those who work in the communications and transportation industries, to those who work in the health service and to those with chronic pulmonary, cardiac and renal diseases. In the years between pandemics vaccination should be restricted to the latter. Only in special circumstances should healthy individuals be vaccinated at these times, although this is now the routine practice of doctors who have the care of those living in semi-closed communities such as military establishments and boarding schools. Routine vaccination is also carried out by some industrial medical officers in attempts to reduce the costly economic effects of absenteeism at the time of epidemics.

Much work is now being carried out to improve the current influenza vaccines. Split vaccines, which contain only part instead of the whole virus particle (Brandon et al., 1969), are now generally available. These vaccines are certainly less toxic but probably no more effective than standard preparations. Vaccination carried out with live attenuated viruses has been shown to be far more effective than the current procedure (Beare et al., 1968). It would, however, be very difficult for commercial companies to produce vaccines of this kind.

Further details on vaccination against respiratory viral disease can be obtained from the excellent review by Hobson (1967).

Antiviral chemotherapy

In spite of intensive efforts even less progress has been made in this field than with vaccines. Of the many substances that have been shown to possess antiviral properties only three, methisazone, idoxuridine and amantadine, are at the moment available for clinical use. The many problems concerned with the development and evaluation of these compounds has been discussed elsewhere (Heath, 1969).

Amantadine is the only one of the above three drugs which has been extensively investigated in respiratory virus disease. In the laboratory it has been shown to be active against some of the recent strains of influenza A virus. Unfortunately clinical trials have not consistently confirmed its effectiveness. Many of the trials have made use of volunteers deliberately infected with influenza viruses. Tyrrell and his colleagues (1965) failed to demonstrate any effect on infections induced by two British 1957 Asian strains, whereas Togo,

Hornick & Dawkins (1970) observed a significant reduction in feverish illness when the A2/Rockville/65 strain was used as challenge virus. Conflicting reports have also been obtaned in prophylactic studies carried out during natural outbreaks. Amantadine was thus found to produce reduction of contact infection due to the last of the Asian strains of influenza in the 1967–68 outbreak (Galbraith et al., 1969a), but the same group in a similar study failed to obtain protection against the Hong Kong variant that was prevalent the next winter (Galbraith et al., 1969b). More recent reports have, however, been more encouraging. A carefully controlled trial in Finland (Oker-Bloom et al., 1970) has shown that amantadine gave a 52 per cent protection against infections caused by the Hong Kong virus. This compound has also been shown to be effective when administered to patients with established disease (Hornick et al., 1969).

Considerable efforts are currently being made to develop compounds which are active against viruses, and some aspects such as the work on interferon and interferon inducers (see Finter, 1970) are of particular interest. In spite of this there are no other compounds which have been evaluated sufficiently to merit further discussion here.

Conclusion

The observation of a cytopathic effect in cultures of adenoid tissue by Rowe and his colleagues in 1953, led to the discovery of the adenoviruses and was to be the first important advance in respiratory virology since the discovery of the influenza viruses some 20 years previously. In the following years application of tissue culture techniques resulted in the discovery of so many new viruses that taxonomists have been hard pressed to keep up. Although we now have a detailed knowledge of the aetiology of these conditions it is unlikely that it is complete.

There are few diseases that are as simple as those caused by the respiratory viruses. In general they produce no more than superficial damage to the respiratory tract which is rapidly repaired. The transient nature of these illnesses is evidence of the powerful antiviral mechanisms which the host is able to call upon. Whilst the majority of these infections are trivial they achieve importance because of their great frequency and also because in our present society, relatively minor incapacity is considered adequate justification for absenteeism from work. It is now becoming apparent that, in countries where a high proportion of the population are elderly and where the air is polluted, these diseases are responsible for an appreciable amount of serious and even fatal illness. Because of this, respiratory viral disease must be regarded as the last of the great pestilences. Eradication is going to be far more difficult than the comparable problem with diseases of single aetiology such as poliomyelitis and smallpox. It seems probable that this will have to be achieved in piecemeal fashion, with influenza given first priority.

References

ANDREWES, C. H., CHAPRONIERE, D. M., GOMPELS, A. E. H., PEREIRA, H. G. & RODEN, A. T. (1953). Lancet, ii, 546.
ANDREWES, C. H., LAIDLAW, P. P. & SMITH, W. (1934). Lancet, ii, 859.
BEARD, C. W. & EASTERDAY, B. C. (1967). J. infect. Dis., 117, 66.

BEARE, A. S., HOBSON, D., REED, S. E. & TYRRELL, D. A. J. (1968). *Lancet*, **ii**, 418.
BEVERIDGE, W. I. B. & BURNET, F. M. (1946). *Spec. Rep. Ser. med. Res. Coun.*, No. 256.
BLANDFORD, G. (1970). *Br. med. J.*, **i**, 758.
BLANDFORD, G., CURETON, R. J. R. & HEATH, R. B. (1971). *J. med. Microbiol.*, **4**, 351.
BRANDON, F. B., COX, F., QUINN, E., TIMM, E. A. & McLEAN, I. W., JR., (1969). *Bull. Wld Hlth Org.*, **41**, 629.
BRIMBLECOMBE, F. S. W., CRUIKSHANK, R., MASTERS, P. L., REID, D. D. & STEWART, G. T. (1958). *Br. med. J.*, **i**, 119.
CECIL, R. L., PLUMMER, N. & SMILLIE, W. G. (1944). *J. Am. med. Ass.*, **124**, 8.
CHANOCK, R. M. (1956). *J. exp. Med.*, **104**, 555.
CHANOCK, R. M., ROIZMAN, B. & MYERS, R. (1957). *Am. J. Hyg.*, **66**, 281.
COATES, H. V. & CHANOCK, R. M. (1962). *Am. J. Hyg.*, **76**, 302.
COLE, G. A. & NATHANSON, N. (1968). *Nature*, **220**, 399.
Commission of Acute Respiratory Disease (1948). *Am. J. Hyg.*, **48**, 263.
DENK, H. & KOVAC, W. (1965). *Arch. ges. Virusforsch.*, **17**, 641.
DINGLE, J. H., BADGER, G. F., FELLER, A. E., HODGES, R. G., JORDAN, W. S., JR., & RAMMELKAMP, C. H. (1953). *Am. J. Hyg.*, **58**, 16.
EADIE, M. B., STOTT, E. J. & GRIST, N. R. (1966). *Br. med. J.*, **ii**, 671.
FAZEKAS DE ST. GROTH, S. (1952). *J. Hyg. Camb.*, **50**, 471.
FINTER, N. B. (1970). *In* "Modern Trends in Medical Virology", 2. Ed. R. B. Heath & A. P. Waterson. London: Butterworths.
FRANCIS, T. & STUART-HARRIS, S. H. (1938a). *J. exp. Med.*, **68**, 789.
FRANCIS, T. & STUART-HARRIS, S. H. (1938b). *J. exp. Med.*, **68**, 813.
FRASER, P. K., HATCH, L. A. & HUGHES, K. E. A. (1962). *Lancet*, **i**, 614.
FRIEDMAN, R. M., BARON, S., BUCKLER, C. E. & STEINMULLER, R. I. (1962). *J. exp. Med.*, **116**, 347.
FRY, J. (1957). *Br. med. J.*, **ii**, 1453.
FULGINITI, V. A., ELLER, J. J., SIEBER, O. F., JOYNER, J. W., MINAMITANI, M. & MEIKLEJOHN, G. (1969). *Am. J. Epidemiol.*, **89**, 435.
GALBRAITH, A. W., OXFORD, J. S., SCHILD, G. C. & WATSON, G. I. (1969a). *Lancet*, **ii**, 1026.
GALBRAITH, A. W., OXFORD, J. S., SCHILD, G. C. & WATSON, G. I. (1969b). *Bull. Wld Hlth Org.*, **41**, 677.
GARDNER, P. S. (1970). *In* "Modern Trends in Medical Virology,". 2 Ed. R. B. Heath & A. P. Waterson. London: Butterworths.
GARDNER, P. S., McQUILLIN, J. & COURT, S. D. M. (1970). *Br. med. J.*, **i**, 327.
GEORGE, R. B. & MOGABGAB, W. J. (1969). *Ann. intern. Med.*, **71**, 1073.
HAMBLING, M. H. (1964). *Br. med. J.*, **i**, 1223.
HAMRE, D. (1968). *Rhinoviruses*. p. 59. Basel/New York: Karger.
HARFORD, C. G., HAMLIN, A. & PARKER, E. (1955). *J. exp. Med.*, **101**, 577.
HEATH, R. B. (1969). *Br. J. hosp. Med.*, **2**, 1807.
HERS, J. F. Ph. (1955). "The Histopathology of the Respiratory Tract in Human Influenza". Leiden: H. Stenpert Kroese.
HERS, J. F. Ph. & MULDER, J. (1961). *Am. Rev. resp. Dis.*, **83**, pt. II, 84.
HERS, J. F. Ph., MULDER, J., MASUREL, N. v. d., Kuip, L. & TYRRELL, D. A. J. (1962). *J. Path. Bact.*, **83**, 207.
HOBSON, D. (1967). *In* "Modern Trends in Immunology," 2. Ed. R. Cruickshank & D. M. Weir. London: Butterworths.
HOORN, B. & TYRRELL, D. A. J. (1965). *Br. J. exp. Path.*, **46**, 109.
HOPE SIMPSON, R. E. (1958). *Practitioner*, **180**, 356.
HORNICK, R. B., TOGO, Y., MAHLER, S. & IEZZONI, D. (1969). *Bull Wld Hlth. Org.*, **41**, 671.

KAPIKIAN, A. Z., MITCHELL, R. H., CHANOCK, R. M., SHVEDOFF, R. A. & STEWART, C. E. (1969). *Am. J. Epidemiol.*, **89**, 405.

KIM, H. W., CANCHOLA, J. G., BRANDT, C. D., PYLES, G., CHANOCK, R. M., JENSEN, K. & PARROTT, R. H. (1969). *Am. J. Epidemiol.*, **89**, 422.

Lancet (1969). Vaccine Against Respiratory Syncytial Virus, **ii**, 311.

LIDWELL, O. M. & SOMMERVILLE, T. (1951). *J. Hyg. Camb.*, **49**, 365.

LIDWELL, O. M. & WILLIAMS, R. E. O. (1961). *J. Hyg. Camb.*, **59**, 309 and 321.

LWOFF, A. (1959). *Bact. Rev.*, **23**, 109.

MILLER, D. L. & LEE, J. A. (1969). *J. Hyg. Camb.*, **67**, 559.

MILLER, L. F., RYTEL, M., PIERCE, W. E. & ROSENBAUM, M. J. (1963). *J. Am. med. Ass.* **185**, 92.

MUFSON, M. A., CHANG, V., GILL, V., WOOD, S. C., ROMANSKY, M. J. & CHANOCK, R. M. (1967). *Am. J. Epidemiol.*, **86**, 526.

MURPHY, B. R. & GLASGOW, L. A. (1967). *Antimicrob. Agents & Chemother*. p. 661.

OGASAWARA, K., AIDA, M. & NAGATA, I. (1961). *J. Immun.*, **86**, 599.

OKER-BLOOM, N., HOVI, T., LEINIKKI, P., PALOSVO, T., PETTERSSON, R. & SUNI, J. (1970). *Br. med. J.* **iii**, 676.

OSWALD, N. C., SHOOTER, R. A. & CURWEN, M. P. (1958). *Br. med. J.* **ii**, 1305.

Report of the Medical Research Council Working Party on Acute Respiratory Virus Infection. (1965). *Br. med. J.*, **ii**, 319.

RITCHIE, J. M. (1958). *Lancet*, **i**, 618.

ROBINSON, T. W. E., CURETON, R. J. R. & HEATH, R. B. (1968). *J. med. Microbiol.*, **1**, 89.

ROBINSON, T. W. E., CURETON, R. J. R. & HEATH, R. B. (1969). *J. med. Microbiol.*, **2**, 137.

RODEN, A. T. (1963). *Post-grad. med. J.*, **39**, 612.

ROSS, J. G. & POTTER, C. W. (1961). *Lancet*, **i**, 81.

ROWE, W. P., HUEBNER, R. J., GILMORE, L. D., PARROTT, R. H. & WARD, T. G. (1953). *Proc. Soc. exp. Biol. Med.*, **84**, 570.

SCHONELL, M. E., GRAY, W., MOFFAT, M. A. J., CALDER, M. A. & STEWART, S. M. (1969). *Br. J. Dis. Chest.*, **63**, 140.

SMITH, W., ANDREWES, C. H. & LAIDLAW, P. P. (1933). *Lancet*, **ii**, 66.

STARK, J. E., HEATH, R. B. & PETO, S. (1964). *Arch. ges. Virusforsch.*, **14**, 160.

STARK, J. E., HEATH, R. B. & CURWEN, M. P. (1965). *Thorax.*, **20**, 124.

STUART-HARRIS, C. H. (1965). "Influenza and Other Virus Infections of the Respiratory Tract," 2nd ed. London: Edward Arnold.

STUART-HARRIS, C. H. & FRANCIS, T. (1938). *J. exp. Med.*, **68**, 803.

STUART-HARRIS, C. H., ANDREWES, C. H. & SMITH, W. (1938). *Spec. Rep. Ser. med. Res. Coun.*, No. 228.

SYDISKIS, R. J. & SCHULTZ, I. (1966). *J. infect. Dis.*, **116**, 455.

TOGO, Y., HORNICK, R. B. & DAWKINS, A. T. (1970). *J. Am. med. Ass.*, **203**, 1089.

TONG, M. J. & FONG, J. (1964). *J. Immun.*, **93**, 35.

TYRRELL, D. A. J. (1952). *Quart. J. Med. n. s.*, **21**, 291.

TYRRELL, D. A. J. (1965). "Common Colds and Related Diseases". London: Edward Arnold.

TYRRELL, D. A. J. & BYNOE, M. J. (1965). *Br. med. J.*, **i**, 1467.

TYRRELL, D. A. J., BYNOE, M. L. & HOORN, B. (1965). *Br. J. exp. Path.*, **46**, 370.

WALSH, J. J., DIETLEIN, L. F., LOW, F. N., BURCH, G. E. & MOGABGAB, W. J. (1961). *Archs intern. Med.*, **108**, 376.

WYNN-WILLIAMS, N. (1961). *Br. med. J.*, **i**, 469.

CHAPTER 7

ALCOHOL DEPENDENCE AND NEURO PSYCHIATRIC SYNDROMES DUE TO ALCOHOL

B. D. HORE

'In the bottle discontent seeks for
comfort, cowardice for courage and
bashfulness for confidence.'

Dr. Johnson

That drinking alcohol may lead to impairment of health and social well being has been recorded since time immemorial, and society has thus varyingly restricted the use of alcohol although at the same time being aware of the enjoyment alcohol brings, and its importance as a social custom. Society's attitudes to its members whose drinking leads them into difficulties have ranged from condemnation to humorous condescension (e.g. the music hall drunk). The medical profession has not been immune from these views; medical texts on alcoholism in the last century and early part of this century reveal a dichotomy between those who view the problem as essentially a moral one, and those who regard the alcoholic as a sick person. It is perhaps only in the last thirty years that an attempt has been made to understand scientifically the reasons behind the behaviour of those people who continue drinking despite obvious medical and social harm. Such people are usually called alcoholics. What actually constitutes an alcoholic, i.e. what is an adequate definition, has been and remains a considerable problem.

The most quoted definition is probably that of the WHO (1952): 'Alcoholics are those excessive drinkers whose dependence on alcohol has attained such a degree that it shows a noticeable mental disturbance or interference with their bodily or mental health, their interpersonal relations, and their smooth social and economic functions; or who show the prodromal signs of such development. They therefore require treatment.'

Besides the irrelevance to the definition of such terms as 'they require treatment' and the obvious anomaly of including the prodromal features of a syndrome in the definition of the syndrome itself more serious problems arise (Seeley, 1959a). These include the term 'excessive drinkers'; 'excessive' compared with whom? This must be a relative term, for it means anyone whose drinking goes beyond the traditional, customary or dietary levels of alcohol used by the community to which the person belongs. A second criticism is the use of social rather than medical criteria as part of the definition with the recognised difficulty of quantifying such variables. There are advantages however in such a definition. The most important is the use of the term 'dependence'. This has been discussed in relation to alcohol by Edwards

(1967). It implies a state in which drinking appears to have become a dominating necessity, one that cannot be broken, and this suggests that alcoholism is comparable to such disorders as dependency on drugs such as heroin and amphetamine. Dependency disorders are those in which there is physical or psychological dependence on a drug. Physical dependence implies that on withdrawal of the drug a characteristic withdrawal syndrome occurs. Dependency in relation to drugs including alcohol can be divided into three groups. In the first, physical dependence is regularly and rapidly produced and the personality of the individual is of secondary importance to the pharmacological effect of the drug. An example is heroin dependence. In the second, physical dependence does not occur but a pharmacological property produces a desired effect in certain personalities leading to psychological dependence. An example is possibly amphetamine. Finally, there are those drugs which produce a combination of physical and psychological dependence.

Alcohol is an example of this last group. The evidence that alcohol can produce physical dependence was afforded initially by Isbell (1955) who showed in a group of prison volunteers given large quantities of concentrated alcohol for periods of 7–87 days that abrupt cessation of intake in those who had taken the drug for 48 days led to severe withdrawal syndromes characterised by epileptic fits and delerium tremens. Mendellson (1964) has more recently, in ten subjects who ingested large quantities of whisky for 24 days, confirmed these findings; eight of the ten subjects showed withdrawal tremor, amnesias and hallucinations. The weight of clinical experience suggests that there are many people who also become psychologically dependent on alcohol, i.e. use alcohol as a way of reducing anxiety, depression. The obvious problem that arises if alcoholism is to be regarded as a dependency disorder is why, if the majority of the populace drink, there are relatively so few alcohol dependent subjects. The reasons for this are complex and are considered below.

Physical dependency on alcohol appears to be associated with two modes of drinking behaviour (Jellinek, 1960). These are 'loss of control' and 'inability to abstain'. In the former, once a drinking bout begins it is only terminated by the patient becoming incapable or by the patient being forced to stop (e.g. imprisonment, admittance to hospital); in the latter there is a daily continuous use of alcohol with the patient being totally unable to abstain. Jellinek (1960) considers social attitudes to drinking and different normal drinking patterns in different countries account for the different frequency in different countries of these patterns. Thus in North America and Great Britain 'loss of control' is the most frequent pattern seen, whilst in France 'inability to abstain' is the rule.

Physical dependence occurs much later than psychological dependence and the difficulty of insisting on it as a criterion for alcohol dependency is that much potentially preventative social harm and morbidity arises from alcohol misuse long before this stage is reached.

Prevalence

The prevalence of alcoholics in any population is controversial. At least two factors are responsible for this (Mellor, 1967); firstly, the difficulty of defining alcoholism, and, secondly, the fact that many alcoholics conceal the fact. There have been several different methods used to measure prevalence, some of which are described below. One of the simplest is the hospital admission rate of patients diagnosed as alcoholics or as suffering from alcoholic syndromes, but all are agreed that this provides a totally inadequate measure as many alcoholic patients never reach hospital. A second method is the use of the Jellinek formula (WHO, 1951). This attempts to estimate the prevalence of alcoholism using the frequency of cirrhosis in a community as an indirect estimate. It assumes the relationship between cirrhosis and alcoholism to be constant. The original formula was as follows. In any given year the total number of alcoholics $A = PD/K$ where PD is the number of deaths from alcoholic cirrhosis and K is the percentage of alcoholics with complications who die from cirrhosis of the liver. Later, when it was realised that there are alcoholics who did not have the complications of those included above but who should be included the formula became $A = R \times PD/K$ where R is the ratio of all alcoholics to alcoholics with complications. Although such a formula would appear to be likely to produce an under-estimate (as death certificates are likely to underestimate alcoholic causes of cirrhosis) and can further be criticised on other grounds (Popham, 1956; Seeley, 1959b) there is evidence that comparing with more direct methods there is considerable agreement. Thus Popham in calculating prevalence (1970) in 16 various areas estimated by the Jellinek and independent methods found excellent agreement in eight, good agreement in three and fair or poor in five. Popham concluded (1970) that the formula is a valuable guide to prevalence if it is used to estimate the total number of alcoholics in one place at a moment of time. The figure for Great Britain using this formula is 360 000 (WHO, 1951) or 11/1000.

Finally, there are the field studies which have been done in either one of two ways. Firstly, in any given community one can use 'key members' of the community (who are likely to be involved with alcoholics) to estimate the number of alcoholics they know. In this country this has been done for example by Parr (1957) using general practitioner postal questionnaires; and by investigators (Rowntree Report, 1963) who obtained data from health visitors and probation officers. Moss & Davies (1967) in a very thorough survey of one country used 13 sources of information. The figures obtained differ with different methods. Thus Parr recorded a rate of 1·1/1000, and Moss & Davies 6·2/1000 males and 1·4/1000 females. All studies record a lower prevalence in general practice and all studies showed a higher prevalence in males. The alternative method is to take a representative sample of the population. A comprehensive example of this was performed by Bailey, Haberman & Alksne (1965) in an area of Manhattan in which a random sample of over 4000 families was obtained and one family member was asked about family drinking habits.

Although there is considerable variation in the methods used, most workers in this country would consider the number of alcoholics in Great Britain by the WHO definition to be at least 200,000. This figure alone is enough to indicate the size of the problem. It should be noted that it considerably exceeds the number of drug dependent subjects and further the present facilities for treatment are clearly inadequate.

Aetiological Theories of Alcohol Dependency

Genetic

Care has to be taken in defining what one believes to be inherited, i.e. in a genetic theory of alcohol dependency is one primarily concerned in the inheritance of a specific (metabolic) syndrome or is one referring to the inheritance of basic personality types particularly vulnerable to alcohol dependence. Genetic research in this field has included attempts to link dependence with colour blindness (Cruz-Coke, 1965, 1966; Cruz-Coke & Varela, 1965), and blood groups (Nordmo, 1959) and also twin studies (Kaij, 1957, 1960; Tienari, 1963). As regards the former two links, evidence has been conflicting (Edwards, 1970). In Kaij's twin study 54·2 per cent of the monozygotic pairs were concordant as were 35 per cent of the dizygotic pairs. In Tienari's twins there were five concordant identical twins and seven discordant. Partanen *et al.* (1966) undertook a painstaking study of the genetics of drinking using 902 male twin pairs and found evidence suggesting that a genetically determined 'appetite for alcohol' may exist. As Edwards (1970) points out the higher concordance rates for identical compared with non-identical twins may relate primarily to genetic factors determining basic personality characteristics (implying 'alcohol prone' personality types) rather than to the inheritance of a metabolic error of genetic origin.

Socioeconomic

Jellinek (1960) has reviewed how socioeconomic factors have at various times been regarded as determining drinking behaviour in a society and possibly the extent of alcoholism. This has been used to explain the high prevalence of alcoholism in France (with society favourable to the use of alcohol as a beverage, drinking being regarded as manly and according to Jellinek almost one-third of the electorate involved in the alcohol industry), and within a country the high incidence in certain groups, e.g., poverty and poor housing, leading to solace for males in public drinking places. It is clear however in either situation that some individual members do not become alcoholics, i.e. an individual propensity must exist.

Metabolic and endocrinological

The idea of a primary metabolic anomaly as the prime cause for alcoholism is a very well known one. Such a theory would require the convincing demonstration of a metabolic anomaly present in the alcoholic and absent in the non-alcoholic. Such an anomaly should also be present in the early stage of alcoholism particularly, as metabolic abnormalities may arise in late stages of alcohol dependence as a consequence of nutritional and metabolic change induced by prolonged drinking. The metabolic anomaly found in the early stages of alcoholism should subsequently correlate with the development of alcoholism. Such evidence has not been forthcoming. One recent example of biochemical differences in a population in relation to alcohol has been the demonstration (Von Wartburg & Papenberg, 1970) that 20 per cent of a Swiss population and 4 per cent of a population sample from London and Liverpool have an active enzyme variant of human liver alcohol dehydrogenase which *in vitro* increases alcohol breakdown. However, as

Von Wartburg points out, the frequency of this variant enzyme is unknown in an alcoholic population.

Psychological theories

Learning theory. These theories have seen alcohol dependency as essentially learnt behaviour and attempted to understand the process in the light of two fundamental learning processes, that is classical and operant (instrumental) conditioning. Classical conditioning refers to the process whereby an organism acquires a new link between a stimulus and response by repeated presentations of the two. Thus in the classical experiments of Pavlov after salivation (unconditioned response) was produced by food (unconditioned stimulus), presenting the animal with a bell (conditioning stimulus) followed by food for a number of trials eventually led to the animal salivating to the bell alone. This new response (absent at the outset of the experiment) was the conditioned response. It is theoretically possible that anxiety relief may occur fortuitously in association with other stimuli surrounding drinking behaviour. The pairing of alcohol and such stimuli may lead eventually to alcohol alone producing anxiety relief.

Operant conditioning is a learning process which obeys the simple law of effect, i.e. an organism will tend to repeat behaviour if that behaviour leads to reward and the reverse holds true. Such a reward could be the known tranquillising effect of alcohol. It is known from animal experiments that a non-regular reward produces the strongest learning of this type, therefore the fact that the alcoholic may not always be anxious when drinking and therefore will not always be rewarded will tend to strengthen drinking behaviour. It is also known that the effect of a reward is higher if given immediately. The alcoholic at the beginning of a drinking bout may gain considerable reward from such processes as anxiety relief and relief of depression. The punishment (or non-reward) of the illness which comes at the end of the drinking bout thus occurs much later and has little effect on the learning process. A variant of the operant conditioning theory considers the prime reason for drinking in the established alcoholic is the fear of withdrawal symptoms (non-reward). To avoid this the patient continually drinks in an effort to stave off the withdrawal symptoms, i.e. he stays in a state of 'permanent reward'.

According to these theories, the fact that only some people become alcohol dependent could lie first in the different individual levels of anxiety and depression, which thus require different degrees of relief. And, secondly, in the availability of alcohol. Finally, different people will approach relief with different attitudes. These attitudes may be dependent on parental training, thus a potential alcohol dependent subject who has been brought up in a strict teetotal family will approach alcohol with a degree of guilt. Although alcohol may relieve anxiety in such a subject the degree of guilt that drinking induces may render the situation non-rewarding. Whilst the above theories seem very plausible and can explain initial reasons for drinking, direct evidence in support is scanty. Knupfer (1963) in a study of drinking patterns in California found that heavy drinkers were those who drank to relieve unpleasant emotions. Kraft (1968) in a very small group of alcoholics who appeared to drink for anxiety relief found that their drinking was reduced considerably when anxiety was relieved by other means. However, Hore (1970) in a small group of alcoholics studied intensively in a prospective follow-up was unable to find significant correlations between drinking behaviour and levels of anxiety, depression and craving for alcohol as measured by subjective rating scales. Further, relapse was not associated with any significant change in these levels in the 14 days preceding the relapse onset.

Psychoanalytical theories These imply that the subject is orally fixated, i.e. the subject requires gratification by oral means. As with other aspects of analytical theory the essential problem of such a view point is that it is not testable.

Alcohol dependency

The most widely held theory (Jellinek, 1960) is that whilst early drinking behaviour is governed by psychological needs, after a period of years physical dependency as well as psychological dependency occurs. The alcohol dependent patient can thus be grouped with patients dependent on other drugs and as stated earlier fits into the intermediate group of dependent drugs, i.e. those where physical dependence can occur but where initially the personality of the subject leads them to experimentation with the drug. The criteria of this physical addictive process (Jellinek, 1960) are the increased tolerance to alcohol, the presence of a withdrawal syndrome, and a drinking pattern characterised by loss of control or inability to abstain.

Jellinek has described the different stages of alcohol addiction. Firstly, there is the predependent stage of symptomatic drinking where the stigma of dependency are absent, and drinking behaviour can be seen as learnt behaviour on the principles outlined above. The consumption of alcohol gradually increases, and leads to the second phase, the prodromal phase of dependency. Here there are behavioural changes such as surreptitious drinking, unwillingness to discuss the problem, the beginnings of feeling of guilt, and the onset of periods of amnesias (Palimpsests) for the drinking period. This phase is followed by the dependent phase proper with the emergence of either loss of control or inability to abstain. The former is usually seen in this country and in North America. With loss of control the drinking of any small quantity of alcohol is felt as a physical demand and drinking continues until either the patient becomes unconscious or is forcibly stopped. The original psychological conflicts, social situations or need to test himself start the new bout of drinking. During this phase there is considerable social disorganisation including increasing alienation of family and disruption of work pattern. The patient may become alcohol centred making sure that he is never without alcohol; each day frequently begins with a drink, one purpose of which is to prevent the withdrawal symptoms, e.g. the tremor following a night's abstinence.

The addictive phase leads to the chronic phase with frequent regular periods of intoxication, social disorganisation and in a minority of cases the appearance of alcoholic psychosis. The ultimate end is the Skid Row alcoholic (Edwards *et al.*, 1966). It is important to realise that this image is often given to all alcoholics both by the general public and physicians, i.e. the only form recognised is the end stage. There is considerable evidence that the earlier stages of the alcohol dependent person are not recognised by the physician due to his image of the alcoholic*, and his unawareness that in the early stages of alcohol dependency, alcohol dependent patients are not socially different from their non-dependent peers (Edwards *et al.*, 1967, Strauss & Bacon, 1951). The view outlined above thus sees alcohol dependency as one of the drug dependency disorders, the condition being a gradual one beginning with psychological dependency leading to physical dependency and progressive physical, mental and social deterioration.

The Patient with a Drinking Problem

One of the physician's contributions to the management of the alcohol dependent person is for him to recognise such a patient. This is not helped by the tendency for the patient to deny any problem with drink. Another problem is that unless the physician is careful the patient and doctor enter into a technical argument about what is an alcoholic. For these reasons some psychiatrists in their practical dealing with the patient prefer the term drinking problem. The physician who considers possibly that one of his patients has a drinking problem is still left to decide by what criterion he judges this and whether to refer the patient for specialist advice. To assess the severity of the drinking problem careful enquiry needs to be made of the following symptoms; regular morning nausea, retching and vomiting, and loss of memory for the night before (these indicate heavy regular drinking in the evening), morning 'shakes' (indicating physical dependency), the presence of hallucinations and past episodes of delerium tremens; epileptic fits, and the presence of amnestic periods during the day. Search should be made for evidence of loss of control and inability to abstain. All the above phenomena indicate that the patient is either dependent on alcohol or will become so shortly. It should be realised however that such symptoms indicate a relatively advanced drinking problem. Many patients when seen will not show such phenomena but will show severe social and interpersonal problems. Assessment of these (often denied by the patient) will frequently require corroboration from other sources, e.g. relatives. Any patient whose drinking behaviour is leading to social, occupational, mental or physical harm and who despite this continues drinking as before, has a drinking problem.

Social complications of alcohol dependency

These are of prime importance. Their frequency and effects far outweigh the medical complications to be outlined below. All areas of the alcohol dependent' life are affected. Usually his work suffers, causing frequent loss of his job, and increasing difficulty in obtaining another. Amongst professional classes it is however noteworthy that dependency may be tolerated for a surprisingly long time. Relations with spouse (often initially neurotically based) deteriorate with repeated quarrelling, episodes of separation and finally desertion and divorce. Excessive spending on alcohol coupled with low earnings lead to financial penury and failure to maintain financial commitments with subsequent loss of habitation. Relationships with relatives, and non-alcoholic friends deteriorate leading to rejection. The patient when seen initially may thus be isolated and without work, money or housing.

* Being only of the Skid Row type (Blane *et al.*, 1963).

Morbidity of the alcohol dependent patient

Although the contribution of alcohol to certain illnesses is theoretically well known the importance of alcohol as a factor contributing to the patient's morbidity is often missed partly because of the patient's unwillingness to inform the physician of his drinking habits, and also by the physician's incorrect stereotype of the alcoholic, and because of lack of systematic enquiry into the patient's drinking habits. The contribution that alcohol makes to certain illnesses has been estimated by Nolan (1965) in the U.S.A. and by Green (1965) in Australia. Nolan (1965) studied 900 consecutive medical admissions to the Grace New Haven Community Hospital in the U.S.A. Every admission was asked systematically about drinking habits. He considered that 13 per cent of patients seen were alcoholics using a definition similar to that of the WHO (1952) and that 10 per cent of admissions were due to diseases in which alcohol had played a major aetiological part, and a further 0·4 per cent due to diseases in which alcohol was probably an aetiological factor. When the alcoholic group was compared with the non-alcoholic group the following illnesses were significantly higher in the former. These were acute bacterial pneumonia, cirrhosis, acute gastritis, acute pancreatitis, epileptic fits and pulmonary tuberculosis. There was also evidence that the alcohol dependent person significantly delayed his admission to hospital compared with the non-alcohol dependent. Management of these medical conditions was interfered with in the alcohol dependent subject in that discharge against medical advice occurred frequently, and some patients had to be treated for the alcohol withdrawal syndrome. Green (1965) assessed 1000 consecutive patients admitted to the medical wards of St. Vincent's Hospital, Melbourne. An alcoholic was defined as someone who was physically, mentally or socially incapacitated by prolonged excessive drinking. There were 12·1 per cent of patients who satisfied this definition and 3·4 per cent of total admissions were for diseases in which alcohol was a definite aetiological factor. A further 2·2 per cent admissions were for diseases in which alcohol was a probable factor. It is of interest that in both surveys the percentage of patients termed alcoholics were identical. The lower incidence of alcohol being a contributory factor to diseases in the Australian study may be accounted for by the less rigorous questioning used in this study re drinking habits. As far as the author is aware there are no comparable studies in the U.K.

Disorders Associated with Alcohol Dependency

Neurological syndromes

These are described in detail by Victor (1962). The account below is only intended to be an outline, further details can be obtained from his excellent review. A more recent review is that of Lees (1967). The syndromes can perhaps be usefully divided as follows (Victor, 1962).

Syndromes due to direct action of alcohol on central nervous system. These include acute intoxication in which the well known changes of disturbance in balance, gait, and speech are accompanied by emotional changes including a shift towards extroversion. It is not recognised enough however that intoxication and subsequent coma may lead to death. Coma in the alcoholic presents a problem in differential diagnosis in that the causes include the direct effect of alcohol, hypoglycaemia, head injury and post epileptic coma. Much less common than ethanol intoxication but likely to occur in Skid Row alcoholics is acute methanol intoxication. This presents with the symptoms of ethyl alcohol intoxication together with abdominal and visual symptoms, the latter being a precursor of bilateral retrotulbar neuritis (Lees, 1967).

Syndromes due to withdrawal effect of alcohol in the alcohol dependent subject. The commonest of these is probably the 'morning shakes'. This refers to the tremulousness of arms, legs and voice especially the former, seen on arising after a night's abstinence and relieved by alcohol. It is an important symptom as it indicates to the physician physical dependency. The full blown withdrawal syndrome is the form of acute organic reaction (toxic confusal state) termed delerium tremens. This has the usual features of the acute organic reaction syndrome, i.e. disorientation, lack of grasp of reality, illusions, visual hallucinations and fear, the development of paranoid ideas and delusions accompanied by restlessness and hyperactivity. In severe cases epileptic fits are not uncommon. On examination there may be a marked tremor. Amnesia for the episode is common. The condition forms part of the differential diagnosis of the acute organic reaction, it is likely to occur when the alcohol dependent patient in the middle of his drinking bout suddenly has his drinking supply cut off, as on admittance to hospital. In the management of this condition phenothiazines have been constantly used. There have been criticism of this however (Edwards, 1967). It has been suggested that the condition should be managed in the same way as in withdrawal syndromes due to other drugs producing physical dependency (e.g. heroin) i.e. the patient should be given either decreasing doses of alcohol or drugs which have cross tolerance with alcohol. These include Chlordiazepoxide and Paraldehyde but not Chlorpromazine.

Syndromes believed to be due to associated nutritional deficiencies. These include the classical neurological syndromes, i.e. Wernicke's Encephalopathy, Korsakov's psychosis and peripheral neuropathy. Large series of the first two syndromes have been described by Victor (1962). It is not uncommon for each syndrome to show evidence of the other, thus for example according to Victor the vast majority of patients with Korsakov's psychosis show evidence of the stigma of Wernicke's Encephalopathy even years later, conversely patients with Wernicke's Encephalopathy may show a mental state similar to that of Korsakov's psychosis. Wernicke's Encephalopathy refers to a triad of confusion, ocular disturbance (most frequently rectus palsy and nystagmus) and ataxia of stance and gait. Korsakov's psychosis is usually regarded as a state of amnesia and confabulation. Victor has emphasised however how the mental state in this condition may be that initially of a confused state and that later when this has subsided, formal psychiatric testing will show a widespread intellectual defect which is not confined to a memory disturbance. The latter disturbance which is however the greatest intellectual defect takes the form of inability to learn new material and inability to remember past events in their correct chronological sequence.

Aetiological nature of these conditions. It appears generally agreed that Wernicke's Encephalopathy represents an acute reversible biochemical disturbance due to thiamine deficiency. In the case of Korsakov's psychosis and peripheral neuropathy and unlike Wernicke's syndrome, adequate vitamin supplements and cessation of alcohol does not always lead to recovery and recovery if it does occur is frequently slow.

Syndromes in which the pathogenesis is uncertain. These include Marchia-fava Bignani disease (primary degeneration of the corpus callosum), central pontine myelinolysis and cerebellar degeneration. All these conditions except the latter are very rare and are described by Victor (1962) and Lees (1967). Cerebellar degeneration is important in that it produces a cerebellar syndrome in middle age characterised primarily by ataxia of gait (with minimal ataxia of arms, speech or ocular movements) which has to be distinguished from that due to carcinoma of the bronchus.

Epilepsy and alcohol. Lees (1967) has given a useful list of the causes of epilepsy in association with alcohol. These include, acute intoxication, as a withdrawal symptom on its own and unaccompanied by the syndrome of delerium tremens ('rum fits'), as part of delerium tremens, hypoglycaemia, cerebral degeneration in association with alcohol dependency, and as a trigger in a patient with epilepsy.

Psychiatric syndromes associated with alcohol dependency

Besides the classic neuropsychiatric syndromes described above, mention must be made of alcoholic hallucinosis, morbid jealousy (the 'Othello syndrome') alcoholic fugue state, and the increased incidence of suicide in the alcoholic.

Alcoholic hallucinosis is an important condition in that it may be confused with a schizophrenic psychosis. Classically, there is the sudden onset of auditory illusions and hallucinations appearing in clear consciousness and forming the basis of a paranoid delusional system. The hallucinations are often offensive and may be of the classic schizophrenic type, i.e. 'third person' or 'running commentary' hallucinations. The clinical picture may be very similar to that of a paranoid schizophrenic illness (Slater & Roth, 1969) but other schizophrenic features, e.g. thought disorder, primary delusions, incongruity of affect; and disturbance of volition are said to be absent and in the patient with alcoholic hallucinosis there may be clinical and psychiatric evidence of intellectual defect absent in schizophrenia. It must be admitted however that in practice cases occur which are indistinguishable from para-noid schizophrenic psychosis, and some authorities have doubted the exis-tence of this as a separate entity, and regard it as a schizophrenic illness precipitated in a potential schizophrenic by the use of alcohol. It is interesting to note further that although the vast majority of cases make a full recovery on stopping alcohol, a minority become schizophrenic. This happened in Benedetti's 1952 series (13 of the 113) and in Victor & Hope's series (1958) (4 of the 16 patients).

Morbid jealousy. In this syndrome the patient develops the fixed idea, often becoming delusional that his spouse or sexual partner is being unfaith-ful. The patient spends much of his time searching for evidence to confirm this belief, and may make thorough searches of his partner's clothing and possessions for evidence. Frequently, the spouse will be followed or the patient will return home at unexpected hours to confirm his belief. The unfortunate spouse will be harangued regularly and denial will not be accepted. Although this syndrome is not confined to the alcoholic it is well recognised in such patients and the beliefs are often reinforced by the spouse's frequent feeling of revulsion towards sexual intercourse with the alcoholic.

Alcoholic fugue states. Fugue states refer to those states where a patient wanders away from familiar surroundings and appears in unfamiliar surroundings unaware of how he arrived there. Such states can arise in depression, epilepsy and hysteria as well as in alcohol dependency. In alcohol dependency they arise during a drinking bout which is followed by amnesia for activities during that bout. They are known colloquially as 'lost weekends'.

Suicide and the alcoholic. Suicide is a genuine hazard in the alcoholic. In Kessel & Grossman's (1961) study in London the suicide rate for alcoholics admitted to two In Patient units was eighty six times as high for men in the same age groups as in the general population. In a study in the poisons unit at Edinburgh 32 per cent of men admitted with self-poisoning had severe alcohol problems (Batchelor, 1954).

Treatment of the Alcohol Dependent Patient

There are difficulties in assessing the outcome of treatment, but in the field of psychiatry they are by no means unique to alcohol dependency. Firstly, there are no really adequate studies on the natural history of alcohol dependency, and no controlled trial in which randomisation of patients has been carried out between treatment and non-treatment control groups (Edwards, 1967). Failing this the most satisfactory method would be to quantify drinking behaviour before and after treatment with a serious attempt being made to render the presence or absence of treatment the only changing variable in the two situations. This however has rarely been done. The usual procedure is to state the drinking behaviour at the end of treatment. When this has been done the results have suggested that approximately one-third of the patients become abstinent, about one-third reduce their drinking and one-third appear unaltered. This is illustrated by the results from studies at well known centres in this country described below.

Glatt (1959), using In Patients treated by group methods, found one-third became abstinent, one-third improved and one-third didn't improve. Davies *et al.* (1956) in a two year follow-up of 50 Maudsley In Patients found 36 per cent fell into the best group (being abstinent for most of the time), 42 per cent into the middle group (indulged in drinking during the period but without gross or long standing impairment of their social efficiency) and 22 per cent did badly (spending most of the two years in a state of social incompetence or in an institution). They made the important point (confirmed later by others) that the prognosis at six months is a reliable guide to drinking behaviour at a later date. Walton *et al.*, in Edinburgh (Walton *et al.*, 1966) using a combination of in patient and out patient treatment found approximately half of the patients abstinent at six months and eighteen months and a third of the total number of patients had been abstinent throughout. At six months, 18 per cent were regarded as improved but still drinking and 23 per cent not improved. Edwards & Guthrie (1966) randomly allocated 40 alcohol dependent men to in patient and out patient treatment. Both groups were followed up for six months and the outcome was assessed by 2 observers separately. No difference was seen in the two groups. The WHO (1952) has advocated the use of out patient facilities primarily in treating dependence and studies such as those above perhaps indicate that initially at least treatment should be attempted as an out patient. Admission would be used as essentially a means of stopping the patient drinking in the middle of a drinking bout, the patient not being able to stop as an out patient. In patient units of course provide for more than this, as they frequently become a therapeutic community where intensive group psychotherapy can be carried out.

Aim of treatment

Alcohol dependence frequently runs a relapsing course and this may occur despite relatively intensive medical support (Hore, 1970). This fact must be clearly appreciated, and despondency not induced in the physician. A relapsing course is frequent in many medical disorders, e.g. rheumatoid arthritis, bronchial asthma, but because of this no physician would regard the patient as not requiring treatment. As Edwards (1967) has pointed out, in realistic terms the work of an alcoholic treatment service is the long term care of people more or less frequently in difficulties. Although it is not strictly true (Davies, 1962, Kendell, 1965) to state that the alcohol dependent patient never returns to normal drinking this is frequently the aim of treatment and there are good psychological reasons why total abstinence is perhaps easier to maintain than controlled drinking.

Methods of treatment

These can be perhaps divided into individual or groups, the former often seen in out patient treatment. Here the patient is offered a relationship and practical help with current life problems. Abstem (citrated calcium carbide) is sometimes added. This substance when taken regularly will produce unpleasant symptoms in the patient if alcohol is taken, and the fear of this may prevent drinking. However, it is evident that this can only have a marginal effect, as the patient who intends to drink can stop his tablets for two days, and drink without fear. For some patients, as an additional deterrent to drinking, it can be a help however. The use of tranquillisers in relieving the anxiety of the patient who stops drinking has been criticised in that the patient may leave his dependency on alcohol and become dependent on tranquillisers instead. The same problem may arise in relation to feelings of depression. Many patients who give up alcohol feel initially miserable; this is not an indication however for automatically giving an antidepressant. Aversion treatment has for many years been used in the treatment of the alcohol dependent subject. This involves the temporal pairing of two stimuli, alcohol and a stimulus producing a continued fear response to alcohol. Chemical aversion (apomorphine) fell into disrepute because accurate pairing frequently was impossible and electrical aversion has been used instead. Undoubtedly, some patients are helped by this method but its superiority over other methods which are less time consuming and require less expertise has still to be shown.

Group methods. These constitute an important method of treating the alcohol dependent subject and are of course well established in treatment of other psychiatric conditions and has parallels with groups with religious and political affiliation (Frank, 1961). Essentially, the group members all have a similar problem, i.e. here it is alcohol dependence. The leader (as in Alcoholics Anonymous (A.A.)) is either an ex-alcoholic or, as in hospital practice, a non-alcoholic, but in the latter case the leader adopts a non-authoritarian interpretative role. In the group there is a discussion of the reasons for drinking and, the alcoholic is not permitted to deny the extent of his problem or his personal inadequacies. Particularly in the A.A. group where all group members have drinking problems is denial not permitted. Group members attempt to understand the reasons behind their drinking, and find ways other than alcohol of solving their problems. In A.A. there is in addition the sponsorship system whereby an ex-alcoholic takes under his wing the new group member, and makes himself available at all times (medical support can obviously not compare with this). In the sponsorship system there is also the advantage that the new member is comforted by someone who has been through the same difficulties which of course the non-alcoholic therapist has not. The exact mechanisms that allow group methods to permit attitude and behavioural change in the group members are not known but it would appear that in all groups whether for treating psychiatric patients or of religious and political nature certain factors are common. First there is the group itself which is committed to a single group idea, in this case becoming abstinent, secondly, there is the element of confession and the group's refusal to allow evasion and denial, thirdly, there is (as well shown in A.A.) demonstrated 'a road back', i.e. another way of coping, and finally there is the considerable degree of support given. One problem which is very real to the alcohol dependent subject is that of 'filling the gap' in his life that becoming abstinent produces. Belonging to a group and spending ones time in group activities provides a means of filling that gap; and in A.A. it is not uncommon to find members spending several evenings a week involved in A.A. activities. A.A. also provides groups for the spouses of alcoholics (Alanon) and children of alcoholics (Aliteen). Further information on the activities of A.A. can be obtained from the headquarters:

Alcoholics Anonymous, Central Services Office,
11 Redcliffe Gardens, London, S.W.10
(Tel. 01-352 9669)

who will also provide a list of regular group meetings throughout the country, which is very useful for any physician involved in trying to help the alcohol dependent patient.

Clinical experience suggests group methods are effective although whether more effective or not than individual methods is not really known. They do have the advantage of requiring less medical and paramedical personnel and of course more patients can be treated per unit time.

Community services. The alcohol dependent subject often requires practical help in terms of housing and work. In recent years in a few areas a system of after-care hostels has been developed in which alcohol dependent patients live together in a community where group psychotherapy is obligatory. Such hostels are often autonomous being run by the members (apart from administration) who control admission to the hostel. An example is the Rathcoole Experiment (Cook et al., 1968). The duration of stay is very variable and it should be realised (Myerson, 1956) that some patients may require support in such a hostel for many years.

The patient refusing help

It is characteristic of the early stage of alcohol dependency that the subject denies his drinking problem and in some patients it appears that considerable personal suffering has to occur before the patient admits to the severity of his problem. This denial may extend over not only months but years. As the genuine desire for help would appear to be of importance for a successful outcome of treatment the physician at times is faced with a difficult problem. Sometimes help has to be confined to the family of the patient, e.g. getting them to join Alanon and Aliteen; and on some occasions the physician has to accept the patients refusal but make it clear that he will always be willing to help if and when the patient wishes this.

The general physician's role in treating alcohol dependency

This is of considerable importance both as regards the physicians general attitude to the problem and the management of individual patients. As regards the former the physician requires a basic understanding of alcohol dependence and the ability to avoid stereotypes of the alcoholic. Moralising is not in the author's view the correct and proper attitude for the physician to take, the alcohol dependent subject needing as much professional concern and interest (if not more) as any other group of patients who consults the physician.

References

BAILEY, M. B., HABERMAN, P. W. & ALKSNE, H. J. (1965). *Qt. Jl. Stud. Alcohol*, **26**, 19.

BATCHELOR, I. R. C. (1954). *J. ment. Sci.*, **100**, 451.

BENEDETTI, G. (1952). *In* 'The Alcoholic Hallucinoses'. Stuttgart: Thieme.

BLANE, H. T., OVERTON, W. F., Jr., & CHAFETZ, M. E. (1963). *Qt. Jl. Stud. Alcohol*, **24**, 640.

COOK, T.. MORGAN, H. G. & POLLOCK, B. (1968). *Br. med. J.*, **1**, 240.

CRUZ-COKE, R. (1965). *Lancet*, **1**, 1131.

CRUZ-COKE, R. (1966). *Archos. Biol. med. Exper.*, **3**, 21.

CRUZ-COKE, R. & VARELA, A. (1965). *Lancet*, **2**, 1348.

DAVIES, D. L., SHEPHERD, M. & MYERS, E. (1956). *Qt. Jl. Stud. Alcohol*, **17**, 485.

DAVIES, D. L. (1962). *Qt. Jl. Stud. Alcohol*, **23**, 94.

EDWARDS, G. (1967). *Hosp. Med.*, **2**, 272.

EDWARDS, G. (1970). *In* 'The Status of Alcoholism as a Disease'. Modern Trends in Drug Dependence and Alcoholism I, Ed. Phillipson R.V. London: Butterworth.

EDWARDS, G. & GUTHRIE, S. (1966). *Lancet*, **1**, 467.

EDWARDS, G., HAWKER, A., WILLIAMSON, V. & HENSMAN, C. (1966). *Lancet*, **1**, 249.

EDWARDS, F., FISHER, M. K., HAWKER, A. & HENSMAN, C. (1967). *Br. med. J.*, **4**, 346.

FRANK, J. (1961). *In* 'Persuasion and Healing'. Baltimore: Johns Hopkins Press.

GLATT, M. (1959). *Lancet*, **268**, 1318.

GREEN, J. R. (1965). *Med. J. Aust.*, **I**, 465.

HORE, B. D. (1970). *In* 'Factors in Alcoholic Relapse'. M. Phil. thesis, Univ. of London (Institute of Psychiatry).

ISBELL, H., FRASER, H. F., WICKLER, A., BELLEVILLE, R. E. & EISENMEN, A. J. (1955). *Qt. Jl. Stud. Alcohol.*, **16**, 1.

KAIJ, L. (1957). *Acta genet.*, **7**, 437.

KAIJ, L. (1960). *In* 'Alcoholism in Twins'. Studies of the Aetiology and Sequel of Alcohol. Stockholm: Almquist and Wiksell.

JELLINEK, E. M. (1942). *In* 'Alcohol addition and Chronic Alcoholism'. New Haven: Yale Univ. Press.

JELLINEK, E. M. (1960). *In* 'The Disease Concept of Alcoholism'. New Haven: College and Univ. Press.

KENDELL, R. E. (1965). *Qt. Jl. Stud. Alcohol*, **26**, 247.

KESSEL, W. I. N. & GROSSMAN, G. (1961). *Br. med. J.*, **2**, 1971.

KNUPFER, G. (1963). *In* 'Factors related to Amount of Drinking in an Urban Community'. (Report No. 6). California Drinking Practices Study, California State Dept. of Public Health, 2151 Berkeley Way, Berkeley, California, U.S.A.

KRAFT, T. (1968). *In* 'Experience in the Treatment of Alcoholism in Progress in Behaviour Therapy'. Ed. H. Freeman. Bristol: J. Wright & Sons.

LEES, F. (1967). *Hosp. Med.*, **2**, 264.

MELLOR, C. (1967). *Hosp. Med.*, **2**, 284.

MENDELLSON, J. M. (1964). *Qt. Jl. Stud. Alcohol*, Suppl. 2.

MOSS, M. C. & DAVIES, E. B. (1967). *In* 'A Survey of Alcoholism in an English County'. Geigy Ltd.

MYERSON, D. J. (1965). *New Engl. J. Med.*, **254**, 1168.

NORDMO, S. M. (1959). *Am. J. Psych.*, **116**, 460.

NOLAN, J. P. (1965). *Am. J. med. Sci.*, **249**, 135.

PARR, D. (1957). *Br. J. Addiction*, **54**, 25.

PARTANEN, J., BRUUN, K. & MARKKANEN, T. (1966). *In* 'Inheritance of Drinking Behaviour'. Helsinki: Finnish Foundation for Alcohol Studies.

POPHAM, R. E. (1956). *Qt. Jl. Stud. Alcohol.*, **17**, 559.

POPHAM, R. E. (1970). *In* 'Indirect Methods of Alcoholism, Prevalence Estimation; a Critical Evaluation. *In* 'Alcohol and Alcoholism'. Ed. R. E. Popham. p. 294. Univ. Toronto Press.

Rowntree Report. (1960–63). *In* 'Chronic Alcoholics'. Ed. G. Fry & Williams. Steering Group on Alcoholism, Joseph Rowntree Social Service Trust.

SEELEY, J. (1959*a*). *Qt. Jl. Stud. Alcohol.*, **20**, 352.

SEELEY, J. (1959*b*). *Qt. Jl. Stud. Alcohol*, **20**, 245.

STRAUSS, K. & BACON, S. (1951). *Qt. Jl. Stud. Alcohol.*, **12**, 231.

SLATER, E. & ROTH, M. (1969). *In* 'Clinical Psychiatry'. 3rd Edition. Balliere, Tindall and Cassell.

TIENARI, P. (1963). *Acta psychiatry, scand.*, Supp. 171, 391. Translated by Radio Copenhagen.

VICTOR, M. & HOPE, J. M. (1958). *J. nerv. ment. Dis.*, **126**, 451.

VICTOR, M. (1962). *In* 'Clinical Neurology'. Ed. A. B. Baker. Vol. 2. Hoeber Harper.

VON WARTBURG, J. P. & PAPENBERG, J. (1970). *In* 'Biochemical and Enzymatic Changes induced by Chronic Ethanol Intake'. Int. Encycl. of Pharmoc. and Section 20, Vol. 1, Chap. 12.

WALTON, H. J. RITSON, E. B. & KENNEDY, R. I. (1966). *Br. med. J.*, **2**, 1171.

WHO. (1951). WHO Tech. Report Series No. 42. Sept. 1951.

WHO. (1952). WHO Tech. Report Series No. 48. Expert Committee on Mental Health, Alc. Sub-Committee 2nd Report.

CHAPTER 8

THE METABOLIC EFFECT OF ALCOHOL IN MAN

M. CLARK

This Chapter deals with the metabolism of alcohol and the organic disease produced by alcohol. The term 'ethanol' or 'alcohol' will be used interchangeably to cover both pure ethyl alcohol and the alcohol found in alcoholic beverages. There is no good evidence that any one form of alcoholic beverage is more harmful than another and most organic diseases found in alcoholics can be reproduced experimentally with pure ethanol.

The consumption of a large amount of an alcoholic beverage leads to a number of immediate effects in which other added substances known as 'congeners' may play a role. The total congener content varies from as low as about 3 g per 100 litres in vodka to 285 g per 100 litres in bourbon; scotch whisky contains 100 g per 100 litres. The bulk of the congeners consist of ethyl acetate and iso-amyl alcohol with significant amounts of iso-butanol. After consumption of equal quantities of either bourbon or vodka there was no difference in the incidence of the nystagmus produced (Murphree, Greenberg & Carroll, 1967). These workers then made 'superbourbon'; in this substance the ethyl alcohol content was kept constant at 80° U.S. proof, while the congeners were selectively increased by distillation. In the doses given to volunteers, superbourbon contained eight times the amount of congeners as in normal bourbon. Superbourbon produced a much greater and longer lasting nystagmus than did bourbon itself and, in addition, the mild E.E.G. changes produced by both drinks persisted longer after superbourbon. It is of interest that the nystagmus persisted after the blood alcohol level had returned to zero.

It is possible therefore that these congeners play some role in the acute intoxication produced by alcoholic beverages, although it is unlikely that the amounts present in most drinks will be sufficient to have much effect. The possible role of these congeners in the aetiology of hangovers is under active investigation.

It is important at this point to be familiar with the different measures used by scientists and the public when alcohol is referred to. In the United Kingdom proof spirit contains 57·1 per cent v/v or 49·2 per cent w/w of alcohol, while in the United States of America proof spirit is 50 per cent alcohol by volume. Measures that are used include 1 oz (U.K.) equalling 28·4 ml, 1 oz (U.S.) equalling 29·6 ml, and $\frac{1}{6}$ gill (standard U.K. single measure) equalling 23·7 ml. Most spirits sold in this country are 70° proof, that is about 40 per cent v/v of alcohol. Since the density of ethanol is 0·79, a standard U.K. measure is equivalent to 7·5 g of ethanol.

Absorption

Ethanol is absorbed predominantly from the stomach and upper jejunum, and it has been shown that increasing the concentration of ethanol in the stomach increases gastric absorption (Cooke & Birchall, 1969). Ethanol distributes itself throughout the body water and thus the effect of alcohol is dependant upon body size and total body water distribution.

Metabolism

Ethanol is metabolised to carbon dioxide and water (Fig. 8.1). The liver is responsible for well over 90 per cent of ethanol oxidation (Thompson, 1956) primarily by the NAD-linked enzyme alcohol dehydrogenase (ADH).

1. $\begin{cases} CH_3\,CH_2\,OH + NAD^+ \xrightarrow{\quad ADH \quad} CH_3\,CHO + NADH + H^+ \\ \qquad\qquad\qquad\qquad\qquad\qquad\qquad Acetaldehyde \\ Ethanol \\ \\ CH_3\,CH_2\,OH + NADPH + H^+ + O_2 \xrightarrow{\quad MEOS \quad} CH_3\,CHO + NADP + 2H_2O \end{cases}$

2. $CH_3\,CHO + NAD^+ + CoA\text{-}SH \longrightarrow CH_3CO\text{-}SCoA + NADH + H^+$
   Acetyl CoA

3. Acetyl CoA $\longrightarrow$ Tricarboxylic Acid Cycle $\longrightarrow CO_2 + H_2O$
   - - - - Fatty Acid Synthesis
   - - - Cholesterol

FIG. 8.1. Metabolism of ethanol.

ADH is a zinc containing cytoplasmic enzyme which has been isolated from a number of species including human liver (von Wartburg, Bethune & Valle, 1964). The physiological significance of this enzyme system has been recently reinvestigated (Krebs & Perkins, 1970). These workers have shown that a small amount of ethanol is normally formed by bacteria in the gastrointestinal tract of animals and this is subsequently metabolised by the liver.

An atypical ADH has been found in human liver (von Wartburg, Papenburg & Aebi, 1965) with different substrate specificities and it has been postulated that this may account for the varying metabolic rates of ethanol.

The oxidation of ethanol produces acetaldehyde and reduced nicotinamide adenine dinucleotide ($NADH_2$) (Westerfield, 1961). Human volunteers who were given 1·5 g or more of ethanol showed on liver biopsy a reduction of NAD^+ and an increase in $NADH_2$ which was maximal after four hours (Cherrick & Leevy, 1965). In these normal volunteers the $NADH_2$ level had returned to control levels after 8 hours but the rapidity of $NADH_2$ reoxidation depends on liver function and is impaired when morphological changes are present. (Leevy, 1967).

The second step in alcohol metabolism namely the oxidation of acetaldehyde is catalysed by aldehyde dehydrogenase with again NAD^+ as a coenzyme. The product acetyl-CoA is the ubiquitous intermediate of carbohydrate and lipid metabolism. Acetate which is formed either from acetyl-CoA or directly from acetaldehyde has been found to increase in the blood after ethanol administration (Lundquist, 1960); it is subsequently metabolised in peripheral tissues mainly muscle (Lindeneg *et al.*, 1964).

The rate of acetaldehyde oxidation is rapid and exceeds the rate of ethanol oxidation (Lubin & Westerfield, 1945) so that little acetaldehyde is detected in the blood after ethanol ingestion. Chronic ingestion of alcohol to human volunteers produced acetaldehyde levels of 0·15 mg per 100 ml (0·03 mM) when the blood alcohol levels ranged from 54 mg per 100 ml (11 mM) to 500 mg per 100 ml (100 mM). (Majchrowicz & Mendelson, 1970). In this study there was no dose or dose time relationship between blood ethanol and blood acetaldehyde levels making it unlikely that acetaldehyde plays a major role in the biological consequence of alcohol consumption.

The acetyl-CoA formed after ethanol oxidation is mainly oxidised to carbon dioxide in the Tricarboxylic cycle, a small proportion sharing the same pathways of 2-carbon fragments originating elsewhere. The complete oxidation of ethanol produces about seven kilocalories per gram (130 kJ), the oxidation of one molecule of ethanol requiring three molecules of oxygen to produce two of carbon dioxide. The energy released during ethanol oxidation may be conserved as 18 molecules of adenosine triphosphate (ATP) formed per molecule of ethanol converted to carbon dioxide (Senior, 1967). The respiratory quotient for oxidation of ethanol is 0·67, very near the 0·7 for the oxidation of fat. Thus ethanol behaves more like a lipid than a carbohydrate, the acetate that is formed giving rise to no net synthesis of carbohydrate.

Recently an hepatic microsomal ethanol oxidising system (MEOS) has been described (Lieber & DeCarli, 1970). This oxidase system has a pH optimum of 7·2 (as opposed to ADH of 10·4) and has as its coenzyme nicotinamide adenine dinucleotide phosphate ($NADP^+$). This microsomal enzyme system can be fully differentiated from ADH both by its cofactor requirements and the effect of inhibitors (Lieber, Rubin & DeCarli, 1970).

Ethanol seems to share, therefore, with a number of drugs such as pentobarbitone, metabolism in a microsomal mixed function oxidase system. Induction of MEOS has been demonstrated with alcohol and a variety of drugs (Rubin & Lieber, 1968) and chronic administration of alcohol to rats increases the hepatic smooth endoplasmic reticulum, the ultrastructural site of this oxidase system (Rubin, Hutterer & Lieber, 1968). Rubin *et al.* (1970) have demonstrated in 3 non-alcoholic volunteers proliferation of smooth endoplasmic reticulum and induction of microsomal oxidase function after 12 days ethanol administration.

The importance of this microsomal enzyme system is at present difficult to assess. Because of the induction of the system that has been demonstrated both *in vitro* and *in vivo* after alcohol, it has been suggested that MEOS is more important in the chronic alcoholic (Lieber, 1970). It has been demonstrated that an enhanced rate of metabolism of a number of drugs occurs in alcoholics (Kater Zieve & Tobin, 1968) and induction of their metabolising enzymes is an attractive mechanism. On the other hand high concentrations of ethanol seem to depress activity of MEOS *in vitro* which would again agree with the findings that intoxicated alcoholics metabolise drugs more slowly (Rubin *et al.*, 1970). Tephly, Tinelli & Watkins (1969) and Khanna & Kalant (1970) have data suggesting that MEOS does not have an important role in alcohol oxidation *in vivo*. The evidence is at present incomplete and at most MEOS could only account for up to 20 per cent of ethanol oxidation.

Physiology

The rate of ethanol disappearance from the body is about 100 mg/kg per hour. The disappearance rate is fairly constant for a given person but varies among individuals from 50 to 100 mg/kg per hour (Thompson, 1956). Ethanol given orally or intravenously to normal human volunteers produces the highest blood alcohol level approximately one hour later; this level then decreases in a linear fashion (Fig. 8.2). Using ^{14}C labelled ethanol it has been shown (Clark & Senior, 1968) that 85 per cent of a single dose is expired as $^{14}CO_2$ in the first 10 hours and 93 per cent or more within 24 hours. Urinary excretion of (^{14}C) ethanol itself was less than 4 per cent in 24 hours and expiration of (^{14}C) ethanol as vapour was less than 2 per cent.

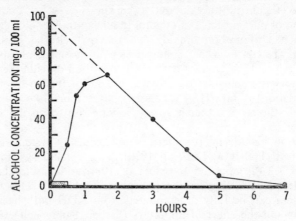

FIG. 8.2. Blood alcohol levels following oral administration of 0·5 g/kg of ethanol (from Clark & Senior, 1968) with permission from authors and Williams and Wilkins Co.

Many attempts have been made to vary this constant rate of ethanol metabolism and there is contradictory evidence on the effects of glucose, thyroid hormones and insulin in both animals and man (Stokes & Lasley, 1967). Fructose is however the only agent that has been convincingly shown to increase the rate of ethanol metabolism in man (Tygstrup, Winkler & Lundquist, 1965). The mechanism whereby fructose enhances ethanol metabolism is unclear but it has been suggested that intermediates of fructose metabolism affect dissociation kinetics of the ADH-NAD complex (see Forney & Harger, 1969; Mendelson, 1970).

The rate limiting step in ethanol metabolism was believed to be specifically dependant upon hepatic ADH activity (Westerfield, 1961); the linear rate of oxidation of ethanol above 10 mg per cent being due to saturation of ADH. *In vitro* studies of ADH initially gave a K_m of one millimolar (mM) (Blair & Vallee, 1966), but further evidence *in vitro* at physiological pH or from the decline in blood levels in man suggest that the K_m is nearer 2 mM or 0·1 mg/ml. In the blood ethanol range from 4 mg/ml (i.e. 80 mM or nearly fatal levels) to 0·5 mg/ml (10 mM or mildly intoxicated), the enzyme would be 98 per cent and 85 per cent saturated respectively. The kinetics would be linear throughout the range described above and thus the enzyme is rate limiting at all ethanol concentrations found in man (Goldstein, 1970). The kinetic studies of Theorell & Chance (1951) have indicated that dissociation of the NADH-ADH complex is by far the slowest reaction in the initial oxidation of ethanol, thus limiting the rate of the process.

An additional rate limiting factor may well be the reoxidation of $NADH_2$. The major system for $NADH_2$ reoxidation (the flavoprotein cytochrome system) is situated within the mitochondria, while ADH is found in the soluble fraction of the cells. Since the mitochondrial membrane is relatively impermeable to $NADH_2$ intermediate carriers such as alpha glycero-phosphate transport the hydrogen from $NADH_2$ formed in the cytoplasm to the mitochondrial flavoprotein cytochrome system. Although other pathways for the reoxidation of $NADH_2$ exist (see Lieber, 1967) the accumulation of $NADH_2$ frequently occurs and this may well be the most important limiting step in the metabolism of alcohol.

Metabolism of alcohol in alcoholics and non-alcoholics

A number of studies have shown that the rate of ethanol metabolism in alcoholics is no different from the rate in non-alcoholics providing that both groups have been abstinent for at least 3 weeks (see Mendelson, 1970). In both non-alcoholics and alcoholics increased metabolism of ethanol has been found after chronic ingestion (Mendelson, Stein & McGuire, 1966) and it has been demonstrated that rates of ethanol metabolism increase as a function of the amount and duration of ethanol ingestion (Mendelson, Stein & Mello, 1965). The rate of ethanol metabolism is on the other hand impaired when overt liver disease is present (Kater, Carulli & Iber, 1969).

Tolerance to alcohol may then in part be related to the increased metabolic rate as the subject continues to drink, however it is likely that increased tolerance is more a behaviour phenomenon rather than a metabolic one.

Nutrition and malnutrition

Alcohol makes up nearly 10 per cent of the daily calorie consumption of the adult population of the United States of America (see Hartroft, 1967). This small amount of alcohol makes very little difference to the overall caloric balance, but if drinking is increased to the level of a bottle of spirits in a day, approximately 2000 extra calories will be consumed. It must be realised that this amount of alcohol is regularly consumed by many so called 'executive drinkers' and as Hartroft (1967) pointed out it is very difficult for such people to continue to take the necessary protein and yet keep their total calorie intake in a reasonable range. You cannot, therefore, lose weight, eat an adequate diet (containing about 12 per cent protein) and still drink more than a small amount.

In the chronic alcoholic of the lower social group, very little attempt is made to take a balanced diet and his food intake is usually limited to minimal carbohydrate and virtually no protein (Leevy, 1962). In a large series of patients hospitalised for complication of alcoholism dietary deficiency was characteristic of 35 per cent (Leevy, 1967). In addition to total calorie deficiency these patients have deficiencies of vitamins particularly of the B complex and ascorbic acid (Leevy & Baker, 1968).

The nutritional status of the alcoholic is however variable, Neville *et al.* (1968) finding no significant malnourishment and vitamin deficiency in a group of alcoholics admitted to a psychiatric ward. The role of malnutrition as opposed to the direct effect of alcohol in producing disease in the alcoholic is hotly debated. We will see that in some instances in the experimental situation it is possible to differentiate and to show that both alcohol and malnutrition play a part. It is probable that in the chronic diseases that we will discuss, both factors are intertwined.

Physical Complications of Alcoholic Excess

The psychological and neurological syndromes have been discussed on pages (216 and 218).

Muscle involvement

Two main clinical entities are recognised both occurring only in chronic alcoholics. The first is an acute myositis following a severe drinking bout and the second consists of muscle wasting involving primarily the lower extremities. (Myerson & Lafair, 1970).

Acute myopathy. These patients are seen with severe muscular swelling with tenderness, fever, raised serum enzymes and sometimes acute renal failure due to the associated myoglobinuria (Hed, Larrson & Wahlgren, 1955). Muscle biopsy shows swollen, pale muscle fibres with intracellular oedema and destruction of mitochondria and myofilaments (Klinkerfuss *et al.*, 1967). It must be remembered in this context that a raised serum aspartate transaminase may not necessarily indicate liver disease in the alcoholic. A concomitant rise in the serum creatine kinase (CK) (derived solely from muscle) and a normal alanine transaminase (solely from liver) will demonstrate the existence of muscle pathology. An additional feature of these patients is the inability to raise the blood lactate after ischaemic exercise (Perkoff *et al.*, 1967). This deficit in lactate production was found in the majority of alcoholics admitted to a large city hospital after an acute binge, even though muscle complaints other than tenderness were absent. Presumably this effect on lactate production from muscle reflects a decreased breakdown in response to the stimulus, since glycogen is present in normal amounts.

Chronic myopathy. In the chronic syndrome, patients seem to develop symptoms over a period of some months. In a study of 10 patients all had muscle weakness and atrophy; the lower extremity and pelvic girdle musculature being most severely affected (Perkoff *et al.*, 1967). In several patients the findings were rapidly progressive, leading to serious disability and these patients were the ones in which muscle tenderness seemed to be prominent. In the remaining patients tenderness was not a prominent feature and stability rather than progression characterised the clinical course. These muscle abnormalities cannot be explained by a neurological deficit, although of course this may be present in the same patient. The muscle biopsy in the chronic stage shows evidence of earlier destruction as in the acute type, but with less intracellular oedema; active regeneration is also a prominent feature (Klinkerfuss *et al.*, 1967). The chronic syndrome may occur following an acute attack, but more commonly there is only a past history of mild muscle tenderness and cramps. Over 60 per cent of patients admitted to one hospital with delerium tremens showed a rise in the CK after 24 hours, indicating that the muscle involvement is more common than is generally realised and should not be overlooked (Myerson & Lafair, 1970).

Haemopoietic Abnormalities

In the chronic alcoholic perhaps the commonest haematological abnormality is multiple vacuoles in white and red cell precursors (Waters, Morley & Rankin, 1966), however the nature of these vacuoles is still undetermined. Recently the presence of 'ring' sideroblasts has been found in about a third of a group of alcoholics studies (Hines, 1969). All these patients had a low serum folate, low serum potassium and low magnesium, and these findings may explain the high incidence of these ring sideroblasts in this particular series. A well recognised entity is megaloblastic change of the bone marrow, and perhaps the commonest abnormality of all is iron deficiency. Finally in this group of haemopoietic disturbances found in the alcoholic we have to consider thrombocytopenia and leucopenia.

Many studies have been performed to establish the mechanisms by which the above findings occur, but it is highly probable that in any individual there is a combination of factors with dietary deficiency playing a major role. It must be emphasised that these changes can occur without severe liver disease and megoblastic changes associated with poor dietary intake can be commonly found in the so called 'social drinker' (Chanarin, 1969).

Direct toxic effect

Firstly we must consider whether alcohol is directly toxic to the bone marrow. Lindenbaum & Lieber (1969) established convincingly that vacuoles could be produced in volunteer subjects by substituting alcohol in doses equalling 46 per cent to 66 per cent of the calorie intake. These were chronic alcoholics who had been in hospital for several months prior to the study period. They were all asymptomatic with normal haematological findings and in normal calorie balance. Through each of the experimental periods they received vitamin supplements including 200 μg of oral folic acid. At the ethanol intake mentioned above, which is $1\frac{1}{2}$ bottles of 70° proof spirit per day, vacuolation of bone marrow pronormoblasts developed and these changes seemed to be dose related (Fig. 8.3). Vacuolation of promyelocytes was seen less consistently and only with the larger doses. In addition to the above findings in half of the subjects the platelet count was depressed after 4 weeks of high dose ethanol intake. In a more recent study (Hines & Cowan, 1970) excessive amounts of alcohol were given to 3 alcoholics who were on an adequate diet except for folate content. All 3 patients developed folate deficiency, hypomagnesaemia and evidence of liver dysfunction. In 2 of the 3 sideroblastic bone marrow abnormalities developed which responded to pyridoxal phosphate. These workers suggest that the differing folate status may be the reason why sideroblasts were not seen in the study of Lindenbaum & Lieber (1969).

Results obtained by Ryback & Des Forges (1970) suggest that alcohol has a direct effect on platelet turnover since thrombocytopenia occurred after

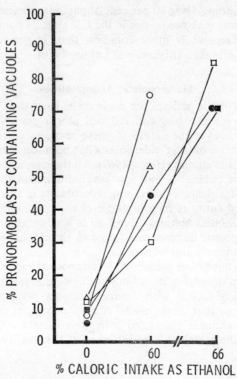

FIG. 8.3. Ethanol given to five chronic alcoholic volunteers, as 60% or 66% of their total calorie intake. 'O per cent' values are from the pre-ethanol period bone marrow (from Lindebaum & Lieber, 1969) with permission of authors and *New Eng. J. Med.*

chronic alcohol intake in 3 well nourished alcoholics. This same group (Post & Des Forges, 1968) had previously shown a fall in platelet count 4–6 hours after an acute infusion of ethanol.

Depressed utilisation of haematinics

Alcohol seems to be directly toxic to the bone marrow but additional effects on utilisation of the various haematinics have also been demonstrated. Sullivan & Herbert (1964) gave alcohol to chronic alcoholics who were in hospital with anaemia. These patients were on a low folate but otherwise normal diet supplemented with 50 μg of folic acid daily; the minimal daily requirement for normal haemopoesis. On this minimal daily amount these workers showed that alcohol suppressed the reticulocyte response but that this suppression could be overcome by giving larger amounts of folic acid, i.e. 150 μg daily (Fig. 8.4). This data was interpreted to show interference with folate utilisation and as the serum iron concentration also increased during the alcohol period interference with iron metabolism was also suspected. This effect on ferrokinetics had been shown earlier and seems to be independant of folate status (Waters *et al.*, 1966).

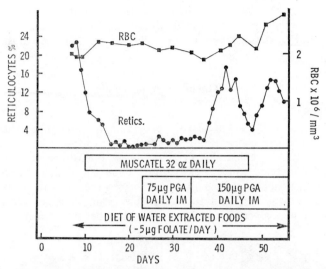

Fig. 8.4. The effect of intramuscular folic acid on red cell and reticulocyte counts in a chronic alcoholic who was on a folate deficient diet and drinking muscatel wine (from Sullivan & Herbert, 1964) with permission of authors and *J. Clin. Invest.*

Malabsorption of haematinics

It has also been shown that malabsorption of tritium labelled folic acid occurs in alcoholics who have recently been drinking (Halsted, Griggs & Harris, 1967). More recently a study of 4 chronic alcoholics showed malabsorption of vitamin B_{12} (Lindenbaum & Lieber, 1969b). An average fall of 41·5 per cent occurred in the absorption of B_{12} after a total alcohol intake of about 200 g given over 1 week. Two of these subjects showed absorption of B_{12} after alcohol in the frankly abnormal range and one of these two showed dilatation of the endoplasmic reticulum and focal cytoplasmic degeneration of the ileal mucosa.

Thus it would appear that diminished haemopoesis has multiple causes in the alcoholic; dietary deficiency of haematinics and a direct toxic effect of alcohol on the bone marrow probably the most significant.

Effect on leucocytes

Leucopenia is often found in the chronic alcoholic, in addition there is inhibition of leucocytosis in response to a toxic agent. McFarland & Libre (1963) found a leucopenic response to bacterial infections in 10 chronic alcoholics admitted to hospital: 3 of these patients also had thrombocytopenia. In response to repeated injection of endotoxin these patients failed to show a normal level of leucocytosis, indicating a diminished granulocyte reserve. Twenty days after admission, with abstinence and hospital diet, the response to endotoxin was normal. Further work in 1965 (Green & Kass) showed that mice treated with 3 ml of 5 per cent ethanol failed to clear administered bacteria from their lungs as quickly as controls. These two pieces of evidence both suggest an effect of alcohol on white cell activity, and more recently a depression in leucocyte mobilisation in response to a stimulus was shown in alcoholics (Brayton *et al.*, 1970). All these effects may well contribute to the increased susceptibility to infection seen in the chronic alcoholic.

Metabolic Derangements

Hypoglycaemia

Clinically hypoglycaemia usually occurs in the alcoholic who is malnourished but it can occur in normal adults after excessive consumption, or in children after accidentally drinking large quantities of alcohol (see Madison, 1968). The frequency of hypoglycaemia is probably underestimated in this country, but it is particularly important that it is recognised, since delay in treatment can lead to irreversible brain damage. Patients with postalcoholic hypoglycaemia can present with either minimal impairment of

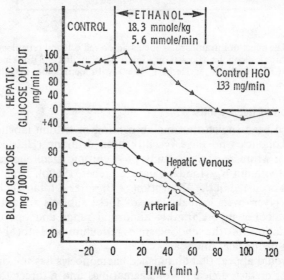

FIG. 8.5. Effect of ethanol on hepatic glucose output (HGO) and peripheral glucose utilisation in a fasted dog (from Madison, 1968) with permission of author and Academic Press who have copyright.

cerebral function or they can be stuporosed or unconscious. These findings can easily be confused with the effect of alcohol itself on cerebral function, so that hypoglycaemia must always be suspected. The lowest blood glucose recorded has been 5 mg/100 ml, and when reviewing 67 cases Madison found that 46 patients had levels below 30 mg/100 ml and 19 below 20 mg/100 ml.

Pathogenesis. Ethanol does not produce hypoglycaemia in man or other animals unless its administration is preceded by a 48–72 hour fast (Freinkel, *et al.*, 1963). Susceptibility to hypoglycaemia as in the clinical situation, is inversely related to the hepatic store of glycogen which may rapidly become depleted. In animal experiments after 2–3 days starvation, alcohol has been shown to lower the hepatic glucose output, and in addition it decreases the peripheral utilisation of glucose. The blood glucose depends on these two above parameters, a fall in blood glucose thus occurs whenever the decreased hepatic output cannot be compensated for by the decreased peripheral utilisation (Fig. 8.5). Under the conditions of these experiments, the hepatic glucose output is derived almost exclusively from gluconeogenesis and it is an inhibition of this process that ethanol produces (see Madison, 1968). Ethanol in man inhibits gluconeogenesis from lactate in both fed and fasted state; hypoglycaemia in the non-fasted state being prevented by glycogenolysis (Kreisberg, Siegal & Owen, 1971).

The inhibition in gluconeogenesis is probably related to the excess $NADH_2$ produced by ethanol oxidation; $NADH_2$ has been shown to inhibit a number of the enzymatic steps involved in gluconeogenesis.

Intravenous injection of methylene blue, a redox dye which is capable of oxidising $NADH_2$ produced an immediate increase in hepatic gluconeogenesis in the experiments performed on the fasted dogs mentioned above, although recent data in rat liver perfusions showed no change in glucose production after methylene blue (Kaden, Oakley & Field, 1969). This excess of reducing equivalents is a unifying concept in much of the metabolic derangement produced by alcohol.

Hyperlipaemia

The effects of ethanol on lipid metabolism will be discussed fully under the mechanisms leading to a fatty liver. In 1957 Allbrink and Klatskin found hyperlipaemia in 5 chronic alcoholics and since then Losowsky et al. (1963) have shown increased serum lipids this being mainly of the triglyceride fraction, with a smaller rise in the plasma phospholipids and cholesterol. The mechanism of this hyperlipaemia is not understood, but may be related to increased lipoprotein release from the liver, and also to a reduction in the rate of clearance of lipoproteins (see Lieber, 1967). Clinically many of the alcoholic subjects that are found to have hyperlipaemia, also have abdominal pain, which in the majority turns out to be pancreatitis (Nestel, 1967). Indeed in 1958, Zieve described a syndrome of hyperlipaemia, jaundice, haemolytic anaemia and pancreatitis occurring in the chronic alcoholic. Since that time a number of investigators have tried to unravel the relationship between hyperlipaemia and pancreatitis (Greenberg et al., 1966), but no firm conclusions have been drawn; it is probable that alcohol can produce hyperlipaemia independent of pancreatitis, although often the sequence of events seems to be pancreatitis first, followed by hyperlipaemia as a sequel. Experimentally alcohol will increase the plasma triglyceride levels in normals (Nestel, & Hirsch, 1965) as well as in chronic alcoholics (Schapiro et al., 1965), and alcohol infusion can raise the plasma FFA when the serum alcohol level is above 200 mg/100 ml. This plasma FFA on chromatography is composed of fatty acids derived from adipose tissue, indicating increased mobilisation (see Isselbacher & Greenberger, 1964). Thus increased fatty acids are delivered to the liver for their subsequent oxidation or incorporation into lipoprotein. As mentioned above, increased release of these lipoproteins or their decreased clearance due to inhibition of lipoprotein lipase, may well be important in alcoholic hyperlipaemia.

Hyperuricaemia

It is usually considered that the consumption of a large amount of alcoholic beverage is a predisposing factor, or a precipitating cause, of gout. Since gouty subjects have increased serum uric acid, it was natural that investigators would study the effect of ethanol on uric acid. Lieber *et al.* (1962) showed that the levels of serum uric acid were elevated in alcoholics admitted when acutely intoxicated. In 5 of 12 subjects the serum levels in the acute stage were well above the normal range. In the remaining seven, although within the normal range initially, they fell to lower levels as the patient recovered from the acute episode; the average decrease was 38 per cent.

In 7 subjects intravenous or orally administered ethanol increased the serum uric acid significantly. Ethanol as discussed earlier, produces on oxidation excess $NADH_2$ and one of the mechanisms for reoxidation of

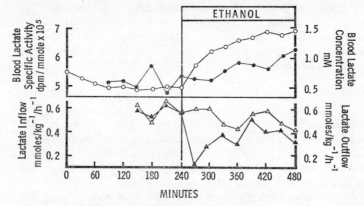

FIG. 8.6. Specific activity-time course curves for blood lactate ●—● and blood lactate concentrations ○—○ during an infusion of [^{14}C] lactate, with calculated lactate inflow ▲—▲ and lactate outflow △—△ Ethanol was administered orally at 9·8 g/h as indicated (from Kreisberg, *et al.*, 1971) with permission from authors and *J. Clin. Invest.*

$NADH_2$ is linked with reduction of pyruvate to lactate. This increased production of lactate by the liver was thought to be the cause of the raised blood lactate levels seen in the acutely intoxicated alcoholic. More recent experiments in man (Kreisberg, Owen & Siegal, 1971), however, have shown that the ethanol induced hyperlacticacidemia is due to decreased lactate disposal rather than increased lactate production (Fig. 8.6). It has also been shown that lactate enhances the reabsorption of uric acid in the renal tubule, although the precise mechanism is not understood. Lieber *et al.*, (1962) finally have shown that the rise in serum uric acid after ethanol is accompanied by decreased urinary uric acid output, and these workers further demonstrated that the same effect could be obtained by the administration of sodium lactate. The role of this effect of ethanol on uric acid metabolism as a factor producing the arthritic features of gout needs to be further evaluated before aetiological conclusions can be drawn.

Steroid metabolism

There is considerable evidence that ethanol increases corticosteroid production by the adrenal gland (see Mendelson, 1970). Studies in animals as well as man show that acute administration of alcohol raises the plasma cortisol level; in man this rise is seen when the blood alcohol level is above 100 mg/100 ml (Jenkins & Connolly, 1968). Most investigators have found this rise in plasma cortisol to occur in non-alcoholics as well as alcoholics, a higher rise occurring in those subjects who developed gastrointestinal symptoms (Mendelson & Stein, 1966). A further study has shown that this rise in cortisol production also occurs during long term administration of ethanol to chronic alcoholics under research ward conditions. The increase in plasma cortisol occurred as soon as the alcohol was given, and roughly paralleled the increase in blood alcohol (see Mendelson, 1970). In this study the highest cortisol levels were observed in those subjects with gastrointestinal symptoms, and withdrawal of alcohol led to a prompt fall in plasma cortisol to the basal level. The mechanism by which this rise in cortisol occurs is mediated via the neuro-pituitary axis since the rise does not occur in subjects with hypopituitarism (Jenkins & Connolly, 1968). Impairment of cortisol catabolism or decreased excretion in the urine could also play a role in the increased cortisol levels observed, although neither are thought to be very significant. The stimulus to the increased cortisol secretion is not known and it could be a direct effect of alcohol. It seems likely, however, that stress plays a role as this is a potent stimulus to adrenal secretion. Increased anxiety and depression has been noted in the alcoholic as he continues to drink (McNamee, Mello & Mendelson, 1968), and it is likely that the emotional stress of vomiting associated with excess alcohol is more important than the physical discomfort. When gastrointestinal symptoms are prominent, fasting is an inevitable accompaniment. Fasting has been shown to produce a lower rate of ethanol metabolism, perhaps related to the shortage of substrates for the reoxidation of $NADH_2$: the higher blood alcohol levels then may stimulate the adrenal cortex via the neuropituitary axis (see Mendelson, 1970). Alcoholism must be excluded as a cause of raised cortisol levels when investigating Cushing's syndrome.

The increased cortisol production may play a role in the adaptive mechanisms to drinking excess alcohol; experiments suggest that adrenalectomised animals are less tolerant to ethanol ingestion. In addition to the the effect of cortisol production, ethanol has been shown to increase aldosterone excretion in the urine and this would explain the low urinary sodium excretion found in some alcoholics (see Mendelson, 1970).

Effect of alcohol on water and electrolyte homeostasis

Alcohol produces a diuresis due to suppresion of antidiuretic hormone (Kleeman et al., 1955). Diuresis is not, however, maintained during chronic ingestion of ethanol, and it would appear that the diuresis occurs when the blood ethanol levels are rising, but that it does not persist when blood ethanol has reached a constant level (Ogata, Mendelson & Mello, 1968). It is this difference between acute and chronic ingestion of alcohol which makes interpretation of the data difficult, the effect of alcohol on electrolytes being particularly susceptible to this difference.

In acute studies a decrease in urinary sodium and chloride excretion has been found in some studies but not in all (Rubini, Kleeman & Lamdin, 1955). With chronic ethanol administration there was a significant decrease in urine osmolality with a concommitant decrease in sodium and potassium excretion (Ogata et al., 1968). The urinary excretion of these electrolytes in this study was well below the normal range and thus may well be biologically important in the alcoholic. The effect of alcohol on serum levels was to increase osmolality with an accompanying rise in serum sodium, the precise reason for the increased osmolality being uncertain. The serum potassium fell in most of the above cases and chronic alcoholics admitted after an acute alcoholic binge have been found to have low serum potassium levels and sometimes accompanying electrocardiographic changes (Vetter, Cohn & Reichgott, 1967).

The serum magnesium is depressed in about 25 per cent of alcoholics admitted after an acute binge (Heaton et al., 1962). This lowered serum magnesium may not, however, indicate total body magnesium deficiency and in one study this depression in serum levels seemed to be infrequently associated with decreased red cell magnesium, decreased muscle magnesium or other evidence of total body magnesium deficit (Sullivan et al., 1969). Inadequate magnesium intake, protein calorie malnutrition, increased loss through vomiting, are all factors leading to magnesium deficiency in the alcoholic. A major contributing factor seems to be the failure of the kidney to conserve magnesium in the presence of a low serum level (Sullivan et al., 1969). The reason for all this is ill understood, the increase in urinary magnesium also being seen after an acute alcohol infusion (Kalbfleisch et al., 1963).

In this acute situation the magnesium excretion was independent of the alcohol induced water diuresis and it was also independent of sodium excretion. In three normal subjects, although ingestion of ethanol increased urinary magnesium initially, this subsided after 6 hours so there was no significant effect on overall magnesium balance over a period of 8 days (Dick, Evans & Watson, 1969). The association of neurological and psychiatric illness with low serum magnesium in the alcoholic is striking in some series, but there seems to be no association with alcoholic liver disease. In many of the subjects studied by Kalbfleisch et al. (1963) there was a similar increase in the excretion of calcium with no major change in phosphate excretion. Markkanen and Nanto (1966) confirmed this increase in calcium excretion, this however was accompanied by a rise in serum calcium and phosphate.

In this brief discussion it can be seen that some of the data is conflicting and needs clarifying with further studies. The importance of these electrolyte disturbances particularly in alcohol withdrawal are uncertain (Mendelson, Ladon & Corbett, 1964), but it is undeniable that following an acute binge the alcoholic needs isotonic fluid replacement. The exact role of magnesium deficiency in this situation and in delerium tremens is being actively investigated (Jones et al., 1969).

Other metabolic disturbances

There is abundant information that acute ethanol administration increases urinary excretion of catecholamines and their metabolites in man (see Mendelson, 1970). Studies on the effect of chronic ethanol ingestion has also shown a similar rise in urinary excretion of these substances. Following withdrawal of alcohol in this chronic study, there was a prompt fall in catecholamines and their metabolites when the subjects had no withdrawal symptoms. After higher doses of alcohol however, withdrawal produced symptoms and the urinary catecholamines remained elevated until these symptoms had ceased. When the urinary metabolites are more closely studied, it is found that there is a fall in vanillyl-mandelic acid with a concomitant rise in methoxy-hydroxy phenylglycol excretion. These changes are due to a shift in catecholamine catabolism from an oxidative to a reductive pathway, and are a result of an increased $NADH_2/NAD^+$ ratio already referred to (Davis et al., 1967a).

A change from oxidative catabolism to reductive catabolism of serotinin has also been found after alcohol. Normally serotonin is metabolised to 5-hydroxyindole acetic acid (5-HIAA); one hour after an injection of ethanol there is a decrease in 5-HIAA excretion, all of which can be accounted for by an increase in urinary 5-hydroxytrophol (Davies et al., 1967b). Similar changes in excretion patterns have been noted in chronic alcoholics while still drinking, but not after one week's abstinence from alcohol. The reported differences in the metabolism of serotonin by the alcoholic can also be found in the non-alcoholic after alcohol and in both instances the changes are due to the increased $NADH_2/NAD^+$ ratio.

Ethanol also effects haem and porphyrin metabolism and acute attacks of porphyria can be precipitated by alcohol (Goldberg & Rimmington, 1962). Ethanol has also been shown to elevate delta-aminolaevulinic acid synthetase, (Shanley, Zail & Joubert, 1968) the rate limiting enzyme of haem biosynthesis. More recently a depression of delta-aminolaevulinic acid dehydrase was found in the blood of man (Moore et al., 1971), this enzyme catalysing the condensation of two molecules of delta-aminolaevulinic acid to form porphobilinogen. Once again this effect on enzyme activity is due to a change in the $NADH_2/NAD^+$ ratio, increasing the redox potential and so altering both cytoplasmic and mitochondrial intermediary metabolism.

Gastrointestinal Complications

Alcohol is associated with a number of gastrointestinal disorders, the best known being the acute gastritis which occurs even in the occasional drinker, and hepatic cirrhosis which occurs in the chronic alcoholic.

Keller (1967) showed an association between cancer of the mouth and pharynx and heavy alcohol consumption; this association was more marked when the patients had alcoholic cirrhosis. In a series from the U.S.A. of carcinoma of the oesophagus, 73 per cent of the patients were chronic alcoholics; this compared to 19 per cent in a similar group of patients with carcinoma of the lower bowel (Kamionkowski & Fleshler, 1965). In 1939 Sir Arthur Hurst published figures showing that in workers in the wine and spirit trade there was a fourfold increase in the incidence of carcinoma of the oesophagus; again, carcinoma of the lower bowel had a similar incidence as in the general population. The aetiological relationship between alcohol and carcinoma of the oesophagus is, of course, unknown, and other factors such as malnourishment may well play their part. Abnormalities of oesophageal motility have been noticed in alcoholic patients who had a peripheral neuropathy; the clinical significance of this is at present uncertain (Winship et al., 1968).

Stomach

When we come to consider the stomach the situation seems much better, there being no evidence that chronic gastritis is more prevalent in the alcoholic. The acute gastritis that can easily develop after too much alcohol quickly subsides, and histological examination of gastric biopsies shows no chronic gastritis or gastric atrophy (Palmer, 1954). In a recent retrospective study (Wolff, 1969) the patients with normal biopsies drank more than those with some evidence of gastritis; perhaps, after all, alcohol has some benefit! Despite this absence of chronic gastritis, Engeset, Lygren & Idsoe (1963) have shown a high incidence of gastric ulcers in alcoholics, duodenal ulcer showing the same prevalence in non-alcoholics as alcoholics.

Mallory–Weiss Syndrome

This eponymous term is used to describe the linear tears that occur in the mucosa at the oesophago-gastric junction (Mallory & Weiss, 1929). The tears occur after excessive vomiting and retching and are much more common in the alcoholic (Holmes, 1966). Similar mucosal tears can be produced at the cardia in the cadaver by distending the stomach to a pressure of 150 mm Hg, a pressure well within the range found when a subject is straining. These experimental findings would fit well with the clinical observation of retching prior to haematemesis (Atkinson, et al., 1961). The diagnosis can be made by a barium meal examination of the stomach, but it can be made more easily by gastroscopy. It must be remembered that sometimes the bleeding can be severe and persistent and surgery may be required.

Malabsorption

Malabsorption of folic acid and B_{12} has been referred to previously. Malabsorption of a number of substances has been demonstrated, but the importance of malabsorption in clinical practice is doubtful since dietary deficiency is so much more common. Malabsorption of the pentose D-Xylose was shown in skid-row alcoholics (Small, Longarini & Zamchek, 1959) and these findings were confirmed by Mezey et al., (1970) who showed malabsorption of Xylose in 24 per cent of a group of alcoholics without overt evidence of malabsorption or malnutrition. This malabsorption of Xylose returned to normal when an adequate diet was instituted despite continuation of alcohol.

Malabsorption of amino acids has also been shown in animals and man. In vitro and in vivo studies in rats have demonstrated malabsorption of the actively transported amino acid L-Phenylalanine (Israel, Salazar & Rosenmann, 1968). Malabsorption of D-Phenylalanine which is not actively transported did not occur at the same ethanol concentration, suggesting that the malabsorption seen was not a non-specific toxic effect. Studies in man using a double lumen perfusion system have demonstrated a 50 per cent decrease in absorption of methionine when the test segment is exposed to 2 per cent ethanol, a concentration that can be found in the upper intestine after moderate alcohol consumption (Israel et al., 1969). These authors postulate that certain syndromes of protein deficiency might be aggravated by the inhibitory effect of alcohol on intestinal amino acid absorption. Finally, surgery is often undertaken on the gastrointestinal tract of patients who are alcoholics; the increased mortality and morbidity has a number of causes which often go unrecognised (see Lowenfels, Rohman & Shibutani, 1970).

Alcoholic Liver Disease

It has been shown that both ingestion of large quantities of alcohol and dietary deficiency produce liver cell damage; the specific contribution of these factors individually in the production of hepatic disease is undecided.

Cirrhosis of the liver is increasing in frequency among the causes of death both in the United States (see Popper et al., 1969) and in Europe (WHO report 1968); alcoholism and alcoholic liver disease being one of the most important economic and social problems in the Western World.

The pathogenesis and clinical recognition of liver disease has been facilitated over the last decade by the wider use of specialised liver function tests and more especially the use of liver biopsy. The liver biopsy permits an accurate diagnosis in many patients who have minimal but definite damage to the liver with normal liver function tests.

Since the advent of more or less routine liver biopsies two types of liver disease have been recognised:

Alcoholic fatty liver. In this condition there is an accumulation of fat in the liver, this varying from minimal, detected only by biopsy, to severe accumulation where there is derangement of liver function in addition to the abnormal histology. A particular form of fatty liver is known as alcoholic hepatitis where the biopsy shows liver cell necrosis usually with marked fat accumulation; however, necrosis without steatosis may be present in some cases.

Cirrhosis. This implies end stage liver disease where there is mesenchymal cell proliferation, fibrosis and eventually lobular distortion. In all cases there is evidence of deranged liver function and in most cases some clinical stigmata of the disease is also present.

Biopsy specimens in 3000 randomly selected alcoholic patients admitted to an American city hospital because of withdrawal symptoms or intercurrent infection, showed a normal liver in 31 per cent, fatty liver or liver cell damage or both in 40 per cent and varying degrees of cirrhosis in 29 per cent (see Leevy, 1967). There was no apparent relationship between the biopsy appearance and the amount of alcohol drunk. All of the patients had an inadequate diet, deficient to some extent in vitamins and proteins, however the degree of deficiency bore no relationship to the histological appearance of the liver.

Pathogenesis

Fatty liver The acute or chronic administration of ethanol will produce an accumulation of fat in the liver. Lieber and co-workers have performed a number of elegant experiments where they have substituted ethanol iso-calorically for carbohydrates (see Rubin & Lieber, 1967, 1968a; Lieber & Rubin, 1969). Initial studies in rats showed a ten-fold increase in hepatic triglycerides when these animals were fed alcohol and subsequent studies in alcoholic and non-alcoholic volunteers have confirmed these findings (Rubin & Lieber, 1968b). It is perhaps worth discussing these experiments in some detail since this is the main evidence that in man ethanol per se is toxic to the liver. The non-alcoholic volunteers were fed a standard American diet with vitamin supplements and suitably diluted alcohol was given in 8 divided doses for up to 14 days. The amount of alcohol given ranged from 68 to 160 g per day (Table 8.1). In addition another 2 subjects received the same regime but their diet was altered to be high in protein and low in fat. Liver biopsies taken at the start of the study showed little or no fat histologically and 4+ amounts at the end of the alcohol period. Hepatic triglycerides were approximately 8 mgs per 100 mg protein beforehand and 62 mgs per 100 mg protein after alcohol. The subjects on the low fat diet showed an increase in hepatic lipid, but this was much less, being in the range of 16 mgs per 100 mg protein after alcohol (Table 8.1). Six more subjects were fed the same 2 diets as above and given 270 g of alcohol over 2 days, simulating weekend drinking. All subjects showed an accumulation of hepatic lipid but this was less marked than in the long-term study; again the subjects on a low fat diet showed less fat accumulation.

TABLE 8.1

THE EFFECT OF ISOCALORIC SUBSTITUTION OF ALCOHOL ON
HEPATIC TRIGLYCERIDES OF NON-ALCOHOLIC VOLUNTEERS

(FROM RUBIN AND LIEBER)

Group	Subjects	Duration of alcohol	Range of alcohol dosage	Mean hepatic triglycerides (mg/100 mg protein)	
		Days (mean)	g/day	Before	After
Standard diet	3	11	68–130	9·2	64·1
High protein low fat diet	2	9	79–158	4·2	15·9
Standard diet	3	2	270	9·3	23·2
High protein low fat diet	4	2	270	9·3	17·4

Electron micrographs of the liver histology showed early swelling and destruction of the mitochondria, increased focal cytoplasmic degradation and an increase in the endoplasmic reticulum. This latter finding of an increase in endoplasmic reticulum is accompanied by an increase in the microsomal oxidase system which may play a role in the metabolism of alcohol (see Lieber, 1970).

The above study would seem to establish the role of ethanol as a direct liver toxin and it should be noted that the amount of alcohol given was not excessive, blood alcohol levels were in the range of 20–80 mg/100 ml.

Porta, Koch & Hartroft (1969) were unable to produce liver damage in rats fed alcohol for as long as 7 months, providing they were given adequate amounts of lipotropic agents. Hartroft has pointed out that giving either alcohol or sucrose as 36 per cent of the total calories produces a serious dietary imbalance with a corresponding disturbance in hepatic structure and function. These same workers have been able to produce in rats as severe a fat accumulation in the liver when sucrose makes up 36 per cent of the total calories as they can with alcohol. On both the sucrose and the alcohol containing diets the lipotropic value of the diet was inadequate, but by giving choline chloride this was corrected and fatty change in the liver did not occur. No increased lipid accumulation was found by the same group when rats were given alcohol and a so-called super diet containing 25 per cent protein with a balanced fat carbohydrate ratio. In the experiments quoted above in human volunteers high protein diet did not prevent the hepatic damage and to date Lieber's experiments have not been repeated.

Lieber and co-workers have shown in man as well as in animals, that the lipids found in the liver after chronic alcohol administration are dietary in origin (see Lieber, 1967). On a low fat diet ethanol does not produce the same degree of hepatic steatosis as when the fat content is 80 g per day. If then the lipids seem to be of dietary origin what leads to their accumulation in the liver after ethanol?

Fat absorption is normal after ethanol ingestion as is chylomicron uptake by the liver (Lieber, Spritz & DeCarli, 1966). The formation or the subsequent release of lipoproteins by the liver may be affected by alcohol. Here the data is somewhat conflicting; certainly ethanol in high concentration can depress secretion of lipoproteins in a perfused liver system (Schapiro et al., 1964) but the administration of alcohol to man produces an increase in blood lipids rather than a decrease (Jones et al., 1963). Formation of lipoproteins in the liver are not impaired by ethanol (Isselacher & Greenberger, 1964), and it seems generally agreed that these two mechanisms can only contribute at best to a small degree to the cause of the hepatic steatosis (see Lieber, 1967). Decreased hepatic oxidation of fatty acids has been demonstrated (Reboucas & Isselbacher, 1961) and it is this effect of ethanol, combined with an increase in endogenously synthesised lipid (Lieber & Schmid, 1961), which Lieber and others (see Lieber, 1967) think is the most likely explanation for the increase in hepatic lipids. Unfortunately some of the data regarding the mechanism of hepatic lipid accumulation is contradictory, but it is impossible to consider all the arguments in this article.

Some workers stress the role of non-dietary lipids in hepatic steatosis (see Isselbacher & Greenberger, 1964). The effect of a single dose of alcohol differs according to the different data, however, by and large a rise in plasma FFA is seen. This finding is interpreted by some workers to be the significant effect of ethanol: an increased supply of FFA is delivered to the liver where they are available to be converted into hepatic lipids. The rise in circulating FFA is due to increased release from adipose tissue (Scheig & Isselbacher, 1965) and when this is prevented by say adrenergic blocking agents (Brodie *et al.*, 1961) hepatic lipid accumulation does not occur. Although the effect on FFA of a single large dose of alcohol seems established, in chronic alcoholic administration the role of increased circulating FFA is much less certain (see Lieber, 1967). The pathogenic role of lipid peroxidation in the production of a fatty liver is still uncertain (see DiLuzio & Hartman, 1967), but it is possible that increases in lipid peroxidation might be responsible for the fat accumulation. Antioxidants inhibit lipid peroxidation *in vivo* and *in vitro* and this could explain their role in modifying hepatic injury after alcohol.

Increased fatty acid synthesis can be demonstrated after ethanol *in vitro* and *in vivo* (Lieber & Schmid, 1961), perhaps related to the increased $NADH_2$ which is necessary for fatty acid synthesis. The importance of this increased synthesis as an important mechanism in the production of a fatty liver seems doubtful, since many substances such as glucose and sorbital will increase fatty acid synthesis without affecting hepatic lipid accumulation (Rebouças & Isselbacher, 1961). Finally the reason for the selective accumulation of triglycerides over other classes of lipid has not yet been adequately explained.

Thus, although this is a controversial field, it seems likely that in man lipid accumulates in the liver due to alcohol *per se*. These lipids seem to be mainly of dietary origin in the chronic situation and probably a number of mechanisms are responsible for their accumulation.

Cirrhosis. Fatty liver has been frequently studied—mainly because it is relatively easy to produce experimentally. Cirrhosis on the other hand has only been produced experimentally on a few occasions (Porta, Koch and Hartroft, 1969). In this study rats were given 37 per cent of their total calories as sucrose or alcohol; after 7 months histological examination of the liver showed excess fat, alcoholic hyaline, fibrosis and true cirrhosis, all the features usually found in the liver in human alcoholic liver disease (Table 8.2). These findings only occurred when the lipotropic content of the diet was low

TABLE 8.2

HEPATIC TRIGLYCERIDES AND PERCENTAGES OF LIVERS WITH FIBROSIS AND CIRRHOSIS. (FROM PORTA, KOCH AND HARTROFT)

	Lipotropic value of diet. (*mg choline per 100 k cal*)	Fluid Intake (ad lib)*	Hepatic triglycerides mg/g	Fibrosis	Cirrhosis
A		25% sucrose – 32% alcohol (w:v)	284·5	25	75
	17				
B		water	309·6	40	60
C		25% sucrose – 32% alcohol (w:v)	3·25	0	0
	200				
D		water	5·57	0	0

* Rats drinking water were given sucrose in their diet in isocaloric amounts to that drunk by the other group.

and they could be prevented by administration of choline despite continuing sucrose and alcohol. These experiments confirm and extend the original observations of Best *et al.* (1949) that the choline content of the diet is important when alcohol is being consumed. The high incidence of malnutrition in chronic alcoholics with cirrhosis and the relative effectiveness of a high protein diet in treating this disease despite continuation of alcohol (Erenglu, Edreira & Patek, 1964) has led many workers to consider that malnutrition is the most significant factor in the production of cirrhosis. Children with severe protein malnutrition do not, however, develop cirrhosis. Ramalingaswami, 1964) and cirrhosis definitely occurs in alcoholics with an adequate dietary intake (Powell & Klatskin, 1968).

Fatty liver and cirrhosis

The relationship between fatty liver and cirrhosis has still not been definitely established and there is no good evidence that fatty change is the predisposing factor in the production of cirrhosis. Fatty liver can be maintained for months experimentally without cirrhosis (Hondler & Dubin, 1946) and it would appear that the presence of necrosis is the crucial factor which leads to cirrhosis. Thus 11 of 16 alcoholic patients observed with fatty liver and marked liver cell damage or necrosis developed cirrhosis within a period of 5 years, whereas cirrhosis did not develop in those with a fatty liver alone (Leevy, 1967).

Susceptibility to liver disease

It is well known that even with ingestion of large quantities of alcohol some patients have normal livers. Indeed as mentioned above, some patients can recover from their liver disease despite continuation of small amounts of alcohol. A number of factors have been suggested to explain this apparent differing in susceptibility but no convincing evidence is available. A suggested inherent factor is supported by the reported association of colour blindness, alcoholism and cirrhosis (Cruz-Coke & Varela, 1966), but so far the evidence is incomplete. Differences in dietary patterns in alcoholics may be important but again discrepancies in the severity of the liver involvement occur. Leevy (1967) has measured $NADH_2/NAD^+$ ratios and ADH activity in liver biopsies of alcoholics after chronic ingestion of ethanol; the results suggesting that the ability of the liver to oxidise alcohol might be a key determinent in the development of liver disease. Probably the key factor however is the amount and duration of the alcohol excess—the form of beverage in which it is taken making no difference (Lelbach, 1968). It has been estimated that there is practically no cirrhosis in a group who drink less than 80 g alcohol per day but above 160 g per day the risk is very high (Pequignot, 1961); similarly the extent of the liver damage has been related to the amount of alcohol drunk in both Germany and Chile (see Ugarte, Iturriaga & Insunza, 1970).

Clinical Features and Management of Alcoholic Liver Disease

It is only intended to mention briefly the various clinical syndromes and some special features regarding management.

Fatty liver

This is a completely reversible lesion and normal histology can be found after one week of adequate dietary intake and no alcohol (Seife, Kessler & Lisa, 1950). On the other hand, diet therapy requires 40 days to restore normal morphology in patients in whom 80 per cent of the liver biopsy is occupied by fat globules: this time interval possibly being shortened by androgenic anabolic steroids, which are known to increase protein synthesis. (See Leevy, 1967.) These drugs have had, however, no substantial clinical trial and would certainly not be needed in most cases of fatty liver.

Alcoholic hepatitis

The clinical features are of an acute illness marked by anorexia, weight loss and jaundice (Green, Mistilis & Schiff, 1963). Alcoholic hepatitis can occur in a chronic alcoholic after an acute binge, or it may present after a long history of steady alcohol intake. The liver biopsy shows liver cell necrosis, acute inflammatory cells, Mallory bodies and usually marked fat accumulation. Reynolds et al. (1969) have demonstrated portal hypertension in this group of patients, the liver biopsy showing centrilobular sclerosis but no true cirrhosis. Alcoholic hepatitis is important, since liver cell necrosis usually leads to fibrosis at a later stage, and thus it bridges the gap between fatty liver and true cirrhosis.

Florid alcoholic hepatitis is a serious condition and carries a high mortality (Hardison & Lee, 1966) and abstinence from alcohol is mandatory in the treatment of this condition. Because of the evidence of inflammation on biopsy and the high mortality, corticosteroids have been given in this condition. In a group of severely ill patients no difference in mortality was noted between the controls and the treated groups (see Ugarte et al., 1970). Two studies have recently been performed (Helman et al., 1971; Porter et al., 1971) to assess the role of corticosteroids in the treatment of alcoholic hepatitis. The results were conflicting but corticosteroids should probably be used in severe cases if only to improve the appetite and well-being of the patient.

Cirrhosis

Morphological abnormalities are not spontaneously progressive in the early stages of alcoholic cirrhosis, and lobular distortion can be prevented. Leevy (1967) and co-workers have studied these patients with alcoholic cirrhosis and they believe that the prognosis of active cirrhosis is directly related to the ability to synthesize nucleic acids and protein required for hepatic regeneration. A 75 per cent survival rate was noted over a 2 year period among alcoholic patients with active cirrhosis and increased in vitro deoxyribonucleic acid (DNA) synthesis. In contrast, 5 patients with identical morphology to the above but lack of in vitro hepatic DNA synthesis died. Complete and life long abstinence from alcohol is needed in patients with cirrhosis. 70 per cent of patients with moderate disease who did not abstain died within 2 years. On the other hand in the same study, 60 per cent of the patients who abstained (a relatively small number) were alive at 2 years (Ugarte et al., 1970).

Adequate nutriment and vitamins should be given but there is no indication for steroid therapy although these drugs have been tried in early cases of cirrhosis.

Hepatic iron overload

McDonald (1961) has found an incidence of alcoholism in 29 to 85 per cent of cases of haemochromatosis, while in England Williams, Scheur & Sherlock (1962) have found that 31 per cent of all patients with haemochromatosis are alcoholics. Haemochromatosis on the other hand occurs in total abstainers and it has been suggested that alcohol merely accelerates the development of haemochromatosis (Dubin, 1955).

In the alcoholic with cirrhosis there is often increased hepatic iron deposition. Powell in 1966 showed that there was a significant increase in the total hepatic iron content in those subjects with a heavy alcohol consumption and over half of a series of patients with alcoholic liver disease showed increased iron content, although this rarely approaches the amount seen in haemochromatosis (Scheur, Williams & Muir, 1962). It is still not clear what part alcohol plays in the transition from haemosiderosis to haemochromatosis.

How may alcohol increase hepatic iron content? Wines contain a high iron content ranging from 6·2 to 2·3 mg/l (McDonald, 1964) mainly derived from utensils used in their preparation. Other alcoholic beverages contain little iron and there is no difference in the amount of hepatic iron in wine drinkers as far as can be established. In many alcoholics with cirrhosis, pancreatic disease is present and this condition may increase iron absorption although some workers have shown that iron absorption is increased in any cirrhosis regardless of its aeteology (Williams et al., 1967). Thus the precise relationship between alcohol and iron overload is uncertain and probably multiple factors are at work.

Pancreatic Disease

In the U.S.A. 17–75 per cent of patients with chronic pancreatitis are alcoholics (see Dreiling, Janowitz & Perrier, 1964); this compares to a figure of 4 per cent for this country. Chronic calcific pancreatitis is almost inevitably associated with alcoholism in the U.S.A. but need not necessarily be so here.

If then there is a strong association between alcoholism and pancreatic disease, how does this occur? As in the case of alcoholic liver disease, a lot of experimental data is available but at the present time no definite mechanism for the establishment of pancreatitis has been achieved (see Schapiro, Wruble & Britt, 1966; Kalant, 1969). The most common explanation is that alcohol increases pancreatic secretion at the same time as producing obstruction of the pancreatic duct or sphincter of Oddi; the combination of these two effects having been shown to produce acute pancreatic necrosis (see Schapiro et al., 1966).

Orally ingested alcohol stimulates pancreatic secretion but this increased secretion is not seen when alcohol is given intravenously (see Dreiling et al., 1964). Likewise alcohol does not stimulate pancreatic secretion when placed directly in the duodenum and it is now agreed that increased pancreatic secretion is a result of alcohol stimulated acid secretion, this in turn causing the release of secretin when it reaches the duodenum. Walton *et al.*, (1965) demonstrated moderate increases in pancreatic duct pressure in dogs but the concentration of alcohol (10–20 per cent) was higher than one would expect to find in the duodenum. Davis & Pirola (1966) showed a reduction in pancreatic secretion after alcohol in patients whose pancreatic secretion was being maximally stimulated by secretin. These two results suggest that ethanol by mouth does increase pancreatic duct pressure. It is suggested that the alcohol that is unabsorbed in the stomach reaches the duodenum where it could cause duodenitis, oedema of the papilla, intense spasm of the sphincter of Oddi, all of which prevent pancreatic flow and elevate intraductal pressure. More recently the effects of chronic ethanol ingestion in the pancreas have been studied. Orrego-Matte *et al.*, (1969) showed a decreased $_{32}P$ incorporation into pancreatic phospholipid after ethanol and a recent ultrastructural study of the pancreas after ethanol has shown large numbers of lipid droplets in acinar cells, swelling of acinar mitochondria and focal cytoplasmic degradation (Darle, Ekholm & Edlund, 1970). It will be remembered that these are similar ultrastructure changes to those found in alcoholic fatty liver and similar conclusions regarding causitive factors have been drawn. Sarles *et al.* (1971) has produced in rats histological changes in the pancreas identical to that seen in human chronic pancreatitis after 20–30 months ethanol intake. The action of ethanol on the pancreas seemed to be related to the dietary ratio of protein and lipids (Sarles, Figarella & Clemente, 1971). Chronic pancreatitis, indistinguishable from the pancreatitis seen in chronic alcoholism, has been described in an adult protein deficient population (Shaper, 1964). Mezey *et al.* (1970) found a decreased pancreatic response to secretin in chronic alcoholics without liver disease; the response returning to normal after an adequate protein diet despite consumption of alcohol. Both these observations suggest that protein malnutrition may play a role in the aetiology of alcoholic pancreatitis.

Alcoholic pancreatitis usually occurs after 8–10 years of alcoholism, attacks of abdominal pain occur which progressively become more severe (Howard & Ehrlich, 1961). After alcoholic pancreatitis has begun, recurrent attacks are the rule, while over half will develop evidence of chronic pancreatic disease (Howard & Ehrlich, 1961). The pancreatitis varies in severity from the acute haemorrhagic type to the more benign oedematous pancreatitis when the peripheral vascular failure is not so severe. Once recurrent attacks of pancreatitis have developed there is a persistence of pathological changes between attacks.

Chronic pancreatitis has 3 distinctive features namely steatorhoea, calcification and diabetes (Comfort, Gambill & Baggenstoss, 1946) but pain is often an additional feature (Sarles *et al.*, 1965); this is sometimes described as relapsing chronic pancreatitis.

Withdrawal of alcohol to prevent the recurring acute attacks may be of value but is valueless when pancreatic insufficiency is the main problem.

Pancreatitis does not occur in all patients with alcoholism but the incidence is probably higher than initially recognised. In patients with alcoholic cirrhosis, abnormal pancreatic function tests have been found in approximately a third of cases (Davies, 1969), the majority of these cases having no overt clinical evidence of pancreatic disease. This figure agrees well with post mortem evidence (Table 8.3) of pancreatitis in about 30 per cent of cases of alcoholic cirrhosis (Marin, Clark & Senior, 1969). It seems likely that the steatorrhoea often seen in patients with alcoholic cirrhosis is usually due to this pancreatic disease.

TABLE 8.3

PANCREATIC LESIONS IN 154 AUTOPSY CASES OF LAENNEC'S
CIRRHOSIS (MARIN et al.)

Pathological lesion	No.	Percentage
Acute pancreatitis	7	4·5
Chronic pancreatitis		
severe	5	3·2
moderate	9	5·8
mild	23	14·9
Total	44	28·4

Alcoholic Heart Disease

Four distinct clinical syndromes have been described in alcoholics with evidence of heart disease.

The first comprehensive description of beri-beri heart disease (Aalsmeer & Wenckebach, 1929) described a syndrome of systolic arterial hypertension, collapsing pulse, rapid circulation, marked peripheral oedema and ascites. This picture of classical beri-beri in the Western hemisphere occurs almost exclusively in alcoholics (see Burch & De Pasquale, 1969). This type of heart disease is the least common form of alcoholic heart disease and is less serious in that it responds well and quickly to thiamine (Brigden & Robinson, 1964). Patients in the second group described by Brigden and Robinson presented with a variety of cardiac arrythmias of which atrial fibrillation and multi-focal ventricular beats were the most common. Spontaneous return to sinus rhythm sometimes occurred, but usually relapse followed further drinking. The electrocardiogram, initially thought to be specific (Evans, 1959), showed variable abnormalities depending on the amount of muscle involvement.

The third group of patients presented with hypokinetic heart failure, cardiomegaly and electrocardiographic evidence of severe myocardial damage. The clinical picture does not differ from other forms of cardiomyopathy and unless the history is carefully taken the story of excessive drinking may be missed. The histological findings are usually focal and minimal and out of proportion to the severity of the clinical picture (Burch & DePasquale, 1969). Varying degrees of vacuolisation of muscle fibres with some atrophied and degenerating muscle fibres are found: inflammatory cells may be present but are unusual. More recently cardiac biopsies have been performed using a Menghini needle. On electron microscopy these biopsies show loss or degeneration of contractile elements, the spaces left being filled by swollen mitochondria, which are devoid of cristae. In addition cystic dilatation of sarcoplasmic reticulum with increased fat deposits are found (see Hudson, 1970). All these electron microscope changes were thought to be specific for alcoholic cardiomyopathy (Alexander, 1966) but are now known to be present in other forms of heart disease.

Treatment of these last two groups consists of digitalis and diuretics, the arrhythmia group usually responding well. The patients with the obvious cardiomyopathy initially respond to therapy but a progressive down-hill course is usually inevitable even if alcohol is withdrawn. Prolonged bed rest for up to one year has been tried in this condition with return of the heart to normal size in 50 per cent of cases (see Burch & DePasquale, 1969). In the patients who initially responded 62 per cent were alive, most with normal size hearts after some years of evaluation (mean 6·25 years), resumption of alcohol was the prime factor leading to progressive cardiac deterioration (see Burch & Giles, 1971).

It is important to realise that alcoholic heart disease often occurs in the well nourished social drinker, and many cases in the U.K. are amongst men

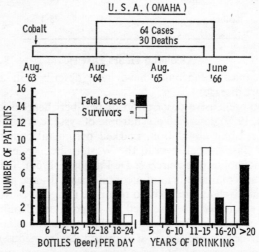

FIG. 8.7. Correlation of the incidence of cardiomyopathy with cobalt addition to beer and the estimated alcohol consumption in the cases seen (from Sullivan *et al.*, 1969) with permission of authors and New York Academy of Sciences.

who work in the liquor trade. In Brigden & Robinsons series one third drank beer alone with an average consumption of 15 pints per day, whilst a quarter drank over a bottle of spirits a day.

The exact relationship between alcohol and the cardiac muscle damage is of course unknown (see Burch & Giles, 1971). Malnutrition, additives to alcoholic beverages have all been blamed, but there seems no good reason for not thinking that ethanol itself is the chief culprit, since ethanol has been shown experimentally to have a deleterious effect on myocardial function (Regan, 1966).

Additives, namely cobalt, however, are thought to have played a role in the cardiomyopathy that was intially described in Quebec (Morin & Daniel, 1967). In both Quebec and Omaha (Sullivan, Egan & George, 1969) the syndrome appeared one month after the addition of cobalt sulphate to beer and no more cases developed one month after this procedure was stopped (Fig. 8.7). A similar relationship between cobalt addition to beer and a cardiomyopathy syndrome developed in Louvain in Belgium (Kestelloot *et al.*, 1966). The cobalt incidentally was added to the beer to improve stability of foam, which is aesthetically pleasing to the customer but difficult to sustain since the introduction of strong detergents for glass washing.

The precise relationship between the cobalt and the severe cardiomyopathy that occurred is still uncertain and largely circumstantial. Since many heavy beer drinkers were unaffected the severity of the disease did not correlate with the amount of beer consumed (Fig. 8.7) and the amount of cobalt added can be taken in some prescribed medicines used for treating anaemia. Cobalt concentrations were elevated ten times over normal in cardiac muscle of patients with cardiomyopathy while magnesium and zinc were decreased; the relationship of these changes to myocardial failure is uncertain (Sullivan, Parker & Carson, 1968).

The pattern of the illness in Omaha and Louvain was similar to Quebec, a slowly emerging epidemic; in Omaha 64 cases developing over 2 years. The cardiomyopathy lead to severe heart failure with a mortality of about 50 per cent in all 3 places. No further cases have been described since cobalt was withdrawn.

References

AALSMEER, W. C. & WENCKEBACH, K. F. (1929). *Wein. arch. inn. Med.* **16**, 193.

ALEXANDER, C. S. (1966). *Am. J. Med.* **41**, 229.

ALLBRINK, M. J. & KLATSKIN, G. (1957). *Am. J. Med.* **23**, 26.

ATKINSON, M., BOTTRILL, M. B., EDWARDS, A. T., MITCHELL, W. M., PEET, B. G. & WILLIAMS, R. E. (1961). *Gut*, **2**, 1.

BEST, C. H., HARTROFT, W. S., LUCAS, C. C. & RIDOUT, J. H. (1949). *Br. med. J.* **2**, 1001.

BLAIR, A. H. & VALLEE, B. L. (1966). *Biochemistry*, **5**, 2026.

BRAYTON, R. G., STOKES, P. E., SCHWARTZ, M. S. & LOURIA, D. B. (1970). *New Engl. J. Med.* **252**, 123.

BRIGDEN, W. & ROBINSON, J. (1964). *Br. med. J.*, **2**, 1283.

BURCH, G. E. & DEPASQUALE, N. P. (1969). *Am. J. Cardiol.* **23**, 723.

BURCH, G. E. & GILES, T. D. (1971). *Am. J. Med.* **50**, 141.

BRODIE, B. B., BUTLER, W. M., HORNING, M. G., MAICKEL, R. P. & MALLING, H. M. (1961). *Am. J. clin. Nutr.* **9**, 432.

CHANARIN, I. (1969). *Br. J. Haemat.* **17**, 515.

CHERRICK, G. R. & LEEVY, C. M. (1965). *Biochem. biophys. Acta.* **107**, 29.

CLARK, C. G. & SENIOR, J. R. (1968). *Gastroenterology*, **55**, 670.

COMFORT, M. W., GAMBILL, E. E. & BAGGENSTOSS, A. H. (1946). *Gastroenterology*, **6**, 239.

COOKE, A. R. & BIRCHALL, A. (1969). *Gastroenterology*, **57**, 269.

CRUZ-COKE, R. & VARELA, A. (1965). *Lancet*, **2**, 1348.

DARLE, N., EKHOLM, R. & EDLUND, Y. (1970). *Gastroenterology*, **58**, 62.

DAVIS, A. E. & PIROLA, R. C. (1966). *Med. J. Aust.* **2**, 757.

DAVIS, A. E. (1969). *Med. J. Aust.* **1**, 508.

DAVIS, V. E., BROWN, H., HUFF, J. A. & CASHAW, J. L. (1967a). *J. Lab. clin. Med.* **69**, 787.

DAVIS, V. E., BROWN, H., HUFF, J. A. & CASHAW, J. L. (1967b). *J. Lab. clin. Med.* **69**, 132.

DiLUZIO, N. R. & HARTMANN, A. D. (1967). *Fed. Proc.* **26**, 1436.

DREILING, D. A., JANOWITZ, H. D. & PERRIER, C. V. (1964). *In* 'Pancreatic Inflammatory Disease'. New York: Hoeber.

DUBIN, I. N. (1955). *Am. J. clin. Path.* **25**, 514.

ENGLESET, A., LYGREN, T. & IDSOE, R. (1963). *Q. Jl Stud. Alcohol*, **24**, 622.

ERENOYLE, E. E., EDREIRA, J. G. & PATEK, A. J. (1964). *Ann. intern. Med.* **60**, 814.

EVANS, W. (1959). *Br. Heart J.* **21**, 445.

FORNEY, R. B. & HARGER, R. N. (1969). *Ann. Rev. Pharm.* **9**, 379.

FREINGEL, N., SINGER, D. L., ARKY, R. A., BLEICHER, S. J., ANDERSON, J. B. & GILBERT, C. K. (1963). *J. clin. Invest.* **42**, 1112.

GOLDBERG, A. & RIMINGTON, C. (1962). *In* 'Diseases of Porphyrin Metabolism'. Springfield, Ill.: Thomas.

GOLDSTEIN, A. (1970). *New Engl. J. Med.* **283**, 875.

GREEN, G. M. & CASS, E. H. (1965). *Br. J. exp. Path.* **46**, 360.

GREEN, J., MISTILIS, S. & SCHIFF, L. (1963). *Archs intern. Med.* **112**, 67.

GREENBERGER, N. J., HATCH, F. T., DRUMMEY, G. D. & ISSELBACHER, K. J. (1966). *Medicine*, **45**, 161.

HANDLER, P. & DUBIN, I. N. (1946). *J. Nutr.* **31**, 141.

HALSTED, C. H., GRIGGS, R. C. & HARRIS, J. W. (1967). *J. Lab. clin. Med.* **69**, 116.

HARDISON, W. G. & LEE, F. I. (1966). *New Engl. J. Med.* **61**, 275.

HARTROFT, W. S. (1967). *Fed. Proc.* **26**, 1432.

HEATON, F. W., PYRAH, L. N., BERESFORD, C. C., BRYSON, R. W. & MARTIN, D. F. (1962). *Lancet*, **2**, 802.

HED, R., LARSSON, H. & WAHLGREN, F. (1955). *Acta med. scand.* **152**, 459.

HELMAN, R. A., TEMKO, M. H., NYE, S. W. & FALLOW, H. J. (1971). *Ann. intern. Med.* **74**, 311.

HINES, J. D. (1969). *Br. J. Haemat.* **16**, 87.

HINES, J. D. & COWAN, D. H. (1970). *New Engl. J. Med.* **283**, 441.

HOLMES, K. D. (1966). *Ann. Surg.* **164**, 810.

HOWARD, J. M. & EHRLICH, E. W. (1961). *Surgery Gynec. Obstet.* **113**, 167.

HUDSON, R. E. B. (1971). *In* 'Cardiovascular Pathology'. Vol. 3. London: Arnold.

HURST, A. (1939). *Lancet*, **1**, 621.

ISRAEL, Y., VALENZUELA, J. E., SALAZAR, I. & UGARTE, G. (1969). *J. Nutr.* **98**, 222.

ISSELBACHER, K. J. & GREENBERGER, N. J. (1964). *New Engl. J. Med.* **270**, 351.

JENKINS, J. S. & CONNOLLY, J. (1968). *Br. med. J.* **2**, 804.

JONES, J. E., SHANE, S. R., JACOBS, W. H. & FLINK, E. B. (1969). *Ann. N.Y. Acad. Sci.* **162**, 934.

KADEN, M., OAKLEY, M. W. & FIELD, J. B. (1969). *Am. J. Physiol.* **216**, 756.

KALANT, H. (1969). *Gastroenterology*, **56**, 380.

KALBFLEISCH, J. M., LINDEMAN, R. D., GINN, H. E. & SMITH, W. O. (1963). *J. clin. Invest.* **42**, 1471.

KAMIONKOWSKI, M. D. & FLESHLER, B. (1965). *Am. J. med. Sci.* **249**, 696.

KATER, R. M. H., CARULLI, N. & IBER, F. L. (1969). *Am. J. clin. Nutr.* **22**, 1608.

KATER, R. M. H., ZIEVE, D. & TOBON, F. (1968). *J. Am. med. Ass.* **206**, 1709.

KELLER, O. Z. (1967). *Cancer*, **20**, 1015.

KESTELLOOT, H., TERRYN, R., BOSMANS, P. & JOOSSENS, R. (1966). *Acta. cardiol.* (Brux). **21**, 341.

KHANNA, J. M. & KALANT, H. (1970). *Biochem. Pharmac.* **19**, 2033.

KLEEMAN, C. R., RUBINI, M. E., LAMDIN, E. & EPSTEIN, F. H. (1955). *J. clin. Invest.* **34**, 448.

KLINKERFUSS, G., BLEISCH, V., DIOSO, M. M. & PERKOFF, S. T. (1967). *Ann. intern. Med.* **67**, 493.

KREBS, H. A. & PERKINS, J. R. (1970). *Biochem. J.* **118**, 635.

KREISBERG, R. A., OWEN, W. C. & SIEGAL, A. M. (1971). *J. clin. Invest.* **50**, 166.

KREISBERG, R. A., SIEGAL, A. M. & OWEN, W. C. (1971). *J. clin. Invest.* **50**, 175.

LEEVY, C. M. (1967). *Fed. Proc.* **26**, 1474.

LEEVY, C. M. (1962). *Medicine*, **41**, 249.

LEEVY, C. M. (1966). *Medicine*, **45**, 423.

LEEVY, C. M. & BAKER, H. (1968). *Am. J. clin. Nutr.* **21**, 1325.

LELBACH, W. K. (1968). *Germ. med. Mon.* **13**, 31.

LIEBER, C. S. (1967). *Ann. Rev. Med.* **8**, 35.

LIEBER, C. S. (1970). *Gastroenterology*, **59**, 930.

LIEBER, C. S. & DE CARLI, L. M. (1970). *J. biol. Chem.* **245**, 2505.

LIEBER, C. S., JONES, D. P., LOSOWSKI, M. S. & DAVIDSON, C. S. (1962). *J. clin. Invest.* **41**, 1863.

LIEBER, C. S. & RUBIN, E. (1969). *New Engl. J. Med.* **280**, 705.

LIEBER, C. S., RUBIN, E. & DE CARLI, L. M. (1970). *Biochem. biophys. Res. Commun.* **40**, 858.

LIEBER, C. S. & SCHMID, R. (1961). *J. clin. Invest.* **40**, 394.

LIEBER, C. S., SPRITZ, N. & DE CARLI, L. M. (1969). *J. Lipid. Res.* **10**, 283.

LINDENBAUM, J. & LIEBER, C. S. (1969a). *New Engl. J. Med.* **281**, 333.

LINDENBAUM, J. & LIEBER, C. S. (1969b). *Nature*, **224**, 806.

LINDENEG, O., MELLEMGAARD, K., FABRICIUS, J. & LINDQUIST, F. (1964). *Clin. Sci.* **27**, 427.

LOSOWSKY, M. S., JONES, D. P., DAVIDSON, C. S. & LIEBER, C. S. (1963). *Am. J. Med.* **35**, 794.

LOWENFELS, A. B., ROHMAN, M., SHIBUTANI, K. (1970). *Surgery Gynec. Obstet.* **131**, 129.

LUBIN, M. & WESTERFIELD, W. W. (1945). *J. biol. chem.* **161**, 503.

LUNDQUIST, F. (1960). *Acta physiol. scand.* **175**, 97.

MACDONALD, R. A. (1961). *Archs intern. Med.* **107**, 606.

MACDONALD, R. A. (1964). *In* 'Haemachromatosis & Haemosiderosis'. Springfield, Ill.: Thomas.

MADISON, L. L. (1968). *Adv. Metab. Dis.*, **3**, 85.

MAFCHROWICZ, E. & MENDELSON, J. H. (1970). *Science*, **168**, 1100.

MALLORY, G. K. & WEISS, S. (1929). *Am. J. Med. Sci.* **178**, 506.

MARIN, G. A. CLARK, M. L. & SENIOR, J. R. (1969). *Gastroenterology*, **56**, 727.

MARKKANEN, T. & NANTO, V. (1966). *Experienta*, **22**, 753.

McFARLAND, W. & LIBRE, E. P. (1963). *Ann. intern. Med.* **59**, 865.

McNAMEE, H. B., MELLO, N. K. & MENDELSON, J. H. (1968). *Am. J. Psychiat.* **124**, 1063.

MENDELSON, J. H. (1970). *New Engl. J. Med.* **283**, 24.

MENDELSON, J. H., LADOU, J. & CORBETT, C. (1964). *Q. Jl Stud. Alcohol*, (Suppl. 2), 108.

MENDELSON, J. H. & STEIN, S. (1966). *Psychosom. Med.* **28**, 616.

MENDELSON, J. H., STEIN, S. & MELLO, N. K. (1965). *Metabolism*, **14**, 1255.

MENDELSON, H. STEIN, S. & McGUIRE, M. T. (1966). *Psychosom. Med.* **28**, 1.

MEZEY, E., JOWE, E., SLAVIN, R. E. & TOBON, F. (1970). *Gastroenterology*, **59**, 657.

MOORE, R. E., BEATTIE, A. D., THOMPSON, G. G. & GOLDBERG, A. (1971). *Clin. Sci.* **40**, 81.

MORIN, Y. & DANIEL, P. (1967). *Canad. med. Ass. J.* **97**, 926.

MURPHREE, H. B., GREENBERG, L. A. & CARROLL, R. B. (1967). *Fed. Proc.* **26**, 1468.

MYERSON, R. M. & LAFAIR, J. S. (1970). *Med. Clins N. Am.* **54**, 723.

NESTLE, P. J. (1967). *Australas. Ann. Med.* **16**, 139.

NEVILLE, J. N., EAGLES, J. A., SAMSON, G. & OLSON, R. E. (1968). *Am. J. clin. Nutr.* **21**, 1329.

NYGREN, A. (1966). *Acta med. scand.* **179**, 623.

ORREGO-MATTE, H., NAVIA, E., FERES, A. & COSTAMAILERE, L. (1969). *Gastroenterology*, **56**, 280.

Ogata, M., MENDELSON, J. H. & MELLO, N. K. (1968). *Psychosom. Med.* **30**, 463.

PALMER, E. D. (1954). *Medicine*, **33**, 236.

PEQUIGNOT, G. (1961). *Munch. med. Wschr.* **103**, 1464.

PERKOFF, S. T., DIOSO, M. M., BLEISCH, V. & KLINKERFUSS, G. (1967). *Ann. intern. Med.* **67**, 481.

POPPER, H., DAVIDSON, C. S., LEEVY, C. M. & SCHAFFNER, F. (1969). *New Engl. J. Med.* **67**, 481.

PORTA, E. A., KOCH, O. R. & HARTROFT, W. S. (1969). *Lab. Invest.* **20**, 562.

PORTER, H. P., SIMON, F. R., POPE, C. E., VOLWILER, W., FENSTER, L. F. (1971). *New Engl. J. Med.* **24**, 1350.

POST, R. M. & DESFORGES, J. (1968). *Blood*, **31**, 344.

POWELL, L. W. (1966). *Australas. Ann. Med.* **15**, 110.

POWELL, W. J. & KLATSKIN, G. (1968). *Am. J. Med.* **44**, 406.

RAMALINGASWAMI, V. (1964). *Nature*, **201**, 546.

REBOUCAS, G. & ISSELBACHER, K. J. (1961). *J. clin. Invest.* **40**, 1355.

REGAN, T. J., KOROXENIDIS, G., MOSCHOS, C. B. & OLDEWURTEL, H. A. (1966). *J. clin. Invest.* **45**, 270.

REYNOLDS, T. B., HIDEMURA, R., MICHEL, H. & PETERS, R. (1969). *Ann. intern. Med.* **70**, 497.

RUBIN, E., BACCHIN, P., GANG, H. & LIEBER, C. S. (1970). *Lab. Invest.* **22**, 569.

RUBIN, E., HUTTERER, F. & LIEBER, C. S. (1968). *Science*, **159**, 1469.

RUBIN, E. & LIEBER, C. S. (1967). *Fed. Proc.* **26**, 1458.

RUBIN, E. & LIEBER, C. S. (1968a). *Gastroenterology*, **54**, 642.

RUBIN, E. & LIEBER, C. S. (1968b). *New Engl. J. Med.* **278**, 869.

RUBIN, E. & LIEBER, C. S. (1968c). *Science*, **162**, 690.

RUBINI, M. E., KLEEMAN, C. R. & LAMDIN, E. (1955). *J. clin. Invest.* **34**, 439.

RYBACK, R. & DESFORGES, J. (1970). *Archs intern. Med.* **125**, 475.

SARLES, H., FIGARELLA, C. & CLEMENTE, F. (1971). *Digestion*, **4**, 13.

SARLES, H., LEBREUIL, G., TASSO, F., FIGARELLA, C., CLEMENTE, F., DEVAUX, M. A., FAGONDE, B. & PAYAN, H. (1971). *Gut*, **12**, 377.

SARLES, H., SARLES, J. C., CAMATTE, R., MURATORE, R., GAINI, M., GUINN, C., PASTOR, J. & LEROY, F. (1965). *Gut*, **6**, 545.

SCHAPIRO, R. H., DRUMMEY, G. D., CHIMIZU, Y. & ISSELBACHER, K. J. (1964). *J. clin. Invest.*, **43**, 1338.

SCHAPIRO, R. H., SCHEIG, R. L., DRUMMEY, G. D., MENDELSON, J. H. & ISSELBACHER, K. J. (1965). *New Engl. J. Md.* **272**, 610.

SCHAPIRO, H. L., WRUBLE, D. & BRITT, L. G. (1966). *Surgery*, **60**, 1108.

SCHEIG, R. & ISSELBACHER, K. J. (1965). *J. Lipid. Res.* **6**, 269.

SEIFE, M., KESSLER, B. J. & LISA, J. (1950). *Archs intern. Med.* **86**, 658.

SENIOR, J. R. (1967). *Postgrad. Med.* **41**, 65.

SHAPER, A. G. (1964). *Br. Med. J.* **1**, 1607.

SHANLEY, B. C., ZAIL, S. S. & JOUBERT, S. M. (1968). *Lancet*, **1**, 70.

SMALL, M., LONGARINI, A. & ZAMCHECK, N. (1959). *Am. J. Med.* **22**, 575.

STOKES, P. E. & LASLEY, B. (1967). *In* 'Biochemical Factors in Alcoholism'. Ed. R. P. Maichel. New York: Pergamon.

SULLIVAN, J. F., EGAN, J. D. & GEORGE, R. P. (1969). *Ann. N.Y. Acad. Sci.* **156**, 526.

SULLIVAN, J. F., PARKER, M. & CARSON, S.E. (1968). *J. Lab. clin. Med.* **71**, 893.

SULLIVAN, J. F., WALPERT, P. W., WILLIAMS, R. & EGAN, J. D. (1969). *Ann. N.Y. Acad. Sci.* **162**, 947.

SULLIVAN, L. W. & HERBERT, V. (1964). *J. clin. Invest.* **43**, 2048.

TEPHLY, T. R., TINELLI, F. & WATKINS, W. D. (1969). *Science*, **166**, 627.

THEORELL, H. & CHANCE, B. (1951). *Acta chem. scand.* **5**, 1127.

THOMPSON, G. N. (1956). *In* 'Alcoholism'. Springfield, Ill.: Thomas.

TYGSTRUP, N., WINKLER, K. & LUNDQUIST, F. (1965). *J. clin. Invest.* **44**, 817.

UGARTE, G., ITURRIAGA, H., INSUNZA, I. (1970). *In* 'Prog. Liver. Dis.' Ed. H. Popper & F. Schaffner, London: Heinemann.

VETTER, W. R., COHN, L. H. & REICHGOTT, M. (1967). *Archs intern. Med.* **120**, 536.

WALTON, B. E., SCHAPIRO, H., YEUNG, T. & WOODWARD, E. R. (1965). *Am. J. Surg.* **31**, 142.

WARTBURG, J. P. von, BETHUNE, J. L. & VALLEE, B. L. (1964). *Biochemistry*, **3**, 1775.

WARTBURG, J. P. von, PAPENBERG, J. & AEBI, H. (1965). *Canad. J. Biochem.* **43**, 889.

WATERS, A. H., MORLEY, A. A. & RANKIN, J. G. (1966). *Br. Med. J.* **2**, 1565.

WESTERFIELD, W. W. (1961). *Am. J. clin. Nutr.* **9**, 426.

WHO Statistics report, 1968. **21**, No. 11, 629, Geneva.

WILLIAMS, R. A., SCHEUR, P. J. & SHERLOCK, S. (1962). *Q. Jl Med.* **31**, 249.

WILLIAMS, R., WILLIAMS, M. S., SCHEUR, P. J., PITCHER, C. S., LOISEAU, E. & SHERLOCK, S. (1967). *Q. Jl Med.* **36**, 1.

WINSHIP, D., CALFLISH, C. R., ZBORALSKE, F. F., HOGAN, W. J. (1968). *Gastroenterology*, **55**, 173.

WOLFF, G. (1970). *Scand. J. Gastro.* **5**, 289.

CHAPTER 9

MANAGEMENT OF CHRONIC RENAL FAILURE

D. N. S. KERR

Prior to 1960 the management of chronic renal failure was a haphazard affair of coping with emergencies as they arose. The introduction of regular haemodialysis and transplantation transformed it into a concerted plan of action (Table 9.1). The execution of this plan calls for an efficient organisation comprising physician, urologist, dietitian, social worker, and dialysis administrator and is therefore best carried out in a renal clinic devoted to the purpose. The ramifications of this clinic must be curtailed by financial or other stringencies. In a typical large American centre (the Colorado General Hospital) dialysis absorbs 7 per cent of the hospital budget (Holmes, 1971) and in Newcastle upon Tyne the dialysis service provides 15 per cent of the laboratory load. Freed from their present restrictions the renal services in these centres—and similar large referral hospitals—would divert an unacceptable proportion of the health budget to 1 per cent of the patients. The need for the fourth step in Table 9.1 will therefore persist in most countries and economic considerations must colour the whole of this description.

TABLE 9.1

PLAN OF MANAGEMENT OF CHRONIC RENAL FAILURE

Investigation of primary disease
Treatment of primary disease
Conservative management of renal failure
Selection for dialysis or/and transplantation

Selected
Preparation for dialysis or
transplantation in good time.
Initiation of dialysis before working
capacity is lost.

Rejected
Giovannetti diet.
Symptomatic treatment.

INVESTIGATION AND TREATMENT OF PRIMARY RENAL DISEASE

Ideally the first symptom or sign of chronic renal disease should lead to full investigation at a time when pyelography is rewarding and renal biopsy simple. However a substantial minority of patients are still allowed to decline into renal failure without such investigation and many present to their doctors for the first time in advanced uraemia. Differential diagnosis is then difficult and the rewards for establishing a correct diagnosis diminish as renal function declines. A description of the diagnostic process in late renal failure has been given elsewhere with an extended list of the causes (Kerr, 1971a). In Table 9.2, I have listed the major causes as judged by referrals to dialysis and transplant centres; systemic diseases causing renal failure are under-represented in such series as they are judged by referring physicians to be unsuitable, but their partial exclusion does not radically alter the situation seen in general medical clinics. In the older age group (over 55), which is scarcely represented in dialysis and transplant statistics, chronic pyelone-phritis and essential hypertension assume greater importance.

Investigation for the cause of late renal failure is justified by the discovery of a tiny minority with lesions which are reversible at a terminal stage. It is obvious from Table 9.2 that the economic returns are meagre; fortunately the most important screening tests—such as taking a drug history—are cheap and innocuous.

TABLE 9.2

CAUSES OF RENAL FAILURE IN SOME SERIES OF PATIENTS
ACCEPTED FOR DIALYSIS OR/AND TRANSPLANTATION

Area	Newcastle	Europe		Australasia	International
Authors	1964–1971	Drukker et al., 1969	Parsons et al., 1970	Australian N.D.R.T.S. 1970	Murray, Barnes & Atkinson, 1971
Patients	213	3140	1362	403	1414
Percentage due to:					
Glomerulonephritis	43	64	55	57	63
Pyelonephritis	20	21	21	17	18
Polycystic disease	9	6	6	4	4
Analgesic nephropathy	1·5	*	3	9	1
Primary hypertension	14·5	1	*	4	4
Hereditary nephritis	0	1	*	1	2
Others	12	7	15	8	15†

* not separately classified.
† published total exceeds 100 per cent as some patients had two diseases.

Chronic glomerulonephritis

There is no specific treatment for any form of primary glomerulonephritis causing renal failure. Proliferative glomerulonephritis is not helped and may be harmed by corticosteroids (Black, Rose & Brewer, 1970) none of the immunosuppressive drugs enjoying a current vogue has proved effective in controlled trials (Cameron, 1971). Membranous glomerulonephropathy is usually unaffected by all forms of treatment; the rare responses to prolonged corticosteroid therapy (Rastogi, Hart-Mercer & Kerr, 1969) are confined to patients with early lesions. Focal glomerulosclerosis is distinguished from the minimal lesion by its resistance to all forms of treatment (White, Glasgow & Mills, 1970).

The diagnosis of chronic glomerulonephritis is therefore made on clinical grounds supported by the presence of proteinuria and an abnormal urinary deposit. Renal biopsy is scarcely justifiable at the stage of renal failure unless it is essential to exclude some other cause.

Chronic pyelonephritis

A history of urinary infection in childhood should be carefully sought since it correlates well with renal scarring in adult life (Asscher et al., 1969, Asscher, 1971). However pyelonephritis in childhood is often silent so a negative history is of little value. The changes which it produces in the intravenous pyelogram are easily recognised (Hodson, 1967); there is inequality between the kidneys in size, shape and time of appearance of the pyelogram; the cortex is scarred in some areas, hypertrophied in others; the calyces are drawn out and clubbed under the scars and they contract sluggishly on the cinepyelogram. Many of these features can be recognised in a high dose pyelogram with tomograms or in a retrograde pyelogram if renal function is too poor for conventional intravenous pyelography.

Striking contraction and distortion of the kidney can also develop when pyelonephritis begins in adult life in an appropriate setting such as the obstructed urinary tract of the paraplegic (Tribe & Silver, 1969). However it is doubtful how often this happens when the urinary tract is initially normal; the few serial observations reported in this situation suggest that scarring does not occur (Hodson, 1970) or is more uniform, without much change in the calyces (Bailey, Little & Rolleston, 1969). A history of urinary infection beginning after puberty is so common in females that it is bound to be elicited from many patients with unrelated renal diseases; about 3–5 per cent of female patients will have bacteriuria when first examined since this is the prevalance of urinary infection in the 'normal' population (see Kerr, 1971b, for review). Diagnosis of pyelonephritis starting in adult life cannot therefore rest so heavily on history and pyelography. It is supported by the absence of heavy proteinuria or cast excretion, by a high leucocyte count in the deposit and by loss of concentrating and acidifying power out of proportion to the decline in glomerular filtration rate (Brod, 1971). (For graphs of concentrating and acidifying power against GFR see Brod & Prat, 1967, and Bengtsson, 1967).

The summation of all this evidence permits a diagnosis of pyelonephritis with reasonable confidence in most cases but some of the tests involved are time consuming, require technical skill and are not often performed even in renal clinics. Fortunately the difficulty of diagnosing adult pyelonephritis with certainty (Brit. med. J., 1971) is of doubtful therapeutic importance. The vogue for treating pyelonephritis (with sterile urine) by prolonged administration of antibiotics has passed without a single controlled trial to demonstrate that it has any effects other than diarrhoea, pruritus ani and skin rash. Persistent urinary infection in pyelonephritis certainly requires treatment and its control does preserve renal function (Brod & Prat, 1967) and permit renal growth (Smellie & Normand, 1968). However it should be detected during the routine screening for urinary infection which forms part of normal conservative management. The only advantage that accrues from knowing that pyelonephritis is present is the ability to predict that infection will recur more frequently and will be harder to eliminate than when coincidental bacteriuria is discovered (see Kerr 1971b, for review). Personally I find it easier to screen all patients with renal failure for urinary infection at each visit than to pursue the diagnosis of chronic pyelonephritis to the limit.

Essential hypertension

Essential hypertension ranks third among the causes of chronic renal failure at Newcastle (Table 9.2). Its infrequency in the other series quoted in Table 9.2 is puzzling and suggests either reluctance to accept patients with this diagnosis for dialysis and transplant, or underdiagnosis.* Papilloedema is not invariably present (Sevitt, Evans & Wrong, 1971) and the glomerular

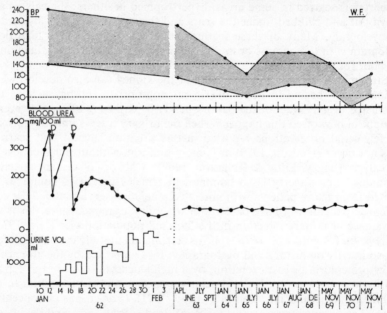

FIG. 9.1. Recovery of renal function after short term haemodialysis in a man aged 32 with essential malignant hypertension.

changes can be mistaken for those of glomerulonephritis. The distinction between the two conditions will become important when prediction of recurrent glomerulonephritis after transplantation (Richardson et al., 1970) becomes an everyday procedure; in the interim it is mainly of prognostic interest. Prolonged survival without dialysis after control of blood pressure is probably commoner in essential hypertension and can sometimes occur even if the patient presents in oliguria with apparently terminal uraemia (Sevitt, Evans & Wrong, 1971) (Fig. 9.1). However prolonged recovery is uncommon even in essential hypertension if the initial plasma urea is ele-

* The format of some of the questionnaire forms discourages this diagnosis.

vated; only half the patients with a plasma urea over 60 mg/100 ml survived 1 year in the large series of Breckenridge, Dollery & Parry (1970).

Features favouring essential hypertension are an appearance of premature senility in young men, normal kidney size on pyelography and rapid improvement in the renal deposit (but with persistent excretion of hyaline casts) after control of blood pressure. Confident diagnosis demands a renal biopsy but this procedure is seldom justified when renal failure is advanced except as part of an assessment for renal transplantation; restoration of normal blood pressure is mandatory whatever the primary diagnosis.

Analgesic nephropathy

The importance of analgesic nephropathy as a cause of renal failure in Britain has only gained recognition in the last 5 years (Prescott, 1966; Bell *et al.*, 1969; Koutsaimanis & De Wardener 1970; Murray, Timbury & Linton, 1970; Murray, Lawson & Linton, 1971). The fact that it still appears high up on the list of diseases leading to dialysis and transplant (Table 9.2) suggests that it is still escaping detection since it is the most reversible of the diseases causing renal failure. Numerous reports now attest the remarkably long survival of patients who cease analgesic intake even at a late stage in renal failure (Fig. 9.2) (Bell *et al.*, 1969; Murray, Lawson & Linton, 1971).

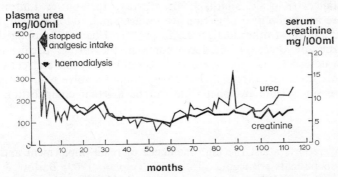

Fig. 9.2. Prolonged survival in chronic renal failure after withdrawal of analgesics in a woman of 34 with analgesic nephropathy. She requires sodium bicarbonate to control acidosis, diuretics to control the resultant sodium overload, allopurinol to prevent secondary gout and has been treated several times for renal osteodystrophy (Fig. 9.10). Nonetheless she works full time and has brought up a young family.

The diagnosis depends on suspicion. Every patient in renal failure should have a full drug history including careful and specific probing about the intake of analgesics and other medicaments which contain (or did until recently contain) phenacetin and related compounds—Tab. Codeine Co., Sonalgin, Saridone, Yeastvite, Beecham's powders, etc. The disease should be suspected if there has been a total intake of phenacetin exceeding 2 kilograms in a patient without obvious cause for renal failure. The intake of aspirin and related drugs should be noted but their role in the production of analgesic nephropathy is controversial and epidemiological evidence suggests that it is small (Bengtsson, 1969; Koutsaimanis & De Wardener, 1970). Although paracetamol is suspect, as a major metabolite of phenacetin, there is so far little evidence that it is nephrotoxic (Kerr, 1970).

The diagnosis can be confirmed with near certainty if calcified papillae are seen on radiographs of the renal tract or if sloughed papillae are passed and identified histologically or are shown as 'ring signs' on infusion or retrograde pyelography. If these signs are absent, as they often are, the diagnosis can be made with less confidence from other suggestive evidence—a history of renal colic in the absence of calculi, prominent polyuria and polydypsia, sterile pyuria, hyperchloraemic acidosis, bilateral and usually symmetrical renal scarring on pyelography and loss of concentrating and acidifying power out of proportion to the decline in glomerular filtration rate (Bengtsson, 1967; Steele, Györy & Edwards, 1969).

Even if the diagnosis rests only on suspicion, nephrotoxic drugs should be totally withdrawn. In the majority of such patients analgesics are taken from force of habit or to relieve headache or psychological symptoms. Total analgesic withdrawal is then possible though relapse is common unless patients are followed indefinitely and questioned at each follow-up visit. A substantial minority of British patients have taken their analgesics on good indications and still require analgesia. They pose a considerable problem since there is some anecdotal evidence that aspirin is nephrotoxic in these circumstances (Kincaid Smith, 1970; Murray, Lawson & Linton, 1971) and there are theoretical objections to paracetamol, indomethacin, flufenamic acid and most other analgesics. In practice I have been obliged to use these drugs on occasion and have not seen the further decline in renal function described by others. However careful follow-up and conservative dosage are obviously essential. Follow-up should involve regular culture of the urine since acute pyelonephritis can be a lethal complication of this disease.

Gout

Many reports attest the high incidence of renal impairment and hypertension in patients with gout (Talbot & Terplan, 1960; Barlow & Beilin, 1968) but the renal disease progresses very slowly (Graham & Scott 1970). Consequently gout does not rank high among the causes of renal failure in young and middle aged adults; it contributed less than 1 per cent of the candidates for dialysis in the European series of Drukker and colleagues (1970) and these were at the upper end of the age range with a mean of 46. The diagnosis is straightforward since renal failure is almost always preceded by joint manifestations. Differentiation from secondary gout may be difficult if the onset of renal disease cannot be dated and it then depends on rather complex tests of urate production and renal handling (Rieselbach et al., 1970). However the distinction is not important since both conditions are treated with allopurinol.

Allopurinol will usually control the joint symptoms (Wilson, Simmonds & North, 1967) but its effect on renal function is less certain. Some reports suggest that it will arrest the progress of renal disease (Levin & Abrahams, 1966) and may even produce a modest rise in glomerular filtration rate (Wilson, Simmonds & North, 1967; Ogden, Briney & Smyth, 1969). These are difficult assertions to prove in a disease with so prolonged a course without treatment, but they encourage the use of allopurinol in a sufficient dose to keep the plasma urate well below 6 mg/100 ml.

Urinary obstruction

Relief of chronic urinary obstruction is often followed by improvement in renal function (Fig. 9.3). Normal renal function (to ordinary clinical testing) can be regained after total anuria for several days from acute-on-chronic obstruction (Abercrombie, Hanley & Joekes, 1970) and some recovery is usual if total unilateral obstruction is relieved within 3 months (Brunschwig, Barber & Roberts, 1964). The fear of missing an unsuspected urinary obstruction has therefore dominated urological management of both acute and chronic renal failure; cystoscopy and retrograde pyelography have been freely and rather indiscriminately used to avoid this mistake. However, these procedures are uncomfortable and not without risk in renal failure so some restriction of their use is necessary. The indications for cystoscopy can usually be obtained by clinical examination for evidence of lower urinary tract obstruction (Clark, 1971).

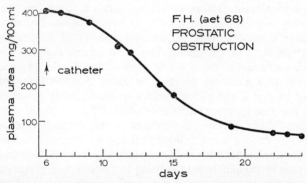

FIG. 9.3. Improvement in renal function, shown by fall in plasma urea, after relief of acute-on-chronic retention of urine in an 80 year old man with benign prostatic hypertrophy. Control of urinary infection and rehydration played a part in the improvement which was more dramatic than that usually seen after relief of retention.

The history should include specific questions about force of micturition, hesitancy and dribbling; where doubt exists the act of micturition should be observed. The bladder should be percussed and palpated before and after micturition and the prostate palpated rectally. Where there is only faint suspicion of lower urinary obstruction its presence can be confirmed without catheterisation by measurement of residual urinary volume either quantitatively by the radio-hippuran technique (Shand et al., 1970) or qualitatively on a post-micturition film after infusion pyelography.

Upper urinary tract obstruction is often silent (Fig. 9.4), but the history should include specific questions about backache and drug therapy of migraine (methysergide being specified by all its names) to detect the reversible condition of periureteric fibrosis (Kerr et al., 1967; Packham & Yates-Bell, 1968; Saxton et al., 1969). However, detection of upper urinary obstruction now depends very largely on the use of infusion pyelography as a routine in patients with unexplained renal failure. The technique and its hazards have been reviewed by Fry and Cattell (1970, 1971). Obstructed kidneys may be visualised only on late films taken up to 24 hours after the injection. If no shadow can be seen after a maximum dose of contrast (about 2 ml/kg of 50 per cent Hypaque or equivalent medium) success may still be achieved if the procedure is repeated after dialysis (Matalon & Eisinger, 1970). An alternative is retrograde pyelography (Chisholm, 1970) (Fig. 9.5). An additional screening method for urinary obstruction is isotope renography; it carries none of the risks of high dose intravenous or retrograde pyelography but its value is detecting chronic obstruction with severely impaired renal function is limited.

CONSERVATIVE MANAGEMENT OF CHRONIC RENAL FAILURE

Control of hypertension

The most important factors governing survival in chronic renal failure are the primary disease and the severity of hypertension. For those patients whose primary disease cannot be arrested control of hypertension is the most important facet of treatment. The great advance of the 1960s was a change in the attitude of the medical profession. At the beginning of the decade it was still common practice to leave hypertension untreated or inadequately treated if the plasma urea was considerably raised, in the fear that a fatal increase in uraemia would follow a fall in blood pressure. It is now recognised that the systemic effects of poorly controlled blood pressure far outweigh any decline in renal function that may occur during drug therapy. This statement applies with particular cogency to patients selected for eventual transplantation or regular haemodialysis; to them a well preserved vascular tree is a much greater asset than a few weeks' prolongation of conservative therapy.

The choice of drug used to be dictated by its supposed effects on renal function; the results of short term studies after parenteral injection were rashly extrapolated to long term treatment. Such short term studies are in practice of limited interest to the clinician. For instance, the latest addition to the range of effective antihypertensives—clonidine—has apparently produced acute changes in GFR varying from a 50 per cent increase to a 50 per cent decrease (Baum, 1966; Bock et al., 1966; Frank and Lowenich-Lagois, 1966; Grabner et al., 1966; Onesti et al., 1971). There is probably a transient fall in GFR in the few hours after parenteral administration if the BP falls abruptly; the conclusion drawn from the individual experiment depends critically on the timing of the post-treatment observations. What is of much greater interest to the clinician is the long term effect of oral therapy which is difficult to disentangle from the natural history of the underlying disease. It appears that clonidine has no adverse effect in these circumstances (Onesti et al., 1969; Raftos, 1969; Macdougall et al., 1970). The same conclusion can be drawn, with greater confidence, in the case of methyl dopa (Luke & Kennedy, 1964) and it probably applies to all the major antihyper-

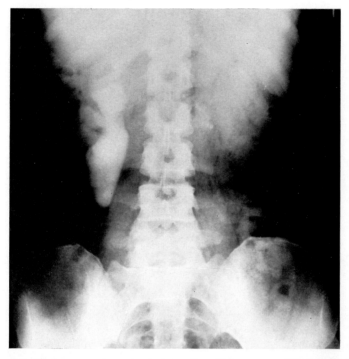

Fig. 9.4. Silent upper urinary tract obstruction. This woman of 38 presented in 1962 with mild chronic renal failure (plasma urea 100 mg./100 ml.) and was diagnosed clinically as inactive chronic pyelonephritis. High dose pyelography 8 years later revealed a hydronephrosis in a single kidney. At no time did she complain of loin pain or other symptoms of hydronephrosis.

[To face p. 264.

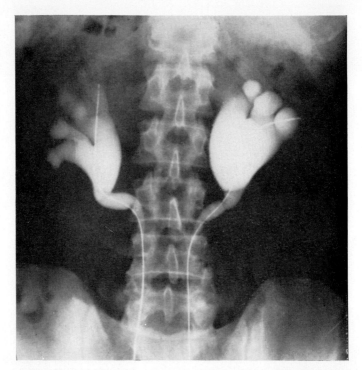

Fɪɢ. 9.5. Silent urinary obstruction due to retroperitoneal fibrosis revealed by retrograde pyelography. The investigation was performed when infusion pyelography failed to show the calyceal pattern in a 45 year old man with unexplained chronic renal failure and remarkably normal urinary deposit. (Courtesy of Dr. P. R. Uldall and Dr. W. Simpson).

tensives in current use.* The selection of a drug can therefore be made on other grounds, particularly the incidence of side effects and tolerance.

Hydrallazine intramuscularly (10–40 mg every 1–4 hours) is my own first choice for the hypertensive emergency but sodium nitroprusside, diazoxide, pentolinium and injections of clonidine, methyl dopa and reserpine all have their advocates. For maintenance therapy the first choice lies between methyl dopa and clonidine. Both drugs lower blood pressure more or less equally in all postures and their commonest limiting side effect is drowsiness. They are therefore unsuitable for patients who drive or fly for a living or have demanding intellectual occupations—one of my patients composes prolifically on guanethidine but cannot write a note on methyl dopa. Clonidine aggravates the dry mouth of uraemia and methyl dopa depresses the already inadequate sexual function particularly of the male uraemic. A sizeable minority of patients with severe hypertension are uncontrolled by tolerable

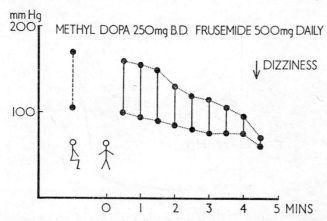

FIG. 9.6. Progressive fall in standing blood pressure in a woman of 60 with chronic renal failure. Her complaint of postural hypotension had been dismissed by some observers as her initial standing blood pressure was high.

doses of either drug or both in combination. Propranolol in doses up to 1 g or more per day is sometimes helpful as adjuvant therapy but, in my experience, it is so seldom effective when used alone in severe renal hypertension that it does not merit consideration as a first line drug. Thiazides have little diuretic effect when the GFR falls to about 20 ml/min (Reubi & Cottier, 1961); at the same time their antihypertensive action largely disappears.

The most powerful antihypertensives for maintenance therapy are the sympathetic blockers guanethidine, bethanidine and debrisoquine. Their great drawback is the considerable postural and exertional hypotension that accompanies their effective use. It is rarely possible to reduce sitting blood pressure to normal with these drugs without at the same time inducing uncomfortable postural dizziness. Blood pressure should always be measured sitting or lying, standing and after standard exercise (a 5 metre climb is suitable) when the dose of these drugs is being adjusted. The standing blood

* List of references to other antihypertensives obtainable from the author on request.

pressure should be taken repeatedly until a plateau is reached or until dizziness occurs; a complaint of postural dizziness is often unjustly dismissed because the initial standing blood pressure is not low (Fig 9.6).

If blood pressure is not controlled by drug therapy, with tolerable side effects, an attempt should be made to control it by adjusting sodium balance. Hypertension in chronic renal failure is accompanied by an increase in total body sodium, an expanded extracellular fluid volume and sometimes an increased blood volume (Blumberg *et al.*, 1967; de Planque, Mulder & Dorhout Mees, 1969; Ledingham, 1971). Removal of the excess sodium restores plasma and extracellular volumes to normal and often corrects the hypertension at the price of a fall in GFR and an increase in uraemia (Levin & Cade, 1965; Berlyne *et al.*, 1968). Sodium depletion can usually be achieved simply by placing the patient on a low-sodium diet; renal conservation of sodium is impaired in nearly all patients with chronic renal disease and a

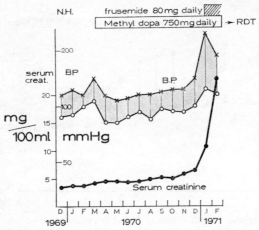

Fig. 9.7. Rapid decline into terminal renal failure in association with the sudden onset of malignant hypertension in a woman of 19 with proliferative glomerulonephritis.

large cumulative deficit of sodium will result if the dietary intake is sufficiently low (10–22 m Eg/day) (Coleman *et al.*, 1966). However, once the excess sodium has been removed, renal sodium excretion falls to a level which, though abnormally high compared with the healthy kidney, still requires rigid sodium restriction (about 22 m Eg/day on average) to maintain balance. When this restriction is added to an already difficult protein-restricted diet the burden is almost intolerable though patients can be persuaded to bear it if the medical-dietetic team is sufficiently dedicated (Berlyne *et al.*, 1968).

An alternative approach is the use of powerful diuretics in high dosage. Frusemide is effective in renal failure down to a GFR of about 3 ml/min (Rastogi *et al.*, 1971). The dose has to be increased as the GFR falls (Allison & Kennedy, 1971) so that very large and expensive doses (500–4000 mg/day) are required in terminal renal failure (Muth, 1968). These enormous quantities are well tolerated; the temporary deafness occasionally seen after massive intravenous therapy (Wigand & Heidland, 1971) has not been reported after oral use. Ethacrynic acid is also effective in renal failure but deafness is a commoner problem and has occurred after oral therapy (Pillay *et al.*, 1969).

In proliferative glomerulonephritis, and to a lesser extent in other chronic renal diseases, the onset of hypertension is often sudden and catastrophic (Fig. 9.7). The interval between follow-up visits at the renal clinic is largely determined by the necessity of detecting the onset of hypertension before irreparable damage is done. In the late stages of glomerulonephritis a month is the maximum safe interval between visits; the time expended by patient and doctor is negligible compared with that demanded by regular haemodialysis.

Control of electrolyte balance

Sodium and water. As GFR declines the kidney adapts by excreting an increased proportion of the filtered sodium (see Allison & Kennedy, 1971, for review). The majority of patients with chronic renal failure therefore remain in sodium and water balance on a free diet for the greater part of the course of their disease. When GFR reaches a critical level, which varies with the individual, sodium and water retention usually occur, leading to hyper-

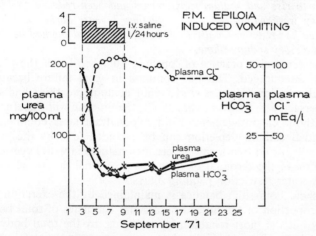

Fig. 9.8. Recovery from acute-on-chronic renal failure in a 25 year old woman with epiloia and the associated renal dysgenesis. On five occasions over 2 years she was admitted with extracellular fluid volume depletion, alkalosis and hypokalaemia following protracted vomiting (? self-induced). She has a mild renal sodium leak when alkalosis is corrected but requires only a small sodium supplement when her extra-renal losses are prevented.

tension (as described in the last section) and eventually to overt oedema. However the inability of the diseased kidney to conserve sodium makes the patient vulnerable to sodium depletion if extrarenal losses occur, e.g. from diarrhoea and vomiting. The response to repletion is gratifying (Fig. 9.8).

A minority of patients, mainly sufferers from pyelonephritis, analgesic nephropathy, obstructive nephropathy, medullary cystic disease and polycystic kidneys, have a profound defect in renal sodium conservation and are susceptible to severe episodes of sodium depletion causing increased uraemia, in the absence of any extra-renal loss. The condition is often overlooked; a considerable rise in plasma urea may occur before the classical signs of extracellular volume depletion are manifest. However patients with this complication are virtually never hypertensive and are usually mildly hypotensive, particularly on sitting or standing up (Polak, 1971). The presence of a sodium leak should be confirmed by measuring sodium concentration while the patient is still depleted and hypotensive. The urinary loss should be estimated again when sodium balance has been restored and dietary supplements administered in the form of sodium bicarbonate (1–4 g per day is usually sufficient to control the acidosis which commonly coexists) and sodium chloride; the latter is most acceptably given as 'Slow-sodium' (Clarkson, Curtis *et al.*, 1971). Careful follow-up is required to prevent relapse and to forestall the onset of hypertension if the sodium leak diminishes as GFR declines.

Case report: *Miss M. A., polycystic disease was admitted with obvious sodium and water depletion, BP 100/70 and plasma urea 550 mg/100 ml. After fluid repletion she stabilised at a BP of 140/80 and a plasma urea of 120 mg/ 100 ml on oral sodium supplements of 215 mEq/24 hr. Within 1 year her BP had begun to rise and sodium supplements had been reduced to 130 mEq/24 hours; they were withdrawn over a further 2 years during which time her plasma urea had risen gradually to 300 mg/100 ml and she had become hypertensive on dietary sodium alone.*

The once popular practice of 'pushing fluids' to lower the plasma urea should be discouraged. Thirst is common in renal failure because of depressed salivary flow (Holmes *et al.*, 1960), acidotic breathing and sometimes renin hypersecretion (Brown *et al.*, 1969); the uraemic will therefore drink to excess without encouragement. Mild hyponatraemia is common in renal failure and if sodium depletion can be excluded (e.g. by the presence of oedema) calls for no treatment. Severe hyponataremia with hypertension is a phenomenon of the terminal oliguric phase of renal failure which must be treated by water restriction pending dialysis.

Potassium. Potassium balance is maintained by the excretion of an increased proportion of the filtered potassium. Estimates of total body potassium vary but the most reliable measurements, by the total body counting technique, have given results in the normal range in renal failure (Boddy *et al.*, 1971). Even mild hyperkalaemia (4·5 to 5·5 mEq/1) is found in less than half of all patients in chronic renal failure and spontaneous elevations above 6·5 mEq/1 are rare (Schwartz, 1955). However there is little reserve capacity for potassium excretion and dangerous hyperkalaemia is easily provoked by potassium-containing medicaments (Keith & Osterberg, 1947). Spironolactone, amiloride and other potassium-sparing diuretics must be used with extreme caution.

Hyperkalaemia can also be precipitated by an exacerbation of acidosis, e.g. during anaesthesia, when the anaesthetist may fail to maintain the hyperventilation to which the patient is accustomed (Goggin & Joekes, 1971).

Emergency treatment for hyperkalaemia is only required if the level is very high, if there are E.C.G. changes (flattened P, widened QRS, peaked T) or if surgery, infection etc. has further depressed renal function. The details of treatment with glucose and insulin, calcium carbonate and sodium bicarbonate intravenously are given by Schwartz & Kassirer (1968) and in standard texts of nephrology. The majority of patients in chronic renal failure can be managed by correcting the cause of the hyperkalaemia and temporary administration of ion-exchange resins. The sodium phase resin (Resonium A) acts fastest but can cause dangerous sodium overload (Berlyne *et al.*, 1966) so it should be changed within a day or two to Calcium Resonium or an aluminium phase resin (Chugh *et al.*, 1968). The continuous use of these occasionally causes hypercalcaemia (Sevitt & Wrong, 1968) or hyperalumi-naemia respectively, but no symptoms have yet been attributed to the latter.

Magnesium. Patients in renal failure follow the general rule that total body stores and plasma concentration of magnesium run parallel with those of potassium. Serum magnesium is usually normal till late in the course of renal failure and a spontaneous rise above 3·5 mg/100ml is unusual (Fig. 9.9).

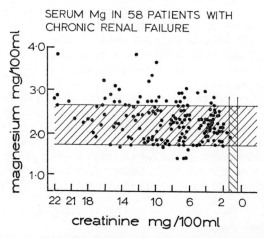

FIG. 9.9. Serum magnesium levels in 58 patients in chronic renal failure, who had not been treated by dialysis and did not admit to consumption of magnesium-containing drugs. The commonest apparent cause of high magnesium levels was vitamin D administration for renal osteodystrophy.

It is doubtful whether these mild elevations play any part in the sympto-matology of uraemia. However magnesium is well enough absorbed from the upper intestine and the colon in renal failure that a further elevation in serum magnesium may follow administration of magnesium-containing antacids, purgatives or enemata (Randall *et al.*, 1964). If the plasma level exceeds 4 mg/100 ml muscle weakness, areflexia, skin irritation, drowsiness and respiratory depression may result. The emergency can be treated by intra-venous administration of calcium gluconate 1–2 g or by haemodialysis.

Hydrogen ion. Metabolic acidosis is an almost invariable accompaniment of renal failure though it may be temporarily reversed by vomiting (Fig. 9.8). Compensation occurs in a predictable manner and the blood pH usually remains within normal limits (7·35 to 7·45) until the plasma bicarbonate falls to about 15 mEq/l (Van Ypersele/de Strihou & Frans, 1970). It is doubtful if any advantage is gained in 'treating the plasma bicarbonate' above that level. However the bicarbonate concentration commonly falls below 15 in the later stages of renal failure and some authorities recommend the administration of alkalis to prevent acidaemia, believing that this delays the onset of renal bone disease. There is no conclusive evidence for this belief but acidosis does promote the loss of calcium carbonate from bone (Lemann, Litzow & Lennon, 1966) and has produced osteomalacia in the absence of renal failure (York and Yendt, 1966). It therefore seems reasonable to correct an acidaemia sufficiently to keep the plasma bicarbonate at or above 15 mEq/l if this can be achieved without producing other complications. Sodium bicarbonate (1–4 g/day) is usually effective but may precipitate hypertension or oedema. Large doses of calcium carbonate are also moderately effective (Clarkson, McDonald & De Wardener, 1966).

Severe acidaemia, with a blood pH below 7·2 and a plasma bicarbonate well below 10 mEq/l is commonly present in episodes of acute-on-chronic renal failure and calls for energetic treatment to relieve hyperventilation, correct hyperkalaemia and improve myocardial function. Sodium bicarbonate intravenously (100–300 mEq over 2–4 hours initially) is rapidly effective but the same object can be achieved with a delay of only 2 or 3 hours, and with less risk of an overshoot, by using equivalent doses of sodium acetate (Feng et al., 1970).

Serum calcium is often very low in patients who require rapid correction of acidaemia. If this is the case calcium should be given prophylactically during and for some hours after the administration of alkali to guard against tetany and grand mal seizures. Calcium gluconate 1 g 8 hourly for the first 24 hours would be a suitable dose for a severely acidotic patient; it should not be given in the same bottle as the sodium bicarbonate. An anticonvulsant (e.g. sodium phenytoin 200 mg IM) should be given as an additional safeguard.

Treatment of bone disease

Bone disease is an uncommon cause of symptoms in renal failure. Only 3 per cent of patients accepted for dialysis and transplant in Boston have bone pain or deformity (Katz, Hampers & Merrill, 1969) and the proportion is similar in Newcastle (Simpson et al., 1971). However the bones are abnormal histologically in virtually all patients dying of renal failure (Follis & Jackson, 1943; Berner, 1944; Ellis & Peart, 1971), and radiological abnormalities are present in a substantial minority. These changes often progress during regular dialysis (p. 285) or after transplantation when steroid therapy is required. The treatment of even asymptomatic bone disease before the start of dialysis has therefore become an important facet of management. A skeletal survey should be carried out at the first hospital visit and serum calcium, phosphate and alkaline phosphatase should be checked at least every 6 months thereafter.

Although changes of osteitis fibrosa, osteomalacia and osteosclerosis, in varying proportions, are present in most patients one or other process often predominates (Stanbury, 1967, 1968; Siddiqui & Kerr, 1971). Osteomalacia is the more important problem in Newcastle and some other centres in Great Britain while hyperparathyroidism is commoner in the United States; the difference has been attributed to the higher dietary intake of vitamin-D and greater exposure to sunlight in America (Lumb, Mawer & Stanbury, 1971).

The standard treatment of osteomalacia is vitamin-D in a dose of 1·25–2·5 mg (50 000–100 000 units) daily. The first active metabolite of vitamin-D, 25-hydroxycholecalciferol, may be preferable (DeLuca & Avioli, 1970) because it has less tendency to cumulate. The second metabolite, 1,25-dihydroxycholecalciferol, which is active without further conversion in the kidney, will presumably be the treatment of choice once it becomes commercially available. The patient should be seen monthly for estimation of serum calcium, phosphate and alkaline phosphatase and for simple tests of renal function so that the hazards of hypercalcaemia and metastatic calcification can be avoided. Calcification may occur predominantly in the arteries (Mallick & Berlyne, 1968), the myocardium (Davidson & Pendras 1967; Terman et al., 1971) or the kidneys; to detect the last, radiographs of the renal tract every few months have been advised but in our experience they have been

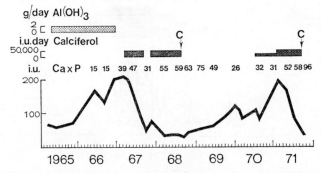

FIG. 9.10. Renal osteodystrophy during prolonged stable chronic renal failure (Fig. 9.2). Biochemical and radiological abnormalities are controlled by vitamin D but relapse occurs within 1–2 years from cessation of therapy.

less useful than observation of plasma urea and creatinine. Vitamin-D should be continued until the serum alkaline phosphatase has been normal for two or three months, then discontinued. The biochemical abnormalities may reappear if the patient survives for long enough (Fig. 9.10) but it is safer to give more than one course of treatment than to risk myocardial calcification. If the serum phosphate is high initially, or rises excessively in response to vitamin-D, it should be brought down to the normal range by oral administration of aluminium hydroxide gel.

Uraemic osteomalacia sufficiently severe to produce symptoms is found mainly in patients with an acidifying defect due to chronic pyelonephritis, analgesic nephropathy, obstruction, calculi or some forms of cystic disease (Cochran & Nordin, 1969; Floyd et al., 1969). It is therefore logical to correct the acidosis (q.v.) but alkalis alone have not been shown to cure the condition. An alternative to vitamin-D is the oral administration of large doses of calcium, as the carbonate if plasma phosphate is high or as the phosphate if it is normal or low. This has been shown to produce a positive balance of calcium and phosphate, suppress parathormone hypersecretion, reduce serum alkaline phosphatase concentration to normal and improve the appearance of bones on radiographs (Clarkson *et al.*, 1970; Curtis *et al.*, 1970). It is said to carry less risk of metastatic calcification than vitamin-D therapy but this assertion has not been tested in controlled trials. Moreover it requires much more patient cooperation than conventional therapy and produces less satisfactory healing on bone biopsy (Eastwood, Bordier & De Wardener, 1971) so it is unlikely to displace vitamin-D.

The bone lesions of hyperparathyroidism also respond to vitamin-D but the risk of metastatic calcification is much greater (Stanbury, 1967; Mallick & Berlyne, 1968). If vitamin D is given, aluminium hydroxide gel should be administered concurrently. Often there is extensive arterial calcification by the time the patient presents with bone disease. If eventual treatment with regular dialysis or transplant is contemplated it is as important to reverse this

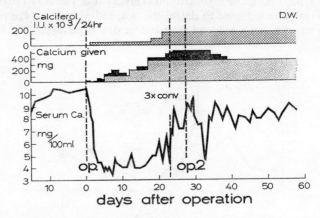

FIG. 9.11. Precipitate fall in serum calcium following parathyroidectomy for secondary hyper-parathyroidism complicating urinary obstruction. Vitamin D was not given pre-operatively because of extensive vascular calcification. The three grand-mal fits resulted in fractures of both femora, many ribs, some vertebrae, one clavicle, humerus and scapula, dislocation of the sterno-clavicular joint and rupture of the quadriceps tendon. His recovery has been surprisingly smooth.

process as to cure the bone disease. For both purposes parathyroidectomy is increasingly popular (Johnson *et al.*, 1969; Hubay *et al.*, 1970; Eilert *et al.*, 1971). A small part of one parathyroid (often described with unjustifiable accuracy as '$\frac{1}{2}$', '$\frac{1}{4}$' or '$\frac{1}{5}$') is usually left behind in the hope that it will function after renal transplant. The operation is followed by a profound and prolonged hypocalcaemia (Fig. 9.11) with the risk of convulsions and pathological fracture. It is probably advisable to give a careful pre-operative course of vitamin-D in the manner recommended for primary hyperparathyroidism (Woodhouse *et al.*, 1971).

Treatment of anaemia

The standard view of the anaemia of chronic renal failure up to the mid-1960s might be summarised 'It is normochromic, normocytic, due to erythropoietin lack rather than uraemia, unresponsive to haematinics except cobaltous chloride which is too toxic. It is a major cause of symptoms in renal failure, requiring intermittent transfusion which must be given cautiously to avoid further deterioration in renal function'. Most of these concepts have been challenged in the last 5 years.

The fear that transfusion might depress renal function by decreasing renal plasma flow was dispelled by Brod & Hornych (1967). Renal function deteriorates only if the patient is precipitated into cardiac failure and this can now be avoided with high dose diuretics. However transfusion has fallen into disfavour for other reasons. It should be avoided whenever possible in patients destined for eventual regular dialysis or transplantation to prevent the introduction of hepatitis into the renal unit (p. 284) and sensitisation against donor kidneys. The extent of the latter hazard is still in dispute; the latest analysis of the European results (Parsons, 1971) has failed to show a clear-cut relationship between transfusion history and graft survival. However the dangers of hyperacute rejection in presensitised subjects are not in dispute (Jeannet et al., 1970; Busch et al., 1971). The renal injury in these patients closely resembles that found in animals experimentally sensitised to leucocytes (Simpson et al., 1970; Matthew et al., 1971). There is little doubt therefore that transfusion will turn out to be a hazard to later transplantation once the statistical artefacts have been eliminated.

Iron deficiency plays an important part in the anaemia of patients on regular haemodialysis (p. 283) and it may also have a role at an earlier stage, particularly in menstruating women. Since the 'normochromic' anaemia of renal failure is in fact manifest by a slightly reduced MCHC, and since serum iron may be depressed by renal infection or heavy proteinuria, the usual criteria of iron deficiency cannot be employed uncritically. Where doubt exists it is worth trying a course of oral iron. Iron absorption is probably impaired in uraemia (Lawson et al., 1971) so a fairly high dose of iron should be employed. Evidence of slight folate deficiency is also present in late renal failure (Siddiqui, Freeburger & Freeman, 1970) but response to this vitamin and to ascorbic acid and the cobalamins is usually negligible. The belief that cobaltous chloride is too toxic for general use is difficult to substantiate from the literature (Hopper, Anderson & Dailey, 1959) and this drug is currently being re-evaluated (Edwards & Curtis, 1971). Androgens have been shown to raise the haemoglobin level of patients on regular dialysis (Richardson & Weinstein, 1970; Shaldon et al., 1971); their effectiveness in late renal failure before dialysis is uncertain, but there is probably a modest rise in haemoglobin (Snyder & Brest, 1966).

The need to dispense with transfusion has shown that it was overused in the past. Most of the blood given to uraemics was directed at their laboratory results rather than their symptoms. Transfusion is hardly ever necessary (except following haemorrhage) at a haemoglobin level above 7 g/100 ml and the great majority of patients adapt well to a haemoglobin between 5 and 7 g. However a significant minority fall below 5 g/100 ml in the last stages of renal failure (Pryor & Joekes, 1969). If they are destined for dialysis or transplant this is an indication for expediting treatment; if only conservative treatment is contemplated intermittent transfusion (with Australia-antigen negative blood) is a worthwhile palliative. Alternatively a Giovannetti diet will often raise the haemoglobin by 1–2 g/100 ml if the plasma urea is reduced, showing that uraemia does play an important role in the anaemia of renal failure (Shaw, 1968).

Low protein diet

The standard treatment for uraemia up to the mid-1960s was a mixed food diet of 40 g protein content which was only moderately effective in lowering plasma urea and reducing symptoms. One reason for its partial failure is that the anorexic patient often responds to a change from his traditional diet by starving himself. The administration of pure carbohydrate calorie supplements as Liquid glucose BPC ("Hycal', Beechams) reduces urea production rate and lowers plasma urea, particularly when protein intakes lower than 40 g are provided (Robson, Kerr & Ashcroft, 1968). Unfortunately the majority of patients find 'Hycal' too sweet and discontinue its use after some weeks or months as outpatients. A less sweet polysaccharide mixture ('Caloreen') which can be sprinkled on food, made into ice cream, etc. was introduced by Berlyne and colleagues (1969) but we have found that patients tire of this too unless they are constantly encouraged.

Gionnavetti & Maggiore (1964) introduced an alternative approach to adequate calorie provision. They pointed out the difficulty of achieving really low protein intakes without cutting down the provision of cereals which are the main calorie source in most diets. They got round this difficulty by using a special flour from which most of the wheat germ had been removed to produce bread, pasta, biscuits, etc. In our experience the continued consumption of these foods requires the same culinary ingenuity by the patient and his family, and the same dedicated perseverance by the dietitian, as the use of 'Hycal' or 'Caloreen'.

A new concept in dietary management was introduced in 1963 by Giordano who showed that a very low nitrogen intake (the equivalent of about 18 g protein) would maintain nitrogen balance if given in a balanced essential amino acid mixture with a synthetic diet. Giordano postulated that the uraemic patient could utilise his own urea to produce non-essential amino acids. This has been confirmed by Giordano and his colleagues (1967) and by Richards and others (1967) using [^{15}N] urea. The main (perhaps the only) mechanism by which this occurs is probably lysis of the urea by intestinal bacteria, reabsorption of the ammonia in portal blood and conversion into amino acids in the liver. A high proportion of the urea production is broken down extra-renally in late renal failure (Robson *et al.*, 1968).

Giovannetti & Maggiore (1964) used this principle in their diet. Having removed second class protein from the cereals they replaced it by first class protein in the form of egg. In this way they were able to achieve nitrogen balance on a protein intake of about 20 g per day, after an initial period of nitrogen depletion. Plasma urea fell dramatically, though other indices of uraemia, e.g. serum creatinine and uric acid were virtually unchanged. Their diet has been modified to suit the taste of Britons (Shaw *et al.*, 1965), Americans (Lonergan & Lange, 1968; Shinaberger & Ginn, 1968) and Germans, and has consistently lowered plasma urea and relieved uraemic nausea and vomiting as the originators claimed. Its effect on other uraemic symptoms has been inconsistent and it remains doubtful how often nitrogen balance is achieved (see Blainey & Chamberlain, 1971, for review). Some of the discrepancies in published results are due to the difficulty of measuring nitrogen balance in uraemic subjects owing to the very slow equilibration on a new diet (Wright, Brereton & Snell, 1970). An equally important problem is the difficulty of ensuring that patients consume all the prescribed diet.

The use of egg as the main source of protein is a major stumbling block to patient acceptance. Several studies have shown that egg is superior to meat, milk and other protein sources (Lonergan & Lange, 1968; Wright, Brereton & Snell, 1970) but others have shown little difference (Ford et al., 1969). The electrolyte content of egg is a problem in patients with very low GFR but this can be overcome by using a dialysed egg powder (Hood et al., 1969) at the price of a further change from traditional food. Egg yolk causes acidosis through metabolism of phospholipids and sulphur-containing amino acids; this can be avoided by using only egg white or countered by administration of calcium carbonate (Franklin et al., 1967). Potatoes contain a good mixture of essential amino acids and have been used as the basis of a Giovannetti-type diet in Germany. Their high potassium content is a disadvantage but this can be corrected by pre-treatment (Tsaltas, 1969).

The contribution that these complicated diets make to patient management is disputed. Personally I have largely abandoned their use. In a two-year period in which we used the Giovannetti diet in an effort to postpone dialysis the average respite gained in 48 patients was less than 3 months. The patient selected for dialysis or transplant is better to start on definitive treatment a few months early than to disrupt his life by major alterations in his diet. This applies particularly to the resistant hypertensive since a Giovannetti diet which is also restricted in potassium and sodium is as near uneatable as anything we ever put in front of patients. The Giovannetti regime should probably be reserved for normotensive patients with slowly progressive disease who have no prospect of dialysis or transplant; in these it can maintain tolerable life until the GFR falls to about 2 ml/min (Shaw et al., 1965; Franklin et al., 1967).

REGULAR HAEMODIALYSIS AND TRANSPLANTATION

These forms of treatment are considered together because it is customary, at the time of writing, to accept most patients for both and to use them interchangeably as circumstances dictate. The patient who receives a transplant is guaranteed a place on dialysis if his graft fails; the patient on regular haemodialysis is offered a cadaver graft whenever a donor kidney of the correct tissue type becomes available even if he is doing well on dialysis. These principles have been established on emotional rather than strictly scientific grounds but their wide acceptance shows how strong the emotional grounds have become. The 'failed transplant' patient may not be the best candidate for the last remaining place on a dialysis programme but having run the gauntlet of medical and social selection once he should know that he is secure and will not be asked to go through it again. The patient who is doing well on regular dialysis has a better chance of surviving the next two or three years by remaining on dialysis than by accepting a transplant (Cameron et al., 1970; Gault & Dossetor, 1970; Gurland et al., 1970), but even when this is honestly put to the patients the great majority opt for a transplant; it appears that the interminable chore of regular dialysis, particularly in the home, is made tolerable by the hope that one will one day win freedom from all its restrictions by a successful transplant.

Selection

At their worst, in the medically unsuitable patient, dialysis and transplantation are a prolongation of death rather than an extension of life. The most important contraindication to both procedures is extensive arterial disease usually the result of long-standing, poorly controlled hypertension. If the patient has had one or two minor strokes, has angina on slight effort (when blood pressure is controlled) or develops ischaemia of the hand if the radial artery is occluded he will probably do badly on both forms of treatment, though there are exceptions to these rules as to most others in medicine.

Most of the other selection criteria that have been used in the past have proved falacious. Youth and age are not a bar to success. Dialysis in the older patient carries a higher mortality than in the young adult, as one would expect, but the difference is not impressive (Cameron *et al.*, 1970; Cohen, Comty & Shapiro, 1970). In the short term children do well on regular dialysis (Cameron *et al.*, 1970; Fine *et al.*, 1970), though whether it is a kindness to the family to prolong the life of a young child for several years with only a small chance of normal development and survival into adult life is a question that is hotly debated every time the decision is called for. Some systemic diseases causing renal failure can be treated successfully. Gout is the outstanding example (Drukker *et al.*, 1970). Diabetes presents fewer problems during dialysis than might have been anticipated (Chazan *et al.*, 1969) but most diabetics in renal failure have other disabilities, particularly blindness, that make them poor dialysis candidates. Goodpasture's syndrome, once considered a strong contraindication to treatment, is now managed successfully by both dialysis and transplant, sometimes with the aid of bilateral nephrectomy (Halgrimson *et al.*, 1971, Nowakowski *et al.*, 1971). Even systemic lupus erythematosus, amyloidosis, Fabry's disease, Wegener's granulomatosis and thrombotic thrombocytopoenic purpura have been treated with success, at least for a few years. An occasional patient with oxalosis has survived a renal transplant but regular dialysis does not prevent the inexorable progression of this very unpleasant disease (Walls, Morley & Kerr, 1969). Malignant hypertension of recent origin is no bar to successful dialysis or transplantation.

Selection is therefore a matter of economics rather than clinical medicine. Estimates of the need for dialysis and transplantation average about 40 per million per year if the age group of candidates is restricted to 15–55 (Branch *et al.*, 1971). The number rises rapidly if the upper age limit is raised. No country has yet provided facilities on this scale though some are planning to do so. In Great Britain about 10 new patients are accepted per million per year. The task of selecting these from the eligible candidates is assigned to the medical staff of the renal unit who usually seek the advice of a medical social worker but do not involve any lay personnel in the decision. The judgement is based on medical suitability, age, family responsibilities and personal qualities: prolonged survival on dialysis calls for a blend of intelligence, self discipline, providence and will to live well above the minimum required of a healthy citizen in a welfare state.

Selection often has to be carried out in a rush because the patient presents for the first time in terminal renal failure. When his disease permits it, however, the decision should be made at least 6 months in advance of the expected onset of terminal uraemia, to allow time for preparation.

Preparation for Dialysis and Transplantation

Dental care. Extractions are difficult once terminal uraemia impairs coagulation or regular dialysis necessitates heparin administration; healthy teeth are desirable before long term steroid therapy is prescribed, following transplantation. As soon as he attends the renal clinic, therefore, the patient with chronic renal disease should be given an appointment with the dentist and encouraged to attend regularly for conservative dental care.

Fertility counselling. Fertility is depressed in chronic renal failure; this may lead to a false sense of security and the neglect of contraceptive precautions. Once the periods become irregular the diagnosis of pregnancy presents problems and immunological tests often give false positives; termination of a non-existent pregnancy has killed at least one patient in renal failure. There is one recorded successful pregnancy which was conceived while the patient was on regular haemodialysis, though with some residual renal function (Confortini *et al.*, 1971). Nonetheless, the chance of success is small (Drukker *et al.*, 1970), the risk to the mother considerable and a young baby is an added burden to a family already struggling with the problems of haemodialysis. All three pregnancies in patients on regular dialysis at Newcastle have therefore been terminated at the parents' request. We now encourage women of child-bearing age to undergo tubal ligation before uraemia is too advanced. Some middle aged husbands opt for vasectomy to spare their wives an operation, albeit minor, but this course should only be adopted if the husband is confident that he would not wish to start another family in the event of his wife's death.

If a live donor transplant is contemplated the situation is a little different. Successful pregnancy after transplantation is no longer rare (Goldby, 1970) and the incidence of foetal abnormality associated with corticosteroid (Bongiovanni & McPhadden, 1960) and other immunosuppressive therapy is much lower than one might have anticipated; none of the 18 children born to mothers after a transplant or the 38 children fathered by transplant recipients, reported by Goldby, was abnormal. It is therefore reasonable for young, childless, women to retain their fertility but they should be well instructed in contraceptive technique so that pregnancy does not occur until the graft is well tolerated and immunosuppression has been reduced to maintenance levels in the second year post-transplant.

Hepatitis screening. All possible candidates for dialysis or transplant should be tested for the presence of Australia-antigen in the blood. The finding of antigen would exclude the patient from either procedure at many centres and would call for special precautions at the others.

Preparation for live donor grafting

If live donor grafting is practiced and the patient is suitable the first task is the screening of family volunteers. A reasonable routine is (1) Interview relatives to ensure that they are true volunteers and are not suffering from any known disease likely to interfere with kidney donation. (2) Check the ABO groups of the recipient and volunteers. Only the donors who are compatible on ordinary transfusion principles need be considered further. If it is suspected that any of the 'volunteers' are acting under duress a fictitious ABO incompatibility is a convenient way of letting them off the hook without fear of recrimination. (3) Carry out full history, examination and renal function studies on all suitable volunteers. Exclude any who have significant risk factors. Reduction of weight to close to the ideal, and cessation of smoking for several months, should be made conditions of 'permission to donate'. (4) Arrange tissue typing of potential donors who have qualified on counts (1) to (3). The immunologist may well ask for tissue typing of other family members to assist in genotyping. (5) Confirm histocompatibility by mixed lymphocyte culture (Bach *et al.*, 1970) or/and exchange of skin grafts in a manner that does not risk presensitisation (Seigler *et al.*, 1970) if these techniques are available locally. (6) Select the closest match from among those that meet the minimum requirements of the centre. Perform IVP to confirm normal renal anatomy. (7) about a fortnight before the proposed operation carry out aortography on the donor. This procedure is left to a late stage so that it is not performed unnecessarily, if the recipient dies or develops a complication that excludes live donor grafting.

Preparation for home dialysis

If live donor transplantation is not practised, or the patient is unsuitable, a long wait for a cadaver graft must be anticipated. The maintenance of a large pool of patients awaiting a transplant is only possible, in current circumstances, if a high proportion of those on regular dialysis perform the operation at home; in July 1971 55 per cent of patients in England and Wales were already established in the home. However the task of getting them home is becoming tougher now that the initial wave of public sympathy has passed its crest. Gordon & Cattell (1970) found that 19 of 33 patients accepted for home dialysis required rehousing or major extensions and the average delay in rehousing was 12 months. It is therefore essential to start negotiations with local authorities, and to proceed to building alterations and the installation of new plumbing, separate electricity meter, water softener etc. long before they are actually required. This is a time-consuming job in a major centre and is the most important function of the home dialysis administrator.

Insertion of arterio-venous fistula. The external teflon-silastic shunt introduced by Quinton & Scribner made regular haemodialysis possible. When they are inserted by a small number of obsessional surgeons and cared for lovingly shunts still give valuable service and at the Royal Free Hospital a remarkable 6 years' function has been obtained from each cannulated limb (Baillod *et al.*, 1969). However most dialysis centres cannot provide a 24-hour a day service from surgeons dedicated to the care of shunts and the general experience is not so happy—the average survival of individual cannulas varies from about 5 to 14 months (Shimizu *et al.*, 1971). The main causes of failure are recurrent thrombosis in the cannulated vessel (Papadimitriou, Carroll & Kulatilake, 1969) and infection around the cannula (Ralston *et al.*, 1971). The latter may lead to septicaemia or recurrent septic pulmonary embolism (Goodwin, Castronuovo & Friedman, 1969). Declotting of shunts has caused fatal cerebral damage (Gaan et al., 1969), possibly from retrograde embolism which has also caused limb ischaemia by occlusion of other peripheral arteries (Rohl, 1970). It is an important source of blood loss, a hepatitis risk, a major disruption of normal life endangering employment and an expensive use of staff time. Anticoagulants have reduced the frequency of clotting episodes (Wing, Curtis & De Wardener, 1967) but they make a major contribution to the high incidence of intra-cerebral and subdural haemorrhage in dialysis patients (Leonard et al., 1969; Drukker et al., 1970; Talalla et al., 1970).

Dissatisfaction with the external shunt led Brescia and his colleagues (1966) to develop the subcutaneous arteriovenous fistula as an alternative. They used a side-to-side anastomosis of radial artery and forearm vein, which remains the most popular technique, though end-to-side and end-to-end anastomosis have their devotees. When the radial and other suitable arteries have already been utilised for external shunts, vein grafts or synthetic grafts have been used to link less accessible vessels (Mozes, et al., 1970) or subcutaneous vein loops have been implanted and attached to deep arteries and veins (Girardet et al., 1970).

Once the fistula has had time to enlarge a leash of arterialised veins appears on the forearm or around the alternative site of anastomosis. A blood supply of about 150–220 ml/min can be obtained for haemodialysis by inserting short wide-bore needles percutaneously, one close to the fistula for the outflow and one more proximally for the return. The development of suitable arterialised veins may take several months in women, so it is advisable to insert the fistula some months before it is needed; the chance of success in creating the fistula is enhanced by using a 'virgin' arm in which the veins have not been used for intravenous therapy. Early insertion of the fistula allows time for the creation of a second fistula in the contralateral arm if the first never produces an adequate flow; cardiovascular complications of the double fistula are not troublesome provided hypertension and anaemia are controlled (Goldsmith et al., 1970). The other complications of the arteriovenous fistula, particularly local infection, septicaemia and bacterial endocarditis (Goodman et al., 1969; Levi, Robson & Rosenfeld, 1970; Ralston et al., 1971) are rarely seen before needling for haemodialysis begins. The patient whose fistula is inserted early therefore incurs little or no penalty during the waiting period before the start of haemodialysis.

Preparation for cadaver grafting

The results of cadaver grafting published to date do not justify using the procedure on patients who still have appreciable renal function and a prospect of independent survival for more than a few weeks. However it smooths the operation of the renal unit if tissue typing of future transplant candidates can be carried out before it is urgently needed. The data on such patients can then be prepared in advance for insertion into the computer (v. inf) and they can be added to the recipient pool as soon as the nephrologist judges that they are approaching the need for haemodialysis.

Patients with rapidly progressive nephritis present a special problem. They should not join the recipient pool at this stage since there is a high risk of recurrence of the disease in a transplanted kidney. This risk is apparently reduced by performing bilateral nephrectomy after haemodialysis has become necessary and waiting for several months while serum complement returns to normal and anti-kidney antibodies disappear from the circulation (Dixon, McPhaul & Lerner, 1969; Richardson *et al.*, 1970). Chronically infected kidneys or those containing calculi are also better removed before cadaver grafting is undertaken.

Live Donor Grafting

Although the ethical problems of performing an operation more major than a conventional nephrectomy on a healthy donor deters many surgeons, this procedure is still widely employed; 40 per cent of the 1473 grafts reported to the Transplant Registry for 1968–9 (Murray, Barnes & Atkinson, 1971) and 25 per cent of the European grafts in 1969–70 (Parsons, Clark & Spoek, 1970) were from living related donors. The reasons are not hard to find. The operation can be planned at leisure and performed in ideal circumstances. The patient can be prepared by intensive dialysis and transfusion of packed cells from Australia-antigen negative blood in the week before the operation. Immediate graft function can be anticipated. The post-operative morbidity suffered by the donors, although not negligible, has not resulted in long term problems in large published series e.g. in the 238 operations reported by Penn and colleagues (1970) only one donor, who has developed calculi in the remaining kidney; need regret his generosity. The best-matched grafts give prolonged survival with excellent rehabilitation and few side effects from the low-dose immunosuppression required. Experience of 40 operations at Newcastle confirms the impression conveyed by the literature that this operation is still justified if it is used discriminately. The problem is, 'what constitutes discriminate use?' Obviously the operation should not be undertaken if the recipient has a short life expectation because of non-renal problems such as severe coronary artery disease or if his pelvic vessels are so diseased that the vascular anastomosis is hazardous. A fairly high standard of histo-compatibility between donor and recipient is a sine-qua-non but it is not easy to lay down rigid rules, e.g. we have accepted a far from perfect match when transplanting the kidney of a widowed mother into her son, fortunately with a good result.

Twenty-five per cent of siblings should turn out to be HL-A identical to the recipient, i.e. they both possess the same 4 genes responsible for the most important histocompatibility antigens. Recipients of HL-A identical grafts have little or no problem with rejection episodes, they require only an easily tolerated dose of azathioprine and can often manage without corticosteroids altogether. Prolonged survival with good renal functions is usual; all the 25 patients in this category at Paris are still surviving, 4 have passed the 5 year mark and one is alive after 11 years (Hors *et al.*, 1971).

Parent-to-child and sib-to-sib grafts with one or more incompatibility give poorer results and necessitate more immunosuppression (Hors *et al.*, 1971). Overall survival from live donor grafting is little different from that during regular haemodialysis (Gurland *et al.*, 1970; Murray, Barnes & Atkinson, 1971). However individual decisions have to be made on the basis of local experience, skill and resources and in some hands live donor grafting is so nearly uniformly successful in the short term, even without HL-A identity (Starzl, Porter *et al.*, 1970), that the operation is likely to remain in use for some years. At Newcastle we are convinced that a live donor graft offers the best prospect of survival for a few years with occupational, social and sexual fulfilment; whether it justifies the risk to the donor is a decision that has to be shared with each family in turn.

Only 20 per cent of the patients screened at Newcastle turn out to have a willing donor who is medically suitable and sufficiently compatible. For the remaining four-fifths the Hobson's choice is regular haemodialysis with or without cadaver grafting.

Cadaver Grafting

There is growing evidence that histocompatibility is as important in cadaver grafting as it is in the related donor operation (Hors *et al.*, 1971). The normal arrangement for cadaver grafting has therefore become the establishment of a large 'recipient pool' i.e. a group of patients on regular haemodialysis who are awaiting transplantation and whose personal details, including ABO group and lymphocyte typing, are stored on a computer. Computers are sited in Leyden for Northern Continental Europe, Paris for France, Copenhagen for Scandinavia, London for most of U.K., Newcastle for Northern England and Southern Scotland, etc. Typical British policy and techniques are described by Branch *et al.*, 1970, Farrow, Fisher & Johnson, 1971, Festen-stein *et al.*, 1971, and Swinney, 1971; the British system which includes about 600 potential recipients—was centralised in Feb. 1972 on a single computer at Bristol. These local sharing schemes are linked by teleprinter and kidneys are now regularly transferred between countries in Europe (Sachs *el al.*, 1971) though the arrangements for transportation still leave a lot to be desired. The majority of the scarce donor kidneys which become available can now be dispatched to recipients who have 3 out of 4 HL-A antigens in common or better.

Interchange of kidneys to obtain close histocompatibility carries two penalties. (1) The recipient centre must take on trust the data supplied, e.g. the suitability of the donor, the length of time that elapsed between death and removal of the kidney ('warm ischaemia time') the maintenance of asepsis and the ABO grouping and tissue typing. In the early days of inter-change there was considerable discrepancy between centres carrying out tissue typing on the same individual but this has been overcome to a remark-able degree. When the kidney is despatched a lymph node or a supply or donor blood is sent with it so that the recipient centre can carry out a 'direct cross match' between the patient's serum and the donor's cells. At the same time it is customary to confirm the HL-A grouping, though this confirmation is not usually available to the surgeon until after the operation. In 31 of 32 international exchanges reported by Sachs and colleagues (1971) there was complete agreement on tissue typing between the centres involved.

(2) The 'cold ischaemia time' between perfusion and cooling of the kidney and its implantation in the patient is inevitably prolonged. In practice this has not turned out to be a major problem in Europe. Kidneys stored by perfusion with balanced electrolyte solutions and suspension in ice-saline slush survive for the 10 hours or so which is necessary for exchange between

most European centres, at least in day-time. The willing cooperation of the armed forces and police of some countries has contributed to the excellent results reported by Sachs and others but will not be proffered indefinitely. The future undoubtedly lies with some form of continuous perfusion of the kidney during the waiting time. Successful preservation of the kidney by pumped perfusion with solutions of plasma proteins or dextrans at temperatures around 10°C has been achieved for 24–72 hours in many laboratories (Belzer, Ashby & Dunphy, 1967; Scott, Morley & Swinney, 1969; Herrman et al., 1970; Cooperman et al., 1971; Sinha et al., 1971). One such system has been adopted by Scandiatransplant and is giving much better results than simple cooling, when the cold ischaemia time is longer than 10 hours (Claes et al., 1971).

Excellent results are being reported from areas where interchange on the European scale is not practicable and where freshness of the kidney appears to compensate for a lower standard of histocompatibility (Myburgh et al., 1970; May et al., 1971). However it is unlikely that these results will be maintained with longer follow-up and it is probable that intercontinental exchange will become the normal method of helping isolated centres once pump perfusion has been established as an every day procedure.

The operation is usually limited to implantation of the kidney in the iliac fossa (Swinney, 1971). The patient's own kidneys are either removed at a prior operation (v. sup) or left in situ. In a minority, hypertension recurs in the postoperative period when corticosteroids are administered in spite of good transplant function; a later planned nephrectomy will usually cure this recurrent hypertension but rejection and stenosis of the artery to the transplant should be excluded first (Papadimitriou, Chisholm & Shachman, 1969).

The pioneers in renal transplant usually removed the spleen in the hope of reducing the recipient's response to foreign tissue. The value of splenectomy has never been established in controlled trial and retrospective analysis does not suggest that it is of value in preventing rejection (Hume et al., 1966). However the use of the operation is increasing again (Murray, Barnes & Atkinson, 1971) and this may reflect the fact that an increasing proportion of recipients have spent many months or years on regular haemodialysis. Slight to moderate splenomegaly is usual in renal failure but the spleen enlarges further during regular dialysis (Magara et al., 1972). This eventually results in leucopenia and even thrombocytopenia which are cured by splenectomy (Bischel et al., 1971), though the operation is rarely required on these indications alone. It is our impression that patients who have been on regular haemodialysis for several years tolerate immunosuppressive drugs poorly and we therefore remove the spleen at or before the transplant operation if there is persistent leucopenia.

Azathioprine remains the mainstay of immunosuppression though cyclophosphamide has re-emerged as an alternative (Starzl et al., 1971). Prednisone is the most valuable drug for suppressing acute rejection crisis; there is no agreement on the best dose regime but the tendency is to use large doses early (Bell et al., 1971) and in rather short courses. Actinomycin C and local irradiation of the graft remain popular additional measures though their value is difficult to assess from the literature. Antilymphocyte globulin (ALG) is a non-standard preparation on which it is dangerous to generalise.

Some batches have proved effective in controlled trials when given prophylactically (Sheil *et al.*, 1971), but it has little or no effect on established
rejection (Mee & Evans, 1970). Platelet and fibrin deposition play a major
part in early rejection and may produce the systemic effects of disseminated
intravascular coagulation (Starzl *et al.*, 1970). This has led to the use of
heparin, coumarins and dipyridamole to suppress rejection reaction (Kincaid-
Smith, 1969) or at least minimise its effects but their value is unproven.

Regular Haemodialysis

The techniques and complications of regular haemodialysis have been the
subject of several recent reviews (Curtis, 1971; Hawe, Goldsmith & Jones,
1971; Kerr, 1971b; Polakoff, 1971; Robinson, 1971; Siddiqui & Kerr, 1971).
They are therefore described here in brief outline only and without reference
to the original literature.

Technique

The methods employed in regular haemodialysis are now virtually standard
through the U.K. and to a lesser extent throughout the world. Dialysis fluid
is made at the bedside or in the home by diluting liquid concentrate with raw,
softened or deionised tapwater (depending on the local water supply) in an
automatic proportioning machine such as the Dylade, Lucas or Drake
Willock. These machines incorporate a conductivity meter which checks the
accuracy of dilution and the latest models incorporate automatic sterilisation
and efficient de-aeration, to improve efficiency of dialysis and prevent 'bubb-
ling' in the blood pathway from diffusion of dissolved gases.

The switch from external shunts to arterio-venous fistulas has involved a
return to blood pumping with the risk of air-embolism; monitors to detect
or prevent this accident are now mandatory.

Non-disposable dialysers remain the 'best buy' even in areas where
labour costs are extremely high. The Kiil which has been the workhouse of
dialysis units for the last decade is being displaced by more efficient designs
such as the Meltec Multipoint and Western Gear Pyramid which are basically
similar to the Kiil but employ different membrane supports. Meticulous care
in avoiding contact with bacterial and other pyrogens is required to prevent
the recurrent problem of febrile reactions early in dialysis, when dialysers are
rebuilt in the hospital or home. For this reason and because of the difficulty
of recruiting sufficient staff, disposable dialysers are gaining popularity in
spite of their formidable cost. The Dow/Cordis Hollow Fiber Kidney, the
Extracorporeal Ex-03 coil, the latest Travenol Coil and the Gambro and Dasco
disposable dialysers all have a performance not far below that of the best
non-disposable dialysers.

A standard regime of 10 hours dialysis 3 times a week has been almost
universally adopted with the Kiil dialyser but it can probably be reduced to
8–9 hours 3 times a week with the newer dialysers.

Complications

Anaemia. The fall in haemoglobin level which characteristically followed
the start of regular haemodialysis in the early days, and demanded transfusion
of 2–4 pints of blood per month, was mainly the result of blood loss in the

dialyser, in excessive blood sampling for laboratory control, in declotting procedures and shunt operations etc. The use of modern dialysers, which can be washed back into the patient with the loss of only 5–10 ml of blood, of thrice weekly dialysis which reduced the need for biochemical monitoring, and of the arterio-venous fistula have drastically reduced these losses and made a 'no-transfusion policy' possible. However blood loss cannot be eliminated altogether and iron deficiency develops sooner or later. This cannot usually be corrected by oral iron which is poorly absorbed in uraemia; a course of 1 g of intravenous iron 2–3 times per year is necessary to maintain iron stores. Folate, ascorbic acid and pyridoxine are all lost by diffusion into the dialysis fluid and obvious depletion of these factors occasionally develops. They are usually given prophylactically in multivitamin supplements. A 60 g protein intake is permitted now that thrice weekly dialysis is standard and this probably contributes to haematopoiesis. Injection of testosterone in large doses (250–500 mg per week) raises the Hb level of many patients by 1–3 g/100 ml.

Hepatitis. Occasional hepatitis epidemics in renal units have been of the short incubation type but the great scourge of the last 5 years has been serum hepatitis. Outbreaks occurred in 72 European centres in 1970 affecting 260 patients and 130 members of staff. The virus is probably introduced into the unit in one of two ways (a) by admission of a carrier to the dialysis programme —uraemic patients are more likely to develop a mild illness and become permanent carriers of the virus than are normal subjects (b) by transfusion of a virus-infected unit of blood or blood-product to a patient. Both these accidents are largely preventable; all blood for transfusion should be tested for Australia-antigen (AA) and discarded if it is positive; until supplies of reagents make this ideal possible, blood intended for renal patients at least should be guaranteed AA negative. This would reduce the incidence of post-transfusion hepatitis by 75 per cent but would not eliminate it altogether, since the present tests for AA are not sufficiently sensitive. Patients who are found to be AA positive should either be refused entry to the dialysis programme or treated in an isolation unit. The former alternative is repugnant but if adequate facilities and staff for isolation are not available it is the only reasonable course of action; a hepatitis outbreak so paralyses the renal service that many other patients are denied treatment.

As an additional safeguard patients and staff are screened regularly for the presence of AA in British dialysis units, so that new cases arising within the dialysis unit can be isolated early and trained for home dialysis if they remain AA positive. This policy seems to be paying off and the disasters of 1969–70 do not appear to be recurring on the same scale.

Hypertension. Hypertension and its sequelae have been the major causes of death in dialysis patients since the technique was introduced. Blood pressure of recent origin can usually be controlled by dietary sodium and water restriction and gentle removal of the excess extracellular fluid by ultrafiltration through the artificial kidney. Strict dietary discipline (sodium intake of about 22 mEq/day, water not more than 500 ml plus urine volume/day) are necessary to maintain this improvement but they can often be relaxed after normotension has been restored for a year or so. A small minority of patients remain severely hypertensive in spite of sodium depletion.

This state is commonly accompanied by extreme hypersecretion of renin and responds well to bilateral nephrectomy; massive fluid replacement is often necessary to prevent hypotension in the 24 hours after the operation.

Bone disease. The differing patterns of bone disease in different dialysis centres is the most puzzling problem in the pathology associated with regular haemodialysis. In many cities, particularly in the United States, hyperparathyroidism progresses during the first year or two of dialysis, producing extensive soft tissue and vessel calcification. Response to parathyroidectomy is gratifying; the precipitate fall in serum calcium that occurs in the few days after operation can be countered by dialysis as well as the more familiar techniques of calcium infusion and vitamin-D administration.

In some other centres hyperparathyroidism, though still present to the extent of maintaining histological change in the bones and a raised plasma parathyroid hormone level, is not conspicuous on radiographs but osteomalacia persists or progresses and the osteosclerosis of untreated uraemia gives way to a progressive osteoporosis. Fractures occur at many sites but particularly the ribs, femoral necks, metacarpals and metatarsals, causing severe disability after a few years of regular dialysis. The bone disease is often accompanied by proximal myopathy. There is no response to calciferol but there are preliminary reports of successful treatment with dihydrotachysterol and 25-hydroxycholecalciferol. No peculiarity of dialysis technique which characterises the centres afflicted with this disease has yet been identified and there are some grounds for believing that it is due, at least in part, to some impurity in the tap water used to manufacture dialysis fluid. Fluoride, which has been under suspicion now appears to play little or no role in the disease. There are preliminary claims that the substitution of deionised or distilled water for tap water in the dialysis fluid may help this otherwise intractable disease.

Other complications. Peripheral neuropathy and pericarditis are largely preventable. They were common when dialysis was postponed to the last possible minute. It is now usual to commence dialysis when the serum creatinine is in the range 10–15 mg/100 ml, at about the time when uraemia is beginning to impair efficiency at work. Sexual function is only partially restored during haemodialysis. There are numerous examples now of men fathering children, but impotence or reduced performance is common, particularly in older males. Pruritis and pigmentation often improve, but may persist in spite of adequate dialysis.

Drug therapy in renal failure. Renal failure, haemodialysis and transplantation all modify the metabolism of drugs. The modifications in antibiotic dosage that are required in these circumstances have been reviewed by Linton & Lawson (1970) and O'Grady (1971). A summary of the effect of renal failure on the metabolism of other drugs (Kerr & Walls, 1971) is available from the author on request.

References

ABERCROMBIE, G. F., HANLEY, H. G. & JOEKES, A. M. (1970). *Br. J. Surg.*, **57**, 511.

ALLISON, M. E. M. & KENNEDY, A. C. (1971). *Clin. Sci.*, **41**, 171.

ASSCHER, A. W., SUSSMAN, M., WATERS, W. E., EVANS, J. A. S., CAMPBELL, H., EVANS, K. T. & EDMUND WILLIAMS, J. (1969). *J. infect. Dis.*, **120**, 17.

ASSCHER, A. W. (1971). *Q. Jl Med.*, **40**, 575.
AUSTRALIAN NATIONAL DIALYSIS AND RENAL TRANSPLANTATION SURVEY (1970).
    First Report by a Subcommittee. *Lancet*, **1**, 744.
BACH, J.-F., DEBRAY-SACHS, M., CROSNIER, J., KREIS, H. & DORMONT, J. (1970).
    Clin. exp. Immun., **6**, 821.
BAILEY, R. R., LITTLE, P. J. & ROLLESTON, G. L. (1969). *Br. med. J.*, **1**, 550.
BAILLOD, R. A., KNIGHT, A. H., CROCKETT, R. E. & NAISH, P. F. (1969). *Proc.*
    Europ. Dialysis Trans. Assoc., **6**, 65.
BARLOW, K. A. & BEILIN, L. J. (1968). *Q. Jl Med.*, **37**, 79.
BAUM, P. (1966). *Atzneimittel-Forsch.*, **16**, 1162.
BELL, D., KERR, D. N. S., SWINNEY, J. & YEATES, W. K. (1969). *Br. med. J.*, **3**, 378.
BELL, P. R. F., BRIGGS, J. D., CALMAN, K. C., PATON, A. M., WOOD, R. F. M.,
    MACPHERSON, S. G. & KYLE, K. (1971). *Lancet*, **1**, 876.
BELZER, F. O., ASHBY, B. S. & DUNPHY, J. E. (1967). *Lancet*, **2**, 536.
BENGTSSON, U. (1967). Proceedings of the Third International Congress of Nephro-
    logy. Vol. 2, 291. Edited by R. H. Heptinstall. Basel: Karger.
BENGTSSON, U. (1969). *Lancet*, **1**, 264.
BERLYNE, G. M., BOOTH, E. M., BREWIS, R. A. L., MALLICK, N. P. & SIMONS, P. J.
    (1969). *Lancet*, **1**, 689.
BERLYNE, G. M., JANABI, K., SHAW, A. B. & HOCKEN, A. G. (1966). *Lancet*, **1**, 169.
BERLYNE, G. M., MALLICK, M. P. & GAAN, D. (1968). *In* 'Fourth Symposium on
    Advanced Medicine'. Ed. O. Wrong. p. 99. London: Pitman.
BERNER, A. (1944). *Helv. med. Acta*, **11**, 961.
BISCHEL, M. D., NEIMAN, R. S., BERNE, T. V., TELFER, N., LUKES, R. J. & BARBOUR,
    B. H. (1971). *Proc. Europ. Dialysis Trans. Assoc.*, **8**, 81.
BLACK, D. A. K., ROSE, G. & BREWER, D. B. (1970). *Br. med. J.*, **3**, 421.
BLAINEY, J. D. & CHAMBERLAIN, M. J. (1971). *Br. med. Bull.*, **27**, 160.
BLUMBERG, A., NELP, W. B., HEGSTROM, R. M. & SCRIBNER, B. H. (1967). *Lancet*, **2**,
    69.
BOCK, K. D., HEIMSOTH, V., MERGUET, P. & SCHÖNERMARK, J. (1966). *Dt. med.*
    Wschr., **91**, 1761.
BODDY, K., KING, P. C., LINDSAY, R. M., WINCHESTER, J. & KENNEDY, A. C. (1971).
    Br. med. J. **1**, 140.
BONGIOVANNI, A. M. & McPADDEN, A. J. (1960). *Fert. Steril.*, **11**, 181.
BRANCH, R. A., CLARK, G. W., COCHRANE, A. L., JONES, J. H. & SCARBOROUGH, H.
    (1971). *Br. med. J.*, **1**, 249.
BRANCH, R. A., COLES, G. A., CROSBY, D. L., JONES, J. H., SUSSMAN, M. & THOMAS,
    W. J. C. (1970). *Br. med. J.*, **1**, 291.
BRECKENRIDGE, A., DOLLERY, C. T. & PARRY, E. H. O. (1970). *Q. Jl Med.*, **39**, 411.
BRESCIA, M. J., CIMINO, J. E., APPEL, K. & HURWICH, B. J. (1966). *New Engl. J.*
    Med., **275**, 1089.
British Medical Journal (1971). Editorial: What is Chronic Pyelonephritis? Vol. **2**,
    61.
BROD, J. (1971). *Br. med. J.*, **3**, 135.
BROD, J. & HORNYCH, A. (1967). *Israel J. med. Sci.*, **3**, 53.
BROD, J. & PRAT, V. (1967). *Proc. 3rd Int. Congr. Nephrol.*, **3**, 37. Ed. E. L. Becker.
    Basel: Karger.
BROWN, J. J., CURTIS, J. R., LEVER, A. F., ROBERTSON, J. I. S., DE WARDENER, H. E.
    & WING, A. J. (1969). *Nephron*, **6**, 329.
BRUNSCHWIG, A., BARBER, H. R. K. & ROBERTS, S. (1964). *J. Am. med. Ass.*, **188**, 5.
BUSCH, G. J., REYNOLDS, E. S., GALVANEK, E. G., BRAUN, W. E. & DAMMIN, G. J.
    (1971). *Medicine, Baltimore*, **50**, 29.
CAMERON, J. S. (1971). *J. Royal College Physicians Lond.*, **5**, 301.

CAMERON, J. S., ELLIS, F. G., OGG, C. S., BEWICK, M., BOULTON-JONES, J. M., ROBINSON, R. O. & HARRISON, J. (1970). *Proc. Europ. Dialysis Trans. Assoc.*, **7**, 25.

CHAZAN, B. I., REES, S. B., BALODIMOS, M. C., YOUNGER, D. & FERGUSON, B. D. (1969). *J. Am. med. Ass.*, **209**, 2026.

CHISHOLM, G. D. (1970). *Proc. Royal Soc. Med.*, **63**, 1242.

CHUGH, K. S., SWALES, J. D., BROWN, C. L. & WRONG, O. M. (1968). *Lancet*, **2**, 952.

CLAES, G., BLOHME, I. & GELIN, L.-E. (1971). *Proc. Europ. Dialysis Trans. Assoc.*, **8**, 307.

CLARK, P. (1971). *Br. med. Bull.*, **27**, 109.

CLARKSON, E. M., CURTIS, J. R., JEWKES, R. J., JONES, B. E., LUCK, V. A., DE WARDENER, H. E. & PHILLIPS, N. (1971). *Br. med. J.*, **3**, 604.

CLARKSON, E. M., DURRANT, C., PHILLIPS, M. E., GOWER, P. E., JEWKES, R. F. & DE WARDENER, H. E. (1970). *Clin. Sci.*, **39**, 693.

CLARKSON, E. M., McDONALD, S. J. & DE WARDENER, H. E. (1966). *Clin. Sci.*, **30**, 425.

COCHRAN, M. & NORDIN, B. E. C. (1969). *Br. med. J.*, **2**, 276.

COHEN, S. L., COMTY, C. M. & SHAPIRO, F. L. (1970). *Proc. Europ. Dialysis Trans. Assoc.*, **7**, 254.

COLEMAN, A. J., ARIAS, M., CARTER, N. W., RECTOR, F. C. & SELDIN, D. W. (1966). *J. clin. Invest.*, **45**, 1116.

CONFORTINI, P., GALANTI, G., ANCONA, A., GIONGO, E., BRUSCHI, E. & LORENZINI, E. (1971). *Proc. Europ. Dialysis Trans. Assoc.*, **8**, 74.

COOPERMAN, A. M., WOODS, J. E., HOLLEY, K. E. & McILRATH, D. C. (1971). *Mayo Clinic Proceedings*, **46**, 193.

CURTIS, J. R. (1971). *Br. med. Bull.*, **27**, 170.

CURTIS, J. R., DE WARDENER, H. E., GOWER, P. E. & EASTWOOD, J. B. (1970). *Proc. Europ. Dialysis Trans. Assoc.*, **7**, 141.

DAVIDSON, R. C. & PENDRAS, J. P. (1967). *Trans. Am. Soc. artif. internal Organs*, **13**, 36.

DELUCA, H. F. & AVIOLI, L. V. (1970). *Archs intern. Med.*, **126**, 896.

DIXON, F. J., McPHAUL, J. J. JR. & LERNER, R. (1969). *Archs intern. Med.*, **123**, 554.

DRUKKER, W., HAAGSMA-SCHOUTEN, W. A. G., ALBERTS, CHR. & SPOEK, M. G. (1969). *Proc. Europ. Dialysis Trans. Assoc.*, **6**, 99.

DRUKKER, W., HAAGSMA-SCHOUTEN, W. A. G., ALBERTS, CHR. & BAARDA, B. (1970). *Proc. Europ. Dialysis Trans. Assoc.*, **7**, 3.

EASTWOOD, J. B., BORDIER, P. & DE WARDENER, H. E. (1971). *Q. Jl Med.*, **40**, 569.

EDWARDS, M. & CURTIS, J. R. (1971). *Lancet*, **2**, 582.

EILERT, J. B., CASEY, D., DEL GRECO, F. & CONN, J. J. R. (1971). *Archs Surg.* **103**, 303.

ELLIS, H. A. & PEART, K. M. (1971). *Nephron.* **8**, 402.

FARROW, S. C., FISHER, D. J. H. & JOHNSON, D. B. (1971). *Br. med. J.*, **2**, 671.

FENG, P. H., WEINBERG, U., REISIN, E., IAINA, A. & ELIAHOU, H. E. (1970). *Israel J. Med. Sci.*, **6**, 732.

FESTENSTEIN, H., OLIVER, R. T. D., SACHS, J. A., BURKE, J. M., ADAMS, E., DIVVER, W., HYAMS, A., PEGRUM, G. D., BALFOUR, I. C. & MOORHEAD, J. F. (1971). *Lancet*, **2**, 225.

FINE, R. N., KORSCH, B. M., GRUSHKIN, C. M. & LIEBERMAN, E. (1970). *Amer. J. Dis. Child.*, **119**, 498.

FLOYD, M., AYYAR, D. R., HUDGSON, P. & KERR, D. N. S. (1969). *Proc. Europ. Dialysis Trans. Assoc.*, **6**, 203.

FOLLIS, R. H. JR. & JACKSON, D. A. (1943). *Bull. Johns Hopkins Hosp.*, **72**, 232.

FORD, J., PHILLIPS, M. E., TOYE, F. E., LUCK, V. A. & DE WARDENER, H. E. (1969). *Br. med. J.*, **1**, 735.

FRANK, H. & LOEWENICH-LAGOIS, K. V. (1966). *Dt. med. Wschr.*, **91**, 1680.
FRANKLIN, S. S., GORDON, A., KLEEMAN, C. R. & MAXWELL, M. H. (1967). *J. Am. med. Ass.*, **202**, 477.
FRY, I. K. & CATTELL, W. R. (1970). *Br. J. Hosp. Med.*, **3**, 67.
FRY, I. K. & CATTELL, W. R. (1971). *Br. J. Radiol.*, **44**, 198.
GAAN, D., MALLICK, N. P., BREWIS, R. A. L., SEEDAT, Y. K. & MAHONEY, M. P. (1969). *Lancet*, **2**, 77.
GAULT, M. H. & DOSSETOR, J. B. (1970). *Am. Heart J.*, **80**, 439.
GIORDANO, C. (1963). *J. Lab. clin. Med.*, **62**, 231.
GIORDANO, C., ESPOSITO, R., DE PASCALE, C. & SANTO, N. G. (1967). *Proc. 3rd Int. Cong. Nephrol.*, **3**, 214. Ed. C. Lovell Becker. Basel: Karger.
GIOVANNETTI, S. & MAGGIORE, Q. (1964). *Lancet*, **1**, 1000.
GIRARDET, R. E., HACKETT, R. E., GOODWIN, N. J. & FRIEDMAN, E. A. (1970). *Trans. Am. Soc. artif internal Organs*, **16**, 285.
GOGGIN, M. J. & JOEKES, A. M. (1971). *Br. med. J.*, **2**, 244.
GOLBY, M. (1970). *Transplantation*, **10**, 201.
GOLDSMITH, H. J., HAWE, B. J., ENGLAND, G. & MANSFIELD, A. (1970). *Proc. Europ. Dialysis, Trans. Assoc.*, **7**, 35.
GOODMAN, J. S., CREWS, H. D., GINN, H. E. & KOENIG, M. G. (1969). *New Engl. J. Med.*, **280**, 876.
GOODWIN, N. J., CASTRONUOVO, J. J. & FRIEDMAN, E. A. (1969). *Ann. intern. Med.*, **71**, 29.
GORDON, P. M. & CATTELL, W. R. (1970). *Proc. Europ. Dialysis Trans. Assoc.*, **7**, 248.
GRABNER, G., MICHALEK, P., POKORNY, D. & VORMITTAG, E. (1966). *Arzneimittel-Forsch.*, **16**, 1174.
GRAHAM, R. & SCOTT, J. T. (1970). *Ann. rheum. Dis.*, **29**, 461.
GURLAND, H. J., HÄRLEN, H., HENZE, H. & SPOEK, M. G. (1970). *Proc. Europ. Dialysis Trans. Assoc.*, **7**, 20.
HALGRIMSON, C. G., WILSON, C. B., DIXON, F. J., PENN, I., ANDERSON, J. T., OGDEN, D. A. & STARZL, T. E. (1971). *Archs Surg.* **103**, 283.
HAWE, B. J., GOLDSMITH, H. J. & JONES, P. O. (1971). *Br. med. J.*, **1**, 540.
HERRMANN, T. J., TURCOTTE, G., SLOAN, C. H. & O'DELL, C. W. (1970). *Investigative Urology*, **7**, 493.
HODSON, C. J. (1967). *Radiology*, **88**, 857.
HODSON, C. J. (1970). *Proc. 4th Intern. Cong. Nephrol.*, Vol. **3**, 282. Ed. N. Alwall, F. Berglund & B. Josephson. Basel: Karger.
HOLMES, J. H. (1971). Personal communication.
HOLMES, J. H., CRANDALL, J. I., DWYER, W. C. & SHORT, W. F. (1960). *Trans. Am. Soc. artif. internal Organs*, **6**, 152.
HOOD, C. E. A., BEALE, D. J., HOUSLEY, J. & HARWICKE, J. (1969). *Lancet*, **1**, 479.
HOPPER, J., ANDERSON, B. G. & DAILEY, M. E. (1959). *Am. J. med. Sci.*, **238**, 66.
HORS, J., FEINGOLD, N., FRADELIZI, D. & DAUSSET, J. (1971). *Lancet*, **1**, 609.
HUBAY, C. A., GONZALEZ-BARCENA, D., KLEIN, L., FRANKEL, V., ECKEL, R. E. & PEARSON, O. H. (1970). *Archs Surg.*, **101**, 181.
HUME, D. M., LEE, H. M., WILLIAMS, G. M., WHITE, H. J. O., FERRE, J., WOLF, J. S., PROUT, G. R., SLAPAK, M., O'BRIEN, J., KILPATRICK, S. J., KAUFFMAN, H. M. & CLEVELAND, R. J. (1966). *Ann. Surg.*, **164**, 352.
JEANNET, M., PINN, V. W., FLAX, M. H., WINN, H. J. & RUSSELL, P. S. (1970). *New Engl. J. Med.*, **282**, 111.
JOHNSON, J. W., WACHMAN, A., KATZ, A. I., HAMPERS, C. L., BERNSTEIN, D. S., WILSON, R. E. & MERRILL, J. P. (1969). *Trans. Am. Soc. artif. internal Organs* **15**, 333.

KATZ, A. I., HAMPERS, C. L. & MERRILL, J. P. (1969). *Medicine, Baltimore*, **48**, 333.

KEITH, N. M. & OSTERBERG, A. E. (1947). *J. clin. Invest.*, **26**, 773.

KERR, D. N. S. (1970). *Br. med. J.*, **4**, 363.

KERR, D. N. S. (1971a). *In* 'Textbook of Medicine'. Ed. P. B. Beeson & W. Cecil-Loeb McDermott. 13th edition. p. 1144. Saunders.

KERR, D. N. S. (1971b). *In* 'Progress in Clinical Medicine'. Ed. R. Daley & H. G. Miller, **6**, 109. Edinburgh and London: Churchill Livingstone.

KERR, D. N. S. & WALLS, J. (1971). *Adverse Drug Reaction Bulletin*, Regional Postgraduate Institute for Medicine and Dentistry, Newcastle upon Tyne. No. 26.

KERR, W. S. J., SUBY, H. I., VICKERY, A. & FRALEY, E. (1967). *Trans. Am. Ass. genito-urin. Surg.*, **59**, 166.

KINCAID-SMITH, P. (1969). *Lancet*, **2**, 920.

KINCAID-SMITH, P. (1970). Analgesic Nephropathy. *Prescribers' Journal*, **10**, 8.

KOUTSAIMANIS, K. G. & DE WARDENER, H. E. (1970). *Br. med. J.*, **4**, 131.

LAWSON, D. H., BODDY, K., KING, P. C., LINTON, A. L. & WILL, G. (1971). *Clin. Sci.*, **41**, 345.

LEDINGHAM, J. M. (1971). *J. Royal College Physicians, Lond.*, **5**, 103.

LEMANN, J. JR., LITZOW, J. R. & LENNON, E. J. (1966). *J. clin. Invest.*, **45**, 1608.

LEONARD, C. D., WEIL, E. & SCRIBNER, B. H. (1969). *Lancet*, **2**, 239.

LEVI, J., ROBSON, M. & ROSENFELD, J. B. (1970). *Lancet*, **2**, 288.

LEVIN, D. M. & CADE, R. (1965). *Ann. intern. Med.*, **62**, 231.

LEVIN, N. W. & ABRAHAMS, O. L. (1966). *Ann. rheum. Dis.*, **25**, 681.

LINTON, A. L. & LAWSON, D. H. (1970). *Proc. Europ. Dialysis Trans. Assoc.*, **7**, 371.

LONERGAN, E. T. & LANGE, K. (1968). *Am. J. clin. Nutr.*, **21**, 595.

LUKE, R. G. & KENNEDY, A. C. (1964). *Br. med. J.*, **1**, 27.

LUMB, G. A., MAWER, E. B. & STANBURY, S. W. (1971). *Am. J. Med.*, **50**, 421.

MACDOUGALL, A. I., ADDIS, G. J., MACKAY, N., DYMOCK, I. W., TURPIE, A. G. G., BALLINGALL, D. L. K., MACLENNAN, W. J., WHITING, B. & MACARTHER, J. G. (1970). *Br. med. J.*, **3**, 440.

MAGARA, L., ULDALL, P. R., SWINNEY, J., TAYLOR, R., ELLIS, H. E., MORLEY, A. M. & KERR, D. N. S. (1972). To be published.

MALLICK, N. P. & BERLYNE, G. M. (1968). *Lancet*, **2**, 1316.

MATALON, R. & EISINGER, R. P. (1970). *New Engl. J. Med.*, **282**, 835.

MATTHEW, T. H., LEWERS, D. T., HOGAN, G. P., RUBIO-PAEZ, D., ALTER, H. J., ANTONOVYCH, T., BAUER, H., MAHER, J. F. & SCHREINER, G. E. (1971). *J. Lab. clin. Med.*, **77**, 396.

MAY, J., SANDS, J., LAWRENCE, J. R., KINCAID-SMITH, P., MORRIS, P. J. & SHEIL, A. G. R. (1971). *Proc. Europ. Dialysis Trans. Assoc.*, **8**, 223.

MEE, A. D. & EVANS, D. B. (1970). *Lancet*, **2**, 16.

MOZES, M., HURWICH, B. J., ADAR, R., ELIAHOU, H. E. & BOGOKOWSKY, H. (1970). *Surgery, St. Louis*, **67**, 452.

MURRAY, J. E., BARNES, B. A. & ATKINSON, J. C. (1971). *Transplantation*, **11**, 328.

MURRAY, R. M., LAWSON, D. H. & LINTON, A. L. (1971). *Br. med. J.*, **1**, 479.

MURRAY, R. M., TIMBURY, G. C. & LINTON, A. L. (1970). *Lancet*, **1**, 1303.

MUTH, R. G. (1968). *Ann. intern. Med.*, **69**, 249.

MYBURGH, J. A., GOLDBERG, B., MEYERS, A. M., VAN BLERK, P. J. P., GECELTER, L., MIENY, C. J., BROWDE, S., SHAPIRO, M., ZOUTENDYK, A. & ANDERSON, C. G. (1970). *Br. med. J.*, **3**, 670.

NOWAKOWSKI, A., GROVE, R. B., KING, L. H. JR., ANTONOVYCH, T. T., FORTNER, R. W., KNEISER, M. R., CARTER, C. B. & KNEPSHIELD, J. H. (1971). *Ann. intern. Med.*, **75**, 243.

OGDEN, D. A., BRINEY, W. G. & SMYTH, C. J. (1969). Abstr. 4th *International Congress of Nephrology*, **1**, 457.

O'GRADY, F. (1971). *Br. med. Bull.*, **27**, 142.

ONESTI, G., SCHWARTZ, A. B., KIM, K. E., SWARTZ, C. & BREST, A. N. (1969). *Circulation*, **39**, 219.

ONESTI, G., SCHWARTZ, A. B., KIM, K. E., PAZ-MARTINEZ, V. & SWARTZ, C. (1971). *Circulation Research*, **28**, Suppl. 2, 53.

PACKHAM, D. A. & YATES-BELL, J. G. (1968). *Br. J. Urol.*, **40**, 207.

PAPADIMITRIOU, M., CARROLL, R. N. P. & KULATILAKE, A. E. (1969). *Br. med. J.*, **2**, 15.

PAPADIMITRIOU, M., CHISHOLM, G. D. & SHACKMAN, R. (1969). *Lancet*, **1**, 902.

PARSONS, F. M., BRUNNER, F. P., GURLAND, H. J. & HARLEN, H. (1971). *Proc. Europ. Dialysis Trans. Assoc.*, **8**, 3.

PARSONS, F. M., CLARK, P. B. & SPOEK, M. G. (1970). *Proc. Europ. Dialysis Trans. Assoc.*, **7**, 15.

PENN, I., HALGRIMSON, C. C., OGDEN, D. & STARZL, T. E. (1970). *Archs Surg.*, **101**, 226.

PILLAY, V. K. G., SCHWARTZ, F. D., AIMI, K. & KARK, R. M. (1969). *Lancet*, **1**, 77.

DE PLANQUE, B. A., MULDER, E. & DORHOUT MEES, E. J. (1969). *Acta med. scand.*, **186**, 75.

POLAK, A. (1971). *J. Royal College Physicians, Lond.*, **5**, 333.

POLAKOFF, S. (1971). *Postgrad. med. J.*, **47**, 501.

PRESCOTT, L. F. (1966). *Lancet*, **2**, 1143.

PRYOR, J. S. & JOEKES, A. M. (1969). *Br. J. Urol.*, **41**, Supplement p. 88.

RAFTOS, J. (1969). *Med. J. Austral.*, **2**, 684.

RALSTON, A. J., HARLOW, G. R., JONES, D. M. & DAVIS, P. (1971). *Br. med. J.*, **3**, 408.

RANDALL, R. E. JR., COHEN, M. D., SPRAY, C. C. JR. & ROSSMEISL, E. C. (1964). *Ann. intern. Med.*, **61**, 73.

RASTOGI, S. P., HART-MERCER, J. & KERR, D. N. S. (1969). *Q. Jl Med.*, **38**, 335.

RASTOGI, S. P., VOLANS, G., ELLIOTT, R. W., ECCLESTON, D. W., ASHCROFT, R., WEBSTER, D. & KERR, D. N. S. (1971). *Postgrad. med. J.*, **47**, April Supplement, 45.

REUBI, F. C. & COTTIER, P. T. (1961). *Circulation*, **23**, 200.

RICHARDS, P., METCALFE-GIBSON, A., WARD, E. E., WRONG, O. & HOUGHTON, B. J. (1967). *Lancet*, **2**, 845.

RICHARDSON, J. A., ROSENAU, W., LEE, J. C. & HOPPER, J. (1970). *Lancet*, **2**, 180.

RICHARDSON, J. R. & WEINSTEIN, M. B. (1970). *Ann. Intern. Med.*, **73**, 403.

RIESELBACH, R. E., SORENSEN, L. B., SHELP, W. D. & STEELE, T. H. (1970). *Ann. intern. Med.*, **73**, 359.

ROBINSON, B. H. B. (1971). *Br. med. Bull.*, **27**, 173.

ROBSON, A. M., KERR, D. N. S. & ASHCROFT, R. (1968). *In* 'Nutrition in Renal Disease'. Ed. G. M. Berlyne. p. 71. Edinburgh: Livingstone.

RÖHL, L. (1970). *Proc. R. Soc. Med.*, **64**, 589.

SACHS, J. A., OLIVER, R. T. D., FESTENSTEIN, H., BLANDY, J. P., SALAMAN, J. R., BALFOUR, I. C., PEGRUM, G. D., WILLIAMS, G. B., HOPEWELL, J. P., MOORHEAD, J. F., BARNES, A. D. & BEWICK, M. (1971). *Lancet*, **2**, 228.

SAXTON, H. M., KILPATRICK, F. R., KINDER, C. H., LESSOF, M. H., MCHARDY-YOUNG, S. & WARDLE, D. F. H. (1969). *Q. Jl Med.*, **38**, 159.

SCHWARTZ, W. B. (1955). *New Engl. J. Med.*, **253**, 601.

SCHWARTZ, W. B. & KASSIRER, J. P. (1968). *Am. J. Med.*, **44**, 786.

SCOTT, D. F., MORLEY, A. R. & SWINNEY, J. (1969). *Br. J. Surg.*, **56**, 688.

SEIGLER, H. F., AMOS, D. B., WARD, F. E., ANDRUS, C. H., SOUTHWORTH, J. G., HATTLER, B. G. JR. & STICKEL, D. L. (1970). *Ann. Surg.*, **172**, 151.

SEVITT, L. H., EVANS, D. J. & WRONG, O. M. (1971). *Q. Jl Med.*, **40**, 127.

SEVITT, L. H. & WRONG, O. M. (1968). *Lancet*, **2**, 950.

SHALDON, S., KOCH, K. M., OPPERMANN, F., PATYNA, W. D. & SCHOEPPE, W. (1971). *Br. med. J.*, **3**, 212.

SHAND, D. G., O'GRADY, F., NIMMON, C. C. & CATTELL, W. R. (1970). *Lancet*, **1**, 1305.

SHAW, A. B., BAZZARD, F. J., BOOTH, E. M., NILWARANGKUR, S. & BERLYNE, G. M. (1965). *Q. Jl Med.*, **34**, 237.

SHAW, A. B. (1968). *In* 'Nutrition in Renal Disease'. Ed. G. M. Berlyne. p. 150. Edinburgh: Livingstone.

SHEIL, A. G. R., KELLY, G. E., STOREY, B. G., MAY, J., KALOWSKI, S., MEARS, D., ROGERS, J. H., JOHNSON, J. R., CHARLESWORTH, J. & STEWART, J. H. (1971). *Lancet*, **1**, 359.

SHIMIZU, A., TRIEDI, H., FAY, W. P. & THOMPSON, G. D. (1971). *J. Am. med. Ass.*, **216**, 645.

SHINABERGER, J. H. & EARL GINN, H. (1968). *Am. J. clin. Nutr.*, **21**, 618.

SIDDIQUI, J., FREEBURGER, R. & FREEMAN, R. M. (1970). *Am. J. clin. Nutr.*, **23**, 11.

SIDDIQUI, J. & KERR, D. N. S. (1971). *Br. med. Bull.*, **27**, 153.

SIMPSON, K. M., BUNCH, D. L., AMEMIYA, H., BOEHMIG, H. J., WILSON, C. R., DIXON, F. J., COBURG, A. J., HATHAWAY, W. E., GILES, G. R. & STARZL, T. E. (1970). *Surgery*, **68**, 77.

SIMPSON, W., KERR, D. N. S., HILL, A. V. L. & SIDDIQUI, J. (1971). *Proc. R. Soc. Med.*, **65**, 477.

SINHA, B. P., ATKINSON, S. M. & PIERCE, J. M. (1971). *Lancet*, **1**, 421.

SMELLIE, J. M. & NORMAND, I. C. S. (1968). *In* 'Urinary Tract Infection'. Ed. F. O'Grady & W. Brumfitt. p. 123. London: Oxford University Press.

SNYDER, D. & BREST, A. N. (1966). *J. Am. Geriat. Soc.*, **14**, 21.

STANBURY, S. W. (1967). *In* 'Renal Disease'. Ed. D. A. K. Black. 2nd Ed. p. 665. Oxford: Blackwell.

STANBURY, S. W. (1968). *Am. J. Med.*, **44**, 714.

STARZL, T. E., BOEHMIG, H. J., AMEMIYA, H., WILSON, C. B., DIXON, F. J., GILES, G. R., SIMPSON, K. M. & HALGRIMSON, C. C. (1970). *New Engl. J. Med.*, **283**, 383.

STARZL, T. E., PORTER, K. A., ANDRES, G., HALGRIMSON, C. G., HURWITZ, R., GILES, G., TERASAKI, P. I., PENN, I., SCHROTER, G. T., LILLY, J., STARKIE, S. J. & PUTMAN, C. W. (1970). *Ann. Surg.*, **172**, 437.

STARZL, T. E., HALGRIMSON, C. G., PENN, I., MARTINEAU, G., SCHROTER, G., AMEMIYA, H., PUTMAN, C. W. & GROTH, C. G. (1971). *Lancet*, **2**, 70.

STEELE, T. W., GYÖRY, A. Z. & EDWARDS, K. D. G. (1969). *Br. med. J.*, **2**, 213.

SWINNEY, J. (1971). *Br. med. Bull.*, **27**, 181.

TALALLA, A., HALBROOK, H., BARBOUR, B. H. & KURZE, T. (1970). *J. Am. med. Ass.*, **212**, 1847.

TALBOTT, J. H. & TERPLAN, K. L. (1960). *Medicine, Baltimore*, **39**, 405.

TERMAN, D. S., ALFREY, A. C., HAMMOND, W. S., DONNDELINGER, T., OGDEN, D. A. & HOLMES, J. H. (1971). *Am. J. Med.*, **50**, 744.

TRIBE, C. R. & SILVER, J. R. (1969). *In* 'Renal failure in paraplegia'. London: Pitman Medical.

TSALTAS, T. T. (1969). *Am. J. clin. Nutr.*, **22**, 490.

WALLS, J., MORLEY, A. R. & KERR, D. N. S. (1969). *Br. J. Urology*, **41**, 546.

WHITE, R. H. R., GLASGOW, E. F. & MILLS, R. J. (1970). *Lancet*, **1**, 1353.

WIGAND, M. E. & HEIDLAND, A. (1971). *Postgrad. med. J.*, **47**, April Supplement 54.

WILSON, J. D., SIMMONDS, H. A., NORTH, J. D. K. (1967). *Ann. rheum. Dis.*, **26**, 136.

WING, A. J., CURTIS, J. R. & DE WARDENER, H. E. (1967). *Br. med. J.*, **3**, 143.

WOODHOUSE, N. J. Y., DOYLE, F. H. & JOPLIN, G. F. (1971). *Lancet*, **2**, 283.

WRIGHT, P. L., BRERETON, P. J. & SNELL, D. E. M. (1970). *Metabolism*, **19**, 201.

YORK, S. E. & YENDT, E. R. (1966). *Can. med. Ass. J.*, N.S. **94**, 1329.

VAN YPERSELE DE STRIHOU, C. & FRANS, A. (1970). *Nephron*, **7**, 37.

CHAPTER 10

CLINICAL PSYCHOPHARMACOLOGY

R. H. S. MINDHAM and MICHAEL SHEPHERD

Despite the early interest of individual workers in the potential value of the chemotherapy of mental disorders it has been pointed out that 'the current phase of the application of chemical substances in mental disease started as part of a group of very disparate procedures largely developed since 1920 and termed physical treatments' (McIlwain, 1957). For some 30 years these physical treatments in psychiatry were associated principally with such crude procedures as malarial fever, insulin coma, electrical convulsions and destructive neurosurgery, but throughout this period a steady interest was maintained in the application of various chemical agents to neuropsychiatric conditions, with particular emphasis on sedatives, anticonvulsants, hypnotics, antibiotics, hormones and sympathomimetic amines. Not until the arrival of a series of novel compounds in the early 1950s, however, did it become necessary to revive the term 'psychopharmacology' to designate a federation of disciplines focussing on old and new psychotropic compounds and drawing on the expertise of chemists, pharmacologists, psychologists, social scientists and clinicians (Shepherd, Lader & Rodnight, 1968).

After an initial period in which high therapeutic expectations were aroused by a host of new psychotropic agents psychopharmacology has entered a more sober phase of progress. In this short review we can do no more than sketch the contours of this large and rapidly expanding subject; the interested reader can consult the numerous books and articles which have appeared in the past fifteen years (Goodman & Gilman, 1970; Kalinowsky & Hippius, 1969; Proceedings of the Collegium Internationale Neuro-Psychopharmacologicum, 1958, 1964, 1965, 1969; the Annual Psychopharmacology Abstracts; Root & Hofmann, 1963, 1965, 1967; Wikler, 1957). The common ground between psychiatry and general medicine is nowhere better illustrated than by this multi-disciplinary area of experimental and therapeutic enquiry.

INVESTIGATION OF THE EFFECTS OF DRUGS

The major advances in psychopharmacology have been initiated by clinical observation rather than by laboratory research. Nonetheless, as with other types of medicaments psychotropic drugs call for a series of investigations in animals and man to establish knowledge on such factors as absorption, distribution, metabolism, excretion, dose-range, mode of action, efficacy, unwanted effects, interactions with other drugs and liability to produce dependence.

Study of Effects of Psychotropic Drugs in Animals

With animals many of the techniques employed are common to the investigation of other drugs and need not be elaborated here. The more important of the behavioural techniques will be briefly outlined.

Behavioural tests

Many drugs, especially those with sedative effects, induce behavioural changes which can be observed with the animal moving in a free environment. These include abnormal postures, immobility, ataxia, loss of righting reflexes, tremor, defaecation, vomiting and convulsions. The differing effect of drugs on several of these forms of behaviour can be recorded at the same time. Alternatively, certain aspects of an animal's activities, e.g. feeding, sleeping, aggression, social and sexual conduct, can be studied selectively by simply observing the animal in a free environment, alone or with other animals, or by using special apparatus. It is, for example, relatively simple to measure the amount of food eaten, the frequency of sexual approaches or the pattern of motor behaviour.

In addition, many special tests of performance have been devised, such as a mouse's ability to cling to a rotating rod to test its motor power and perseverance. Tests in which animals have to show that they can distinguish between materials which are very similar, for example water and a dilute solution of alcohol, permit of an assessment of the acuteness of perception. Learning and memory can be tested by a variety of maze-running tests which usually yield quantitative data and make it possible to measure the differing effects of individual drugs.

A number of tests are used which measure the effects of drugs on *conditioned learning*. In the Pavlovian sense of learning a neutral stimulus is paired with a stimulus which always produces a particular (unconditioned) response, until the response is produced by the neutral (conditioned) stimulus alone. Pavlov's original experiments concerned salivation in dogs produced first by the sight of food (the unconditioned stimulus) and the sound of a bell, and later by the bell (the conditioned stimulus) alone. The effects of drugs on the learning and forgetting of this type of behaviour can be studied objectively.

In *avoidance conditioning* animals are taught to avoid noxious stimuli, which are heralded by innocuous signals, by responding to the innocuous stimuli before the noxious stimuli are given. This type of learned behaviour is more sensitive to the effects of drugs than the classical Pavlovian type and is consequently of greater value in testing drugs.

In *operant conditioning* a particular aspect of random behaviour is selectively rewarded. The reward may be given regularly or irregularly, and with each response or only after a certain number of responses. Animals are commonly taught to press or peck levers and are rewarded with food. This type of behaviour can be readily quantified and the effects of drugs upon it measured with some precision.

Prediction of Psychotropic Drug-Effects in Man from Animal Experiments

Abnormal states in animals which are homologous to illnesses in man have been of great value in the investigation of drugs intended for use in many physical disorders. Unfortunately animal responses must be regarded as no more than analogues to most mental disorders and even when there are striking similarities there is no certainty that they are produced by similar mechanisms. In consequence, prediction of the effects of drugs in man from the results of experiments in animals presents great problems. Three main method are used in attempting to overcome this obstacle.

1. Attempts have been made to establish similarities between abnormal behaviour in man and behaviour in animals by breaking down complex patterns of behaviour to their constituent parts. The selected animal behaviour is then modified by the administration of drugs. There is, for example, some similarity between aggressive behaviour in animals and irritability in man so that a drug which reduces aggression in animals might be expected to reduce irritability in man. In practice, the taming effect of chlordiazepoxide was observed in many animals and proved to have a calming effect in man also.

2. Efforts to study 'model illnesses' in animals have also been made, and are best exemplified by neurotic and depressive reactions. Pavlov's 'experimental neurosis' in dogs was obtained by taking animals which were trained to salivate in response to a particular conditioned stimulus (then presenting an ambiguous stimulus), until a state of aberrant behaviour was produced which continued outside the experimental situation. The resulting state has been described as 'conflict between previously learned patterns for securing a specific reward and a concurrently induced fear of the repetition of a disruptively traumatic experience while receiving the expected gratification' (Masserman, 1960). The condition is accompanied by some of the physiological and behavioural changes associated with some forms of neurosis in man, namely tachycardia, trembling, inactivity, disorganisation of skills and fearfulness. Animals in this state have been used in testing the effectiveness of drugs in relieving symptoms and for comparing the effects of one drug with another.

The administration of reserpine to a variety of animals induces a condition showing some resemblance to retarded depression in man: a general reduction in the level of activity, including the slowing of movements, reduced responsiveness to stimulation and a neglect of activities such as feeding and sexual behaviour (Brodie, 1965). This type of preparation has been widely used in testing the anti-depressant properties of drugs, since drugs which have the effect of reversing the effects of reserpine in animals often prove to have anti-depressant properties in man. The case for regarding this state as a 'model illness' is supported by the knowledge that reserpine can induce a depressive illness in man which is indistinguishable from the natural condition.

3. A more empirical technique is to draw up a profile of the effects of a drug in animals and to compare this with the profiles of drugs of known effectiveness in man. However, many of the items included in the profile may have no direct relationship with the desirable clinical effects. The method assumes that two drugs showing similar effects in animals will show similar effects in man, although the actual effects studied in man and animals may be quite different. While this assumption is likely to hold true in chemically related drugs it is possible for the favourable characteristics of a new drug to be missed simply because its profile of activity in animals is unlike those of drugs known to be clinically effective in man.

In practice, where a large number of drugs are being investigated for psychotropic effects simplified screening procedures are used, most attention being directed towards a principal effect, for example, sedation, stimulation, prevention of fits or reversal of the effects of reserpine. Promising compounds can then be investigated in more detail.

Study of Effects of Psychotropic Drugs in Man

Methods for the study of psychotropic drugs in man also depend on many of the basic techniques of general pharmacology, toxicology and neurophysiology. Behavioural techniques which have been developed to supplement these investigations include such measures of sensory threshold as sensitivity to pain and two-point discrimination; tests of perception such as the frequency of flicker fusion; tests of psychomotor skills such as peg-board games; tests of the ability to learn new material; and changes in physiological functions such as pulse rate and skin conductance induced under conditions of stress. All these investigations furnish quantitative data.

Reliable methods of assessing the mental state are of particular importance for the evaluation of drug-effects in psychiatry. A large number of rating scales have been designed for this purpose with varying degrees of success. They may be designed to give an overall assessment of the mental state or be directed to a particular feature, such as anxiety, depression or the side-effects of drugs. The rating scales in common use have generally been tested in a large patient population and have been shown to have acceptable standards of validity and reliability. Rating scales can be used to assess objective or subjective features of the mental state and may be administered by nurses, psychologists, occupational therapists and the patients themselves, as well as by doctors (provided that the administrator be trained in their use by an experienced person). The scales are generally designed for a particular mode of administration to give information on a particular aspect of the mental state.

Specific and Non-specific Factors in Pharmacological Treatment

Several factors are capable of modifying the course of an illness, and even with physical disease it is comparatively rare for improvement to be attributable to a single element in a patient's treatment. Most mental illnesses are multi-causal and aetiology is poorly understood; many conditions pursue a fluctuating course and a variety of factors are capable of contributing to remission or recovery (Marley, 1959). In such circumstances it is frequently difficult to distinguish between the specific and non-specific effects of treatment. The specific effects of a drug may be defined as those arising directly from its pharmacodynamic properties.

The non-specific effects of drug administration are determined by three main factors: those related to the personal characteristics of the patient; those due to the personality of the doctor prescribing the treatment; and those arising from the environment or 'milieu' in which the treatment is given. The tendency of many patients to respond to treatment even when it has no specific therapeutic action has been widely used in medical practice. The effect of the doctor's personality on treatment is a complex one, but it is well-known that some physicians favour particular forms of treatment from which they obtain better results than others who are less enthusiastic about them. The setting in which treatment is given also exerts an important influence on its effect; a drug given in hospital, for example, may be more effective than the same drug given at home, and external forces such as occupational therapy, work therapy and social activities may affect a patient's progress.

Probably most recent work on non-specific therapeutic responses has been focused on the 'placebo effect' (Loranger, Prout & White, 1961) which has been defined by Shapiro (1967) as 'the psychological, physiological or psychophysiological effect of any medication or procedure given with therapeutic intent, which is independent or minimally related to the specific effect of the procedure and which operates through a psychological mechanism.' The word 'placebo' originates from the practice of giving an inert preparation 'to please' the patient in conditions where no specific treatment is available. Several authorities consider that the tendency to respond to placebo is a fixed element in the personality, some patients showing it to a marked degree, some not at all (Joyce, 1959); others believe that the propensity is very widespread and dependent upon the particular circumstances of an illness, the personality of the doctor and the nature of the treatment given (Liberman, 1964). In addition, the nature of an illness, the patient's expectation of its course and of the effects of treatment all alter the response to medication. The prescription of treatment is in itself an important element of the transaction between the doctor and patient, acknowledging as it does the patient's status as a 'sick' person (Mechanic, 1966).

Evaluation of Psychotropic Drugs

From what has already been said on the specificity of therapeutic effects it follows that the pharmacological effects of drugs can easily be obscured by other aspects of treatment. Few treatments in psychiatry have such clear-cut effects that the benefits they bestow are self-evident. The multiplicity of effects on the course of an illness can not only obscure the value of a treatment but may also prevent recognition of its ineffectiveness. Proper assessment almost always involves carrying out a carefully designed comparison between the effects of the treatment and those of an inactive or a well-established treatment. In this way it is usually possible to distinguish between the specific and non-specific aspects of therapy.

The ethics, purposes, design, conduct and analysis of clinical trials have been fully documented (Hill, 1950, 1960, 1963, 1965); however, there are certain aspects of clinical trials which need special emphasis when they are applied to psychiatric conditions. These may be listed as follows.

1. Though the patient population must be clearly defined so as to furnish a group which is as homogeneous as possible, diagnostic criteria in psychiatry are ill-defined and frequently controversial. This difficulty can be overcome in some measure by adopting an operational definition of the condition being studied, thereby avoiding theoretical considerations.

2. The initial assessment of the type and severity of the illness and assessment during treatment generally involves the use of rating scales. It is important that these should be used within their limitations and not be expected to provide information for which they were never intended.

3. It is necessary that the prejudices of the investigators and subjects are

not allowed to bias observations made on the effects of treatment. This is usually prevented by using the 'double-blind' method of assessment, where neither the patient nor the assessor is aware of the allocation of the treatment regimes. It is essential that every effort be made to preserve the 'blindness' of a study: remarkably subtle differences between treatments can impair this aspect of the design.

4. As the effects of many psychotropic drugs are closely dependent upon the dosage employed, a comparison can only be made between treatments when they are given in equivalent dosage: for this to be effected it may be necessary to carry out some investigation to allow the appropriate dosages to be determined.

5. The methods by which the results are to be analysed should be closely related to the design of the trial and should involve a simple method of comparison. All too often in psychiatry too little thought is given to this question until a study is completed.

Unwanted Drug Effects

No drug is free of some 'unwanted' effects, defined as the effects of a drug which do not contribute to the therapeutic effects sought. Unwanted effects of drugs are usually closely related to their pharmacological characteristics and are usually unavoidable if the drug is given in a sufficient dosage to produce its clinical effects. When a drug is used for more than one purpose, the unwanted effects in the treatment of one condition may be the therapeutic effects in another. With reserpine, for example, the hypotensive effects are unwanted when the drug is used as a sedative: but when the drug is used as a hypotensive agent it is the sedative effects which are unwanted. Lader (1971) has drawn a useful distinction between three types of unwanted effects. First, there are those which occur when the dosage of the drug is just above that necessary to achieve a therapeutic effect: these effects may be avoidable by reducing the dosage, but this is difficult to achieve in practice as the plasma concentrations of drugs vary so much in the intervals between administration, being either well above or well below the level required to give unwanted effects. Secondly, there are those which occur at dosage levels below those required to produce the therapeutic effect: these are unavoidable and a decision has to be made as to whether the beneficial effects of the medication outweigh the unwanted effects. The third type reflect the biological characteristics of the patient; such idiosyncratic effects include skin rashes, anaphylaxis and gastro-intestinal disturbances.

Many drugs used in both psychiatry and general medicine bring about changes in the mental state which must be regarded as 'unwanted effects'. Intoxication with many drugs, especially in ill patients, can cause confusional states which usually present as rapidly fluctuating symptoms, including disorientation in time and place, disturbed behaviour, disturbances of consciousness and attention, and a variety of abnormalities of perception which often include visual hallucinations. The knowledge that the drugs given are capable of inducing disturbances of this kind is an important aid in diagnosis. A number of drugs are known to be capable of causing depression and many others have come under suspicion: the effect of reserpine in this respect is well known and its mechanism of action to some extent understood, but the well-authenticated depressant effect of other drugs, such as pro-gestational contraceptives and phenobarbitone, are less readily explained. Cases of hypomania have been described in patients receiving L-dopa (Bunney *et al.*, 1970) but cases of depression are also reported (Jenkins & Groh, 1970). Disturbances of the mental state associated with the corticosteroids include both depression and elation as well as confusional episodes (Michael & Gibbons, 1963). The psychoses resembling schizophrenia which can be induced by LSD and amphetamines sometimes continue after the drugs have been withdrawn. Dementia has been described following the administration of ergot for migraine (Bradshaw & Parsons, 1965).

The special problems of drug dependency have been omitted from this review for want of space (Isbell and Chruściel, 1970).

CLASSIFICATION OF PSYCHOTROPIC DRUGS

The various generic terms such as 'tranquillisers' and 'neuroleptics' are of more metaphorical than scientific interest and will not be used here. A truly adequate classification of these drugs has yet to be constructed (Shepherd, 1972). Besides the traditional pharmacological distinction between compounds which 'stimulate' and 'depress' the central nervous system, may be added those which are only psychotomimetic and an inevitably miscellaneous group. In this context the term 'depressant' indicates a substance which has the effect of diminishing a particular physiological or psychological function and a 'stimulant' drug is a substance which enhances one or more of these functions.

Centrally Acting Drugs with a Primarily Depressant Action

The control of psycho-motor overactivity has always figured prominently in the management of mentally disturbed patients. Many methods have been used for this purpose, including a variety of drugs such as morphia, paralde-hyde, chloral, alcohol and the bromides. The use of opiates has been super-seded by newer drugs which are more effective and less dangerous. The use of paraldehyde has also greatly declined, partly on account of its limited efficacy, its unpleasant smell and taste and, not least, because of the risk of abscess formation following its injection; it is still used by some workers in the treatment of status epilepticus because of its rapid onset of action. The bromides were never very effective in the control of fits or insomnia, and their serious unwanted effects have led to their abandonment in therapeutics. Alcohol is unreliable as a hypnotic or sedative but chloral has retained a place as an effective and safe hypnotic, especially useful in the young and elderly, in spite of its unpleasant taste.

Barbiturates

Among older drugs with a primarily depressant effect on the central nervous system, the barbiturates have been used most widely in four different ways: to sedate and allay anxiety in small doses; to induce sleep in larger doses; to prevent or control convulsive behaviour in epilepsy; and to control violent behaviour often associated with the psychoses.

Pharmacology. All the barbiturates share the same general formula; the chemical structure of three common derivatives are shown. The barbiturates are readily absorbed from the gut, are widely distributed in the tissues including the brain, and are inactivated largely by metabolism in the liver but partly by excretion in the urine. Tolerance to the administration of the barbiturates develops rapidly, largely due to an increase in the rate of breakdown in the liver brought about by the potentiation of the relevant enzyme systems. The barbiturates have a predominantly depressant effect

GENERAL FORMULA of BARBITURATES

AMYLOBARBITONE

PHENOBARBITONE

on the brain, first reducing the activity of the neo-cortex and then affecting the brain-stem and spinal cord with larger doses. Small doses of barbiturates release the cortex from inhibition by the reticular formation. This effect can be recognised by an increase in electrical activity and by behavioural changes. Larger doses have a depressant effect on both the cortex and the reticular formation which is accompanied by drowsiness or even sleep. Behaviourally, the administration of barbiturates results in a decline in the level of activity and in the precision with which more complex tasks are performed.

Clinical effects. Barbiturates have been widely used as hypnotics and have been shown to be more effective than placebo in this respect. The concept of long and short-acting drugs has been questioned and it seems that the duration of action is more likely to be related to dosage and potency than to differences in the rate of metabolism. Barbiturates are also used in the control of anxiety; controlled studies have confirmed their value in the treatment of chronic anxiety states (Raymond *et al.*, 1957; Weatherall, 1962; Reynolds *et al.*, 1965).

In epilepsy phenobarbitone has retained its position as one of the most important anticonvulsants in spite of the appearance of many newer drugs; it is more effective in grand mal and focal epilepsy and less effective in petit mal. Barbiturates can be used to control tension, agitation and violence. However, when a patient is violently disturbed the degree of sedation produced by the high dose of drugs required to control the behaviour may be so great as to induce sleep or drowsiness which render normal activities impossible. They also have the disadvantage that the effects are short-lived, depending on the continued administration of the drugs for the control of symptoms.

Intravenous barbiturates can be used to facilitate interviews by allowing patients to disclose unpleasant information. The drugs are given by slow intravenous injection; the effect appears to result from a drug-induced decline in the patient's reluctance to talk about his problems. Drugs commonly used for this purpose are thiopentone sodium (Pentothal) and amylobarbitone sodium. Both drugs are given in a dosage ranging from 100–500 mg, the actual dosage and speed of injection depending upon the progress of the interview.

Adverse effects. Apart from sensitivity reactions such as rashes, the main disadvantages of the barbiturates are: (1) the drowsiness often associated with the therapeutic effects; (2) the rapid rise in dosage required to achieve and maintain a particular effect; (3) the serious risk of dependency developing if the drugs are prescribed over any period of time, and the associated risk of fits when the drug is withdrawn; (4) the common use of barbiturates for suicidal attempts which may be successful. Patients taking barbiturates may show the clinical picture of mild intoxication with impairment of mental functions, slurring of speech, ataxia and nystagmus.

Non-barbiturate sedatives and hypnotics

It is apparent from the foregoing account that there is a need in psychiatry and general medicine for drugs with the sedative and hypnotic actions of barbiturates but without their adverse effects. Such claims have been advanced on behalf of several newer compounds.

Essig (1969) has warned against the too ready acceptance of substitutes for barbiturates. He shows that many of the drugs introduced to replace the barbiturates are capable of producing states of intoxication and dependency very similar to those produced by the barbiturates themselves. He recommends that care should be exercised when sedatives are prescribed; prolonged medication, increases in dosage, drug combinations and the switching from one drug to another in the mistaken belief that the risk of dependency is thereby reduced, should all be avoided.

Meprobamate (Equanil) was developed from the drug mephenesin, which has muscle relaxant properties, and introduced as a sedative for the treatment of anxiety in 1954. It is rapidly absorbed from the gut, widely distributed in the tissues and rapidly inactivated by hydroxylation and conjugation. The pharmacological actions of meprobamate closely resemble those of the barbiturates: it has a depressant effect on the central nervous system, induces sedation and muscle relaxation, and has some anti-epileptic action.

After an initial phase of widespread use, it became apparent that the evidence on the efficacy of meprobamate was conflicting. Some studies have shown it to be better than a placebo in the relief of anxiety, and others have shown it to be superior to phenobarbitone (Black, 1969). A great difficulty in evaluating such studies is that the dosage of the substances compared is so important a factor. Meprobamate is usually given in a dose of 400 mg 3 times a day when used as a sedative, and in a larger dose when used as a hypnotic.

MEPROBAMATE

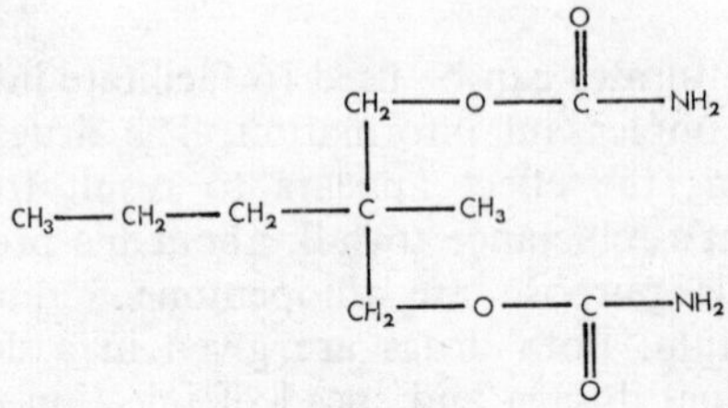

$$CH_2\!-\!O\!-\!C\!-\!NH_2$$

$$CH_3\!-\!CH_2\!-\!CH_2\!-\!C\!-\!CH_3$$

$$CH_2\!-\!O\!-\!C\!-\!NH_2$$

Meprobamate has slight advantages over barbiturates as regards adverse effects, but these have proved to be very similar to those induced by the barbiturates. The drug induces a state of intoxication with drowsiness, incoordination and slurred speech; it is capable of producing dependency; and its abrupt withdrawal results in an abstinence syndrome with insomnia, vomiting, tremors, ataxia, anxiety and frequently fits (Essig, 1966). It has been used successfully in suicidal attempts.

A variety of new hypnotics and sedatives have been produced in the past few years. The history of thalidomide is too well known to require repetition; it is, however, a reminder that all medication should be avoided unless it is really required.

Glutethimide (Doriden) is chemically related to the barbiturates; it has been shown to have hypnotic effects but, like the barbiturates and meprobamate, can give rise to dependency and its withdrawal leads to an abstinence syndrome including fits. It is prescribed in a dosage of 250–500 mg.

Mandrax, another popular new tablet contains a new substance methaqualone and an antihistamine, diphenhydramine. It is an active hypnotic but, like the barbiturates and other drugs, potentiates the effects of alcohol and can induce dependency.

Benzodiazepines. In recent years the benzodiazepines have come into widespread use as sedatives and hypnotics. The structural formulae of chlordiazepoxide (Librium) and diazepam (Valium) illustrate the chemical basis of this class of compounds.

CHLORDIAZEPOXIDE

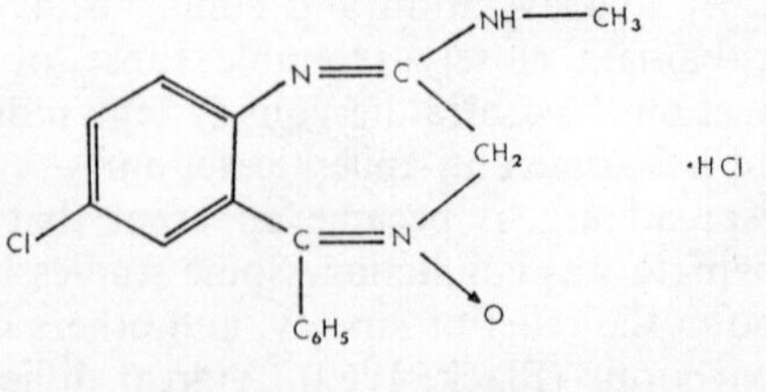

DIAZEPAM

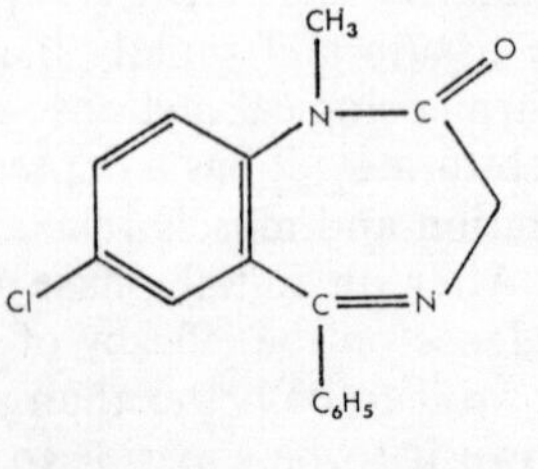

·HCl

Apart from their sedative effects the benzodiazepines are muscle relaxants, anti-convulsants and appetite stimulants. Although they vary in potency, diazepam being two to three times more potent than chlordiazepoxide, their pharmacodynamic actions are generally similar. They have been shown to have a taming effect in a variety of animals.

Clinical trials have shown varying results, but some evidence suggests that they are about as effective as barbiturates in the treatment of anxiety (Capstick *et al.*, 1965; McDowall, Owen & Robin, 1966). Their main advantage lies in their relative safety; ingestion of large doses has been followed by survival (Hines, 1960; Tobin, 1964).

Diazepam and chlordiazepoxide can be used in most circumstances in which a mild sedative is required. As a sedative chlordiazepoxide is prescribed in a dosage of 10–20 mg tds and diazepam 2–10 mg tds. An additional dose at night may help to induce sleep in tense patients. Diazepam is also widely used as an anticonvulsant and can be given by intravenous injection in status epilepticus (Lombroso, 1966). Nitrazepam (Mogadon) is used mainly as a hypnotic in a dosage of 5–10 mg.

Adverse effects include rashes, drowsiness, lapses of attention, confusional episodes, ataxia, slurred speech, and excessive weight gain. Physical dependence can be produced and withdrawal is followed by an abstinence syndrome which includes fits (Hollister, Motzenbecker & Degan, 1961).

In their actions the benzodiazepines resemble the barbiturates in many respects. It is wise to warn patients of the likelihood of drowsiness, the danger of driving and the potentiating effect of alcohol.

Phenothiazines

The discovery and development of the phenothiazine derivatives have constituted a major advance in the chemotherapy of mental illness. Chlorpromazine (Largactil, Thorazine) was the product of a systematic examination of these compounds in France during the late 1940s. It was first used as a pre-medication for general anaesthesia and was later found to be useful in sedating disturbed patients. Delay and his colleagues described its value in the management of excitement, and subsequently Delay & Deniker (1952) evaluated the drug more systematically in a variety of psychiatric conditions. Many other phenothiazines have since been developed. They are frequently referred to as 'tranquillisers', as opposed to 'sedatives', because of their property of controlling hyperactive and aggressive behaviour without impairment of consciousness and withdrawal phenomena.

Pharmacology. All the phenothiazine compounds are modifications of the basic molecule. The drugs vary in their potency, sedative effects, antihistamine effects and unwanted effects. The substitution of the chlorine atom in position 2 of the phenothiazine molecule by a fluorine atom greatly increases its potency; similarly, the replacement of the side-chain in chlorpromazine, position 10, by a piperazine side-chain results in an increase in potency and a corresponding increase in extra-pyramidal effects. The drugs fall into three main groups, depending on the nature of the side-chains:

1. Those compounds with an aliphatic side-chain terminating in a dimethylamine group in position 10. Chlorpromazine is the best-known drug of this type.
2. Those compounds with a piperadine ring at the end of the side-chain in position 10, represented by thoridazine (Melleril).

3. Those compounds with a piperazine ring at the end of a side-chain in position 10, represented by trifluoperazine (Stelazine).

Although the different side-chains alter the potency of the molecules, the pharmacodynamic actions are sufficiently similar for them to be outlined together.

GENERAL FORMULA of the PHENOTHIAZINES

CHLORPROMAZINE

THIORIDAZINE HYDROCHLORIDE

TRIFLUOPERAZINE

The phenothiazine derivatives are rapidly absorbed when given by mouth. They are widely distributed in all the tissues and reach relatively high concentration in all parts of the brain, but particularly in the mid-brain. Chlorpromazine is metabolised to a large number of substances, some of which may be biologically active in their own right. The processes involved are sulphoxidation, hydroxylation, demethylation, n-oxidation and conjugation to form glucuronates. Some unchanged drug is excreted in the urine and faeces. There is wide individual variation in the precise routes of metabolism and the speed at which it occurs. Phenothiazine drugs, to varying degrees, exhibit the following properties; sedation, anti-emetic effects, and some antagonism to adrenaline, acetyl-choline, 5-hydroxytryptamine and to histamine.

Whereas barbiturates depress the responsiveness of the reticular formation in the cat to direct stimulation, chlorpromazine induces minor changes of this kind but brings about a marked rise in the threshold to auditory stimuli. Bradley (1963) has suggested that chlorpromazine selectively depresses the effect of afferent impulses on the reticular formation. Conversely, Killam (1962) has suggested that chlorpromazine increases the flow of afferent impulses to the reticular formation but at the same time increases the selectivity of the filtering mechanisms within the reticular formation, leading to a reduction in efferent impulses. This worker also suggests that chlorpromazine can cause 'cortical blockade' although it appears to have little direct effect on the cortex itself. It will probably be necessary to study the effect of chlorpromazine on different parts of the brain separately before being able to understand its overall effect. Chlorpromazine is capable of suppressing 'sham-rage' in cats in which the brain has been sectioned above the hypothalamus, suggesting that it can act at that site (Dasgupta *et al.*, 1954). In epileptic patients chlorpromazine increases the frequency of paroxysmal discharges and wave and spike complexes.

Clinical effects. At the time of its introduction chlorpromazine was used mainly to control the behaviour of violently disturbed patients, whether suffering from schizophrenia, affective states, acute and chronic brain syndromes or behaviour disorders. The phenothiazines are still prescribed for a variety of disorders but are of greatest importance in the treatment of acute and chronic schizophrenia and of mania. They are also employed in the treatment of some non-psychiatric conditions.

The schizophrenias. The action of phenothiazines on the schizophrenias should probably be regarded as non-specific and symptomatic rather than as a specific 'anti-psychotic' effect. There is, nevertheless, considerable evidence in favour of the efficacy of phenothiazines in the treatment of some forms of schizophrenia. For example, in the large-scale double-blind study of newly admitted acute schizophrenics conducted by the United States Psychopharmacology Service Center Collaborative Study Group (1964) groups of patients were treated with chlorpromazine, another phenothiazine or a placebo on a flexible dosage schedule. At the end of 6 months the global assessments of progress which were carried out on the patients remaining in the trial showed that they all tended to be improved but of those on the drugs 75 per cent were rated as 'much' or 'very much' improved, whereas fewer than 40 per cent of those on the placebo were so rated. In addition, those patients who deteriorated proved to be on the placebo while none of the drug treated group were worse. These global improvements were supported by a more detailed study of the changes in individual symptoms.

The advantages of continued phenothiazine treatment in chronic schizophrenia have been less clear-cut. Factors other than drug taking can bring about improvements in the social activities of chronic patients (Wing & Freudenberg, 1961). Symptoms do not always return or worsen if drugs are withdrawn but there is some evidence that maintenance therapy with drugs allows some patients to lead a more normal life. One study, for example, has shown that patients receiving a placebo for 6 months suffered from more hallucinations and delusions, were less well orientated, had less coherent speech, and performed more rituals than patients receiving drugs for some part of that period (Good, Sterling & Holtman, 1958). Another investigation has suggested that patients receiving an active drug were out of hospital for longer than those receiving a placebo and that the advantage increased with time (Pasamanick *et al.*, 1964).

A recent study, performed under the auspices of the Medical Research Council, of patients who had recovered from a schizophrenic illness showed that during the first year of follow-up those given a phenothiazine had a lower chance of recurrence than those receiving placebo (Leff & Wing, 1971). It should be noted, however, that this study was carried out on a selected group of patients; patients were excluded if they were so much at risk that they could not be given the placebo or so well that the risk of recurrence did not justify continued medication.

Controlled studies have indicated that among the various phenothiazine derivatives trifluoperazine is more effective than chlorpromazine in the treatment of paranoid as opposed to undifferentiated schizophrenia (Childers & Therrien, 1961) and also of withdrawn schizophrenics (Gwynne et al., 1962). Thioridazine has been shown to be as effective as chlorpromazine without inducing as much extra-pyramidal symptomatology (Herman & Pleasure, 1963). However, the U.S. Psychopharmacology Centers Collaborative Study showed no differences between chlorpromazine, fluphenazine (Moditen) and thioridazine in the treatment of acute schizophrenics when a flexible dosage schedule was employed (1964).

Other psychiatric conditions. Chlorpromazine and other phenothiazines can be helpful in mania and hypomania (Lehmann, 1954) and can also be helpful in other states where agitation and overactivity are prominent, such as agitated depression (Hollister, 1967). Phenothiazines have also been used to manage delirium tremens and the withdrawal of dependence-inducing drugs and alcohol, and to stimulate appetite in anorexia nervosa.

Non-psychiatric conditions. Phenothiazines have been used as sedatives in a variety of conditions. Chlorpromazine and thioridazine are the best drugs for this purpose; a dosage of 25–75 mg tds will generally be adequate.

Chlorpromazine has proved to be of value in the treatment of tetanus on account of its muscle relaxant properties (Laurence & Webster, 1963). Phenothiazines are also useful as anti-emetics, especially prochlorperazine (Stemetil) which can be given orally, by injection, or rectally as a suppository, and may be particularly helpful for patients having irradiation. Chlorpromazine in a dose of 50 mg by intra-muscular injection can be invaluable in the suppression of intractable hiccough, even when this is caused by malignant tumours invading the phrenic nerves.

Phenothiazines are widely used as an adjunct to analgesic therapy. Chlorpromazine is used with a variety of opiates in terminal malignancy and can be given orally or by injection. Promazine (Sparine), a very weak phenothiazine drug, is administered by intravenous injection with pethidine to facilitate forceps delivery with pudendal block but without general anaesthesia. It should be noted that phenothiazines given with analgesics, particularly opiates, may produce severe hypotension which might carry a serious outcome in conditions such as myocardial infarction where the blood pressure can already be depressed.

Paradoxically, chlorpromazine can be effective in some cases of hemibalismus and senile chorea.

Adverse effects. Although there is some variation in the severity of particular unwanted effects induced by therapeutic doses of particular preparations, in their major unwanted effects the phenothiazines resemble each other.

Central nervous system. Drowsiness is common and is most frequently produced by chlorpromazine and thioridazine. This effect generally declines after a few days administration of the drug.

A Parkinsonian state can be induced by all phenothiazine compounds when they are given in sufficiently large doses. In therapeutic dosage thioridazine is less likely to produce this effect. Other extra-pyramidal syndromes associated most frequently with the administration of drugs closely related to trifluoperazine include akathisia, in which there is uncontrollable restlessness and movements of the limbs, and dystonic reactions in which grimacing, jerky non-repetitive movements of the face, limbs and tongue and abnormal postures of neck, head and limbs are seen. The suggestion that the phenothiazines act by inducing a Parkinsonian syndrome, with slowing of thought and action, and that the appearance of these symptoms is essential to their therapeutic effect is not generally supported (Cole & Clyde, 1961). Extrapyramidal syndromes associated with the phenothiazines are generally reversible, but cases of dyskinesias persisting after the withdrawal of drugs have been reported (Uhbrand & Faurbye, 1960). These cases of 'tardive dyskinesias' have mainly occurred in female patients with brain damage, occasionally due to leucotomy.

Chlorpromazine is known to increase synchronisation in the electroencephalogram, with an increase in paroxysmal discharges, and can induce fits, especially in patients with a history of epilepsy (Rickels, 1963).

Autonomic nervous system. The phenothiazines can induce hypotension and tachycardia, both effects being attributed to anti-adrenergic effects of the drug. The inhibition of ejaculation associated with thioridazine is probably due to the same mechanism.

The frequently observed anti-cholinergic effects include blurring of vision, constipation, dryness of the mouth and retention of urine. These effects should be remembered in the presence of prostatic hypertrophy and in glaucoma.

Miscellaneous. The various endocrine effects which occasionally result from the administration of phenothiazines include disturbances of menstruation, galactorrhoea and impotence.

Electro-cardiographic changes have been reported and resemble those seen after quinidine administration. Cases of sudden death have been recorded which are probably related to the cardiovascular effects of the drugs (Hollister & Kosek, 1965).

Lenticular and corneal opacities as well as pigmentation of the retina can occur when administration is long continued.

The jaundice reported in association with chlorpromazine and other phenothiazines is usually accompanied by pyrexia, nausea and eosinophilia. It is believed to be a hypersensitivity reaction resulting in obstruction of the small bile ducts through the swelling of the lining cells and to be unassociated with widespread cellular damage. Clinical recovery usually occurs in about one month, but it may take longer for pathological tests to return to normal.

Blood dyscrasias have been reported and may affect various series of blood cells.

A sensitivity of the skin to sunlight frequently develops during the course of administration of the phenothiazines. Skin sensitivity may develop among the staff who handle phenothiazines. Protection from the drug by the wearing of gloves is the only effective prophylactic measure.

Dependency does not occur.

Administration. The phenothiazines are administered for a variety of psychiatric conditions but are particularly important in the treatment of the schizophrenias. As these drugs can obscure the clinical features of a mental illness they should be prescribed whenever possible only after a definite diagnosis has been made, unless there are pressing reasons for doing otherwise. Caution is particularly important when a diagnosis of schizophrenia is being considered, as it carries such serious implications for prognosis and further management. While the depressant action of the phenothiazines is of value in the management of other psychiatric syndromes such as agitation, delirium and severe tension states, these compounds are best avoided in the milder psychiatric conditions for which equally effective alternatives are available, often carrying a lower risk of unwanted effects.

In general, chlorpromazine and thioridazine are the drugs of choice in controlling excited patients. They can be given by mouth or injection, according to the clinical requirements. The usual dosage is 25–100 mg tds but much larger doses can be prescribed when necessary. In the excited patient 50–100 mg of either drug by intra-muscular injection is quickly effective and can be repeated.

Trifluoperazine (1–10 mg tds) and fluphenazine (1–4 mg bd) are more suitable for the withdrawn apathetic schizophrenic. They are, in general, unsuitable for the excited patient.

In the long-term treatment of schizophrenia it is common practice to administer phenothiazine drugs for a period of six to twelve months. Towards the end of this period the drug is gradually withdrawn. If symptoms recur as the dosage is reduced it may be necessary to continue medication for a longer period, but it should be remembered that some patients suffer from recurrent schizophrenic episodes with prolonged periods of remission.

For those patients who appear to require continuous medication over a long period it is worth considering the use of the recently introduced long-acting phenothiazines. Their main advantage is to ensure that the patient has received the drug, but they are less satisfactory than more frequently administered medication in achieving good control of symptoms in acute conditions. The drugs now available are derivatives of the very potent drug, fluphenazine: they are fluphenazine enanthate (Moditen enanthate) and fluphenazine decanoate (Modecate). These drugs are given by deep intra-muscular injection in sesame oil in doses of 12·5–25 mg every 2–4 weeks. The long duration of action is attributed to two factors: the drug is slowly released from an oil-tissue depot and then de-esterification slowly releases the free fluphenazine base. Several workers have compared the effects of these drugs, administered as described, with several phenothiazines given orally, and have shown them to be comparable in effect with other drug treatments and superior to a placebo (Bankier, Pettit & Bergen, 1968; Ravaris, Weaver & Brooks, 1965; van Praag *et al.*, 1970). They are of special value in the long-term management of chronic schizophrenic patients, many of whom are known to be unreliable in taking drugs, especially when their illnesses have paranoid features (Wilson & Enoch, 1967). Precautions are necessary in their use: they should only be given to patients who have responded to fluphenazine without serious side-effects, and provision should be made for continued psychiatric supervision, rehabilitation and social support. Recently cases of suicide have been attributed to the action of these drugs and although the relationship is tenuous this possibility should be borne in mind (de Alarcon & Carney, 1969).

It is a matter of personal preference whether to prescribe anti-Parkinsonian drugs routinely or only when side-effects demand them. When a new patient is receiving phenothiazines for the first time in large doses, alarming and unexpected side-effects might make subsequent treatment more difficult: for these patients it is probably best to give a drug such as orphenadrine hydrochloride (Disipal) 50 mg 3 times a day, benztropine methanesulphonate (Cogentin) 1–2 mg twice daily, procyclidine hydrochloride (Kemadrin) 5 mg 3 times a day or benzhexol (Artane) 1–2 mg 3 times a day from the beginning. All these drugs can be administered parenterally in the treatment of severe dystonic symptoms of acute onset. In patients with chronic illness receiving small doses of drugs, remedies for Parkinsonism may be unnecessary. In the case of long-acting phenothiazines troublesome Parkinsonism may occur in the few days after the injection, and anti-Parkinsonian drugs given from the second to the tenth day may be quite sufficient. There is a tendency for the Parkinsonism induced by a fixed dosage of drugs to diminish as time passes.

Rauwolfia derivatives

For many years substances derived from the plant *Rauwolfia serpentina* have been used in India to treat a variety of illnesses. In Western medicine a purified alkaloid derivative, reserpine, has been used since the 1950s in the treatment of hypertension and as a 'tranquilliser' in psychiatry. More recently synthetic reserpine-like compounds have been produced, of which the best known is tetrabenazine, a benzoquinolizine derivative.

Pharmacology. The main effect of reserpine in the brain is to bring about a depletion of amines over the course of a few weeks (Lewis, 1963). Some workers hold that sedation only occurs when indole amines are reduced in concentration (Brodie *et al.*, 1960). Others claim that catecholamine depletion is more important in causing sedation and support this claim by showing that the effect of reserpine on the brain amines can be reversed by the administration of dihydroxyphenlalanine, a precursor of the catecholamines (Carlsson, Lindquist & Magnusson, 1957). It has become customary to use animals in which the brain amines have been depleted by reserpine administration for a variety of pharmacological experiments, mainly relating to the anti-depressant drugs. The hypotensive effect of reserpine may be caused by the effect of the decline in brain amine concentration in the sympathetic centres. Other autonomic effects are common and include brachycardia, flushing, nasal congestion and diarrhoea. Reserpine has a taming effect on a variety of animals.

Tetrabenazine resembles reserpine in all its actions but it is much less potent in reducing the concentration of brain amines, although it acts more quickly.

Clinical effects. As a hypotensive agent reserpine is giving way to newer and more effective preparations with less severe unwanted effects. In the

RESERPINE

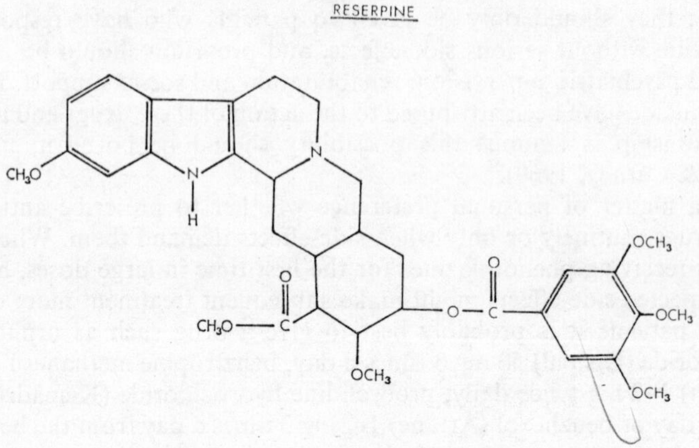

CH_3O N   H   N

CH_3O-C O $O-C$ OCH_3 OCH_3 OCH_3

OCH_3

TETRABENAZINE

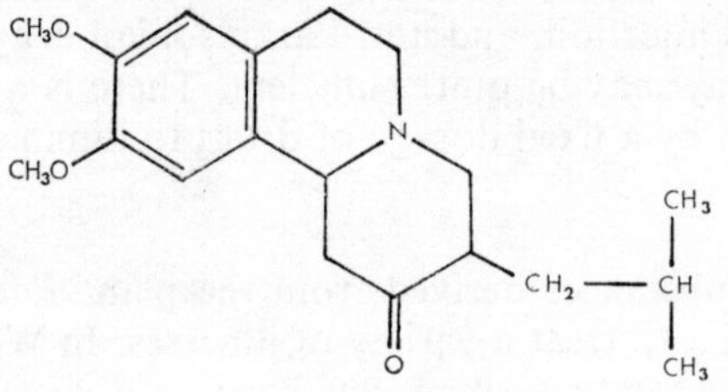

CH_3O
CH_3O N   O CH_2-CH CH_3 CH_3

practice of clinical psychiatry the use of reserpine has greatly diminished but it has retained scientific interest for a number of reasons, mainly arising from its adverse effects.

In man reserpine has a calming effect which has been used in psychiatry in the treatment of schizophrenia, particularly in controlling over-activity, restlessness and violence, and in other psychiatric conditions with similar symptoms. Apart from the problems raised by its unwanted effects, reserpine has been shown to be generally less effective in the treatment of schizophrenia than the phenothiazines (Shepherd & Watt, 1956).

Both reserpine and tetrabenazine reduce choreiform movements and have been found to be valuable in the management of movement disorders. Reports have been made of their use in Huntington's chorea (Brandrup, 1969; Sattes, 1960) and more recently they have been given successfully in a variety of dystonic conditions, including dystonia musculorum deformans and those following chronic phenothiazine administration. Tetrabenazine appears to be more effective than reserpine, producing a greater degree of improvement and being effective in a larger proportion of cases.

Adverse effects. Apart from the autonomic effects of reserpine which may be unpleasant, the principal unwanted effects are depression and Parkinsonism. The administration of reserpine can be followed by severe depression (Muller *et al.*, 1955) and there is evidence from the examination of the brains of people who have committed suicide that depletion of brain amines can accompany naturally occurring depression in man (Shaw, Camps & Eccleston, 1967). Parkinsonism is a common unwanted effect and, like naturally occurring Parkinson's Disease, may also be associated with a depletion of amines in the brain stem. Thus the two main unwanted effects of reserpine appear to be closely related to its major pharmacological action. The adverse effects of tetrabenazine are very similar.

Butyrophenones

Pharmacology. The butyrophenones are chemically related to pethidine. Their properties clearly resemble those of the phenothiazines. They have very few autonomic effects but they induce hypotension and brachycardia.

HALOPERIDOL

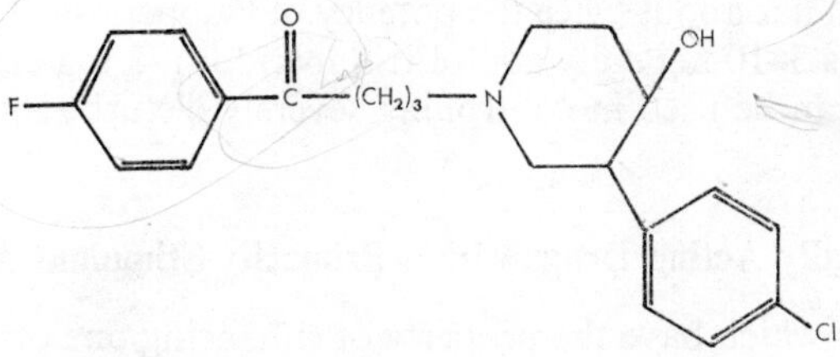

TRIFLUPERIDOL

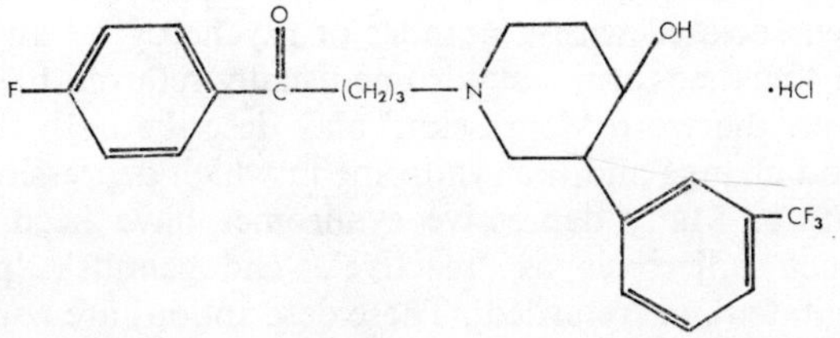

Clinical effects. Haloperidol (Serenace) has been shown to be comparable in clinical effects to chlorpromazine (Kristjansen, 1966). Early hopes that the drugs would be especially effective in mania have not been fulfilled. Haloperidol compares favourably with chlordiazepoxide when used in the treatment of anxiety states (Greenberg, 1970). The butyrophenones have also been shown to be effective in the treatment of tics in adolescent patients and to be superior, in this respect, to diazepam and a placebo (Connell et al., 1967).

Butyrophenones can be used to produce a state of quiescence and 'psychic indifference' which allows minor operative procedures to be performed without general anaesthesia. This state has come to be known as 'neuroleptanalgesia'. In the technique, the drug droperidol is given by slow intravenous injection with an opiate such as pethidine. Assisted respiration is frequently necessary during the procedure and it is necessary to block the cardio-vascular effects of the drug with atropine. The method is still being evaluated (Shephard, 1965).

Adverse effects. Both haloperidol and trifluperidol (Triperidol) frequently induce Parkinsonism which can be relieved by anticholinergic drugs or by reducing the dose. The butyrophenones potentiate the effects of many sedative drugs, including barbiturates and opiates. There have been many reports of the butyrophenones precipitating depression; this possibility should always be borne in mind, especially when the drugs are used in the treatment of affective disorders (Gerle, 1964). Hypotension is a common unwanted effect. Rashes, agranulocytosis and jaundice have been reported less commonly.

Administration. The indications for the use of the butyrophenones are very similar to those for the phenothiazines: they are particularly useful in the treatment of schizophrenic patients who are sensitive to phenothiazine drugs.

Trifluperidol has about twice the potency of haloperidol. The normal dose of haloperidol is 3–10 mg daily and of trifluperidol 1–3 mg daily, but a much higher dosage can be used in controlling severely disturbed patients.

Centrally Acting Drugs with a Primarily Stimulant Action

Although drugs which have the property of enhancing one or more functions of the central nervous system have come to be widely employed in clinical practice, the use of the term 'depression' can give rise to great confusion. In its pharmacological connotation it signifies a reduction in the activity of an organ or function. As a clinical concept it denotes a morbid change in mood which may be associated with a number of psychological and physiological changes which together form a syndrome usually referred to as a depressive illness. However, the word 'depression' may describe both the symptom of depressive mood change and the syndrome in which depression of mood is a prominent feature. Many depressive syndromes have been described and labelled by such adjectives as 'reactive', 'endogenous', 'puerperal', 'involutional', 'agitated', or 'retarded'. These descriptions are based on different aspects of the condition, sometimes a prominent aetiological factor, sometimes the age group affected, and sometimes the leading clinical features. Depressive states also occur in association with other psychiatric conditions such as schizophrenia, obsessional illness, and organic conditions. In view of these observations it is not surprising that controversies have occurred over the classification of depressive disorders which, in turn, lead to difficulties in assessing treatments of them.

Amphetamines

The amphetamines have been used for many years in combating fatigue in service personnel and in the treatment of various medical disorders.

Pharmacology. A number of preparations have been used of which amphetamine and methylamphetamine are the most common. The D-isomers are the more active.

AMPHETAMINE SULPHATE   METHYLAMPHETAMINE

$$\text{CH}_2\text{—CH—NH}_2 \cdot \tfrac{1}{2}\text{H}_2\text{SO}_4 \qquad\qquad \text{CH}_2\text{—CH—NH—CH}_3 \cdot \text{HCl}$$

The drugs appear to have a directly stimulating effect on the ascending reticular activating system. They cause tachycardia, a rise in blood pressure and mydriasis; they suppress appetite, probably by a direct action on the hypothalamus. Amphetamines potentiate the tricyclic and monoamine oxidase-inhibiting antidepressants and reverse the effects of reserpine. Behaviourally, the amphetamines induce restlessness, over-activity and elation of mood, and they increase both physical performance and endurance.

Clinical effects. Though the amphetamines have long been used alone and in combination with barbiturates for the treatment of mild depressive disorders, such as those which occasionally follow virus infections, a collaborative trial in which amphetamine (10–15 mg daily) was given to acutely depressed patients seen in general practice, showed it to be no better than a placebo (General Practitioner Clinical Trials, 1964). The amphetamines have also been prescribed as anorexics; to help in the disclosure of unpleasant material in abreactive or psychotherapeutic interviews; in the treatment of nocturnal enuresis; and for their paradoxical sedative effect in overactive children and some psychopathic disorders. The amphetamines facilitate conditioned learning but the learned behaviour is more readily extinguished (Turner & Young, 1966). Amphetamines have also been used in the treatment of narcolepsy for some years (Prinzmetal & Bloomberg, 1935): because of the serious unwanted effects (*vide infra*) and the absence of an effective alternative, this is probably the only condition in which their therapeutic use is now justifiable.

Adverse effects. The amphetamines induce anxiety, irritability, restlessness, insomnia, shaking, dryness of the mouth, palpitations, headache, impotence and anorexia. As the effects of the drugs wear off, activity decreases and the subject experiences a lowering of mood which may be unpleasant. Large doses of amphetamines can induce a psychotic illness with hallucinations and paranoid delusions, which is clinically indistinguishable from acute schizophrenia (Connell, 1958). Some of these psychoses persist after withdrawal of the drugs.

The greatest recent advance in knowledge of the characteristics of the amphetamines has been the full realisation of their addictive properties (Kiloh & Brandon, 1962). The dangers of dependency and of serious withdrawal effects have been greatly increased by the popularity of the amphetamine/barbiturate mixtures in the treatment of affective disorders prior to the introduction of the tricyclic and monoamine oxidase inhibiting antidepressant drugs. Attempts are being made to reduce the manufacture and stocking of the amphetamines in some areas by a voluntary ban on prescriptions, thereby reducing the risk of theft. It has recently been shown that voluntary restraint of this kind can lead to a reduction in the rate at which new addicts present for treatment (Wells, 1970).

Administration. When administration is indicated the amphetamines are generally given in a dosage of 5–10 mg twice daily, with one dose on waking and one at midday. Slow release capsules of 15 mg given in the morning may be found to be convenient for some patients.

Methylamphetamine for intravenous injection is no longer generally available.

Other stimulants

Cocaine. Cocaine was used by the Peruvian Indians to increase physical endurance. In its use as a stimulant it has been superseded by other drugs on account of its addictive properties.

Caffeine occurs naturally in tea and coffee and has been used in some analgesic tablets although it is not an analgesic itself. It possesses mild stimulant properties but has no application in psychiatry.

The anti-depressants

Until the mid-1950s the principal forms of physical treatment in general use for depressive illness were electro-convulsive therapy (E.C.T.) and one or other of the amphetamine preparations. In these circumstances the discovery of several new drugs with supposedly anti-depressant properties was widely welcomed. The anti-depressant drugs are of two main types: the tricyclic drugs and the monoamine oxidase inhibiting drugs.

Tricyclic anti-depressant drugs

In 1948 the possible antihistaminic, sedative and anti-Parkinsonian properties of the substituted iminodibenzyls were first investigated. Later, when the therapeutic properties of the phenothiazines were discovered there was further interest in these compounds, which resemble chlorpromazine chemically. A trial of imipramine hydrochloride (Tofranil) in chronic psychotic patients was carried out by Kuhn who unexpectedly reported that some patients showed an elevation in mood. Subsequently Kuhn (1958) administered imipramine to a large number of depressed patients and confirmed his earlier observation of its effect on mood. His observations have been fully confirmed by subsequent work and demonstrate the value of meticulously executed, open, uncontrolled trials in the early evaluation of new treatments.

Pharmacology. Among the most commonly used tricyclic antidepressants are *imipramine hydrochloride* (in desipramine one CH_3 group is replaced by H) and *amitriptyline* (in nor-triptyline one CH- radicle is replaced by H). The drugs are rapidly and completely absorbed when given by mouth, reach high levels in the plasma, are widely distributed in the tissues, and attain a relatively high concentration in the brain. In the plasma the drugs are approximately 90 per cent bound to protein, almost irrespective of concentration. The drugs are metabolised in the body and only a small percentage of the unchanged drug is excreted in the urine and faeces (Sjöqvist *et al.*, 1967). Imipramine is metabolised by demethylation, hydroxylation and conjugation to form glucuronates (Crammer, Scott & Rolfe, 1969). Of the metabolites of imipramine desmethylimipramine is certainly active pharmacologically. The metabolism of other tricyclic drugs has been less fully studied. Brodie's hypothesis (1965) that responders to imipramine metabolise imipramine more slowly and consequently excrete less of its metabolites in the urine has not been confirmed (Elkes, 1968).

IMIPRAMINE HYDROCHLORIDE

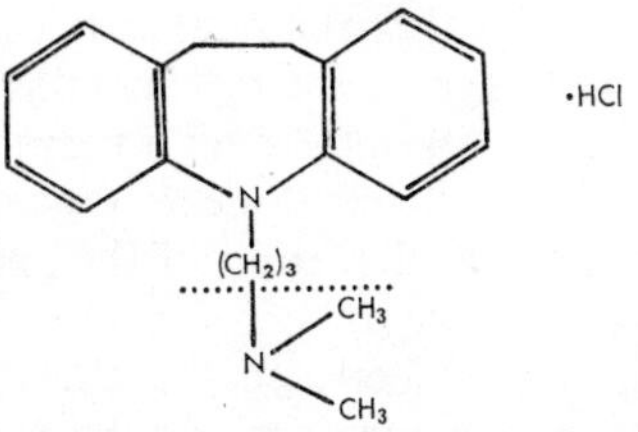

AMITRIPTYLINE

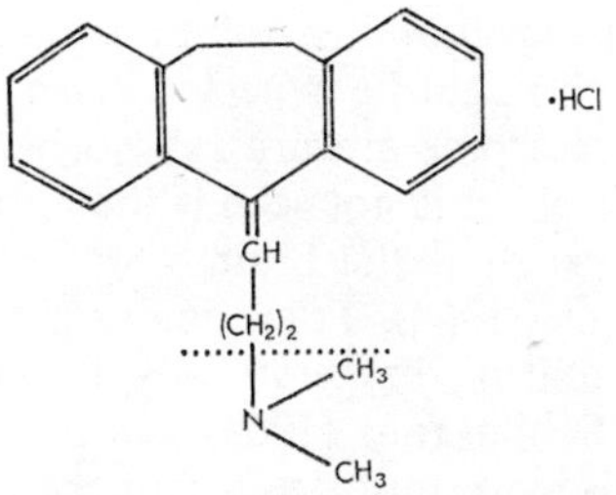

DESIPRAMINE HYDROCHLORIDE

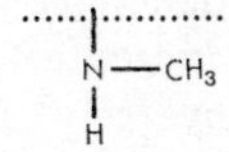

NORTRIPTYLINE HYDROCHLORIDE

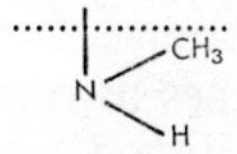

In many of their properties the tricyclic anti-depressants resemble chlorpromazine; they all have anticholinergic effects similar to those of atropine and potentiate the effects of many other substances, such as nor-adrenaline, amphetamine and lysergic acid.

Studies of the plasma levels of tricyclic anti-depressants have been of two main types; those using a loading dose and studying its subsequent elimination, and those studying the 'steady state' plasma levels of the drugs. Haydu, Dhrymiotis & Quinn (1962) claimed that a high plasma level following a loading dose was associated with rapid excretion and a poor therapeutic response; conversely, a low plasma level was associated with a low rate of excretion and a good therapeutic response. These findings have not been generally confirmed. Sjöqvist and his colleagues have found a forty-fold variation in the nortriptyline plasma levels of depressed patients: they have shown a direct relationship between plasma levels and the severity of side-effects, but so far have been unable to show a direct relationship between plasma levels and therapeutic effects. In one of their studies a knowledge of the plasma level of the drug was useful in one patient in that it revealed so low a level as to preclude therapeutic effects; in another patient a very high plasma level indicated a risk of serious adverse effects (Åsberg et al., 1970). Walter (1971) and Braithwaite et al. (1972) found higher plasma levels of tricyclic drugs in responders than in non-responders. In general, however, the results of the studies of plasma levels of these drugs have demonstrated no clear pattern.

A number of observations have suggested that tricyclic anti-depressants alter the permeability of the cell membrane and that this reduces the uptake of nor-adrenaline from the extracellular space. A variety of tricyclic anti-depressants have been shown to inhibit the absorption into the brain tissue of labelled nor-adrenaline injected into the ventricles of rats (Glowinski & Axelrod, 1964). Other studies have demonstrated that desipramine and protriptyline prevent the accumulation of nor-adrenaline, but not of dopamine, in the brain following a dose of dopa, after the intracellular storage sites had first been blocked with reserpine and the breakdown of accumulated amine by nialamide (Carlsson, 1966).

When reserpine is administered by injection to rats previously treated with desipramine, the animals exhibit hyperactivity instead of the sedation which might be expected. This observation suggests that the amines released by reserpine are not reabsorbed because of a change in the cell membrane. This effect is not seen if the reserpine is given in small doses over a period of hours, or if the brain stores of amines are first depleted (Sulzer, Bickel & Brodie, 1964). Tricyclic drugs do not appear to cause depletion of the amine content of the nerve cells themselves (Carlsson, 1966).

Schildkraut (1969) has reviewed the relationship between the effects of anti-depressant drugs and the biochemical changes which accompany them. In this field there are three well authenticated facts: all drugs which are effective anti-depressants bring about changes in the biochemistry or physiology of the brain; all drugs which elevate mood also increase the levels of biogenic amines at receptor sites in the brain and, conversely, drugs which depress the mood reduce these metabolites; deficiencies of serotonin, nor-adrenaline and their metabolites occur in some patients with affective disorders. However, although there appears to be good evidence that the tricyclic anti-depressant drugs do bring about changes in the movement of amines in the brain, this may not be their only effect, or even the one by which the anti-depressant effect is mediated.

Clinical effects. The results of over 100 trials have shown a variable but definite anti-depressant effect of the tricyclic drugs (Wechsler, Grosser & Greenblatt, 1965) and these have been confirmed by a large scale study conducted by the Medical Research Council. It has been claimed that the beneficial effects of tricyclic drugs are due to a non-specific sedation and are no more effective than those of thioridazine (Hollister et al., 1967; Paykel et al., 1968). It has since been shown that the drugs are only comparable in effect in the anxious and hostile patients and that retarded patients do better on tricyclic drugs. When effective, the action of imipramine on depressed mood generally develops slowly, sometimes taking four weeks to become evident. Individual variation of response is marked: some patients respond well, some partially and others not at all (Kuhn, 1958).

Several studies have attempted to discover whether continued administration of tricyclic drugs to patients who have recovered from a depressive illness prevents a recurrence of symptoms (Seager & Bird, 1962; Imlah, Ryan & Hamilton, 1964; Hordern et al., 1964; Kay, Fahy & Garside, 1970). They have all pointed to the relative benefits of patients on 'maintenance' treatment but in none of these studies was the advantage attributable solely to the effects of the drugs taken. A study conducted under the aegis of the Medical Research Council's Committee on Clinical Trials in Psychiatry has shown a clear advantage, in respect of the risk of relapse, to patients receiving an active drug in the 6 months following complete remission of symptoms, as compared with those receiving a placebo (Mindham, Howland & Shepherd, 1973).

Many new tricyclic compounds, chemically related to the earlier drugs, continue to appear. They have similar anti-depressant properties but induce different degrees of sedation. In general, amitriptyline (Tryptizol) and its congeners exert a more sedative action than those compounds closely related to imipramine. It is frequently claimed that new drugs act more quickly than the older ones; this has never been satisfactorily demonstrated, possibly because of the methodological difficulties in doing so (Edwards, 1965). A study of the treatment of depression in general practice has demonstrated that those patients who eventually responded to amitryptyline showed some improvement after only one week of treatment; however, the patients receiving amylobarbitone exhibited a similar degree of improvement after one week, suggesting that the improvement at that stage of treatment was largely attributable to a sedative rather than to an anti-depressant effect (Blashki, Mowbray & Davies, 1971).

Adverse effects. The most frequently reported unwanted effects are due to the anticholinergic properties of the tricyclic compounds. Åsberg *et al.* (1970) have shown the severity of unwanted effects of nor-triptyline (Allegron) to be directly related to the plasma levels of the drug. Dryness of the mouth, difficulty with visual accommodation, difficulty in initiating micturition, constipation, palpitations and postural hypotension are often encountered. Retention of urine, paralytic ileus and heart failure have been reported. Occasionally electrocardiographic changes resembling those produced by quinidine are seen. Recently cases of sudden death in patients with heart disease receiving amitriptyline have been recorded (Coull *et al.*, 1970).

Amitriptyline and related drugs often cause drowsiness but this usually becomes less troublesome after the first few days of administration. Imipramine can also induce drowsiness, but more often causes insomnia.

The tricyclic anti-depressants very occasionally precipitate excitement or even hypomania (Leyberg & Denmark, 1959). Visual hallucinations can occur, probably as the first symptoms of a toxic confusional state. Other effects include excessive sweating, dizziness, tremor, ataxia, Parkinsonism, lactation and oedema. Occasionally skin rashes and rarely agranuloctosis have been reported. Tricyclic anti-depressants are frequently taken in suicidal attemps which may be successful.

Monoamine oxidase inhibitors (MAOI's)

After the introduction of isoniazid and iproniazid in the treatment of pulmonary tuberculosis it was observed that the administration of both drugs could be associated with a euphoriant effect (Robitzek, 1952). Zeller & Barsky (1952) originally reported that iproniazid inhibited the action of monoamine oxidase enzymes and suggested that the stimulant effect of the drugs was due to a rise in brain amine concentration consequent upon a slowing down of their destruction. Since this time the monoamine oxidase inhibitors have been widely used in clinical psychiatry.

Pharmacology. There are two main groups of monoamine oxidase inhibitors, the hydrazine and non-hydrazine derivatives, of which iproniazid and tranylcypromine may be taken as respective representatives. Nialamide, isocarboxazid and phenelzine are chemically related to iproniazid.

IPRONIAZID   TRANYLCYPROMINE SULPHATE

Parnate

The drugs are rapidly absorbed, widely distributed and rapidly metabolised and excreted. They induce an increase in the amines in the brain, counteract the effect of reserpine in reducing brain amines and potentiate the action of amines or their precursors when they are given in the diet or by injection. Iproniazid causes over-activity, mydriasis and vaso-constriction in animals. Some of the effects of reserpine in animals, e.g. inactivity, fall in body temperature, hypotension and bradycardia are either reversed by iproniazid or prevented if the drug is administered before reserpine. The effects of tryptamine or tyramine are potentiated when these compounds are given to animals which have previously received iproniazid (Tedeschi, Tedeschi & Fellows, 1959).

Tranylcypromine has a chemical formula which closely resembles that of amphetamine and is both a stimulant and a monoamine oxidase inhibitor. However, the amphetamine-like actions are not marked until the dosage is well above that required for inhibition of monoamine oxidases.

Clinical effects. Controlled trials of the effects of monoamine oxidase inhibitors in depression have not upheld the exuberant early claims, and the firm evidence for the drugs being effective in the treatment of depression is unimpressive (see p. 320). Iproniazid (Marsilid), tranylcypromine (Parnate) and phenelzine (Nardil), a hydrazine derivative, appear to be the most pharmacologically active compounds (Bates & Douglas, 1961).

It has been suggested that the effects of the monoamine oxidase inhibiting drugs is mainly stimulant (Wittenborn et al., 1961). This is to some extent supported by the knowledge that tranylcypromine, which is both an active monoamine oxidase inhibitor and an amphetamine-like stimulant, has been shown to be superior to placebo in the treatment of reactive depression (Batholomew, 1962), whereas the evidence in favour of the effectiveness of those drugs with no amphetamine like action is less convincing. Several groups of workers have shown a potentiation of the effects of monoamine oxidase inhibiting drugs by amino-acids (Pollin, Cardon & Kety, 1961; Pare, 1963; Coppen, Shaw & Farrell, 1963). However attempts to demonstrate a direct correlation between the anti-depressant action of the drugs and their potency as monoamine oxidase inhibitors have not been successful (Pare & Sandler, 1959).

Claims have been made for the efficacy of the monoamine oxidase inhibiting drugs in the treatment of 'atypical' depressive states—characterised by phobias, hysterical conversion symptoms, a worsening of symptoms in the evenings and a failure to respond to electro-convulsive therapy (West & Dally, 1959)—and in the treatment of phobic anxiety states (Kelly *et al.*, 1970). These claims are all based on uncontrolled, retrospective studies.

Adverse effects. The monoamine oxidase inhibitors are associated with a number of autonomic unwanted effects, including blurring of vision, dry mouth, warm extremities, constipation, and difficulty in initiating micturition. Headaches, exacerbations of migraine, and oedema are occasionally seen. Some of the drugs induce drowsiness, others states of excitation, with restlessness, pressure of speech and insomnia. Liver damage, occasionally fatal, may be caused by hydrazine derivatives.

Drug interactions of the monoamine oxidase inhibitors with many compounds is well established and can be of great clinical importance. The actions of such widely prescribed drugs as barbiturates, opiates (especially pethidine), and sympathomimetic drugs, for example, can be potentiated. The practice of using monoamine oxidase inhibiting drugs with tricyclic anti-depressants, which has been claimed to be effective in the treatment of some refractory cases (Gander, 1965), can result in a state of excessive excitation.

The so-called 'cheese reaction' follows the ingestion of a variety of foodstuffs, including cheese, after an interval varying from 10 minutes to over 2 hours. The patient at first experiences a thumping of the heart and a throbbing of the blood vessels in the neck which is followed by severe pulsating headache of sudden onset, at first localised but soon spreading to involve the whole of the head. During the attacks patients may feel flushed, perspire freely, experience photophobia, feel nauseated, vomit, or complain of stiffness in the neck. The attacks last from a few minutes to several hours. The blood pressure rises rapidly in the attacks, the systolic pressure generally exceeding 200 mm Hg when headache is experienced. Recovery is generally complete but in some patients there is bleeding into the subarachnoid space which may be accompanied by neurological changes and occasionally causes death.

Since it was first observed many aspects of this reaction have been elucidated by clinical and pharmacological studies (Blackwell, 1963; Blackwell *et al.*, 1967). The reaction can occur in patients taking a variety of monoamine oxidase inhibitors in conjunction with many amine containing foods: it was reported in 4·3 per cent of a group of monoamine oxidase inhibiting drugs takers in one study and is five times more likely to occur with tranylcypromine than with phenelzine, though there is no known way of picking out those patients who are likely to have the attacks. Animal experiments have shown that the attacks are caused by pressor amines, such as tyramine, being absorbed directly from the gut. Normally these amines are metabolised in the gut wall by monoamine oxidases, but when the enzymes are inhibited by a monoamine oxidase inhibitor they can pass into the blood stream unchanged. Cheese, beer, yeast, meat extracts and broad beans are among the large number of foodstuffs containing amines capable of inducing this reaction and patients receiving monoamine oxidase inhibitors should be warned against them. The attacks can generally be aborted by the slow intravenous injection of up to 10 mg of phentolamine mesylate (Rogitine).

Comparison of effects of anti-depressant treatments

The action of the amphetamines on mood is transient and there appears to be no effect on the general course of depressive disorders. The newer anti-depressant drugs have a much slower onset of action but a much more sustained effect, although it is not clear whether they terminate an attack or merely suppress the symptoms until the illness has run its course.

Of the various studies which have compared the effects of drugs with each other and also with the effect of electro-convulsive therapy, the most impressive is that carried out under the aegis of the Medical Research Council which compared imipramine, phenelzine, electro-convulsive therapy and a placebo in the treatment of some 250 moderately severely depressed patients (MRC, 1965). While electro-convulsive therapy proved to be the most effective treatment in the short term, over a longer period the results with imipramine were very similar; about two thirds of the patients responded to both treatments, although it should be emphasised that some patients who failed to respond to imipramine subsequently recovered with electro-convulsive therapy. This result compares with a response rate of about one third among the patients receiving phenelzine or the placebo. Such evidence, taken in conjunction with the conflicting and never impressive results of trials of the monoamine oxidase inhibitors, suggests strongly that the tricyclic compounds are the more effective drugs in the treatment of moderately severe depression. Electro-convulsive therapy, however, remains the treatment of choice for more severe depressive illness.

Use of anti-depressant drugs in general medicine

All doctors see patients who have become depressed in association with physical disease. Depression may follow infections such as influenza; it may enter into the clinical picture of prolonged and painful illnesses such as rheumatoid arthritis or of debilitating conditions following accidents and operations where the pattern of life has been suddenly and drastically changed. Other patients will become depressed during the course of a terminal illness. The course of physical disease may bear a close relationship to psychological factors, as is well illustrated by many gastro-enterological conditions (Lennard-Jones, 1971). Depression following the death of a spouse or close friend is also common. Tricyclic anti-depressants will be the most useful drugs in the management of most of these cases, although some of them may prove to be very resistant to pharmacotherapy.

Many patients in good physical health are referred to general physicians because of somatic complaints. Some hypochondriacal disorders of this type, which can be very protracted and lead to multiple referrals, are associated with a disturbance of mood which may respond to anti-depressant medication even when the disturbance of affect is not conspicuous. General physicians will also see patients who have become depressed as a result of taking medication such as reserpine or corticosteroids. The depression in these cases may not be relieved by discontinuation of the offending drug; it can require anti-depressant treatment and admission to a psychiatric unit.

Many women with primarily affective disorders are referred to obstetricians and gynaecologists. The commonest symptoms are irritability and depression, often experienced pre-menstrually, and best treated with either sedatives or hormone treatment, rather than with anti-depressant drugs (Tonks, 1968). An unwanted pregnancy is often associated with an affective disorder: anti-depressants may be indicated but it is unwise to give them, or any other psychotropic drug, in the first 3 months of pregnancy as their effect on the foetus is so uncertain. Among puerperal psychiatric disorders depressive reactions are most frequent: some of these patients will require anti-depressant treatment but many of the minor affective disorders at this time require no medication. It has been estimated that about one woman in 500 requires inpatient treatment following confinement (Pitt, 1968).

Tricyclic anti-depressant drugs, although themselves capable of producing Parkinsonism, have been used successfully in the treatment of Parkinson's disease (Laitinen, 1969). This effect may be due to their anticholinergic properties, to their anti-depressant effects, or to both.

Several tricyclic anti-depressants have been used in the treatment of nocturnal enuresis in children. The effectiveness of imipramine as compared with a placebo was clearly demonstrated in a double-blind trial in which dosage was based on body area (Shaffer, Costello & Hill, 1968). Relapse commonly occurred when medication was stopped but there was a good response when it was recommenced.

Beneficial effects from monoamine oxidase inhibitors have been claimed in the treatment of angina pectoris, Raynaud's disease and peripheral circulatory disease and the effect attributed to a blockage of pain fibres by the drugs (Cesarman, 1959). These findings have not been generally confirmed.

Administration of anti-depressant drugs in depressive disorders

It should be stressed that the administration of drugs is only one aspect of the management of the depressed patient. Once the diagnosis of a depressive illness has been made and treatment initiated, it is necessary to follow the patient's progress and to look out for changes in his condition which may lead to suicide. Where a patient is treated at home it is essential that the relatives should fully appreciate the morbid nature of the patient's condition, be able to supervise his drug taking and be instructed to look out for signs of deterioration. Relatives can also play an important part in the patient's rehabilitation.

Where a patient is seriously suicidal or psychotic, admission to hospital is often indicated. The care of the patient will then fall to the psychiatrist who will have to decide between drug treatment and electro-convulsive therapy. In less severely ill patients, treatment with drugs will be the more usual course. The choice of a particular drug for the treatment of a depressed patient is to some extent a matter of personal preference, but there are a few general principles that help in selecting the most appropriate drug and its dosage. In the moderately severely depressed patient displaying a persistent morbid change in mood—possibly associated with feelings of guilt, self-depreciation, retardation of thought and action, disturbance of sleep and appetite, hypochondriasis and agitated behaviour, but *not* serious suicidal intentions—the choice is from one of the tricyclic drugs. When the patient is agitated, a drug like amitriptyline or nortriptyline is to be preferred because of their more sedative properties. Where lack of energy, listlessness and inertia are the dominant clinical features imipramine or desipramine is the more suitable drug.

In view of the mode of action of the tricyclic anti-depressants *it is essential to use a sufficient dosage for a sufficient period of time.* With most of these drugs 150 mg a day is an average dose but the optimum dosage is so variable that in each patient the dosage should be increased to the maximum that can be reasonably tolerated. Many doctors find it helpful to start with a modest dosage such as 25 mg 3 times a day and build it up over the course of the first week; others prefer to start with the full dosage. In some patients a dosage in excess of 300 mg a day may be required though, with elderly people especially, some caution is required because of the liability to develop a toxic confusional state on quite small doses. In the case of the more sedative tricyclic anti-depressant drugs a proportion of the daily dose can be given at night, thereby avoiding the addition of a hypnotic.

Once treatment is started it should be continued in full dosage for at least 4 weeks before the drug is abandoned unless serious deterioration demands that electro-convulsive therapy be given. When a patient fails to respond to a drug there is little point in switching to one which is closely related chemically, e.g. from imipramine to desipramine. Patients who suffer from recurrent illnesses tend to respond to the same drug each time and patients who are blood-relatives tend to respond to the same drugs (Angst, 1961). It has been shown that there is an hereditary factor in the control of plasma levels of nor-triptyline which may account for this finding (Alexanderson, Price Evans & Sjöqvist, 1969).

In *mild depressive disorders* a variety of regimens can be used. Where there is a fluctuating mental state, with an admixture of affective symptoms, a sedative drug like diazepam can be more useful than an anti-depressant. Some psychiatrists use the monoamine oxidase drugs for this type of condition, especially where phobias are part of the clinical picture. In clinical practice there do appear to be a small number of patients of this type who respond well to monoamine oxidase inhibiting drugs and it may be that these form so small a proportion of the total that they are obscured in clinical trials. However, in view of the serious toxic effects of the monoamine oxidase inhibitors and their very limited therapeutic efficacy it is probably un-justifiable to use them routinely for these mild depressive conditions. Where depression is deeper, a tricyclic drug is more appropriate. When the choice lies between a tricyclic drug and a monoamine oxidase inhibitor it is preferable to use the tricyclic drug first because the change to a monoamine oxidase inhibitor can be made immediately; when, on the other hand a monoamine oxidase inhibitor is prescribed first, 10 to 14 days must be allowed to elapse before the patient is given a tricyclic drug because of the possibility of a dangerous interaction.

A number of preparations are available which contain two or more psychotropic drugs in the same capsule or tablet, often a tricyclic anti-depressant combined with a benzodiazepine or a phenothiazine. Although these preparations have some advantage in respect of convenience of administration, it is generally better to use as few drugs as possible in a patient's treatment and to concentrate on administering the main therapeutic drug in optimal dosage. Where additional medication is required this can be prescribed separately and only for so long as necessary.

When any of the anti-depressant drugs are administered patients should be warned of their dangers. The tricyclic compounds may cause drowsiness which makes driving dangerous, and this effect is greatly enhanced by small amounts of alcohol. The dietary restrictions for patients on monoamine oxidase inhibitors should be explained in detail: recently attention has been drawn to the doctor's responsibility in informing the patient of them (*British Medical Journal*, 1970).

Psychotomimetic Drugs

Although many centrally acting drugs can occasionally precipitate psychotic reactions when administered in excessive dosage or to susceptible individuals, there is a group of drugs which, in relatively small dosage, more regularly induce marked changes in perception, mood and thought. Unlike the other psychotropic drugs the so called psychotomimetic drugs are primarily of interest because of their capacity to provoke mental abnormalities rather than to suppress them. The readiness with which the drugs induce changes in perception, states of ecstasy and mystical insight has led to their widespread use in religious ceremonies and by para-religious cults of various kinds. Many of the compounds occur naturally in various parts of the world and in some cases their psychological effects have been known for centuries. The best known psychotomimetic compounds are mescaline, lysergic acid diethylamide (Lysergide, L.S.D.), psilocybin, and phencyclidine. The pharmacological effects of an extract of the cactus peyotl was discovered by Lewin in 1888, and subsequently its active constituent, mescaline, was isolated. Lysergide was discovered in 1943 (Hofmann, 1959).

The resemblance between the states produced by the psychotomimetic drugs and naturally occurring psychiatric conditions, especially schizophrenia, has led to their use in research into the possible causes and treatment of the psychoses. In pursuing possible chemical causes of the psychoses it was suggested that substances with actions similar to those of the psychotomimetic drugs might be produced in the brain in the course of various diseases and give rise to mental symptoms. Chemical similarities between some metabolites of the catechol amines and mescaline prompted the adrenochrome hypothesis of the causation of schizophrenia (Hoffer, Osmond & Smythies, 1954). A number of naturally occurring substances which might be capable of producing hallucinations have been investigated but, so far, a satisfactory chemical basis for the symptoms of schizophrenia remains elusive. The states produced by the psychotomimetic drugs can also resemble a variety of other psychoses, including both the depressive and manic forms of the affective psychoses, epileptic psychoses and psychoses associated with structural brain damage, as well as the psychoses induced by other chemical agents.

On the supposition that substances which antagonise the effects of the psychotomimetic drugs in animals would be effective against the symptoms induced by the drugs in man, it was hoped that psychotomimetic drugs might be used to induce 'psychotic' behaviour in animals which would then be used to test the effects of various drugs. This expectation is to some degree fulfilled in that phenothiazines like chlorpromazine are usually effective in controlling the acute psychosis induced by lysergide as well as the symptoms of acute schizophrenia, but the method has been of less general use than might have been expected when applied to animals.

Pharmacology. The psychotomimetic drugs are of several clinical types: the phenylethylamines, of which mescaline is the best known; the lysergic acid derivatives, of which lysergic acid diethylamide is the best known; and the indoleamines, represented by psylocybin. There are, in addition, several other drugs of similar action but differing chemical structure. The relationship between structure and activity has been closely studied in the case of the piperidyl benzilate group and a high potency for psychological effects shown to be associated with the short aliphatic side-chains.

MESCALINE SULPHATE

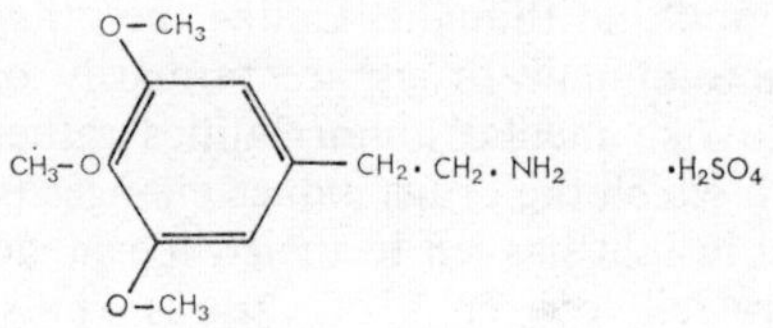

LYSERGIC ACID DIETHYLAMIDE

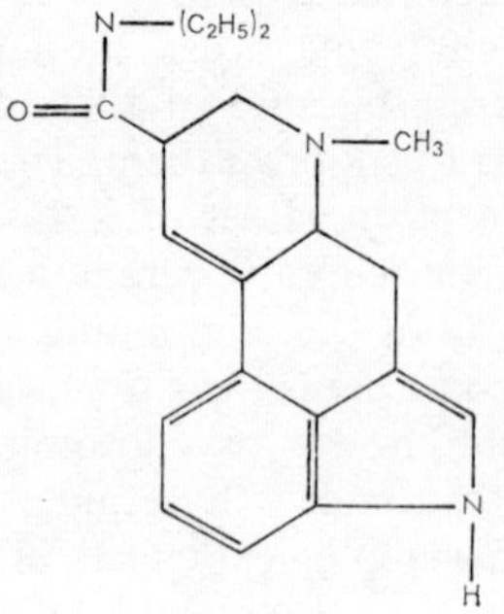

PSILOCYBIN

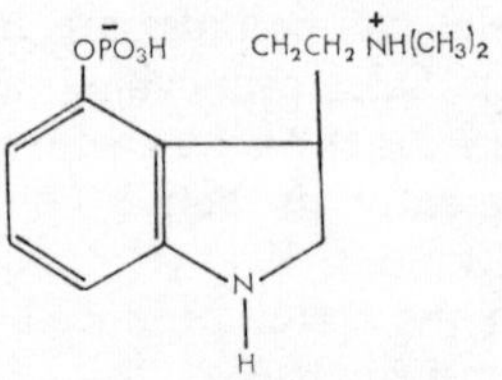

The psychotomimetic drugs share many of their pharmacological properties in spite of their differing chemical formulae. The following account refers principally to the actions of mescaline and lysergide, as these are the most commonly encountered members of the group. Peripherally, the drugs have a stimulant effect on smooth muscle and bring about a constriction of small blood vessels. Centrally, they stimulate sympathetic centres, causing tachycardia, mydriasis and elevation of blood pressure. Although most of the psychotomimetic drugs have strong anticholinergic effects, these do not appear to bear a direct relationship to the psychological effects. Observations of the effects of the drugs on the electroencephalogram are contradictory: experiments have variously suggested central and peripheral origins for the electrical discharges associated with visual hallucinations. When given the drugs many animals show a disturbance of behaviour which has been regarded as a disintegration of both innate and learned patterns of behaviour. Experiments have included studies of the effects of the drugs, generally mescaline or lysergide, on the web-building activities of spiders, the postures of fish, the movement of snails and 'waltzing' in mice. Some animals demonstrate excitability after receiving the drugs; others exhibit a calming reaction.

Clinical effects. Though the actions of all the psychotomimetic drugs are similar, in many respects the clinical effects mentioned here are principally those of mescaline and lysergide. Both mescaline and lysergide induce physiological changes which may be accompanied by changes in affect, perception and cognition. However, the effects produced are very variable, even in the individual patient, and are particularly dependent upon the social circumstances in which the drugs are given. The following account is given in the sequence in which the effects are generally experienced.

The physical effects come on about thirty minutes after oral administration of the drug. There may be nausea, anorexia, vomiting, chest pains, dizziness, headache, sweating, tremor, incoordination, ataxia and alternating feelings of heat and cold. Autonomic effects include palpitations, blurring of vision, urinary frequency, papillary dilation, tachycardia and a rise in blood pressure. The somatic symptoms may be followed by a state of great anxiety and dread. As this dies away a state of euphoria or emotional lability may ensue. Thinking processes may be slowed or accelerated and are irrational and loosely related. Perceptual changes occur in about half the subjects taking the drugs: there may be changes in perspective and distortion of images; colours may appear to be more vivid, textures exaggerated, sounds distorted; the experience of body image and of time are often disturbed. Hallucinations can occur in any sensory modality; these are frequently abstract in form. The subject may feel detached from his environment and changed in himself, as with depersonalisation experiences. Performance in tests of memory, attention and dexterity declines. As the dosage of drug is increased the changes in mental state come to resemble an acute confusional state more closely.

The psychotomimetic drugs have been used in the treatment of a variety of mental illnesses. Busch & Johnson (1950) found L.S.D. to be of value in neurotic states where they 'disturbed the barriers of repression' and allowed patients to relive long past events 'with frightening realism'. The use of L.S.D. has been extended to group psychotherapy as well as individual therapy, and is claimed to allow expression of unpleasant material and to enable a patient to have insight into his emotional problems. Lysergide is claimed to be of value as an adjunct to psychotherapy in the treatment of phobias, sexual neuroses and some psychopathic states (Sandison, 1964). At the same time attention is drawn to the need for an experienced team to look after the patients receiving the drug and to the dangers associated with its use The published evidence suggests that psychotomimetic drugs have no established place in the treatment of mental illness. Their use is better restricted to experienced research workers.

Adverse effects. In the acute phase of intoxication the subject may be a danger both to himself and to others; cases of suicide and even homicide have been recorded (Ungerleider, Fisher & Fuller, 1966). When the acute effects of intoxication have died down, abnormalities may persist which were not present before the drugs were taken; these include depersonalisation, visual hallucinations and other disorders of perception, anxiety, depression, mood swings and paranoid beliefs, and may last for a few days or be so prolonged as to be indistinguishable from naturally occurring mental illness (Department of Health and Social Security, 1970). The acute effects can generally be terminated by giving chlorpromazine, 50–100 mg by intramuscular injection. Electro-convulsive therapy may be useful in cases resistant to treatment (Hatrick & Dewhurst, 1970).

Concern that the illicit taking of lysergide might spread has led to the restriction of its manufacture in Great Britain.

Miscellaneous Drugs

Lithium salts

Lithium salts have been used for a variety of medicinal purposes. In the nineteenth century they were prescribed for arthritis and gout, in this century as a salt substitute and for manic-depressive disease.

Pharmacology. Lithium has chemical properties similar to those of sodium. It is in the same group in the periodic table of the elements but with a smaller atomic weight; it is widely distributed in the body and is capable of substituting for sodium in nerve cells and skeletal muscles; it is removed from the nerve cell at one tenth the rate of sodium (Keynes & Swan, 1959), and depresses its electrical activity (Grundfest, Kao & Altamirano, 1954). Cade (1949) reported drowsiness in guinea pigs following intra-peritoneal injection of lithium salts.

Coppen & Shaw and their colleagues using isotope dilution techniques have demonstrated changes in the distribution of sodium in depressed and manic patients. 'Residual sodium' (intracellular sodium and a small amount of exchangeable bone sodium) increased by 50 per cent in depressions and by an average of 200 per cent in mania. In a small number of patients, 'exchangeable sodium' (body sodium with which the isotope mixes) and residual sodium were measured before and during lithium administration and it was found that the administration of lithium was associated with a marked fall in both values (Coppen, 1967). Coppen and his colleagues believe that the changes in the distribution of sodium which they report are probably caused by changes in the cell wall permeability brought about by the presence of lithium ions.

Clinical effects. After Cade's report that lithium salts had a calming effect on manic patients Schou (1954) studied the effects of lithium salts in mania and reported a 'good' response in 14 of 38 patients. Maggs (1963) carried out a double-blind cross-over comparison between lithium salts and a placebo in the treatment of 28 manic patients. He found lithium salts to be superior but not markedly so. Seven patients had to be withdrawn on account of toxic effects and disturbed behaviour.

The role of lithium salts in the treatment of mania is now widely accepted. It has a slower onset of action than some other treatments and is not effective in a high proportion of cases. However, it may be of value for patients resistant to other forms of treatment and for patients who have responded to it in previous attacks of mania.

Hartigan (1963) and Schou (1963) suggested that lithium salts might exert a prophylactic effect in patients who had suffered from mania. This claim has since been extended to include the prophylaxis of certain forms of depressive disorder although there is no convincing evidence that lithium is effective in the treatment of depression itself. The use of lithium salts in the prophylaxis of affective disorders remains controversial and is the subject of several large scale trials in different parts of the world. Until recently these claims have only been supported by open trials with retrospective or no controls and the need for properly designed clinical trials is apparent (Blackwell & Shepherd, 1968; Baastrup *et al.*, 1970; Coppen *et al.*, 1971; Hullin *et al.*, 1972; Cundall *et al.*, 1972).

Unwanted effects. Unwanted effects are very common and include nausea, vomiting, diarrhoea, tinnitus, drowsiness, ataxia, giddiness, blurred vision, thirst, polyuria and trembling of the hands. Confusion, coma, muscular twitching, nystagmus and fits can occur in more severe degrees of intoxication. Electrocardiographic changes are relatively common with flattening of inversion of the T-waves. Renal damage can result in a water-losing nephritis; in the early stages this may be reversible but soon becomes irreparable. As many as a quarter of 104 patients on lithium were found to have a transient proteinuria (Glesinger, 1954). A vasopressin-resistant, diabetes-insipidus-like state has been reported (Angrist *et al.*, 1970). At least six deaths have been reported from lithium intoxication although some of these resulted from the use of lithium as a salt substitute.

In the event of serious toxic effects administration should be stopped. As sodium displaces lithium in the body, so long as renal function remains adequate large quantities of salty fluids should be given. Renal dialysis may be required for severe oliguria. High serum levels of lithium can precede serious side effects (Maggs, 1963) and it is now generally recommended that administration of the drug be discontinued when the serum level exceeds 2 mmol/litre.

The development of thyroid complications has been described in patients receiving lithium. Twelve of 330 patients receiving lithium developed a goitre but remained euthyroid (Schou, 1968). Discontinuation of the drug led to disappearance of the goitre, and normal thyroid function continued.

In a report of cases where it was known that the mother received lithium in the first trimester of pregnancy, abnormalities were noted in 2 of 40 children. One of the abnormal children exhibited club feet, meningocoele and spina bifida, the other a defective auricle and meatal atresia. Registers are being kept of congenital deformities in Denmark and California (Schou & Amisden, 1970).

Administration. Lithium is usually prescribed as the carbonate since the other salts are hygroscopic. It is given in a dosage of 125–150 mg twice a day with a gradual increase in dose until a steady serum level of 0·8 to 1·2 mmol/litre is attained. The maintenance dosage is in the range 600–1700 mg of lithium carbonate daily. Serum estimations are recommended once or twice weekly until a steady state is achieved and should then be performed occasionally (Schou *et al.*, 1970c). The therapeutic and toxic doses of lithium salts are sufficiently close to render it advisable for medical supervision to be close and continuous.

There are many other drugs including carbamazepine, the alleged cerebral vasodilators, methysergide and l-dihydroxyphenyl alanine which have important effects on mental functioning. Discussion of these drugs has been omitted for lack of space to cover them adequately.

CONCLUSIONS

The last decade has produced relatively few new types of psychotropic drug but there has been a great increase in the knowledge and experience of the drugs developed from the discoveries of the 1950s. Perhaps the most important lesson emerging from psychopharmacology in recent years, however, is the caution required in evaluating the efficacy of new treatments. It is clear that each new drug or treatment needs full evaluation at an early stage. Though the release of a new drug for general use should not be unnecessarily delayed, any claim on its behalf should be substantiated by well designed studies, performed in a number of centres by experienced workers.

The fundamental mechanisms of the mode of action of most of the drugs in current use remain obscure despite a large volume of work. The search continues for drugs with a rapid onset of action, proven efficacy, and few unwanted effects. Meanwhile it would be of great practical help to know which of the available drugs is likely to help the individual patient. Advances of this type are to some extent dependent on refinements in the assessment of symptoms, diagnosis and classification of mental disorders. Attempts have been made to delineate the type of patient who is suitable for particular drugs both clinically and pharmacologically but even with the anti-depressants, on which most of the work has probably been conducted, the clinical indications are still very crude, and the choice is limited by the small number of effective alternatives.

The chances of new drugs being discovered and coming into therapeutic use might be increased in several ways:

1. There is a need for better animal models of human disease and for further understanding of the use and limitations of those already available.
2. There is a need for full advantage to be taken of opportunities to observe the effects on the mental state and behaviour of substances administered to human subjects in the course of medical treatment. This is well illustrated by the opportunities presented by the use of l-dopa in the treatment of Parkinson's disease.
3. Since most important discoveries in psychopharmacology have been made by chance observation rather than by systematic investigation, medical and non-medical workers should be aware of the possible importance of unexpected observations made in the course of all aspects of medical practice. Samuel & Blackwell (1968) give an interesting account of the way the 'cheese reaction' to monoamine oxidase inhibiting drugs was discovered. It is clear from their remarks that any observation on the actions or interactions of substances and their effects on the mental state should not be lightly dismissed.
4. Drugs already known to influence the mental state should be more systematically investigated by trained clinical psychopharmacologists.
5. The effects of drug combinations differ in important respects from those of their constituents, and observation of their effects can make important contributions to clinical psychopharmacology (Shepherd, 1965).

References

ALEXANDERSON, B., PRICE EVANS, D. A. & SJÖQVIST, F. (1969). *Br. med. J.*, **4**, 766–768.
ANGRIST, B. M., GERSHON, S., LEVITEN, S. J. & BLUMBERG, A. G. (1970). *Compr. Psychiat.* **2**, 141–146.

ANGST, J. (1961). *Psychopharmacologia*, **2**, 381.

ÅSBERG, M., CRONHOLM, B., SJÖQVIST, F. & TUCK, D. (1970). *Br. med. J.*, **3,** 18.

BAASTRUP, P. C. & SCHOU, M. (1967). *Archs gen. Psychiat.*, **16**, 162.

BAASTRUP, P. C., POULSEN, J. C., SCHOU, M. THOMSEN, K. & AMDISEN, A. (1970). *Lancet*, **2**, 326.

BANKIER, R. G., PETTIT, O. E. & BERGEN, B. (1968). *Dis. nerv. Syst.*, **29**, 56.

BARTHOLOMEW, A. A. (1962). *Med. J. Aust.*, **15**, 655.

BATES, T. J. N. & DOUGLAS, A. D. McL. (1961). *J. ment. Sci.*, **107**, 538.

BLACK, A. A. (1969). *Br. J. hosp. Med.*, **2**, 1453.

BLACKWELL, B. (1963). *Lancet*, **2**, 849.

BLACKWELL, B., MARLEY, E., PRICE, J. S. & TAYLOR, D. (1967). *Br. J. Psychiat.*, **113**, 349.

BLACKWELL, B. & SHEPHERD, M. (1968). *Lancet*, **1**, 968.

BLASHKI, T. G., MOWBRAY, R. & DAVIES, B. (1971). *Br. med. J.*, **1**, 133.

BRADLEY, P. B. (1963). *In* 'Physiological Pharmacology'. Ed. W. S. Root & F. G. Hofmann, Vol. **1**, p. 417. New York: Academic Press.

BRADSHAW, P. & PARSONS, M. (1965). *Q. Jl Med.*, **34**, 65.

BRAITHWAITE, R. A., GOULDING, R., THEANO, G., BAILEY, J and COPPEN, A. (1972). *Lancet*, **1**, 1297.

BRANDRUP, E. (1960). *Nord. Med.*, **8**, (31), 968.

BRAZIER, M. A. B. (1963). *In* 'Physiological Pharmacology'. Ed. W. S. Root & F. G. Hofmann. Vol. **1**, p. 219. New York: Academic Press.

BRITISH MEDICAL JOURNAL (1970). **3**, 354.

BRODIE, B. B., FINGER, K. F., ORLANS, F. B., QUINN, G. P. & SULSER, F. (1960). *J. Pharmacol.*, **129**, 250–256.

BRODIE, B. B. (1965). *In* 'The Scientific Basis of Drug Therapy in Psychiatry'. Ed. J. Marks & C. M. B. Pare. p. 127. Oxford: Pergamon.

BUNNEY, W. E., MURPHY, D. L., BRODIE, H. K. H. & GOODWIN, F. K. (1970). *Lancet*, **1**, 352.

BUSCH, A. K. & JOHNSON, W. C. (1950). *Dis. nerv. Syst.*, **11**, 241.

CADE, J. F. J. (1949). *Med. J. Aust.*, **2**, 349.

CAPSTICK, N. S., CORBETT, M. F., PARE, C. M. B., PRYCE, I. G. & REES, W. L. (1965). *Br. J. Psychiat.*, **111**, 517.

CARLSSON, A., LINDQUIST, M. & MAGNUSSON, T. (1957). *Nature*, **180**, 1200 C.

CARLSSON, A. & WALDECK, B. (1965). *J. Pharm. Pharmac.*, **17**, 243 C.

CARLSSON, A. (1966). *Pharmac. Rev.*, **18**, 541.

CESARMAN, T. (1959). *Ann. N.Y. Acad. Sci.*, **80**, 988.

CHILDERS, R. T. & THERRIEN, R. (1961). *Am. J. Psychiat.*, **118**, 552.

COLE, J. O. & CLYDE, D. J. (1961). *Rev. canad. Biol.*, **20**, 565.

CONNELL, P. H. (1958). *In* 'Amphetamine psychosis'. London: Oxford University Press.

CONNELL, P. H., CORBETT, J. A., HORNE, D. J. & MATHEWS, A. M. (1967). *Br. J. Psychiat.*, **113**, 375.

COPPEN, A., SHAW, D. M. & FARRELL, J. P. (1963). *Lancet*, **1**, 79.

COPPEN, A. (1967). *Br. J. Psychiat.*, **113**, 1237.

COPPEN, A. (1970). *Scientific Basis of Medicine, Annual Reviews*, p. 189. London: Athlone Press.

COPPEN, A., NOGUERA, A., BAILEY, J., BURNS, B. H., SIRANI, M. S., HARE, E. H., GARDNER, R. and MAGGS, R. (1971). *Lancet*, **2**, 275.

COULL, D. C., CROOKS, J., DINGWALL-FORDYCE, I., SCOTT, A. M. & WEIR, R. D. (1970). *Lancet*, **2**, 590.

CRAMMER, J. L., SCOTT, B. & ROLFE, B. (1969). *Psychopharmacologia*, **15**, 207.

CROCKET, R., SANDISON, R. A. & WALK, A. (eds.). (1963). *In* 'Hallucinogenic Drugs and their Psychotherapeutic Use'. London: Lewis.

CUNDALL, R. L., BROOKS, P. W. & MURRAY, L. G. (1972). *Psychol. Med.*, **2**, 308.
CURRY, S. H. (1968). *Analyt. Chem.*, **40**, 1251.
DASGUPTA, S. R. & WERNER, G. (1954). *Br. J. Pharmacol.*, **9**, 389.
DE ALARCON, R. & CARNEY, M. W. P. (1969). *Br. med. J.*, **3**, 564.
DELAY, J. & DENIKER, P. (1952). *Le Congrès de Psychiatrie et de Neurologie de Langue Française*, Ed. Masson. p. 503. Luxembourg: Masson et Cie.
DENIKER, P. (1960). *Comprehens. Psychiat.*, **1**, 92.
DEPARTMENT OF HEALTH AND SOCIAL SECURITY (1970). Reports on Public Health and Medical Subjects No. 124 H.M.S.P. London: H.M.S.O.
EDWARDS, G. (1965). *Br. J. Psychiat.*, **111**, 889.
ELKES, A. (1969). *In* 'Mode of Action of Imipramine'. MD Thesis, Univ. London.
ESSIG, C. F. & AINSLIE, J. D. (1957). *J. Am. med. Ass.*, **164**, 1382 C.
ESSIG, C. F. (1966). *J. Am. med. Ass.*, **196**, 714.
ESSIG, C. F. (1969). *In* 'Abuse of central stimulants'. Ed. Sjöqvist F. & M. Tottie. Stockholm: Almqvist & Wikell.
GANDER, D. R. (1965). *Lancet*, **2**, 107.
GENERAL PRACTITIONER CLINICAL TRIALS (1964). *Practitioner*, **192**, 151.
GERLE, B. (1964). *Acta psychiat. scand.*, **40**, 65.
GERSHON, S. & YUWILER, A. (1960). *J. Neuropsychiat.*, **1**, 229.
GLESINGER, B. (1954). *Med. J. Aust.*, **1**, 277.
GLOWINSKI, J. & AXELROD, J. (1964). *Nature*, (Lond.), **204**, 1318 C.
GOOD, W. W., STERLING, M. & HOLTZMAN, W. H. (1958). *Am. J. Psychiat.*, **115**, 443.
GOODMAN, L. S. & GILMAN, A. (1970). *In* 'The Pharmacological Basis of Therapeutics'. New York: Macmillan.
GOTHELF, B. & KARCZMAR, A. G. (1963). *Int. J. Neuropharmac.*, **2**, 39.
GREENBERG, A. (1970). *Amer. med. Ass. Annual Convention*, 3–11, Chicago, Illinois.
GRUNDFEST, H., KAO, C. Y. & ALTAMIRANO, M. (1954). *J. gen. Physiol.*, **38**, 245.
GWYNNE, P. H., HUNDZIAK, M., KAVTSCHITSCH, J., LEFTON, M. & PASAMANICK, B. (1962). *J. nerv. ment. Dis.*, **134**, 451.
HARTIGAN, G. P. (1963). *Br. J. Psychiat.*, **109**, 810.
HATRICK, J. H. & DEWHURST, K. (1970). *Lancet*, **2**, 742.
HAYDU, G. G., DHRYMIOTIS, A. & QUINN, G. P. (1962). *Am. J. Psychiat.*, **119**, 574.
HERMAN, E. & PLEASURE, H. (1963). *Dis. nerv. Syst.*, **24**, 54.
HILL, A. B. (1950). *Br. med. Bull.*, **7**, 278.
HILL, A. B. (1960) *In* 'Controlled Clinical Trials'. Oxford: Blackwell.
HILL, A. B. (1963). *Br. med. J.*, **1**, 1043.
HILL, A. B. (1965). *Proc. R. Soc. Med.*, **58**, 295.
HINES, L. R. (1960). *Curr. ther. Res.*, **2**, 227.
HOFFER, A., OSMOND, H. & SMYTHIES, J. (1954). *J. ment. Sci.*, **100**, 29.
HOFMANN, A. (1959). *Acta physiol. pharmac. neerl.*, **8**, 240.
HOLLISTER, L. E., MOTZENBECKER, F. P. & DEGAN, R. O. (1961). *Psychopharmacologia*, **2**, 63.
HOLLISTER, L. E. & KOSEK, J. C. (1965). *J. Am. med. Ass.*, **192**, 1035.
HOLLISTER, L. E., OVERALL, J. E., SHELTON, J., PENNINGTON, V., KIMBELL, I. & JOHNSON, M. (1967). *Archs gen. Psychiat.*, **17**, 486.
HORDERN, A., BURT, C. G., GORDON, W. F. & HOLT, N. F. (1964). *Br. J. Psychiat.*, **110**, 641.
HULLIN, R. P., MCDONALD, R. & ALLSOPP, M. N. E. (1972). *Lancet*, **1**, 1044.
IMLAH, N. W., RYAN, E. & HARRINGTON, J. A. (1964). *Proc. 4th Int. Congr. Neuropharmacol. Birmingham*, Elsevier, Amsterdam, **1965**, 438–442.
ISBELL, H. & CHRUŚCIEL, T. L. (1970). *In* 'Dependence Liability of "Non-Narcotic" Drugs', Bull. Wld. Hlth. Org., Suppl. to Vol. 43.
JENKINS, R. B. & GROH, R. H. (1970). *Lancet*, **2**, 177–180.
JOYCE, C. R. B. (1959). *Br. J. Pharmac.*, **14**, 512–521.
KALINOWSKY, L. B. & HIPPIUS, H. (1969). *In* 'Pharmacological, convulsive and other somatic treatments in psychiatry'. New York: Grune & Stratton.

KAY, D. W. K., FAHY, T. & GARSIDE, R. F. (1970). *Br. J. Psychiat.*, **117**, 667.

KELLY, D., GUIRGUIS, W., FROMMER, E., MITCHELL-HEGGS, N. & SARGANT, W. (1970). *Br. J. Psychiat.*, **116**, 387.

KEYNES, R. D. & SWAN, R.C. (1959). *J. Physiol.*, **147**, 626.

KILLAM, E. K. (1962). *Pharmac. Rev.*, **14**, 175.

KILOH, L. G. & BRANDON, S. (1962). *Br. med. J.*, **2**, 40.

KLERMAN, G. L. & COLE, J. P. (1965). *Pharmac. Rev.*, **17**, 101.

KLINE, N. S. & SACKS, W. (1963). *Am. J. Psychiat.*, **120**, 274.

KRISTJANSEN, P. (1966). *Clin. Trials, J.*, **3**, 385.

KUHN, R. (1958). *Am. J. Psychiat.*, **115**, 459.

LADER, M. H. (1971). *Psychol. Med.*, **1**, 150.

LAITINEN, L. (1969). *Acta neurol. scand.*, **45**, 109.

LAURENCE, D. R. & WEBSTER, R. A. (1963). *Clin. Pharmac. Ther.*, **4**, 36.

LEFF, J. P. & WING, J. K. (1971). *Br. med. J.*, **3**, 599.

LEHMANN, H. E. & HANRAHAN, G. E. (1954). *Archs neurol. Psychiat.*, **71**, 227.

LENNARD-JONES, J. E. (1971). *Practitioner*, **206**, 64.

LEWIS, J. J. (1963). *In* 'Physiological Pharmacology. A Comprehensive Treatise'. Ed. W. S. Root & F. G. Hofmann. Vol. **1**, p. 479. New York: Academic Press.

LEYBERG, J. T. & DENMARK, J. C. (1959). *J. ment. Sci.*, **105**, 1123.

LIBERMAN, R. (1964). *J. Psychiat. Res.*, **2**, 233.

LING, T. M. & BUCKMAN, J. (1963). *In* 'Lysergic acid (LSD25) and Ritalin in the treatment of neurosis'. London: Larribonde Press.

LOMBROSO, C. T. (1966). *Neurology, Minneap.*, **16**, 629.

LORANGER, A. W., PROUT, C. T. & WHITE, M. A. (1961). *J. Am. med. Ass.*, **176**, 920.

McDOWALL, A., OWEN, S., ROBIN, A. A. (1966). *Br. J. Psychiat.*, **112**, 629.

McILWAIN, H. (1957). *In* 'Chemotherapy and the Central Nervous System'. London: Churchill.

MAGGS, R. (1963). *Br. J. Psychiat.*, **109**, 56.

MARLEY, E. (1959). *J. ment. Sci.*, **105**, 19.

MASSERMAN, J. H. (1960). *In* 'Drugs and Behaviour'. Ed. J. H. Masserman & J. G. Miller. New York: Wiley.

MECHANIC, D. (1966). *Soc. Psychiat.*, **1**, 11.

MEDICAL RESEARCH COUNCIL (1965). *Br. med. J.*, **1**, 881.

MICHAEL, R. P. & GIBBONS, J. L. (1963). *Int. Rev. Neurobiol.*, **5**, 243.

MINDHAM, R. H. S., HOWLAND, C. & SHEPHERD, M. (1973) (In press.)

MULLER, J. C., PRYOR, W. W., GIBBONS, J. E. & ORGAIN, E. S. (1955). *J. Am. med. Ass.*, **159**, 836.

NATIONAL INSTITUTE FOR MENTAL HEALTH (1964). *Archs gen. Psychiat.*, **10**, 246.

OVERALL, J. E., HOLLISTER, L. E., MEYER, F., KIMBELL, I. & SHELTON, J. (1964). *J. Am. med. Ass.*, **189**, 605.

PARE, C. M. B. & SANDLER, M. J. (1959). *J. Neurol. Neurosurg. Psychiat.*, **22**, 247.

PARE, C. M. B. (1963). *Lancet*, **2**, 527.

PASAMANICK, B., SCARPITTI, F. R., LEFTON, M., DINITZ, S., WERNERT, J. J. & McPHEETERS, H. (1964). *J. Am. med. Ass.*, **187**, 177.

PAYKEL, E. S., PRICE, J. S., GILLAN, R. U., PALMAI, G. & CHESSER, E. S. (1968). *Br. J. Psychiat.*, **114**, 1281.

PITT, B. (1968). *Hosp. Med.*, **1**, 815.

POLLIN, W., CARDON, P. V., KETY, S. S. (1961). *Science*, **133**, 104.

PRINZMETAL, M. & BLOOMBERG, W. (1935). *J. Am. med. Ass.*, **105**, 2051.

PROCEEDINGS OF THE COLLEGIUM INTERNATIONALE NEURO-PSYCHOPHARMACOLOGI-CUM. Various Editors: 1958, 1964, 1965, 1969. New York: Academic Press.

PSYCHOPHARMACOLOGY ABSTRACTS. National Institute for Mental Health, U.S.A.

RAYMOND, M. J., LUCAS, C. J., BEESLEY, M. L., O'CONNELL, B. A. & FRASER ROBERTS, J. A. (1957). *Br. med. J.*, **2**, 63.

RAVARIS, C. L., WEAVER, L. A. & BROOKS, G. W. (1965). *Dis. nerv. Syst.*, **26**, 33.

REES, W. L. & BENAIM, S. (1960). *J. ment. Sci.*, **106**, 193.

REYNOLDS, E., JOYCE, C. R. B., SWIFT, J. L., TOOLEY, P. H. & WEATHERALL, M. (1965). *Br. J. Psychiat.*, **111**, 84.

RICKELS, K. (1963). *J. nerv. ment. Dis.*, **136**, 540.

ROBITZEK, E. H., SELIKOFF, I. J. & ORNSTEIN, G. G. (1952). *Q. Bull. Sea View Hosp.*, **13**, 27–51.

ROOT, W. S. & HOFMANN, F. G. (1963, 1965, 1967). *In* 'Physiological Pharmacology. A Comprehensive Treatise'. New York: Academic Press.

SAMUEL, G. & BLACKWELL, B. (1968). *Hosp. Med.*, **1**, 942.

SANDISON, R. A. (1964). *Practitioner*, **192**, 30.

SATTES, H. (1960). *Psychiat. Neurol.*, **140**, 13.

SCHILDKRAUT, J. J. (1969). *New Engl. J. Med.*, **281**, 197, 248, 302.

SCHOU, M., JUEL-NIELSEN, N., STRÖMGREN, E. & VOLDBY, H. (1954). *J. Neurol. Neurosurg. Psychiat.*, **17**, 250.

SCHOU, M. (1963). *Br. J. Psychiat.*, **109**, 803.

SCHOU, M. (1968). *J. psychiat. Res.*, **6**, 67.

SCHOU, M. & AMDISEN, A. (1970). *Lancet*, **1**, 1391 C.

SCHOU, M., BAASTRUP, P. C., GROF, P., WEIS, P. & ANGST, J. (1970c). *Br. J. Psychiat.* **116**, 615.

SEAGER, C. P. & BIRD, R. L. (1962). *J. ment. Sci.*, **108**, 704.

SERRY, D. (1969). *Lancet*, **1**, 417 C.

SHAFFER, D., COSTELLO, A. J. & HILL, I. D. (1968). *Archs Dis. Childh.*, **43**, 665.

SHAPIRO, A. K. (1959). *Am. J. Psychiat.*, **116**, 298.

SHAW, D. M., CAMPS, F. E. & ECCLESTON, E. G. (1967). *Br. J. Psychiat.*, **113**, 1407.

SHEPHARD, N. W. (ed.). (1965). *In* 'The Application of Neuroleptanalgesia in Anaesthetic and other Practice'. Oxford: Pergamon.

SHEPHERD, M. & WATT, D. C. (1956). *J. Neurol. Neurosurg. Psychiat.*, **19**, 232.

SHEPHERD, M. (1965). *Proc. R. Soc. Med.*, **58**, 964 (Symp No. 7).

SHEPHERD, M., LADER, M. & RODNIGHT, R. (1968). *In* 'Clinical Psychopharmacology' London: English Universities Press.

SHEPHERD, M. (1971). *Psych l. Med.* **2**, 96.

SJÖQVIST, F., HAMMER, W., IDESTRÖM, C-M., LIND, M., TUCK, D. & ÅSBERG, M. (1967). *Excerpta med. (Amst.) int. Congr. Serv. No.* **145**, 246.

SULZER, F., BICKEL, M. H. & BRODIE, B. B. (1964). *J. Pharmac. exp. Ther.*, **144**, 321.

TEDESCHI, D. H., TEDESCHI, R. E. & FELLOWS, E. J. (1959). *J. Pharmac. exp. Ther.*, **126**, 223.

TOBIN, J. M., LORENZ, A. A., BROUSSEAU, E. R. & CONNER, W. R. (1964). *Dis. nerv. Syst.*, **25**, 689.

TONKS, C. M. (1968). *Hosp. Med.*, **1**, 383.

TURNER, R. K. & YOUNG, G. C. (1966). *Behav. Res. Ther.*, **4**, 225.

UHBRAND, L. & FAURBYE, A. (1960). *Psychopharmacologia*, **1**, 408.

UNGERLEIDER, J. T., FISHER, D. D. & FULLER, M. (1966). *J. Am. med. Ass.*, **197**, 389.

VAN PRAAG, H. M. *et al.* (1970). *Psychiat. Neurol. Neurochir.*, **73**, 165.

WALTER, C. J. S. (1971). *Proc. R. Soc. Med.*, **64**, 282.

WECHSLER, H., GROSSER, G. H. & GREENBLATT, M. (1965). *J. nerv. ment. Dis.*, **141**, 231.

WELLS, F. O. (1970). *Br. med. J.*, **2**, 361 C.

WEST, E. D. & DALLY, P. J. (1959). *Br. med. J.*, **1**, 1491.

WEATHERALL, M. (1962). *Br. med. J.*, **1**, 1219.

WIKLER, A. (1957). *In* 'The Relationship of Psychiatry to Pharmacology'. Baltimore: Williams & Wilkins Co.

WILSON, J. D. & ENOCH, M. D. (1967). *Br. J. Psychiat.*, **113**, 209.

WING, J. K. & FREUDENBERG, R. K. (1961). *Am. J. Psychiat.*, **118**, 311.

WITTENBORN, J. R., PLANTE, M., BURGESS, F. & LIVERMORE, N. (1961). *J. nerv. ment. Dis.*, **133**, 316.

ZELLER, E. A. & BARSKY, J. (1952). *Proc. Soc. exp. Biol., (N.Y.)*, **81**, 459.

CHAPTER 11

POPULATION SCREENING

JOCELYN CHAMBERLAIN

There has been an increasing interest in recent years in screening as a means of preventing or controlling some of the chronic diseases which have come to be such important causes of morbidity and mortality in developed countries. The reasoning behind this particular form of medical care is that by early detection and treatment it will be possible to nip the pathological process in the bud and prevent its progression to a full-blown disease with possibly serious morbidity and eventual death.

Screening can be defined as the presumptive identification of unrecognised disease or risk of disease by medical investigation which does not arise from a patient's request for advice for specific complaints. This definition includes two points made previously by the U.S. Commission on Chronic Illness (1957) and by the Nuffield Provincial Hospitals Trust's Working Group on Screening in Medical Care (1968). The first of these is that the screening test is intended only to sort out people who probably have the disease from those who probably do not, and is not intended to make a firm diagnosis. A positive result to a screening test always needs to be confirmed by definitive diagnostic procedures. The second point is that screening is initiated by the doctor and is offered to the individual (who in this context is not a patient) as a form of care which will benefit him. The assumption that early detection and treatment must necessarily be of benefit sounds reasonable on the face of it, but closer examination shows that it is not as simple as it seems and detailed knowledge is essential in four main areas to be sure that screening is justified.

Firstly, it is necessary to understand the epidemiology and natural history of the condition—what is its incidence in the population, what sort of people does it attack, what is its aetiology, how long does the disease process take to develop, are there any presymptomatic warning signs and, if so, at what level of these can the diseased be split off from the normal? Secondly, it is necessary to know the efficiency of the screening test—does it give many false results, is it reproducible between different observers and at different times and is it acceptable to the people most at risk from the disease? Thirdly, it is necessary to know the effectiveness of the treatment which is to be offered—does it, in fact, prevent or retard the disease process, is it acceptable (remembering that it is frequently a life-long burden), does it have serious side-effects or complications?

The last area in which extra knowledge is required is the practical but often controversial one of resources and costs. It is frequently postulated that screening makes sound economic sense because by treating the disease early, later expensive treatment will be avoided, and the costs of maintaining the screening service will be more than offset by this subsequent saving. In fact this hypothesis too can only be tested by long-term population studies which compare the resources used by people whose disease was detected by screening, with those who sought medical care in the ordinary way. Although frequently the necessary information is not available, a balancing of costs versus effectiveness is an ideal requisite for the decision on whether or not to provide a screening service. This is obviously of particular importance in a system which offers equal health care to all, when the relative priority of different methods of care has to be assessed in order to give the most effective use of resources.

PURPOSES OF SCREENING

Before going on to examine these different areas for research in detail, it is useful to look at the reasons for development of screening and the various forms it can take.

Protection of Public Health

An early example of screening was that employed in the nineteenth century by the U.S. Public Health Service which vetted would-be immigrants to the United States at their port of arrival and, on the basis of what must have been a very arbitrary medical examination, refused entry to those who were considered diseased. The objective behind this form of screening was to protect the health of other people in the community and it was obviously of negative value to the person diagnosed as having a disease for which he might be deported. This form of screening as a public health protection measure has since been developed to a much more sophisticated level for various infective diseases. In this country the best example is the mass X-ray screening service for the diagnosis of tuberculosis; although, over the years the emphasis of this has altered from protecting the public to helping the individual, its principal original purpose was to control the spread of the disease by identifying cases at an early stage and removing them from the community.

Antenatal and Child Health Care

Another early development of screening was in the antenatal and child welfare field. This form of early detection is much more akin to the population screening for chronic disease now under consideration, since here the purpose of screening is to benefit the individual mother and her baby. Although screening in antenatal care has long been firmly established, it has not in fact been evaluated in the way suggested below for the newer screening procedures; there is, however, much circumstantial evidence that regular antenatal screening is of benefit for the prevention of conditions such as pre-eclampsia (Butler & Bonham, 1963), and Rhesus haemolytic disease of the newborn (Walker, 1959). Similarly, in the case of child health screening, controlled trials have not been done but there can be little doubt that the early diagnosis and treatment of developmental abnormalities such as deafness, or congenital dislocation of the hip, is of benefit. The main doubt remaining about these procedures is that the validity of many of the tests used under service conditions has not been tested and there may be a proportion of false results (Knox, 1968a).

Surveillance of Disease

A third form of screening or surveillance is that which is part of the follow-up of an illness which has presented in a symptomatic way. Examples of this are in the monitoring of patients who have had a hydatidiform mole in whom excretion of gonadotrophins can give early warning of choriocarcinoma, or regular examination of the thyroid state of patients who have had thyroidectomy. Although many of the problems of recall and of record-keeping in this form of surveillance are similar to those of general population screening, the essential difference is that the high-risk group being screened in this instance is identified as a result of their original illness. They are not selected from a well population, and surveillance is regarded as an essential part of the treatment.

Research

Another use of screening is in epidemiological research, where it is a necessary method for determining the total extent of a disease in a population, often a more useful measure than that obtained from, for example, the selected group of patients who reach hospital. Such research carries with it the same ethical responsibility to the people who are being investigated as any other form of medical research. While they should be told that the primary purpose of the screening test is to further medical knowledge, naturally every effort will be made to make sure that the people found to have disease will get the necessary help. One of the principal purposes of epidemiological research in chronic diseases is to find out if screening is of value.

Prescriptive Screening

Finally, we come to the topic of this Chapter, population screening as a method of case-finding offered to people as a service, whose primary objective is to detect and treat a chronic disease before the patient has spontaneously sought medical care. The Working Group on Screening in Medical Care, set up by the Nuffield Provincial Hospitals Trust (1968), has named this 'prescriptive screening' and has underlined the particular ethical responsibility of those who offer this form of care to people who have not presented with any complaint. They point out that when the doctor or health authority takes the initiative in investigating uncomplaining people, there is a presumptive undertaking, not only that any abnormality present will be detected, but also that those affected will benefit from treatment. Unfortunately, in screening for chronic diseases, the treatment which can be offered often means life-long drugs or, in the case of cancers, surgery; both these forms of therapy have their complications and side-effects, which make it impossible to be sure that no person will suffer a disadvantage as a result of screening. It is therefore important to be sure that the total benefit of screening should exceed any possible harm done (Wilson, 1970). Before introducing a screening service, its benefits, hazards and costs should be weighed up as carefully as possible, firstly from the medical aspect and then economically.

NATURAL HISTORY OF THE DISEASE

In this process of evaluation, it is necessary to have a detailed knowledge of the epidemiology of the particular condition. Its full extent in the population before screening must be clear for any assessment of the value of early intervention to be made. The first essential is that the natural history of the condition be fully understood from the earliest stage at which an individual may be identified as being at risk, through the stage of early, perhaps presymptomatic, disease, to overt disease, disability and death.

In the chronic diseases against which prescriptive screening is aimed, unravelling the natural history usually requires prospective surveys of large populations continued over several years. Although, in patients already suffering from the disease, possible risk factors can be identified, their contribution to the development of the condition can only be determined in prospective inquiries in which assessments of risk factors are made on the apparently healthy whose subsequent experience of the disease is then measured. Through identification of the causes and early warning signs of later disease, such studies are of practical importance in suggesting appropriate stages at which screening might be introduced in order to prevent or retard the disease process.

Ischaemic Heart Disease

A great deal of work has been done in elucidating the many factors involved in the natural history of ischaemic heart disease, in several prospective incidence studies of this condition (e.g. Stamler et al., 1960; Kannel et al., 1962). As well as the obvious factors of age and sex, numerous others including family history, physical inactivity, obesity, cigarette smoking, saturated fatty acids and carbohydrates in the diet, competitive personality, raised serum cholesterol, raised blood pressure, and E.C.G. changes have been incriminated by their association with subsequent ischaemic heart disease. The predictive value of many of these factors has been studied by Morris et al. (1966) who examined a sample of 667 middle-aged London bus drivers and conductors and have been measuring subsequent occurrence of ischaemic heart disease. Seven per cent of men, all of whom were free of disease at the start of the study, developed it within 5 years of their initial examination. As expected the incidence was higher in later than in early middle age, in men with a bad family history, in drivers as compared to conductors who are more active and perhaps less subject to stress, in cigarette smokers and in the obese. Discriminant function analysis, used to isolate the risk factors which, independently of the others, make the biggest contributions to predicting ischaemic heart disease, showed that raised casual systolic blood pressure and raised casual serum cholesterol are much the most important predictors of subsequent disease. Seventy per cent of the new cases occurred in the 40 per cent of men whose levels of systolic blood pressure and/or cholesterol were in the top quarter, although only one out of 7 men identified in this way were affected by ischaemic heart disease within 5 years. These findings were corroborated in the Framingham study (Truett, Cornfield & Kannel, 1967) which also used discriminant function analysis to separate the effects of the different factors. Morris and his co-workers suggest that the natural history of ischaemic heart disease can be described in terms of the *causes*, (age, obesity, smoking, etc.) which, operating separately or together, lead to the *precursors*, raised blood pressure and raised serum cholesterol, which in turn lead to overt disease.

The natural history of ischaemic heart disease has been studied in greater depth than any other chronic disease and, although the search for more specific causes and precursors continues, intervention studies have now been started in which people identified by screening as being at risk are being randomly allocated to treatment or control groups. Possible methods of control now being evaluated are treatment by clofibrate (Morris & Gardner, 1969), treatment by antihypertensive drugs (U.S. Veterans Administration, 1970), modification of diet (Turpeinen *et al.*, 1968), and specific health education about smoking (Reid, personal communication) and about diet and exercise, (Rose, 1970). However, until the results of such studies appear, no improvement in prognosis can be promised to people identified by screening as being at risk.

The Borderline Problem

A problem frequently encountered in studying natural history is that of establishing the dividing line between health and disease. In a population many variables of bodily function are distributed in a unimodal distribution

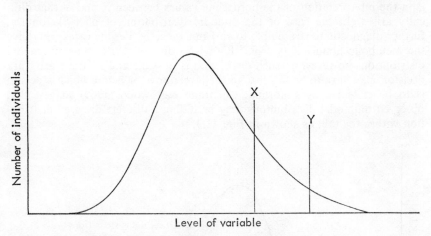

FIG. 11.1. Unimodal distribution curve, e.g. blood sugar.

curve, usually slightly skewed to the 'diseased' side of the population mean. This sort of distribution applies to measurements frequently used as tests for disease, such as blood pressure, body weight and blood sugar. More rarely, the distribution of a measurement is bimodal, such as the blood phenylalanine level used to identify phenylketonuria. Examples of these are shown in Figs. 11.1 and 11.2.

In both these distributions we can usually recognise a part of the population in which the test level is clearly within the bounds of health (to the left of X on the arbitrary scale of the diagrams); while at the other extreme (to the

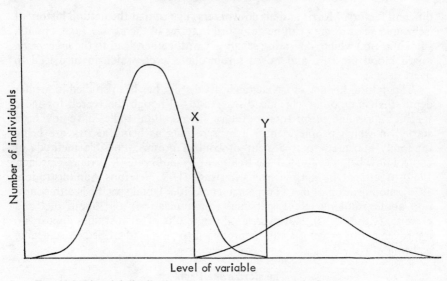

FIG. 11.2. Bimodal distribution curve, e.g. serum phenylalanine.

right of Y) there is an area we could certainly declare indicative of disease. It is in the interpretation of the borderline values between X and Y that difficulty arises. In the case of the bimodal distribution of phenylketonuria, further diagnostic tests are able to sort out those borderline cases who have the metabolic abnormality from those who do not. With many unimodal distributions however, no such distinction is possible and a purely arbitrary decision may have to be taken as to the level above or below which a person is to be classified as abnormal. Cochrane & Elwood (1969) suggest that observed unimodal distributions may be hiding a discrete diseased distribution within the tail, as shown in Fig. 11.3.

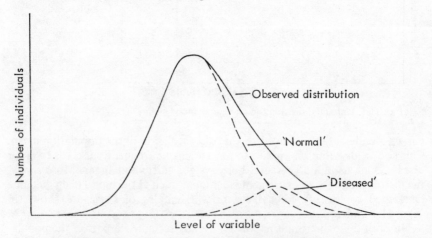

FIG. 11.3. Statistical model of 'Normal' and 'Diseased' distribution within an observed unimodal distribution (Cochrane & Elwood, 1969).

Distinction Between Health and Abnormality

A convenient measure of 'normality' often used is the range of plus or minus two standard deviations from the mean value of a variable for a whole (healthy and diseased) population. Five per cent of values (2·5 per cent at either end of the distribution) are thus classified as 'abnormal'. Such calculation is however only applicable to variables which have a statistically normal distribution, (that very simply is a bell-shaped distribution with an equal number of values on either side of the mean) and these are unusual, most physiological variables being markedly skewed (Elveback, Guillier & Keating, 1970).

It is also recognised that the range of normal for any test result varies with age and sex and a number of other extraneous factors. A diastolic blood pressure of 90 mmHg, for example, might be an appropriate dividing line between normality and hypertension in a young man, but would be an inappropriate level in a woman of 80. Different ranges of normality are required for different age-groups.

Murphy & Abbey (1967) in a discussion on the misuse of the 'normal range', point out that in addition to factors causing variability between and within the individuals being tested, there is also variability in the clinical value of a certain level of the index being measured which depends on the disease for which one is looking. For example, the leucocytosis in appendicitis is slight, the disease common, and accurate early diagnosis of great importance in its management. These three considerations suggest that the minimum diagnostic level should be set low. In contrast, the level should be set high in a condition such as primary malignant neoplasm of the liver, which is uncommon, often associated with a very high leucocytosis, and in which diagnosis does not lead to any improvement in prognosis. They point out the absurdity of using the same diagnostic level of white cell count (perhaps taken as two standard deviations above the mean value for a whole population) in seeking for those two conditions and suggest that it would be more reasonable to record the 'range in disease', different ranges being given for the same test in different diseases.

When applying a battery of tests as in automated biochemical screening to a population not suspected of any particular disease, the number of 'ranges in disease' which should be considered in distinguishing the healthy from the diseased could be enormous since there will doubtless be different interactions between many of the test variables occurring in different diseases. It is apparent that whether one is looking for a 'normal range' or a series of 'ranges in disease', much more work is still needed in definition. Perhaps the most satisfactory cut-off point for determining 'normality' is that defined by Cochrane & Elwood (1969) as 'the level below which treatment does more harm than good'.

Randomised Controlled Trials

The only satisfactory method whereby such a cut-off point can be defined is a randomised controlled trial. People whose level of the variable has been measured are randomly divided into a study group which is given the appropriate treatment and a control group which is not. Subsequent development of the disease in both groups is compared and hence the effect of treatment in altering prognosis can be assessed, and, if the numbers are large enough, can be determined for varying levels of the test result. As well as giving essential information about the effectiveness of treatment, long term follow-up of the control group in a randomised controlled trial provides an accurate description of the natural history of the disease in the same way as the prospective incidence studies described previously in relation to ischaemic heart disease.

TABLE 11.1

PERCENTAGE OF BORDERLINE DIABETICS WHO EXPERIENCED A CARDIOVASCULAR EVENT DURING SEVEN YEARS.

Adapted from a report of the Bedford trial of tolbutamide in the treatment of early diabetes (Keen & Jarrett, 1970).

	Placebo No diet	Placebo + Diet	Tolbutamide No Diet	Tolbutamide + Diet
All Entrants n = 248	37·0	38·0	29·5	25·0
High-risk Entrants n = 75	66·6	50·0	54·2	47·0
Low-risk Entrants n = 173	30·2	30·6	13·5	17·0

The Bedford study of early diabetes (Keen, 1966) is a good example of such a trial. 248 adults, found by screening to have blood sugar levels between 120 and 199 mg/100 ml, 2 hours after a loading dose of 50 g of glucose, have been randomly allocated into four groups, given tolbutamide or a placebo, and restricted or normal diet. All groups have been regularly examined and the development of complications recorded. Subjects have been classified into low and high-risk groups, the latter coming into the trial either with clear clinical or E.C.G. evidence of cardiovascular disease or with clinically significant hypertension.

As shown in Table 11.1, over a 7 year period the effect of tolbutamide was not significantly different from that of a placebo in the group as a whole, but, combined with dietary restriction it has been followed by a significant reduction in the occurrence of cardiovascular events in low-risk subjects (Keen and Jarrett, 1970). This study is continuing and may eventually show a significant long-term benefit from treating the whole group, perhaps also defining a screening level of blood sugar below which treatment is ineffective.

Inadequate Knowledge of Natural History

Screening has been introduced for some conditions without an adequate knowledge of the natural history of the disease, and this inevitably raises problems in determining the effectiveness of screening. In such cases knowledge of the course which the disease would have followed without screening has to be deduced indirectly, by comparison of the effects of the disease in a population in which screening has been practised, with another in which it has not. Such control populations are necessarily removed either in time or space, and the disadvantage of 'before and after' or 'here and there' comparisons is that the course of the disease may be affected by so many social and medical variables that conclusions about the value of a particular measure applied in one population, but not the other, are fraught with uncertainty. Some of these variables, such as a different age structure of the populations being compared, can be determined and the rates standardised to allow for this, but there can still remain many unsuspected differences between the the populations. The great advantage of the randomised controlled trial is that here the groups to be compared are taken from the *same* population, and are then randomly allocated into study and control. Hence they should be subject to the same influences, known or unknown.

In the recent past a full screening service has been introduced for two conditions, phenylketonuria (Wilson, 1968) and carcinoma in situ of the cervix (Knox, 1966), on inadequate formal evidence of the course which the abnormality would follow if left untreated.

Phenylketonuria

In this condition, inherited through an autosomal recessive gene, the basic biochemical defect of a failure of phenylalanine hydroxylase to convert phenylalanine to tyrosine leads to accumulation of phenylalanine in the blood and excretion of phenylpyruvic and phenylacetic acids in the urine. The most important characteristic of the disease is severe mental retardation and it is postulated that keeping the blood phenylalanine low from a very early age by means of a low phenylalanine diet leads to normal intelligence and development. The basic abnormality can be detected by the Guthrie bacterial inhibition test on a dried blood specimen, which has now replaced the less sensitive Phenistix urine test, and is performed routinely on all infants within the first week of life. There is a proportion of false positive results to this test, since transient hyperphenylalaninaemia sometimes occurs from other causes in early life, but about 1 child in 10 000 is eventually diagnosed as having the disease.

It has been shown that a low phenylalanine diet can lower blood phenylalanine (Bickel, 1953) but its effectiveness in preventing mental retardation has never been tested in a randomised controlled trial. Many treated phenylketonuric children have developed with normal intelligence which certainly suggests that the diet is effective, but it has also been demonstrated that intelligence may be normal or only slightly impaired in the present of a high blood phenylalanine level (Mabry, Denniston & Coldwell, 1966). Hence it is impossible to be certain that normal intellectual development in treated children necessarily results from the treatment. A study of the natural history, to determine what proportion of children with the biochemical defect suffer from mental retardation or the other stigmata of the disease has not been done and now, on ethical grounds, would be unacceptable. However, it has recently been shown (Levy et al., 1970) that the prevalence of phenylketonuria among a 'normal' teenage and adult population is extremely low.

Carcinoma-in-situ of the Cervix

Here, the value of cervical screening is based on the histological finding that the cells seen in carcinoma-in-situ show loss of stratification, loss of differentiation, and nuclear abnormalities, similar to those in invasive cancer; and on the suggestion that a sequential change in the histology can be followed from non-cancerous dysplasia through carcinoma-in-situ and micro-invasive carcinoma to invasive squamous carcinoma (Govan *et al.*, 1966).

However, direct evidence on the progression of the cellular abnormality and hence on its natural history is impossible because the method of diagnosis (biopsy) usually entails complete removal of the lesion; unless its entire border with normal tissue can be seen, it cannot rightly be termed pre-invasive, and therefore the whole lesion must be removed (Knox, 1968b). It might have been possible several years ago to conduct a randomised controlled trial of screening versus not screening, and from comparison of the subsequent development of invasive carcinoma in both groups, to draw conclusions about the proportion of carcinoma-in-situ which would have become invasive and over what time period this would have occurred. The opportunity to do such a study was missed and it would now be regarded as unethical to offer screening to some women but withhold it from others.

Because of this attempts have been made to show the effect which cervical screening has had on the mortality from cervical carcinoma in populations in which it is widely practised compared with those in which it is or was not. Such comparisons have so far provided no conclusive evidence that cervical screening has reduced mortality (Ahluwalia & Doll, 1968; Hammond, 1971) although it is of course possible that an effect will become apparent later when a greater proportion of women have been screened and when the time interval taken for in-situ lesions to progress to death from invasive carcinoma has expired. Using an approach suggested by Dunn (1953) and Knox (1966), data on incidence of carcinoma-in-situ and of invasive carcinoma in British Columbia (Fidler, Boyes & Worth, 1968), have been analysed, and it has been found that many more women have carcinoma-in-situ than apparently would eventually develop invasive carcinoma, suggesting that many of the carcinomas-in-situ regress. This analysis however is cross-sectional—that is, it is comparing women in different age-groups; a study of incidence in the same cohort of women followed over many years should be able to give more firm evidence, but in the absence of a randomly chosen group of unscreened controls, it would still not be possible to be positively certain of the natural history of carcinoma-in-situ.

SCREENING TESTS

The second main area for research into the value of screening concerns the efficiency of the screening tests themselves. Cochrane & Holland (1971) list the criteria by which screening tests should be judged. Since the tests are to be applied to large numbers of people they should be quick and easy to perform, reasonably cheap, acceptable, and safe. They should give a true measure of the attribute being investigated and should produce few false results. It is difficult to find a single test that fulfils all the criteria and so compromises may have to be made. The U.S. Commission on Chronic

Illness (1957) in its definition of screening stressed that the screening test is not intended to be diagnostic and that persons with positive or suspicious findings should be referred for further diagnosis to establish the need for treatment.

Sensitivity and Specificity

The false results which may be given by a screening test are measured by its *sensitivity* and *specificity*, often together referred to as its *validity*. Sensitivity is defined as the ability of a test to classify as positive all persons with the disease; if a test has a sensitivity of 90 per cent this means that 10 per cent of the diseased people screened by it will give false negative results and will be missed by screening. Specificity, the converse, is defined as the ability of a test to classify as negative all persons without the disease; if a test has a specificity of 90 per cent, 10 per cent of non-diseased persons screened by it will give false positive results and will be wrongly referred for follow-up as a result. The classification of sensitivity and specificity is shown in Table 11.2 taken from Thorner & Remein (1961).

TABLE 11.2

CLASSIFICATION OF SCREENING TEST RESULTS

Screening test results	True Diagnosis		Total
	Diseased	Not diseased	
Positive	a	b	$a + b$
Negative	c	d	$c + d$
Total	$a + c$	$b + d$	$a + b + c + d$

a = true positives. c = false negatives
b = false positives. d = true negatives.

Sensitivity is calculated by $a/(a + c) \times 100$, the percentage of people with the disease who were detected by the test. Specificity is calculated by $d/(b + d) \times 100$, the percentage of people without the disease who had a negative result to the test.

The importance of these concepts is obvious. An insensitive test allows many diseased people to slip through the net, decreasing the efficiency of the screening programme in the prevention of ill-health and perhaps giving the individuals a false sense of security which may delay their seeking help when symptoms do appear. A non-specific test on the other hand causes many well people to be referred for further tests with all the worry, inconvenience and cost that entails to the individual, as well as possible iatrogenic complications of management, and a great overloading of resources in dealing with these unnecessary referrals.

The validity of a test is obviously closely related to the natural history of the disease. With tests which measure a continuous variable in the population it is possible to vary the sensitivity and specificity by changing the level at which the test is considered positive.

In Fig. 11.4, if the prevalence of true disease is represented by the shaded distribution within the tail of the larger healthy population, and the vertical line X represents the level of the variable regarded as best separating diseased from non-diseased, the area *a* represents the true positive results, *b* the false

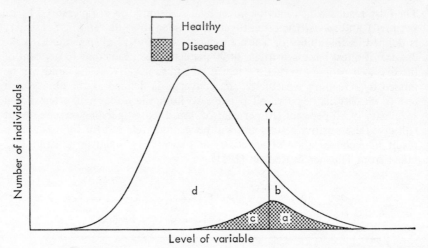

FIG. 11.4. Classification of screening test results (Thorner & Remein, 1961).

positives, *c* the false negatives and *d* the true negatives. By moving the dividing line to the left, *c* becomes smaller thus reducing the number of false negatives and improving the sensitivity, while *b* becomes larger thereby decreasing the specificity. The reverse happens if the test level is moved to the right.

Validity Studies

The method of determining sensitivity and specificity is by means of a survey which, as well as screening a population, also examines the whole population definitively by the best diagnostic methods available to determine the true prevalence of the disease. The population chosen for such a study should ideally approximate as closely as possible to the population for whom screening is ultimately intended. Estimation of the sensitivity and specificity of a test in a population of hospital inpatients, for example, will give answers which almost certainly do not apply to a general population.

One of the best examples of a study of screening test validity is that carried out by Graham & Hollows (1966) in the Ferndale glaucoma study. Over 4000 people between the ages of 40 and 75, living in three Welsh mining villages, were screened for chronic simple glaucoma by applanation and Schiotz tonometry. In addition they all underwent slit-lamp microscopy examination and ophthalmoscopy, and one third had a visual field test. Out of 14 previously unknown cases of glaucoma found in this survey, 7 were missed by tonometry screening, having an intra-ocular pressure of less than 21 mmHg—the commonly accepted cut-off point between healthy and glaucomatous people. The sensitivity of tonometry as a screening test for glaucoma in this population therefore was only 50 per cent. The specificity was more satisfactory, with only 6 per cent of non-glaucomatous people having false positive results, though since this applies to the major part of the population examined, the actual number of false positives all of whom require specialist assessment is large. The authors concluded that tonometric screening, although widely practised, is the least effective of the methods they used to detect glaucoma. Ophthalmoscopy proved the best but this needs to be carried out by trained ophthalmologists and hence would be impractical for population screening. Visual field screening is more sensitive than tonometry but is non-specific. Its high false positive rate, twice that of tonometry, puts it out of court as a practical screening test—the diagnostic follow-up of 12 per cent of the population screened would swamp the ophthalmic services to the detriment of all else.

Predictive Value

Another useful index of a screening test is the predictive value or diagnostic precision of a positive test, which is defined as the proportion of positive test results which represent true disease. It is a measure of the accuracy of the test in detecting the disease at which it is aimed. The predictive value of a positive test is represented in Table 11.2 by $a/(a + b) \times 100$. The size of b, the false positive results, may be large in relation to the total positives, indicating a low predictive value, but this does not imply that its relation to the total numbers of non-diseased persons, the specificity, is also low because, in diseases with a low prevalence the denominator is relatively very large compared with the numerator. This is illustrated in Table 11.3 which is derived from the study by Shapiro, Strax & Venet (1971) of palpation and mammography as screening tests for breast cancer. What these tests in fact detect is an abnormality in the breast, which under screening circumstances as an indicator of carcinoma, has a predictive value of only 20 per cent. This means that out of every 5 women biopsied only one is found to have cancer. But although the predictive value is low, out of over 56 000 screening examinations only about 500 biopsy recommendations turned out to be

TABLE 11.3

VALIDITY OF SCREENING TESTS FOR BREAST CANCER

Adapted from Shapiro *et al.*, 1971.
The false negative results to screening (c) were not determined in this study.

	Confirmed carcinoma	No carcinoma	Total
Biopsy performed as a result of screening	127	497	624
Negative to screening	c	$55\,977 - c$	$55\,977$
Total	$127 + c$	$56\,474 - c$	$56\,601$

negative, giving a specificity of the order of 98 per cent. (The exact figure cannot be given in this case because the false negative rate (c) is not known and so all cells in Table 11.3 cannot be filled in; when the prevalence is so low however (about 2 per 1000 screened), variation in the false negative rate (sensitivity) makes little difference to the specificity.)

In Fig. 11.4 the predictive value is shown by the relationship between the area a and the whole area, a + b, to the right of the dividing line between health and disease. If the prevalence can be increased by selection of a high-risk group for screening (based on knowledge of aetiological factors in the disease which have been determined by study of its natural history) there will be an increase in true positives proportional to the increased prevalence (Thorner & Remein, 1961). The predictive value of the test is thus increased, while the sensitivity and specificity remain unchanged. This is an important point in practice since clearly the cost of screening per case detected is lower the higher the disease prevalence and this is indicated by the predictive value of the test but not by sensitivity. Specificity however, as an index of the cost of follow-up does provide helpful information on the economic aspect of screening.

Reproducibility

Another important attribute of a screening test is its ability to give consistent results when used on the same subject at different times or by different observers. This is called the reproducibility, repeatability, or precision of a test. It can be affected by biological variation of the index measured, by variation between and within observers, and by variation within the test instrument or technique. The method of evaluating reproducibility consists of obtaining a series of paired measurements of the same person made by the same or different observers. It is calculated as the proportion of all results which are agreed, or as the proportion of all positive results which are agreed. The latter proportion is preferred because there is more often disagreement about the positive test results, but when the prevalence is low the proportion of all agreed results is heavily weighted with negatives and hence important differences in the positives can be masked.

Much work has been done on the reproducibility of blood pressure measurement as a screening test. Rose, Holland & Crowley (1964) discuss the different causes of variability in blood pressure readings. Firstly, there are measurement errors, some of which may be due to the sphygmomanometer; cuffs of different widths and lengths can lead to different readings. Secondly, there are important measurement errors arising in even the best trained observers; some of these may be connected with factors such as auditory acuity, reaction-time and the difficulty of reading a moving column, but there are two less obvious sources of error, terminal digit preference and prejudice against certain values. When, as in most clinical situations, the blood pressure is recorded to the nearest 5 mmHg, at extreme ends of the pressure range it has been shown that more values ending in 0 are recorded than would occur by chance, indicating that observers are preferring 0 values to 5 values. Even when pressure is recorded in 2 mmHg steps, different observers taking several pressures have their own particular terminal digit preferences. It has also been shown that where a particular value is thought to represent the dividing line between 'health' and 'disease' (for example, a diastolic blood pressure of 90 mmHg), too few of these values are recorded; the prejudice against them may be because the observer consciously or unconsciously makes the decision as to the subject's disease status and records for him a value which classifies him firmly as either healthy or diseased. This prejudice against the border-line values also occurs in other measurements and, in the case of intra-ocular pressure, was responsible for the mistaken theory that this variable had a bimodal distribution in the population (Graham & Hollows, 1966).

The third source of variability which influences test results is biological. In the case of blood pressure there is very wide biological variation within an individual caused by several known factors such as emotional state, recent activity, posture, and temperature of surroundings, and probably by unknown factors as well. In a survey of 700 men examined annually in four successive years, Armitage *et al.* (1966) using a specially designed sphygmomanometer which eliminates terminal digit preference and prejudice against dividing values, found that the standard deviation for individual subjects between separate occasions was 9·1 mmHg for systolic pressure and 7·2 mmHg for diastolic pressure. Using the mean of the four annual pressures as a standard, they calculated that if a single examination had been used to separate the 'hypertensives' from the 'normotensives', there would have been 35 per cent false positive and 5 per cent false negative classifications. They concluded that the reproducibility and validity of blood pressure as a screening test can be considerably improved if more than one reading is taken, and that case-finding, with the implication of subsequent drug treatment, should not be based on a single reading. Although the variability of blood pressure estimation may be greater than that of many other screening tests it serves to underline the importance of a test that gives reproducible results.

Acceptability

It is of obvious importance to ensure that a screening test is reasonably acceptable to the public and in particular to the people who are most at risk of developing the disease. Acceptability may be affected by personal factors, such as perception of need, and the convenience of attending for screening; and by factors intrinsic to the test, such as the discomfort it causes, and the place where it is performed.

An indication of acceptability is given by the response rate when screening is offered to a population. The cervical smear test for carcinoma-in-situ of the cervix is acceptable to large numbers of women but apparently not to older women of low socio-economic group who are consistently under-represented in statistics of women screened, and who are the group at particularly high risk. Offering different methods of testing, such as providing a domiciliary service, are one way of improving acceptability. Domiciliary testing by district nurses of women on a 'risk register' of problem families has been shown to increase the acceptability in high risk groups, and hence also to increase the yield of disease detected by screening (Osborn & Leyshon, 1966). Figs. 11.5 and 11.6, derived from their data, show firstly that home testing was accepted by a greater proportion of women in social classes IV and V than attended the clinic service, and secondly that the proportion of positive

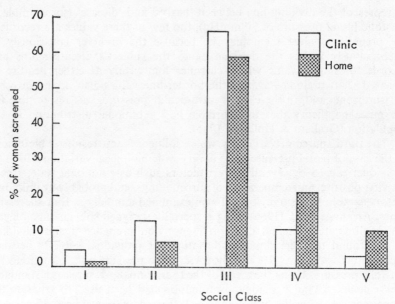

FIG. 11.5. Social Class Distribution of Women Screened (Osborn & Leyshon, 1966).

smears found was much higher among women tested at home than those tested at clinics.

Another alternative is to devise different test methods, and this has been done in cytology by Koch & Stakemann (1962) and Davis & Kurz (1962) who have developed a vaginal irrigation pipette which can be used by the woman

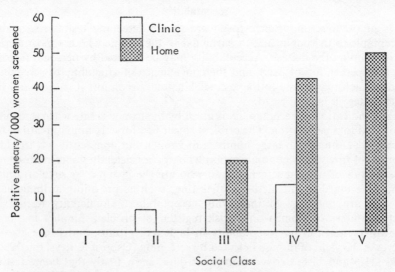

FIG. 11.6. Social Class Distribution of Women with positive smears (Osborn & Leyshon, 1966).

herself to wash out cells from the cervix. The validity of this method compared with cervical smears has been tested and found reasonably satisfactory (Husain, 1970) and it has been shown to be acceptable in the United States by Davis & Jones (1966). Its acceptability in Great Britain has been reported as somewhat unsatisfactory by Macgregor, Fraser & Mann (1966). A randomised trial comparing the acceptability of the vaginal pipette with that of the cervical smear is at present in progress in this country (Carruthers, personal communication).

Organisation

Improving acceptability and response is only one aspect of the problem of organising resources to provide a screening test or series of tests for the public. The needed scale of provision is likely to be large and operational studies of how this can best be achieved are desirable before a service is introduced, although they have seldom been done in the past. The information needed from such studies include the best geographical siting of screening to make it easily available; the training and deployment of staff; the provision of services for follow-up; and the method of recording test results to ensure both that the result is notified to the appropriate authority; and that the individual can be recalled for later screening where this is necessary. It is likely that computers will play an increasing role in the recording of screening procedures and will provide a method of linking the screening record with subsequent screening tests and with other health records.

The cost of providing a screening service is another area for investigation. Not only does the cost of the screening process itself need to be recorded, but also the cost of the campaign to persuade people to attend, of the clerical work involved and of the record system. The cost of follow-up procedures is also important, particularly when the specificity of the test is low.

Safety

The safety of the screening procedure is of such obvious importance that it hardly seems necessary to mention it. When contemplating new screening tests their possible dangers are usually taken into consideration; for example, the possible danger of an accumulating dose of radiation from repeated mammography is an aspect of breast cancer screening that obviously needs expert study. Risks from screening procedures need to be seen in perspective; for techniques of accepted value small risks must inevitably be taken. Subjecting virtually all newborn infants to a heel prick to obtain blood for a Guthrie test will probably cause some morbidity, a very small proportion of which may be serious—known instances include a broken tibia from rough handling of the infant, and osteomyelitis of the calcaneum resulting from infection introduced at the time of the test. Nevertheless where, as in this form of screening, the prevalence of the condition sought is extremely low, continuing surveillance of the dangers of the test is needed to ensure that the drawbacks do not outweigh the advantages.

MANAGEMENT OF THOSE WHO SCREEN POSITIVE

The third and perhaps most important area in evaluation of screening concerns the fate of individuals who have a positive result to the test. The importance of this cannot be over-stressed for it is only by study of these people that the effectiveness of early detection can be shown, and it is also in these people that most harm resulting from screening is likely to occur. Commonly reports of screening are given which claim to show its value simply by a tally of the abnormalities found, as though having got to the point of diagnosis, there were no further problems. In fact the problems raised by treatment for chronic disease are large and important, and it is only by long-term follow-up of treated patients that the true effect of early diagnosis and treatment can be determined.

Possible harmful effects of screening often quoted are the danger of encouraging hypochondria and the danger of inducing a false sense of security; probably of much greater importance is the danger of submitting symptomless people to a treatment regime which may well have unpleasant or even dangerous side effects when there is no certainty that they will benefit from it. Therefore it is essential, first to be certain that each person submitted to treatment would in fact eventually develop the disease. This, as has already been seen, means defining the test level which separates those who will develop the disease from those who will not, and eliminating false positive results to the test by further diagnostic procedures. Secondly it is essential to prove, by means of randomised controlled trials, that the treatment does in fact improve the long-term prognosis of the condition.

Trials of the Effectiveness of Treatment

Virtually all screening of adults aimed at detecting presymptomatic abnormality also picks up people with overt symptomatic disease who for one reason or another have not sought medical care through the usual channels. This particularly applies to the elderly who seem to accept many potentially remediable disabilities, such as deafness, visual disability, and foot disorders, as a necessary part of ageing. For these overt conditions, and indeed for some presymptomatic conditions where there is an ethical obligation to treat all cases (for example, cancers), the effectiveness of the treatment itself cannot

TABLE 11.4

INCIDENCE OF MAJOR COMPLICATIONS IN THE TREATED AND CONTROL GROUPS
IN THE VA TRIAL OF TREATMENT OF SYMPTOMLESS
HYPERTENSION.

Pre-randomisation Diastolic B.P. (mmHg)	Control Group			Treated Group		
	Number rando-mised	Number with complica-tions	% incidence	Number rando-mised	Number with complica-tions	% incidence
115–129	70	27	38·6	73	1	1·4
105–114	110	35	31·8	100	8	8·0
90–104	84	21	25·0	86	14	16·3

usually be tested, but the effectiveness of screening may be found by comparing a screened with an unscreened population.

Thus two types of trial of effectiveness are possible; the first compares a treated group of abnormalities detected at screening with an untreated group and the second compares a screened group with an unscreened. Similar rules apply to both types of study, of which the principal ones are firstly that the groups should have been chosen from a single population which has been randomly divided into a study group and a control group, and secondly that the effectiveness of the intervention measure should be assessed by positive end-points, such as reduced mortality from the conditions, rather than merely a conversion of the test result to 'normal'.

Hypertension

An example of a randomised controlled trial of treatment of a condition found at screening, is the U.S. Veteran's Administration Co-operative Study of Hypertension (1970). In this study 523 male hospital inpatients with an average age of 50, who as an incidental finding were discovered to have symptomless hypertension with diastolic levels between 90 and 129 mmHg, were the subjects of a double-blind randomised controlled trial of treatment with hydrochlorothiazide, reserpine and hydralazine. The entire group was followed up and all deaths and major cardiovascular complications recorded. Table 11.4 taken from Freis (1970) shows the results.

The average follow-up period for the most severe group was only 1·6 years because the difference between the two groups was so striking that it was considered unethical to withhold treatment from the control group any longer. The remainder were followed for an average of 3·3 years. The complications which were reduced in the treated group were principally cerebrovascular accidents and no difference in the rate of acute myocardial infarction was found between the groups. It is interesting to note that in treated men with an initial pressure below 115 mmHg, in all of whom the length of follow-up was presumably the same, the rate of complications was higher in those with lower pressures. This phenomenon might be due to a higher rate of myocardial infarction among those with moderate hypertension, as has been suggested by Breckenridge, Dollery & Parry (1970).

This study is one of the few which has shown positive benefit from treating a symptomless condition in adults, and provides evidence in favour of screening middle-aged men for this condition and treating those confirmed to have raised diastolic blood pressure down to a level of 105 mmHg. There may be some reservations about its applicability to a well population rather than a population who were already in hospital for some other condition, but faced with the results of this trial few would consider it ethical not to treat such men. The situation regarding treatment of symptomless hypertension in younger (or older) men, and in women, remains unproven but studies of these groups in well populations are now in progress. It is hoped that these studies, particularly in younger men, may show some effect in reducing myocardial infarction as well as cerebrovascular accidents.

Breast Cancer

An example of a randomised controlled trial of screening is the large breast cancer study in the Health Insurance Plan of Greater New York, (Shapiro,

Strax & Venet, 1971) in which 62 000 women aged 40–65 have been studied. The Insurance Plan provides medical care for its 700 000 members in a number of group practices throughout New York, and keeps accurate statistical records of utilisation of all services, thus providing an excellent population base for large epidemiological studies of this type.

The women in the breast cancer study were randomly divided into a study group and a control group; the 31 000 in the study group were offered breast cancer screening by palpation and mammography annually for four successive years. Their subsequent experience of breast cancer is being compared over at least ten years with that of women in the control group who have received no special provision, and the results of screening are being assessed by a comparison of mortality and a comparison of survival rates in the two groups.

TABLE 11.5

PRELIMINARY MORTALITY RESULTS FROM BREAST CANCER
SCREENING STUDY (SHAPIRO *et al.*, 1971)

Age at death	Number of deaths from breast cancer	
	Study Group	Control Group
40–49	15	17
50–59	10	28
60–64	6	7
Total	31	52

During the four years of screening, 246 histologically confirmed cases of breast cancer were found in the study group compared with 199 in the control group. Of the study group cases, 127 were detected at screening, 63 between screening examinations and 56 in women who had refused screening. Out of more than 56 000 screening examinations, 906 biopsies were recommended and 624 performed in order to detect the 127 cancers. 70 per cent of these had no evidence of axillary node involvement compared with 44 per cent of those in the control group. Preliminary mortality results from this study cover the period up to the end of October 1969 at which time every woman had been in the study for at least four years. During this time there were 31 deaths from breast cancer in the study group compared with 52 in the control group. The difference was restricted to women who had been in the study for at least two years and as shown in Table 11.5 seemed to apply only to women in the fifth decade.

The favourable effect of screening suggested by these results cannot yet be regarded as conclusive since the follow-up is short in relation to the natural history of the disease and it is possible that, while the duration of survival has been prolonged by early diagnosis and treatment, subsequent mortality may remain unaffected. The apparent restriction of benefit to women in a single decade also raises questions as to whether this is a true biological finding, which may be answered as more information becomes available.

TABLE 11.6

CASE FATALITY RATES $3\frac{1}{2}$ YEARS FROM DIAGNOSIS IN BREAST CANCER SCREENING STUDY (SHAPIRO *et al.*, 1971)

	Percentage of cases dead within $3\frac{1}{2}$ years
Total Study Group	18·1
Detected at screening	7·6
Presented between screenings	30·7
In women who refused screening	27·8
Control Group	33·7

The New York study has also examined the survival experience of women with breast cancer, to determine if those detected at screening have a longer period of survival, with the results shown in Table 11.6. The apparent clear advantage to cases detected by screening, however, also needs to be treated with caution. There are two difficulties in using survival rates as indicators of the effectiveness of screening. The first of these is the lead time gained by

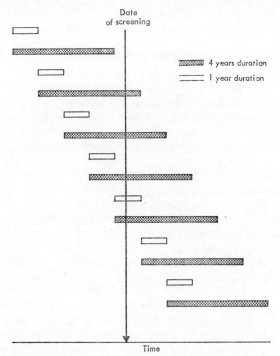

FIG. 11.7. Selection of longer duration cases by screening (Feinleib & Zelen, 1969).

earlier diagnosis. It is obvious that quite independently of any treatment given, early detection automatically improves a survival rate taken from time of diagnosis, improving it by the interval between the early diagnosis and the time it would have been diagnosed if screening had not been performed—the so-called lead time. If the lead time were known, a more accurate measure of effectiveness could be obtained by comparison of survival from time of early detection plus lead time in the screened group, with survival from time of diagnosis in the control group. Hutchison & Shapiro (1968) have calculated that the average lead time gained by early detection of breast cancer is one year, and this has, in fact, been allowed for in Table 11.6.

The second difficulty concerns the selection of longer duration cases by screening. Feinleib & Zelen (1969) have illustrated this by the model shown in Fig. 11.7. In this model, the bars indicate preclinical disease and usual diagnosis occurs at the end of the bar. If the course of preclinical disease is of varying length (in this example varying between 1 and 4 years) the longer cases tend to be over-represented at any point in time, and thus are over-represented among the cases detected by screening. Since long duration of preclinical disease may well be correlated with long duration of the clinical phase, improved survival after screening, even after accounting for lead time, may simply be due to a preponderance of more benign disease among the cases discovered at screening. If the screening could be repeated at intervals equal to the shortest preclinical phase this possible bias could be eliminated but the lead time problem would remain. Feinleib & Zelen conclude that the only method of assessing the effectiveness of screening which will safeguard against these difficulties is the comparison of total mortality in the entire screened population with that in a randomly selected control population.

Complications of Treatment

Controlled trials of effectiveness should also show up any dangers or serious complications of treatment, provided that they are continued to an end-point which is a firm indicator of health. With cancers it is obvious that one cannot assume the disease has been eliminated simply by removal of the primary tumour; but there is a danger, with drug treatments which convert the test index to a 'normal' level, of thinking that benefit necessarily accrues to the patient from this change.

The University Group Diabetes Program (1971), has found that of a group of diabetics randomly assigned to treatment with insulin, oral anti-diabetic drugs or a placebo, those on oral drugs had a significantly greater mortality over an 8 year period than those on either insulin or a placebo. At the start of the trial, all these patients were more ill than those likely to be found by screening, so that this result does not necessarily invalidate the use of these drugs in controlling early diabetes but it does indicate the need for an end-point which shows overall benefit. This particular finding conflicts with that of Keen & Jarrett (1970) who as we have already seen found that in people with borderline values of blood sugar detected at screening, over a 7 year period, tolbutamide with dietary restriction may have reduced the number of cardiovascular events in subjects without a prior history of arterial disease, although in the group as a whole its effect did not differ significantly from that of the placebo.

Where screening has been introduced without a controlled trial of its effectiveness, the extent of iatrogenic consequences of the method of treatment can only be found by a special case-control study. It is likely also that difficulty will be experienced in obtaining a comparable control group, since the people who attend for screening, and of them, the sub-group found to be diseased, may well differ in possibly important respects from the general population.

Acceptability of Treatment

Of equal importance to the acceptability of the screening test and of the definitive diagnostic procedure is acceptability of the treatment offered, if screening is to be an effective means of reducing morbidity. Most drug treatments have side effects and while these may not be so large as to cause measurable changes in health, they may well cause sufficient discomfort to the patient to make him give up the treatment. The annoyance of constant pill-taking, and ordinary forgetfulness, must also play a part in reducing response. It is always difficult to be sure of the extent to which patients observe a particular drug regime, but some studies have been done in which pills have been marked with agents detectable in urine or blood, and subsequently measured. In the Veteran's Administration study of hypertension, for 3 months before any drug treatment was started, the entire group of eligible men was put on a placebo containing riboflavine which, excreted in urine, fluoresces under ultraviolet light. It was found that about half of the men were not taking the pills and so these were eliminated, and the remainder then randomly allocated to treatment or placebo groups to take part in the trial. If as much as a half of all people offered a treatment do not take it as directed, and if some of the remainder drop out because of unpleasant side effects or the boredom of long-continued therapy, the total benefit of early treatment will be very much less than its potential value. It is also possible that those dropping out may belong to a special category whose prognosis may differ from the remainder. The answers to this problem lie in education of the patients in the importance of continued treatment, and to a lesser extent in developing pleasanter and longer acting forms of the drug which may not have to be taken so frequently.

MULTIPLE SCREENING

Multiple screening and a sub-group of it, automated biochemical and haematological screening, are two forms which present particular problems from the point of view of evaluation.

Multiple Screening

Multiple tests may be used in screening for single conditions, such as the several individual tests included in the Stycar test for evaluating infants' hearing, or the use of palpation, mammography, and thermography in screening for breast cancer. The reason for including more than one test for any disease is that the yield of cases found is thereby increased. In ischaemic heart disease, for example, screening by smoking history, exercise history, blood pressure, E.C.G., serum cholesterol, and blood sugar gives a greater yield, and where individuals screen positive to more than one test, a greater predictive value than any of these tests in isolation; it will be noticed, however, that included in this series of tests are at least 3 which screen for other diseases as well, (smoking history for risk of chronic bronchitis and lung cancer, blood pressure for risk of cerebrovascular disease, blood sugar for diabetes) and this series has thus become multiple screening for multiple diseases.

Multiple or multiphasic screening in which a number of tests screen for a number of conditions has been used for many years in antenatal care and in serial examinations of infants and children. In its application to adults, which has developed over the last 20 years, it can be conveniently divided into screening of the elderly which is aimed at detecting overt unreported disability and disease (Sheldon, 1948, Williamson *et al.*, 1964) for which there are accepted methods of treatment, and screening of the middle-aged which is aimed at detecting presymptomatic abnormalities and, by early treatment of these, preventing later disease. It is with the latter group that this section is principally concerned.

The main reason for grouping a battery of tests together is economic; having got an individual to attend for screening it saves time and expense to test him for as many conditions as possible during this one attendance. Considerable work has been done, particularly in the United States, on the organisation of multiple screening including the use of computers in this field. Collen (1966) gives an excellent description of a purpose-built automated multiple screening clinic in which up to 100 000 people per year can undergo 25 different tests, including questionnaires on physical and psychological health. Similar automated multiple health testing facilities are increasing in most developed countries.

The selection of tests for inclusion in such clinics however often seems to be based more on the diagnostic techniques which are available than on proven value of early treatment for the conditions being sought. In an ideal situation every screening procedure included should have been subjected to the lengthy process of evaluating the test, the treatment and its effect on the natural history of the condition, which has already been described. In practice—even in the long-established forms of multiple screening in antenatal and child care—no multiple screening system can at present be said to have conclusively proved its value to those being screened.

Several studies now in progress, investigating the effect of early intervention in individual diseases, will be helpful in completing the evaluation of multiple screening, although they will not be able to determine interactions of the different tests used, nor of the different treatments which may be prescribed for individuals found to have more than one presymptomatic abnormality. There is, as far as is known, at present only one randomised controlled trial of the effect of multiple screening on the health of a middle-aged population. In this study (Trevelyan, personal communication) men and women between the ages of 40 and 64 on the lists of 2 group practices are randomly divided into 2 groups, one of which is invited to attend for multiple screening initially and again after 2 years, and the other acts as a control group. The tests include a health questionnaire, blood pressure, electrocardiogram, chest X-ray, respiratory function, visual acuity and visual fields, audiometry and examination of a specimen of blood for haemoglobin, blood sugar, serum cholesterol, protein-bound iodine, blood urea, and serum uric acid. At a subsequent visit to the doctor, women are screened for cervical and breast cancer, and abnormal results to the other tests for both sexes are confirmed or rejected by more definitive diagnosis.

Various facts about the subsequent health experience of both study and control groups are being measured for several years after the initial screening. As well as comparing the mortality in both groups, information is also collected about the contacts with medical services in and out of hospital, diagnoses made, periods off work, and an assessment of the costs of providing care for both groups. This study should thus eventually provide much needed information about the effect of multiple screening on people's health, the utilisation of health services in the screened compared with the un-screened, and an approximate estimation of the money spent or saved as a result of screening.

Biochemical and Haematological Screening

The examination of a specimen of blood for a number of different biochemical and haematological variables is frequently included in multiple screening clinics and has also in Sweden been used with a minimum of supporting tests as a method of multiple screening of a population (Jungner, 1966). The development of this form of screening has been well described by Wilson (1969) who points out the sequence of events which led to its introduction. The tremendous increase in laboratory test requests in hospital has stimulated the development of automation in laboratory equipment and in the handling and processing of laboratory data; automation has made it possible to carry out many more tests than was formerly possible, and it is possible to offer more tests for a lower cost than in a non-automated system. From here, it is a simple step to perform more tests than have been requested. There is little doubt that the incentive for developing this form of screening came not from the necessity to control disease but from the technological achievements which made it possible to perform many tests on many people. The tests available in automatic analysers have been primarily provided to meet the needs of hospital clinicians and comprise the usual range of diagnostic tests which lend themselves to being automated; their use as screening tests is secondary.

The value of this form of screening is still far from proved, but its use in screening of hospital patients and in patients consulting their general practitioner is under study. Whitehead, Carmalt & Widdowson (1967) have studied the effect of multiple analysis of one specimen of blood, taken soon after a patient is admitted to hospital (an 'admission profile') on several factors, including the length of the patient's stay, and the number of new diagnoses made. Carmalt (1969) reported that no difference had been shown in length of stay in profile patients compared with a randomly selected control group. In 8·3 per cent of patients, however, results of tests which would not normally have been requested led to a new or additional diagnosis, about half of these being mild diabetes and iron deficiency anaemia. When 'profiling' was extended to patients attending their general practitioner, the proportion of diagnostic results rose to 10 per cent, partly because of the inclusion of haemoglobin and erythrocyte sedimentation rate among the tests. These diagnostic results were of varying clinical importance and an attempt to classify them by their effect on the management of the patient has not been reported.

The results which were of diagnostic value, however, were not nearly so frequent as results of unrequested tests for which no explanation could be found. When reviewed within one week of the profile, 36 per cent of patients had unexpected unexplained results to tests which had not been requested. A follow-up of a randomly selected group of these patients at least one year later, indicated that in 15·5 per cent of the original group, the result was still unexplained. Whether or not these 'abnormalities' are indicative of pre-symptomatic disease is still an open question.

Barnett, Civin & Schoen (1970) in a general review of biochemical multiple screening conclude that although the laboratory problems in testing are still formidable, they are being solved far more rapidly than are the problems relating to the medical usefulness of the test results. These workers argue against the assumption that the production of huge volumes of screening information will by itself contribute to human knowledge or health and stress the need for restraint in this form of screening until more concrete evidence of its value can be shown.

USE OF MEDICAL CARE RESOURCES

Once a particular form of screening, whether it be for a single condition or multiple, has been subjected to medical evaluation and found to be effective, it is then necessary to study possible methods of organising it as a service and to estimate the costs and resources which will be required balancing these against its level of effectiveness. The assumption that costs in both money and manpower will be saved has sometimes provided the principal impetus for introducing a screening service, the reasoning being that the costs of initiating and maintaining a screening service and of providing treatment for all the illness found will be less than the costs which would have been incurred if the illness had been allowed to develop into a later state. If the later need for expensive hospital inpatient treatment could be averted by treatment of early pathological change money might be saved.

In any assessment of cost-effectiveness, the costs to the people being screened also need to be considered. Expenses may be incurred in taking time off work to attend for screening and, in cases with positive test results, in attending medical services for further diagnosis. These, and the costs of subsequent treatment of the individuals found to be diseased, need to be set against the costs which would have arisen if the disease had been allowed to follow an uninterrupted course, which might include loss of productivity, social support to dependants and a number of other economic factors affecting a person's family and work which may differ between someone who is alive and well and one who is dead or chronically ill.

The use of screening as a means of conserving scarce medical manpower for its primary role of looking after the sick has also been put forward, particularly in the United States where there has long been a belief in the value of the 'annual physical' examination as a means of staying healthy. With increasing expectations of the public and increasing specialisation of doctors it is now recognised that there are not enough general practitioners or internists to provide this sort of personal service for all who would like and could pay for it, and 'automated multiphasic health testing' using paramedical personnel has developed as an alternative. It has also been encouraged by public health authorities as a means of bringing medical services to those unable to afford them, though publicly financed screening for the indigent often appears to lack the necessary back-up of treatment facilities for all the latent and overt disease detected by it.

The theory that the total use of resources and costs will be reduced by screening remains to be proved and there are good reasons for thinking that the reverse may be true. The costs of setting up and maintaining a screening service for a large population are highly demanding in staff, equipment, and record handling. All screening tests give a certain proportion of false positive results, all of which will use further diagnostic services. The treatment offered may be no different from that which would have been given had the disease presented later, only the follow-up is longer. It is also likely, particularly in the elderly, that screening will reveal need for treatment of conditions, such as deafness or foot disorders, which in the absence of a screening service would not have been brought to medical attention.

An illustration of the scale of resources is provided by a rough estimate of what might be required each year in England and Wales if breast cancer screening by palpation and mammography were found to be effective, if the operational problems surrounding it were solved, and if the American findings were exactly duplicated in this country. In order to screen women between 45 and 64, assuming that 65 per cent of them responded, 400 screening clinics would be needed with at least 3 full-time screening staff, and with mammography equipment, the whole costing between £3 000 000 and £4 000 000 per annum. For reading the mammography films, staff equivalent to nearly 200 radiologists would be needed; as there are only 500 radiologists in the country, paramedical staff would obviously need to be trained for this task. In addition there would be costs arising from the complicated record and recall system which would be necessary, and from the surgical and pathological facilities needed to cope with extra biopsies, as well as the costs of treating the cancers found. For a cost-effectiveness study all these costs need to be balanced against the costs and the outlook for the patients which would have occurred if screening had not been carried out. If much expensive palliative treatment of late cancers could be averted, it could even be that the balance of costs turned out to be in favour of screening. As a result of screening women between 45 and 64, up to 850 lives might be saved each year.

Within any medical care system the total amount of money and resources is limited and some form of rationing inevitable. The purposes of cost-effectiveness and cost benefit studies which balance the total costs calculated in this sort of way against the effectiveness measured in terms of reduced mortality or morbidity, are to predict the resources required for obtaining a stated result, to decide between alternative methods of dealing with a health problem, and to make the more difficult decision on the priority to be given to control of one particular condition as against effort in other areas of medical care competing for the same limited resources. Screening, as a relatively new form of medical care in which many evaluative trials are being carried out, provides a useful opportunity for study of cost-effectiveness, though even in this field there is still a hampering lack of the needed data.

SUMMARY OF PRESENT POSITION

In their well-known review 'The Principles and Practice of Screening for Disease', Wilson & Jungner (1968) concluded that we are still at a very early and comparatively primitive stage in the systematic detection and treatment of early disease. Further research was needed in all of the many chronic conditions which they examined. Similarly, the Nuffield Provincial Hospitals Trust (1968) publication on Screening in Medical Care found that of 10 conditions reviewed, only 4 (*tuberculosis, deafness in children, Rhesus haemolytic disease of the newborn* and *phenylketonuria*) stood up to critical evaluation as conditions for which screening was worthwhile.

In terms of conclusive evidence of the value of screening, there has been little change since then, largely because studies of the effect of screening are necessarily of long duration. The present position regarding the various conditions used to illustrate this chapter can be summarised as follows.

Ischaemic heart disease. There is as yet no conclusive evidence that treatment can alter the course of this disease, but several intervention trials, employing diet, cholesterol-lowering drugs, or advice about smoking and exercise, are now in progress (Turpeinen et al., 1968, Morris & Gardner, 1969, Rose, 1970). If the results of any or all of these trials show that the incidence of myocardial infarction can be reduced by these preventive measures, development of a test which can predict those who are going to be attacked more accurately than the present tests for precursor abnormalities will be needed.

Diabetes mellitus. Again, evidence of the effectiveness of treatment in people with symptomless hyperglycaemia is inadequate. Results which have so far been published from the Bedford trial (Keen & Jarrett, 1970) seem to indicate that oral antidiabetic drugs may be of benefit to certain individuals at low risk of cardiovascular disease, but this finding conflicts with that of the University Group Diabetes Program (1971) which reported a greater mortality from cardiovascular disease in patients treated by oral hypoglycaemic agents than in those receiving insulin or a placebo. Further follow-up in these trials may give more positive results, but at present there is no justification for widespread screening for this condition.

Phenylketonuria. A national service to screen all newborn infants already exists. But evidence of the effectiveness of treatment by low phenylalanine diet, although suggestive is not conclusive (Bickel, 1953). A few individuals with the untreated biochemical defect develop normal intelligence (Mabry, Denniston & Coldwell, 1966) so that in the absence of a randomised controlled trial, it is impossible to be sure that normal intelligence in a treated child is necessarily the result of treatment.

Carcinoma-in-situ of the cervix. Here again a national screening service has been introduced on inadequate evidence, particularly in relation to the proportion of in-situ carcinomas which would become invasive if left untreated (Knox, 1968b). A reduction in mortality from carcinoma of the cervix, which could be attributed to a cervical screening programme, has not yet occurred in any of the areas where screening has been widely practised.

Glaucoma. Tonometry is not sufficiently sensitive for use as a screening test, and the effectiveness of long-term treatment of raised intra-ocular pressure in preventing blindness has not been demonstrated (Cochrane, Graham & Wallace, 1968).

Hypertension. In a selected group of middle-aged males, screening and early treatment of symptomless hypertension has been shown to be of value in preventing cerebrovascular disease (U.S. Veterans Administration, 1970). Research is still required into the effectiveness of treatment in other age/sex groups. Operational trials of methods of organising screening for hypertension, and of keeping symptomless people under treatment are now needed in this country.

Breast cancer. Screening by palpation and mammography has been shown in the short term to be effective in reducing mortality from breast cancer (Shapiro, Strax & Venet, 1971). While awaiting confirmation of this finding in the longer term, some of the formidable problems which would arise in providing resources for mass screening by mammography need to be tackled through operational studies.

Other conditions. Thus it is only in the last two conditions that there is any definite evidence of the value of early detection and treatment. Screening has been advocated for other conditions which have not been mentioned here, but, certainly in adults, its value has not been proved. The biggest problem is always in demonstrating, by a randomised controlled trial, that early intervention alters the natural history of the disease. Trials of early intervention have failed to show a significant benefit in *lung cancer* (Brett, 1968), *bronchitis* (Medical Research Council, 1966), and *iron deficiency anaemia* (haemoglobin levels between 12 g and 8 g/100 ml) (Elwood & Hughes, 1970). Further study is needed before the effect on prognosis of screening schoolchildren for *bacteriuria* in preventing pyelonephritis can be determined. As already mentioned, the effect of *multiple screening* of middle-aged people and *automated biochemical and haematological screening* of patients attending hospitals and general practitioners also needs further assessment.

FUTURE RESEARCH IN SCREENING

For many other chronic conditions, no studies are yet in progress as far as is known. One large problem to which this applies is the screening of elderly people where many surveys have demonstrated a high yield of unreported but overt disability. Since there are recognised treatments for many of these disorders, it is generally accepted that early detection must be beneficial. This hypothesis has not been tested however and it is important both to find out if early detection and treatment really keeps an old person more independent rather than less, and to estimate the resources needed for treatment. For example, the N.H.S. hearing-aid service, which is struggling to maintain even the present level of provision, would be quite unable in its present form to cope with the estimated 900 000 elderly people with untreated hearing problems. Similar considerations almost certainly apply to other services such as chiropody and dentistry.

In addition to the obvious areas of evaluating the tests, the results of treatment and the resources required, research is needed into the incidence of most conditions in order that, for those who screen negative, the interval between successive examinations can be decided, and services rationally planned to cope with the load of disease which will arise within a given time period. If the incidence of the condition falls, the screening service will become uneconomic as is now the case in this country with tuberculosis.

Related to this concept of screening not as a 'one-off' procedure but as a continuing service, is the problem of recording results to ensure that the results of one examination can be linked with those of subsequent tests. Automation will undoubtedly play an important part in the future in developing record systems which enable successive measurements of different indices of health to be available to the family doctor and others involved in the care of the patient, provided that the problems associated with confidentiality of personal demographic and medical records can be satisfactorily solved.

Another important but relatively unexplored area, relevant to the advancement of knowledge of the value of screening, is health education. This can contribute to the control of chronic diseases in three ways, firstly by educating people against the particular behaviour patterns which make them liable to the disease, such as smoking or over-eating; secondly by educating them to report symptoms to their doctor, since screening may well be an inefficient method of detecting conditions when the patient is already aware of discomfort; and thirdly by educating people to be screened for conditions in which the value of this form of care has been proved. Trials of the effectiveness of health education in these three ways are needed.

A similar area for research is the psychological consequence of screening. The public in general seems to be in favour of 'health checks', albeit on the unproved assumption that they are of benefit, and in people who screen negative the sense of reassurance may in itself be of value to health. On the converse side, the worry caused to people found to have signs of early disease may well be disproportionate to the severity of their condition. Christie (personal communication) found that of 404 people referred to their general practitioner as a result of screening, with previously unrecognised hypertension or diabetes, 1·5 per cent had severe psychological reactions to the knowledge of their illness which required drug treatment or referral to a psychiatrist; and an additional 6 per cent suffered milder anxiety. Assessment of the possible psychological harm resulting from false positive results to screening, is particularly important.

But perhaps the most important area for further research relating to early intervention in disease is in the clinical field of developing more effective, safe and pleasant methods of treating chronic disease, rather than in increasing the technological sophistication of diagnosis.

References

AHLUWALIA, H. S. & DOLL, R. (1968). *Br. J. prev. soc. Med.*, 22, 161.
ARMITAGE, P., FOX, W., ROSE, G. A. & TINKER, C. M. (1966). *Clin. Sci.*, 30, 377.
BARNETT, R. N., CIVIN, W. H. & SCHOEN, I. (1970). *Am. J. clin. Path.*, 54, 483.
BICKEL, H. (1953). *Lancet*, 2, 812.
BRECKENRIDGE, A., DOLLERY, C. T. & PARRY, E. H. O. (1970). *Q. J. Med.*, 39, 411.
BRETT, G. Z. (1968). *Thorax*, 23, 414.
BUTLER, N. R. & BONHAM, D. G. (1963). *In* 'Perinatal Mortality'. p. 60. Edinburgh: Livingstone.

CARMALT, M. H. B. (1969). *In* 'Fifth Symposium on Advanced Medicine'. p. 268. London: Pitman.

COCHRANE, A. L., GRAHAM, P. A. & WALLACE, J. (1968). *In* 'Screening in Medical Care'. p. 81. Published for the Nuffield Provincial Hospitals Trust by the Oxford University Press, London, New York, Toronto.

COCHRANE, A. L. & ELWOOD, P. C. (1969). *Lancet*, **1**, 420.

COCHRANE, A. L. & HOLLAND, W. W. (1971). *Br. med. Bull.*, **27**, 3.

COLLEN, M. F. (1966). *In* 'Surveillance and Early Diagnosis in General Practice'. p. 10. Office of Health Economics.

DAVIS, H. J. & KURZ, L. (1962). *Dan. med. Bull.*, **9**, 121.

DAVIS, H. J. & JONES, H. W. (1966). *Am. J. Obstet. Gynec.*, **96**, 605.

DUNN, J. E. (1953). *Cancer*, **6**, 873.

ELVEBACK, L. R., GUILLIER, C. L. & KEATING, F. R. (1970). *J. Am. med. Ass.*, **211**, 69.

ELWOOD, P. C. & HUGHES, D. (1970). *Br. med. J.*, **3**, 254.

FEINLEIB, M. & ZELEN, M. (1969). *Archs envir. Hlth.*, **19**, 412.

FIDLER, H. K., BOYES, D. A. & WORTH, A. J. (1968). *J. Obstet. Gynaec. Br. Commonw.*, **75**, 392.

FREIS, E. D. (1970). *Bull. Int. Soc. Card.*, **11**, 6.

GOVAN, A. D. T., HAINES, R. M., LANGLEY, F. A., TAYLOR, C. W. & WOODCOCK, A. S. (1966). *J. Obst. Gynaec. Br. Commonw.*, **73**, 883.

GRAHAM, P. A. & HOLLOWS, F. C. (1966). *In* 'Glaucoma'. Proceedings of a Symposium held at the Royal College of Surgeons of England, p. 103. Edinburgh: Livingstone.

HAMMOND, E. C. (1971). *In* 'The Early Diagnosis of Cancer of the Cervix', p. 1. University of Hull.

HUSAIN, O. A. N. (1970). *Am. J. Obst. Gynec.*, **106**, 138.

HUTCHISON, G. B. & SHAPIRO, S. (1968). *J. nat. Cancer Inst.*, **41**, 665.

JUNGNER, G. (1966). *In* 'Surveillance and Early Diagnosis in General Practice', p. 14. Office of Health Economics.

KANNEL, W. B., KAGAN, A., DAWBER, T. R. & REVOTSKIE, N. (1962). *Geriatrics*, **17**, 672.

KEEN, H. (1966). *Proc. R. Soc. Med.*, **59**, 1170.

KEEN, H. & JARRETT, R. J. (1970). Proceedings of the Second International Symposium on Atherosclerosis, p. 435. Springer-Verlag, New York, Heidelberg, Berlin.

KOCH, F. & STAKEMANN, G. (1962). *Dan. med. Bull.*, **9**, 127.

KNOX, E. G. (1966). *In* 'Problems and Progress in Medical Care 2', p. 277. Published for the Nuffield Provincial Hospitals Trust by Oxford University Press, London, New York, Toronto.

KNOX, E. G. (1968a). *In* 'Screening in Medical Care', p. 55. Published for the Nuffield Provincial Hospitals Trust by the Oxford University Press, London, New York, Toronto.

KNOX, E. G. (1968b). *In* 'Screening in Medical Care', p. 43. Published for the Nuffield Provincial Hospitals Trust by the Oxford University Press, London, New York, Toronto.

LEVY, H. L., KAROLKEWICZ, V., HOUGHTON, S. A. & MacCREADY, R. A. (1970). *New Engl. J. Med.*, **282**, 1455.

MABRY, C. C., DENNISTON, J. C. & COLDWELL, J. G. (1966). *New Engl. J. Med.*, **275**, 1331.

MACGREGOR, J. E., FRASER, M. E. & MANN, E. M. F. (1966). *Lancet*, **1**, 252.

MEDICAL RESEARCH COUNCIL (1966). *Br. med. J.*, **1**, 1317.

MORRIS, J. N., KAGAN, A., PATTISON, D. C., GARDNER, M. J. & RAFFLE, P. A. B. (1966). *Lancet*, **2**, 553.

MORRIS, J. N. & GARDNER, M. J. (1969). *Am. J. med.*, **46**, 674.

MURPHY, E. A. & ABBEY, H. (1967). *J. chron. Dis.*, **20**, 79.

NUFFIELD PROVINCIAL HOSPITALS TRUST (1968). *In* 'Screening in Medical Care'. Published for the Nuffield Provincial Hospitals Trust by the Oxford University Press, London, New York, Toronto.

OSBORN, G. R. & LEYSHON, V. N. (1966). *Lancet*, **1**, 256.

ROSE, G. A., HOLLAND, W. W. & CROWLEY, E. A. (1964). *Lancet*, **1**, 296.

ROSE, G. A. (1970). *Trans. Soc. occup. Med.*, **20**, 109.

SHAPIRO, S., STRAX, P. & VENET, L. (1971). *J. Am. med. Ass.*, **215**, 1777.

SHELDON, J. H. (1948). *In* 'The Social Medicine of Old Age'. London: Oxford University Press.

STAMLER, J., LINDBERG, H. A., BERKSON, D. M., SHAFFER, A., MILLER, W. & POINDEXTER, A. (1960). *J. chron. Dis.*, **11**, 405.

THORNER, R. M. & REMEIN, Q. R. (1961). *Publ. Hlth. Monogr.*, **67**, (P.H.S. publication, No. 846).

TRUETT, J., CORNFIELD, J. & KANNEL, W. (1967). *J. chron. Dis.*, **20**, 511.

TURPEINEN, O., MIETTINEN, M., KARVONEN, M. J., ROINE, P., PEKKARINEN, M., LEHTOSUO, E. J. & ALIVIRTA, P. (1968). *Am. J. clin. Nutrition*, **21**, 255.

U.S. COMMISSION ON CHRONIC ILLNESS (1957). *In* 'Chronic Illness in the United States', Vol. I. Cambridge, Mass: Harvard University Press.

U.S. VETERANS ADMINISTRATION CO-OPERATIVE STUDY GROUP ON ANTIHYPERTEN-SIVE AGENTS (1970). *J. Am. med. Ass.*, **213**, 1143.

UNIVERSITY GROUP DIABETES PROGRAM (1971). *Diabetes*, **19**, Suppl. 2.

WALKER, W. (1959). *Br. med. Bull.*, **15**, 123.

WHITEHEAD, T. P., CARMALT, M. H. B. & WIDDOWSON, G. M. (1967). *In* 'Automation in Analytical Chemistry', Vol. II, p. 77. New York: Mediad Inc.

WILLIAMSON, J., STOKOE, I. H., GRAY, S., FISHER, M., SMITH, A., MCGHEE, A. & STEPHENSON, E. (1964). *Lancet*, **1**, 1117.

WILSON, J. M. G. (1968). *In* 'Screening in Medical Care', p. 97. Published for the Nuffield Provincial Hospitals Trust by the Oxford University Press, London, New York, Toronto.

WILSON, J. M. G. & JUNGNER, G. (1968). *Public Health Papers, No.* 34. Geneva: World Health Organization.

WILSON, J. M. G. (1969). *In* 'Fifth Symposium on Advanced Medicine', p. 253. London: Pitman.

WILSON, J. M. G. (1970). *Ann. Soc. belge Med. trop.*, **50**, 4, 489.

CHAPTER 12

DISEASES OF HAEMOGLOBIN SYNTHESIS

E. R. HUEHNS

Department of Clinical Haematology,
University College Hospital Medical School, London W.C.1.

There are several reasons why the study of abnormalities in the synthesis of haemoglobin is important in medicine. The first is that some of these conditions lead to severe clinical abnormalities which are relatively common in some parts of the world. The second is that the study of a number of the rarer abnormalities has led to the diagnosis of some forms of congenital haemolytic anaemias and to the further understanding of the control of erythropoiesis. Finally, since their first discovery, the abnormal haemoglobins have been a 'model' system, illustrating the various abnormalities of protein synthesis presumed to be present in the other inborn errors of metabolism. In Fig. 12.1 the various types of disease which can be caused by abnormalities

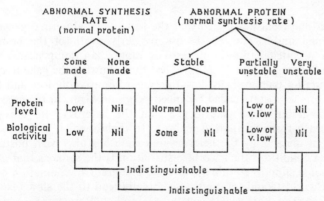

FIG. 12.1. Diagrammatic representation of the main genotypes and phenotypes in inherited protein abnormalities. (Taken from Bennett & Huehns, 1970). In haemoglobin, abnormal synthesis rate of normal protein gives rise to the thalassaemias; normal synthesis rate of abnormal protein gives rise to the abnormal haemoglobins, some unstable, some with abnormal function.

of protein synthesis are outlined. A similar classification can also be applied to haemoglobin (Table 12.1), as with other protein diseases there are two main groups. In the first, the rate of protein synthesis is reduced and any protein made has a normal amino acid sequence; this group gives rise to the thalassaemias. In the second group, the protein synthesised is abnormal, and this gives rise to the abnormal haemoglobins. As with most other inherited disorders one might have expected the incidence of the pathological haemoglobin abnormalities to be extremely low, but the frequency of these disorders

365

has been distorted by genetic selection (see Allison, 1964) leading to the common occurrence of sickle cell disease and the various forms of thalassaemia.

TABLE 12.1

ABNORMALITIES OF HAEMOGLOBIN SYNTHESIS

A Diminished rate of synthesis:

α-Thalassaemia

β-Thalassaemia

B Abnormalities of Haemoglobin Structure:

Sickle cell haemoglobin	Homozygous sickle cell disease and other sickle cell syndromes.
Homozygous haemoglobinopathies	Hb–C disease, Hb–E disease, Hb–D Punjab disease.
Haemoglobins with abnormal function	Haemoglobins with a high O_2 affinity: familial polycythaemia; haemoglobins with a low oxygen affinity; haemoglobin M diseases.
Unstable haemoglobins	These cause haemolytic anaemia and often abnormalities of oxygen dissociation.

It has long been postulated that the loss of the abnormal genes causing thalassaemia and sickle cell disease by early death of the homozygotes (giving a Mendelian fitness of zero) is more than compensated for by a survival advantage of the heterozygotes, thus allowing the gene frequency to increase until a balance is achieved between homozygote loss and heterozygote advantage, a state called balanced polymorphism. In the case of sickle cell haemoglobin there is evidence that the heterozygotes are protected against death from falciparum malaria. In thalassaemia, protection against death from malaria by the heterozygote state has also been postulated. In both these conditions their world distribution is the same as that of malaria lending some support to this hypothesis. The gradual elimination of malaria from the world would, of course, eventually lead to the slow (exponential) disappearance of both sickle cell disease and thalassaemia; a reduction of heterozygote frequency of 20 per cent to 10 per cent would take about 300 years, and this is thought to account for the difference in the frequency of sickle cell trait in America compared to that found in West Africa.

The present review will deal mainly with those abnormalities of haemoglobin synthesis which are of clinical interest, and the reader is referred to a number of other published reviews which deal with some aspects not covered by this paper (structure of haemoglobin: Schroeder & Jones, 1965, Perutz, 1971a and b; genetics: Huehns & Shooter, 1965; abnormal haemoglobin structure: Carrell & Lehmann, 1969, Perutz & Lehmann, 1968; development: Huehns & Beaven, 1971). An outline of the genetic control of haemoglobin synthesis and of the structure and function of normal haemoglobin is given in Appendix 1. The details of various types of pathological haemoglobin abnormalities are listed in Appendix 2.

THE THALASSAEMIAS*

Classification and causes

The thalassaemias are due to an inherited defect in the rate of synthesis of one of the globin chains, the protein made (if any) having a normal amino acid sequence. The situation is complicated because of the subunit structure of the haemoglobin molecule, the developmental changes and the fact that with some genes no synthesis of the affected chains occurs, whilst others allow the continued synthesis of some protein. Only lack of the synthesis of the chains forming Hb–A, namely the α- and β-chains, is important, and there are two main groups of thalassaemias: α-thalassaemia due to lack of α-chain synthesis, and β-thalassaemia due to lack of β-chain synthesis. As the

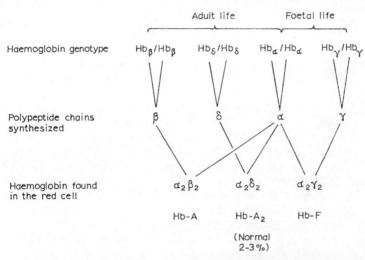

Fig. 12.2. Genetic control of the synthesis of Hb-A, Hb-A₂ and Hb-F. Note that the α-chains for all three haemoglobins arise from the same metabolic pool. There is evidence for a duplicate γ-chain locus and the possibility of a duplicate α-chain locus has also been raised (see appendix 1). There are also loci controlling the synthesis of the embryonic haemoglobin chains, the ε-chains and ζ-chains (see Huehns & Beaven, 1971).

genetic loci controlling the synthesis of haemoglobin (Fig. 12.2) are autosomally inherited, both conditions can occur in the heterozygous (one abnormal and one normal gene) or homozygous form. Clinically, three main types of thalassaemia are found (Table 12.2): thalassaemia minor, which corresponds to the heterozygous forms of the disease, thalassaemia major, which corresponds to the homozygous state, and thalassaemia intermedia, with an intermediate severity, probably due to the interaction of genes only causing partial suppression of the synthesis of either the α- or the β-chains. The exact genetic constitution of these individuals is often not understood.

* More detailed reviews of thalassaemia have been published by Weatherall, & Clegg, 1972; Huehns, 1965; Bannerman, 1972. There has also been a conference on this subject (Fink, 1969).

TABLE 12.2

CLINICAL FEATURES OF THALASSAEMIA

	Major	Intermedia	Minor
Haemoglobin (g/100 ml)	< 6	6–10	> 10
Reticulocytes (%)	2–15	2–10	< 5
Nucleated red cells	+ + + +	+ + + to 0	0
	particularly following splenectomy		
Abnormal red-cell morphology	+ + + +	+ + +	+
Jaundice	+ +	+ 0	0
Splenomegaly	+ + +	+ +	±
Skeletal changes	+ + + to + +	+ + + to 0	0
Transfusion requirement	+ + + to +	+ to 0	0

From the clinical point of view, the lack of chain synthesis is not the whole explanation for the disease, and several factors have to be taken into account:

1. Severity of impairment of chain synthesis. The depression of synthesis of either polypeptide chain leads to some, but not proportionate, reduction in the amount of haemoglobin found in each red cell, that is, a low Mean Cell Haemoglobin (MCH). As the red cell size, Mean Cell Volume (MCV), is also reduced the Mean Cell Haemoglobin Concentration (MCHC) is relatively less affected.

2. Properties of the excess α- or β-chains formed. In β-thalassaemia excess α-chains are formed, and these are very unstable, precipitating in the red cell precursors in the bone marrow forming inclusion bodies. These inclusion bodies are removed from the cells by the pitting phenomenon causing damage to the cell membrane. In the trait form the cell membrane damage is small, and haemolysis is not a feature of the disease. In the homozygous condition cell damage is severe and leads to intramarrow destruction of the red cells, called ineffective erythropoiesis. In α-thalassaemia the excess β- (or γ-chains) formed are more stable and are in some cases, mentioned below, found in the peripheral blood. The presence of Hb–β_4 (Hb–H) may lead to intracellular precipitation and inclusion body formation and thus to haemolysis.

3. Compensatory effects. (a) Bone marrow expansion. The presence of anaemia from any cause leads to tissue hypoxia and increased erythropoietin production. As a consequence, the marrow expands and red cell production is increased until a balance is achieved. In thalassaemia minor, red cell production need only be increased two or three fold and compensation is good with only slight anaemia. However, in β-thalassaemia major the presence of marked ineffective erythropoiesis makes the achievement of the steady state difficult, if not impossible, and marrow expansion due to erythropoietin production is extreme. This causes the well known bone changes of thalassaemia (see page 374).

(b) Continued production of foetal haemoglobin (Hb–F, γ-chains). This is only of importance in β-thalassaemia major; in this condition the more

Hb–F, in absolute terms, is produced the milder the clinical disease caused (see also later).

α-Thalassaemia

In α-thalassaemia, there is a reduction in the number of α-chains synthesised. As has already been pointed out, the α-chains for Hb–F and Hb–A synthesis are controlled by the same genetic locus (Fig. 12.2) and are therefore derived from the same metabolic pool. For this reason, any defect of α-chain synthesis affects the synthesis of both Hb–F and Hb–A and is already manifest at birth, when it is apparently more marked. It might be expected that the reduction of α-chain synthesis would directly lead to an appropriate number of uncombined non-α-chains, i.e. γ- or β-chains, in the cells. However, this is not so, because there is normally a slight excess of α-chain synthesis over β-chain synthesis, and there may be some mutual adjustment in the relative rates of synthesis of the various chains to each other. For these reasons, free non-α-chains (γ or β) are found only in certain situations and never amount to the expected proportion. Another factor affecting the type of free chains found is that α-chains combine preferentially with β-chains to form Hb–A than with γ-chains to form Hb–F. In other words, when γ-chains are being synthesised, Hb–$γ_4$ (also called 'Hb–Bart's' or 'Fast Foetal Haemoglobin') is found. The various different forms of α-thalassaemia will now be described and are summarised in Table 12.3.

There are probably three different α-thalassaemia genes. The *α-thal-1* gene (Na-Nakorn *et al.*, 1969) completely suppresses the α-chain production normally controlled by the affected chromosome whereas the *α-thal-2* and *α-thal-3* (McNeil, 1971) genes only partially suppress α-chain production. The *α-thal-1* and *α-thal-2* genes occur commonly in the Mediterranean and South East Asian populations. *α-thal-1* also occurs in persons of African extraction. These genes occur in the heterozygous, homozygous and doubly heterozygous form. Interaction with α-chain haemoglobin variants also occurs. Clinically, the only important types are α-thalassaemia-1 trait and Hb–H disease.

More recently, a number of workers have been looking at the various forms of α-thalassaemia and have suggested that these would be more easily explained by assuming more than one structural locus controlling the synthesis of α-chains (Lehmann, 1970; Wasi, 1970). If only one locus is assumed to explain the variability of α-thalassaemia, several genes which depress α-chain synthesis to a variable degree are postulated. A similar hypothesis is used to explain the variability of β-thalassaemia and in this case it is known that there is only a single structural locus controlling the synthesis of β-chains. The second possibility is that there are two structural loci controlling α-chain synthesis, and these could be either linked or unlinked. The main difficulty in accepting the two loci hypothesis is that in Hb–Q—H disease all individuals described so far carry no Hb–A. On the two unlinked loci hypothesis some such individuals should show Hb–A. The proportion of Hb–Q in Hb–A+Q heterozygotes should also show a triphasic distribution, but there are not enough data available to test this. On the other hand, two linked loci presuppose that the Hb–Q-gene is closely linked to one for α-thalassaemia. This assumes that the two structural loci

TABLE 12.3

TYPES OF α-THALASSAEMIA

	Haemoglobin abnormalities at birth	Haemoglobin abnormalities during adult life	Clinical Picture
α-thalassaemia-1: completely suppresses α-chain synthesis controlled by the affected chromosome.			
α-thal-1 heterozygote	5–10% Hb-γ_4	No abnormal haemoglobins, Hb-A_2 and Hb-F not increased. Occasional cells may show Hb-H type inclusions.	Thalassaemia minor
α-thal-1 homozygote	85% of Hb-γ_4 c. 15% of Hb-Portland 1 Foetus dies at about 32 weeks gestation.	—	—
α-thal-1 × Hb-Q	Not described, presumably c. 30% Hb-γ_4 with Hb-QF ($\alpha_2{}^Q\gamma_2$) and Hb-Q ($\alpha_2{}^Q\beta_2$).	Clinically Hb-Q–H disease: Hb-Q($\alpha_2{}^Q\beta_2$) Hb-β_4 (Hb-H) 10% and Hb-Q($\alpha_2{}^Q\delta_2$). Hb-H inclusions.	Thalassaemia intermedia.
α-thalassaemia-2: partially suppresses α-chain synthesis controlled by the affected chromosome.			
α-thal-2 heterozygote	1–2% Hb-γ_4	None	None
α-thal-2 homozygote	Similar to α-thal-1 trait clinically not diagnosable	10–20% Hb-β_4 (Hb-H), low Hb-A_2, Hb-H inclusion bodies.	Thalassaemia minor
α-thal-1 × α-thal-2 double	25–30% Hb-γ_4		Hb-H disease
α-thal-2 × Hb-I	Not described	80% Hb-I, 20% Hb-A (simple Hb-I heterozygote has 70% Hb-A, 30% Hb-I)	Thalassaemia minor
α-thalassaemia-3: partially suppresses α-chain synthesis controlled by the affected chromosome, (more severe than α-thal-2)			
α-thal-3 heterozygote	c. 3% Hb-γ_4	No abnormal haemoglobins	Mild red cell changes
α-thal-3 homozygote	20–30% Hb-γ_4	10–20% Hb-H	Hb-H disease

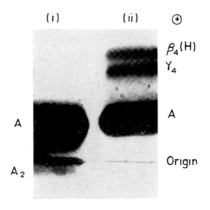

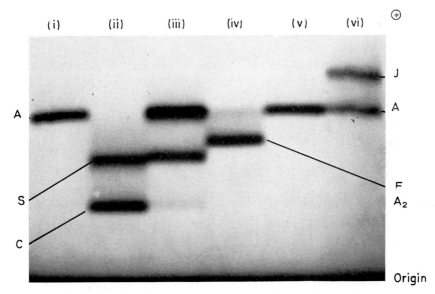

Fig. 12.3. Starch gel electrophoresis of haemoglobin.

    A) Phosphate buffer pH 7.4
      i) normal haemolysate
      ii) haemolysate from Hb-H disease
    B) Tris-EDTA buffer pH 8.6

      i) Hb-A
      ii) Hb-S + C
      iii) Hb-A + S (+ A$_2$)
      iv) Cord blood, Hb-F + A
      v) Hb-A
      vi) Hb-A + J

Taken from Huehns *et al.*, 1960 and Huehns & Shooter, 1964.

[*To face p.* 370.

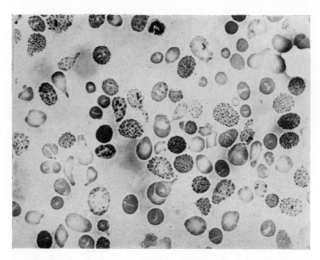

FIG. 12.4. Inclusion bodies in the red cells of Hb-H disease following incubation with brilliant cresyl blue. In α-thalassaemia trait only very occasional cells show inclusion bodies. (Photograph by courtesy of Dr. J. C. White). (× 1000).

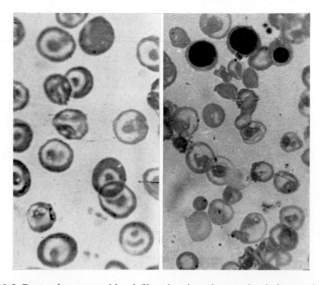

FIG. 12.5. Post splenectomy blood film showing changes in thalassaemia intermedia. In thalassaemia major the changes are similar but more marked, whilst in thalassaemia minor correspondingly milder red cell changes occur. (× 1000).

controlling α-chain synthesis are closely linked. The family where a duplication of the α-chain locus has been demonstrated does not indicate close linkage (see Appendix 1). Thus, it can be seen that the genetic interpretation of α-thalassaemia is not clear and depends on defining the number of loci controlling normal α-chain synthesis (see Appendix 1). A critical appraisal of the pertinent data in relation to thalassaemia is given by Wasi (1970).

α-Thalassaemia 1 Trait

This is a mild form of thalassaemia minor found in the Mediterranean region and South East Asia with a frequency of up to 5 per cent. Clinically, the diagnosis can only be made by exclusion because there are no detectable haemoglobin abnormalities in the adult, Hb–A_2 and Hb–F not being increased (see also β-thalassaemia minor). There may be Hb–H inclusion bodies present in very occasional red cells on supravital staining.

Hb-H Disease

This is a form of thalassaemia intermedia with haemoglobin levels of 8–10 g/100 ml. There is usually splenomegaly. The patients are not very ill, unless the anaemia is exacerbated by pregnancy or some other cause. Hb–β_4 (Hb–H) is found in the cells. This haemoglobin is unstable and should be looked for by electrophoresis in fresh haemolysate on any of the more sensitive supporting systems such as starch gel, cellogel or acrylamide gel (Fig. 12.3a, b). The red cells also form inclusion bodies which can be seen after staining with brilliant cresyl blue (Fig. 12.4). Hb–β_4, like other unstable haemoglobins, precipitates in the red cell, causing haemolysis. This is exacerbated by methaemoglobin-inducing drugs, such as nitrites, sulphona-

TABLE 12.4

CHEMICAL AGENTS REPORTED TO CAUSE HAEMOLYSIS IN PATIENTS WITH GLUCOSE-6-PHOSPHATE DEHYDROGENASE DEFICIENCY AND THESE PRESUMABLY CAN ALSO SIMILARLY AFFECT THE UNSTABLE HAEMOGLOBINS

(Taken from Maizels et al., 1968)

8-aminoquinolines	Primaquine	
	Pamaquine	
	Pentaquine	
Sulphonamides	Sulphanilamide	
	Sulphamethoxypyridazine	
	Salicylazosulphapyridine	
	Sulphacetamide	
Sulphones	Sulphoxone	
	Thiazosulphone	
Nitrofurans	Nitrofurantoin	
	Nitrofurazone	
	Furazolidine	
Acetylphenylhydrazine		Naphthalene derivatives
Acetanilide		Methylene blue
Acetophenetidin		Ascorbic acid
Antipyrine		Probenecid
Amidopyrine		Quinidine
Acetylsalicylic acid		Trinitrotoluene
Paraminosalicylic acid		

mides, etc. (Table 12.4), and these should be avoided in patients with Hb–H. As red cells with haemoglobin precipitates are destroyed in the spleen, splenectomy may improve the haemoglobin level in the more severely affected patients (Rigas & Koler, 1961). However, careful assessment of each individual patient by ^{51}Cr red cell survival and organ scanning is needed. This disease can also be recognised at birth, when 25–30 per cent Hb–γ_4 is found.

The interaction of α-thalassaemia with α-chain abnormal haemoglobins has been described. The most common is Hb–Q—H disease, which is clinically similar to Hb–H disease. The interaction of α-thalassaemia with β-chain abnormal haemoglobin also occurs and leads to a reduced proportion of the abnormal haemoglobin.

β-Thalassaemia

In β-thalassaemia there is a reduction in the number of β-chains synthesised, and although the situation is similar to that of α-thalassaemia, it is a little more complex because there are two types of non-α-chains besides the β-chain (Fig. 12.2); these are the γ- and δ-chains, which form Hb–F ($\alpha_2\gamma_2$) and Hb–A_2 ($\alpha_2\delta_2$) respectively. Because the main non-α-chain synthesised before birth is the γ-chain leading to the formation of Hb–F, the newborn infant is (virtually) unaffected by β-thalassaemia, and any disease only becomes manifest *after the first three months of life*. Again, the disease can occur in the heterozygous and homozygous form, and as with α-thalassaemia there are a number of different genes. In some the β-chain synthesis due to the affected chromosome is completely lacking; in others the δ-chain, the non-α-chain of Hb–A_2, is also affected, producing so called $\beta\delta$-thalassaemia. Genes causing partial lack of β-chain synthesis also occur. Another factor to be taken into account is that some genes, as well as suppressing β-chain synthesis, also partially maintain γ-chain synthesis, and this has an important bearing on the severity of the homozygous condition.

β-Thalassaemia Trait

This is one form of thalassaemia minor. Thalassaemia minor is important in the differential diagnosis of hypochromic anaemia, and the determination of the genetic type may be important from the genetic counselling point of view. The usual way these patients present is with mild hypochromic anaemia, haemoglobin *c.* 10 g/100 ml, and failure to respond to iron. There are no specific physical signs, except occasionally the spleen is palpable. Most patients are of Mediterranean, South East Asian or African extraction, but this need not be so. The diagnosis is made on the blood count. The mild anaemia is associated with small red cells. The MCHC may be normal, while the MCH is low. The blood film shows mild to moderate variation in size and shape of the red cells, with mild hypochromia; target cells are often present; the reticulocyte count is usually normal. These findings, in particular the low MCH, together with a normal or raised serum iron, make the diagnosis of thalassaemia minor but do not distinguish α-thalassaemia trait from β-thalassaemia trait. In β-thalassaemia trait haemoglobin electrophoresis shows a raised Hb–A_2 (normal level = 2–3 per cent of total haemoglobin) either with or without a raised Hb–F (normally not detectable or less than 2 per cent). In $\beta\delta$-thalassaemia trait the Hb–A_2 level is normal, while Hb–F may be either raised or normal. The presence of a trace of Hb–F during pregnancy may not be significant as it often occurs in normal red cells at that time. The failure to find any haemoglobin abnormality indicates either α-thalassaemia trait (see page 371) or more rarely βδ-thalassaemia trait without a raised Hb–F. These two types of thalassaemia minor, without a raised Hb–A$_2$ or Hb–F, make up about 20 per cent of all cases of thalassaemia minor. In this connection it is important to know that iron deficiency lowers the level of Hb–A$_2$ and may mask the finding of a raised Hb–A$_2$ in some cases. There is no treatment indicated in thalassaemia minor. Iron is contra-indicated except when the serum iron is low.

β-Thalassaemia Major and Intermedia

This group of diseases is caused by the inheritance of two genes determining lack of β-chain synthesis, and patients may be homozygous or doubly heterozygous for genes determining β-thalassaemia. The classification of the disease is on clinical grounds. In *β-thalassaemia major* the haemoglobin is less than 6 g/100 ml, and the red cells show marked changes on the blood film with severe hypochromia; nucleated red cells are often present, particularly after splenectomy. There is usually a reticulocytosis. In *β-thalassaemia intermedia* a higher haemoglobin level is maintained, and the red cell changes are less severe (Table 12.2). In both forms, splenic enlargement is always found. In making the diagnosis the ethnic origin and history of onset of the disease after the first few months of life are important. The blood count shows anaemia and variable, but distinctive, red cell appearances (Fig. 12.5). Electrophoresis of the haemoglobin shows increased amounts of Hb–F and/or Hb–A$_2$. The amount of foetal haemoglobin can vary from about 10 to 100 per cent of total haemoglobin.

The severity of any disease after the first few months of life is controlled by two factors: firstly, by the degree of depression of β-chain synthesis by the particular genes involved and, secondly, by the amount of compensation achieved by the continued production of γ-chains. Many β-thalassaemia genes completely suppress the β-chain synthesis controlled by the chromosome involved, while others allow reduced synthesis of β-chains. A measure of the β-chain production remaining is given by the amount of Hb–A present in the double heterozygotes for β-thalassaemia and a β-chain abnormal haemoglobin but such subjects are only rarely available. The continued synthesis of significant amounts of Hb–A leads to some forms of β-thalassaemia intermedia. With some β-thalassaemia genes there is partial failure to turn off Hb–F (γ-chain) production, as well as failure to activate the β-locus. In this context, the percentage of Hb–F found in the homozygote β-thalassaemia major is very misleading, because in cases where no β-chains are made, the production of only a few γ-chains may result in the presence of virtually only Hb–F in the viable cells. If there is genetically determined continued synthesis of Hb–F then this is measured by the amount of Hb–F seen in the adult heterozygote. Thus, a number of β-thalassaemia genes occur. The most severe are those which lead to the complete suppression of β-chain (Hb–A) synthesis with little or no (genetic) activation of γ-chain synthesis. The corresponding homozygotes will show virtually only Hb–F in the cells but will have the most severe form of β-thalassaemia. If there is some continued synthesis of γ-chains (Hb–F) in the heterozygotes, then even if there is total suppression of β-chain synthesis, the corresponding homozygotes will be less severe. A good example of this type has recently been described: in this family, the heterozygote had 7 per cent Hb–F, while the three homozygotes carried only Hb–F, but their disease was of intermediate severity. At the other extreme of the clinical spectrum is the so called 'high-Hb–F' gene. In this condition, c. 25 per cent of the haemoglobin is Hb–F in the trait form, while in the homozygotes only Hb–F is found, β-chain (Hb–A) synthesis being completely suppressed, but compensation is so good that no anaemia is found, and only mild red cell abnormality is seen on the blood film.

Another feature of the disease is the gross marrow expansion and erythropoiesis seen in the bones of the skull, hands etc., and this leads to the typical bone X-ray changes seen. The fingers of young children may show a peculiar form of dactylitis associated with the 'invasion' of the phalanges by the bone marrow. Most of the red cells made in the bone marrow are destroyed *in situ*, a process called 'ineffective erythropoiesis'. Investigation of the synthesis of haemoglobin in β-thalassaemia has shown that α-chains are made at a normal rate and that these excess, uncombined α-chains precipitate in the cell. It is these precipitates which cause the destruction of so many cells in the bone marrow. Clearly those cells which have least β-chain or compensatory γ-chain production will have the largest α-chain precipitates and will be destroyed in the marrow. Thus, only the cells with the highest tetramer (functional) haemoglobin content will reach the circulation, and even these are often few in number with a much reduced haemoglobin content.

Summary of the Laboratory Diagnosis of Thalassaemia

Thalassaemia minor

The presence of mild anaemia with a low MCH in the absence of a reduced serum iron indicates thalassaemia trait. A raised Hb–A_2 and/or Hb–F by haemoglobin electrophoresis indicates a form of β-thalassaemia. Occasionally traces of Hb–γ_4 (Hb–Bart's) or Hb–β_4 (Hb–H), or some red cells with inclusion bodies on staining with brilliant cresyl blue will be formed and indicate α-thalassaemia trait. If no haemoglobin abnormality is found α-thalassaemia trait or $\beta\delta$-thalassaemia will be present but can only be distinguished by family studies.

Thalassaemia intermedia or major

In these cases some haemoglobin abnormality is always present: a raised Hb–F or Hb–A_2 indicating β-thalassaemia, while Hb–β_4 or Hb–γ_4 indicates α-thalassaemia. The red cell appearances are diagnostic.

Treatment of Thalassaemia

There is no specific treatment for thalassaemia, and nothing needs to be done for patients with thalassaemia minor or patients with milder forms of thalassaemia intermedia except to ensure that they are not iron or folate deficient. It is unusual for iron deficiency to develop in thalassaemia, but when it does the patients tend to react more severely to it than do normal individuals.

In the most severe forms of thalassaemia, the only treatment is blood transfusion, and an important question is at what level a regular transfusion regime should be started. Patients with a haemoglobin of approximately 7 g/100 ml often adapt extremely well, and in this group transfusion is only used to tide patients over intercurrent disease. For those cases which require regular transfusion in order to lead acceptable lives the haemoglobin level should be kept over 10 g/100 ml. Usually transfusions have to be given every 6 weeks. In this way, general development becomes fairly normal. The extreme marrow expansion seen in these cases is also reduced with definite changes in the X-ray appearances of the bone. Follow up of patients treated in this way has shown that they do well for a time, but suffer from severe iron overload after a few years and finally die. (For discussion of this 'high transfusion' regime see Fink, 1969.) To overcome this, the iron chelating agents, diethylenetriaminepentaacetate (DPTA) and desferrioxamine, have been used, and thus the rate of development of iron overload can be considerably slowed up. As there is very active erythropoiesis in thalassaemia, the effect of these drugs does not peter out as quickly as in haemachromatosis, and a careful trial of the long term use of these drugs appears warranted.

Another form of treatment used is splenectomy. Splenectomy itself does not influence the course of the disease but is indicated for either hypersplenism, as shown by a more frequent transfusion requirement, or gross splenic enlargement, causing discomfort to the patient.

The treatment of Hb–H disease has already been discussed (see page 371).

Genetic Cause of Thalassaemia

The basic abnormality in thalassaemia is not yet known, but recent work suggests that it is due to the reduced production of the mRNA (messenger RNA), coding for the affected polypeptide chain. How this is brought about is not known. This very important area of molecular pathology has been reviewed elsewhere (Weatherall & Clegg, 1972).

Besides the above cause of thalassaemia there are some abnormal haemoglobins associated with a clinical picture of thalassaemia, and these are found in a low proportion in the cell. The first of these are the Lepore haemoglobins. This group has the β-chain replaced by a new polypeptide chain, consisting at the N-terminal end of the amino acid sequence of the δ-chain (the non-α-chain of Hb–A$_2$, $\alpha_2\delta_2$) while the remainder has the sequence of the β-chain. Various types of Hb–Lepore have different relative amounts of δ- and β-chain sequence. All these haemoglobins have an electrophoretic mobility like Hb–S; they are made in small amounts in the cells and clinically behave like β-thalassaemia, the trait form giving rise to a mild hypochromic anaemia, while interaction with other β-thalassaemia genes or the homozygous state gives rise to thalassaemia intermedia. The converse polypeptide chain, i.e. β-chain sequence followed by δ-chain sequence, giving rise to Hb–Miyada, has also been described (Yanase et al., 1968). These haemoglobins are thought to be due to unequal crossing over between chromosomes.

Another group of abnormal haemoglobins mimics (or causes) α-thalassaemia. These are two minor (less than 5 per cent of total haemoglobin) haemoglobins which migrate on starch gel electrophoresis between the origin and Hb–A$_2$. These haemoglobins have been seen in Greece and in Chinese-Jamaicans. Structural studies of these haemoglobins show that they have more than the usual 141 amino acids, c. 30 being attached to the C-terminal end of a normal α-chain, the extra piece being shorter in the second component. This new piece of chain has a 'nonsense' sequence which does not correspond to a known sequence in another protein (Milner, Clegg & Weatherall, 1971). The precise genetic cause of this abnormality is not known, but it is possible that this may be a mutation of the usual chain termination codons. If this is so, it may indicate that mRNA is longer than necessary to code for the sequence of the protein-chain being synthesised, and it would be interesting to know the normal function of this extra piece of mRNA sequence. Clinically, these abnormal haemoglobins give rise to α-thalassaemia and interact with other α-thalassaemia genes to give rise to Hb–H disease. A haemoglobin with 10 extra amino acids attached to the C-terminal end of the β-chain, called Hb–Tak, has also been described (Flatz et al., 1971), but is not associated with any clinical abnormality.

THE ABNORMAL HAEMOGLOBINS

There are several groups of abnormal haemoglobins; these are listed in Table 12.1 and their electrophoretic separation is shown in Fig. 12.3. The most common abnormality is sickle cell disease, followed by the homozygous haemoglobinopathies. The other diseases caused by the abnormal haemoglobins are relatively rare but are important in that they lead to a clearer understanding of the factors affecting haemoglobin function and those maintaining protein structure.

Sickle Cell Disease

Sickle cell disease is a severe haemolytic disorder caused by the homozygous occurrence of the abnormal haemoglobin, Hb–S. As this haemoglobin has abnormal β-chains, the disease appears only 3–6 months after birth, when γ-chain (Hb–F) synthesis is replaced by β-chain synthesis, in this case β^S-chains giving rise to Hb–S. In the steady state the haemoglobin is c. 8 g/100 ml, PCV 25 per cent, MCHC 31 g/100 ml, reticulocytes about 10 per cent, ^{51}Cr red cell survival c. 8 days (normal c. 28 days). The life expectancy in this disease is very much related to the economic circumstances of the patient. In Africa many patients with sickle cell disease die during infancy and only some, mostly from the higher economic groups, reach adult life, while in North America, the West Indies and Europe the number of adult sicklers is much greater. The most important aspects of the disease are:

   (i) haemolytic process
   (ii) painful crises, etc.
   (iii) low oxygen affinity of the blood.

All these are related to the sickling of the red cell. This process occurs only in the deoxygenated state of the haemoglobin; it increases the mechanical fragility of the cells and it also prevents them deforming sufficiently easily to allow them to pass through the capillaries. As only deoxygenated cells sickle, this will be maximal on the venous side, and unsickling will occur in the lungs where the blood is again oxygenated; any cells remaining sickled are liable to be destroyed when they reach the capillary bed. There is *in vitro* and *in vivo* evidence that repeated sickling and unsickling of the cells damages the cell membrane and causes the formation of irreversibly sickled cells (ISC). These ISCs are rapidly haemolysed, particularly in the spleen, if still present. The time taken for cells to become ISCs after release from the marrow is about 6 days. If stasis of the blood occurs, sickle cells will form in the blood vessels of the area affected and because these are unable to pass through the capillaries, an infarct will form. This process is exacerbated by the local drop in pH and the increase in PCV that often occur. If these infarcts occur in bone they cause the painful crises so often noted in the disease. Multiple infarction will exacerbate the rate of haemolysis, but this only rarely causes increased anaemia. Anaemic crises, however, often occur and are due to depressed response of the marrow by, for example, intercurrent infection, folate or iron deficiency, etc. Other complications caused by the sickling process are leg ulcers and, more rarely, priapism. As explained later (page 380), the sickling process also causes the low oxygen affinity found in the red cells. This last finding is of some benefit to the patient, because as the haemoglobin passes from the arteries to the veins more oxygen per gram of haemoglobin will be given off as the percentage oxygen saturation at the mean venous P_{O_2} will be lower due to the reduced oxygen affinity. Simple calculation from the oxygen dissociation curves in sickle cell anaemia shows that the increased oxygen release in the tissues is greater than any arterial desaturation that may be present. Thus, the low oxygen affinity prevents the tissue hypoxia which the degree of anaemia present would imply. Another effect of the increased oxygen release to the tissues is to decrease the erythropoietin mediated drive to the bone marrow which regulates the degree of compensation seen in haemolytic anaemias. In this sense, the low oxygen affinity, being primary, is the cause of the low red cell mass (see pages 386, 393; Huehns & Bellingham, 1969). In this way the low oxygen affinity benefits the patient by reducing the viscosity of the blood without reducing the oxygen supply to the tissues. Stunted growth, such as occurs in severe β-thalassaemia associated with chronic tissue hypoxia, is not seen in sickle cell disease; although there is gross anaemia, the increased oxygen release per gram of haemoglobin prevents tissue hypoxia. On the other hand, as the sickling process depends on the proportion of deoxyhaemoglobin S in the cells (see page 379), and the low oxygen affinity increases the proportion of deoxyhaemoglobin present at any particular partial pressure of oxygen, the liability of the cells to sickle *in vivo* will be increased.

The Mixed Sickle Cell Syndromes

These syndromes are important because they are also quite common severe haemolytic disorders. They are due to the interaction of a sickling gene with an abnormal gene—either determining β-thalassaemia or a β-chain abnormal haemoglobin, such as Hb–C, etc. The sickle cell gene is common in Africa, in some parts of Greece and other parts of the Mediterranean area. As β-thalassaemia is also found in these areas, sickle cell disease β-thalassaemia is found. In America this interaction is also relatively common because of the presence of β-thalassaemia in the population derived from the Mediterranean immigrants, while in the West Indies β-thalassaemia in the ex-Chinese population is a factor. Haemoglobin–C is only found in West Africa and populations derived from there; thus Haemoglobin–S+C disease is found in West African, West Indian and American Negroes.

Sickle cell β-thalassaemia disease

If this involves a β-thalassaemia gene which completely suppresses Hb–A production, the disease is usually clinically indistinguishable from homozygous sickle cell disease. In cases where there is a low MCHC the haemoglobin level found will be higher. This is due to the marked haemoglobin–S concentration dependence of oxygen affinity of sickle cells, the relatively higher oxygen affinity leading to less release of oxygen to the tissues per gram of haemoglobin and greater erythropoietin drive to the marrow. On haemoglobin electrophoresis the major haemoglobin found is Hb–S, with some Hb–F and Hb–A$_2$. Unfortunately, the proportion of Hb–F does not distinguish this mixed syndrome from the homozygous condition as the amount found in both conditions is similar. The level of Hb–A$_2$, if raised, is diagnostic, but if it is normal due to the presence of $\beta\delta$-thalassaemia, only family studies will distinguish this condition from homozygous sickle cell disease. If a mild β-thalassaemia gene only partially suppressing β-chain production is involved some Hb–A will be present in the red cells and a milder clinical picture will be found. In this connection it is important to remember that Hb–A can be detected in the blood after blood transfusion for more than the 120 days' average red cell survival, and this sometimes causes diagnostic confusion.

Hb–S+C disease

This is another common variant of sickle cell disease, with a considerably milder clinical picture than that found in homozygous sickle cell disease. The haemoglobin is $c.$ 10 g/100 ml and an intermediate shift in the oxygen dissociation curve is found. It is common for patients with this disorder only to be diagnosed during some intercurrent illness or during routine antenatal care. In this condition retinal changes are often seen, but they are also found in the other sickle cell syndromes.

Sickle cell trait, Hb–A+S

This condition only leads to pathology under special circumstances (Levin, 1958), when the tissue oxygen tension drops to very low values, such as might occur during anaesthesia, cardiac failure, or flight in unpressurised aircraft. Some renal involvement may also occur. There is no haemolysis. This condition is recognised by the electrophoretic demonstration of Hb–A+ S in the haemolysate at a ratio of about 60:40. i.e A>S.

Interaction of other β-chain haemoglobins with Hb–S has been described. Hb–S+O, a severe type of sickle cell disease (Ramot *et al.*, 1960, Milner *et al.*, 1970), Hb–S+E (Aksoy & Lehmann, 1957), Hb–S+D (Ringelhann *et al.*, 1967), and Hb–S+J (Charache & Conley, 1964) lead to mild variants of sickle cell disease.

Interaction with α-chain haemoglobins also occurs and leads to the formation of multiple major haemoglobin species (Huehns & Shooter, 1965).

The interaction with Hb–Memphis (Kraus *et al.*, 1966) gives rise to a milder form of the disease.

Irreversibly sickled cells

It was first noted by Diggs that some red cells in the circulation are permanently sickled, and these can be seen on the ordinary stained blood film. The formation of the irreversibly sickled cells (ISC's) is due to damage of the red cell membrane by the sickling process, each red cell only being able to unsickle a limited number of times. This damage to the cell membrane is one of the major causes of the reduced red cell survival in the disease. These cells are removed from the circulation by the spleen and liver, but as the spleen gradually fibroses in sickle cell disease (auto-splenectomy) the splenic mechanisms of destruction of the ISC's are not usually operative in adults. The haemoglobin in these irreversibly sickled cells can still oxygenate and deoxygenate, and the oxygenated cell does not contain any tactoids, the sickle shape of the erythrocyte in this case being due to rigidity of the cell membrane (Bertles & Döbler, 1969). Another feature of these cells is that they have a very high MCHC and hence a very low oxygen affinity (Seakins *et al.*, 1972). The proportion of these cells in the blood is of some clinical importance, because their number is related to the severity of sickle cell disease in those patients who no longer have a spleen.

Molecular Abnormality in Sickle Haemoglobin

In sickle haemoglobin the β-chains are abnormal, and it was shown by Ingram that the glutamic acid at the 6th position from the N-terminus was replaced by valine. This amino acid is on the surface of the molecule. The structure of the molecule can be written $\alpha_2\beta_2^{6\,Val}$ or $\alpha\beta^{6\,Val}\alpha\beta^{6\,Val}$.

Sickling process

Sickling of the red cells is caused by the formation of long aggregates of the Hb–S molecules, several (probably six) of which twist together to form the stiff tactoids which deform the red cell. The primary aggregation of the molecules occurs because in the deoxy-conformation, the two new valine residues in each Hb–S molecule (presumably) form apolar contacts with adjacent molecules. In order for this to be stable, both valines must fit precisely into some, as yet unidentified, sites on the adjacent molecules. When sickle haemoglobin is oxygenated and assumes the oxy-conformation, the fit no longer takes place (Fig. 12.6) and the polymer is broken up. The presence of other haemoglobins, i.e. Hb–A, Hb–C or Hb–F in the cells, reduces the propensity of the cells to sickle, and in this context the amount of the other haemoglobin in the cell may be important. This is well illustrated by the effect of different amounts of Hb–F or Hb–A found in different patients with sickle cell disease or sickle cell disease-β-thalassaemia, the individuals with more Hb–F or Hb–A having a milder disease. Furthermore, in any patient with sickle cell disease the Hb–F distribution is not uniform in the cells, and it has long been known that those cells with the most Hb–F have the longest survival. Recently, it has been shown that some haemoglobin besides deoxy-Hb–S can be included into Hb–S tactoids, and this is presumably because they fit into the tactoid although they are not incorporated into one of the polymers. Hybrids of the type Hb–$\alpha\beta^S\alpha\beta^X$ also occur in the cell and these would prevent an individual Hb–S polymer from lengthening. However, as several (perhaps six) such strands twist together to make the tactoid, lateral forces could allow the tactoid as a whole to lengthen although individual strands may have breaks in them. An interesting, but unexplained, finding is that deoxy Hb–F is excluded from the Hb–S tactoid. With other β-chain abnormal haemoglobins which interact with Hb–S the difference in severity of the various syndromes may be accounted for by the stability of their hybrid haemoglobins and how well they fit into the Hb–S tactoid. Another observation which needs explaining is that patients with identical haemoglobins in their cells may differ in clinical severity, and other unknown

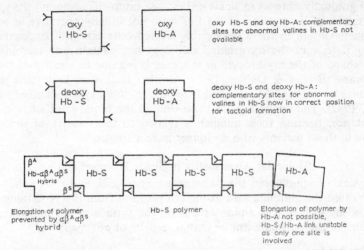

FIG. 12.6. Scheme for the aggregation of sickle haemoglobin. The oxygenated form of Hb–S cannot take part because the complementary sites to the abnormal valines of Hb–S are not in the exact position to allow the necessary fit. The interference of Hb–A and Hb–A/S hybrid ($\alpha\beta^A\alpha\beta^S$) with elongation of polymers is also illustrated. (Modified from Perutz, 1971b).

factors must play a part. One of these may be silent (uncharged) amino acid substitutions in other parts of the molecule. That this may be important is indicated by the finding that the presence of an α-chain abnormality, Hb–Memphis, as well as Hb–S in the cell, or of Hb–C–Harlem, where the Hb–S β-chains have a second amino acid substitution, produces a milder form of the disease. Unfortunately, the understanding of these processes needs a greater knowledge of the precise mechanism of the molecular interaction than is presently available. Although the position of the two new valines in the Hb–S molecule is known from the work of Perutz in Cambridge, the complementary binding site involved in the formation of polymers of Hb–S molecules is not yet known, and even less is known of the detailed structure of the tactoids. Any hypothesis on the mechanism of the sickling process must necessarily be preliminary.

Oxygen affinity. The cause of the low oxygen affinity of the red cells is also directly related to the molecular interaction taking place. Recent studies have shown that the low oxygen affinity of sickle cells is present in cells depleted of 2,3-diphosphoglycerate and that the oxygen affinity is markedly concentration-dependent, as would be expected of a protein-protein interaction. Thus, the molecular interaction in sickle cell disease, which only takes place in the deoxy-conformation, tends to maintain the haemoglobin molecules in this low affinity state and reduces the oxygen affinity measured in the red cells. These results explain the discrepancy between the low oxygen affinity seen in red cells and the normal oxygen affinity reported in haemolysates.

Treatment of Sickle Cell Disease

At the present time, there is no real treatment of sickle cell disease. The obvious approach to treatment is to lessen the propensity of the cells to sickle, and this has been attempted in various ways. It is known that sickling is exacerbated by acidosis and dehydration, and these complications should be avoided. Other factors precipitating crises are infection and malaria, and it has been shown that patients improve by long term antibiotics and anti-malarials (Warley *et al.*, 1965). It is also well known that the socio-economic situation of the patient has a bearing on the severity of the disease, and this is due to relative freedom from infections and better nutrition. Any factor, such as iron deficiency or folate deficiency, which might limit the marrow response would make the anaemia more severe, and may lead to delayed puberty. Iron deficiency is relatively uncommon in sickle cell disease, because of the increased absorption usually associated with marrow hyperplasia. On the other hand, folate deficiency is more common due to the increased need and may be present in subclinical form (that is, without megaloblastic changes in the bone marrow). Treatment of such cases with folic acid may cause the rapid development of secondary sex characteristics.

Crises. A very important aspect of the therapy of sickle cell disease is the treatment of crises and other acute complications. Attempts to make the pH of the blood more alkaline have been used without much success. Another approach has been to convert some of the haemoglobin to either the met-form (Beutler, 1961) or the carbonmonoxy derivative (Sirs, 1963) but neither of these has proved to be clinically useful. An obvious approach has been to attempt to raise the tissue P_{0_2} by allowing the patient to breathe pure oxygen; again this has been unsuccessful. More recently, hyperbaric oxygen has been used in the treatment of sickle cell crises but without consistent success, and this treatment needs further clinical evaluation (Lazlo, Obenour & Saltzman, 1969). Another treatment regime proposed has been the infusion of magnesium glutamate together with alkanisation (Hugh-Jones, Lehmann & McAlister, 1964), but this is ineffective. The use of acetolazamide (Hilkovitz, 1957) also has no effect on the course of the disease. Various other approaches to the treatment of sickle cell disease have been reviewed by Raper (1968).

Urea therapy. Recently, it has been suggested that the new apolar bonds formed during the sickling process could be broken by high concentrations of urea (Nalbandian and co-workers, 1970, 1971a, b, c) and that sickle cell crises could be aborted by the intravenous infusion of urea 30 g/100 ml in sugar solution together with Ringer's solution to raise the blood urea to 150–200 mg/100 ml. This treatment causes massive diuresis, and dehydration of the patient is a real danger. Although under carefully controlled conditions it appears relatively safe, more data are needed before it can be accepted as routine therapy for sickle cell disease (McCurdy & Mahmood, 1971). Another form of treatment is an attempt to prevent the occurrence of crises by oral administration of urea to raise the blood urea to *c.* 60 mg/100 ml. It is difficult to see how the latter regime can prevent the sickling process by the above mechanism as much higher concentrations of urea must be achieved in order to cause enough conformational disturbance of the Hb–S molecules to stop the sickling process. Nevertheless, these authors (Nalbandian *et al.*, 1971b) report clinical improvement in their patients as measured by absent or decreased number of crises, increased haemoglobin levels and sense of well being. Red cell life span is not significantly affected by oral (or intravenous) urea (Bensinger *et al.*, 1971). No beneficial effect of I.V. urea was found by Opio & Barnes (1972). These forms of treatment, therefore, need considerable further evaluation before they can be generally applied.

Cyanate therapy. One group (Cerami & Manning, 1971) has suggested that the good effect of urea reported was not due to the urea itself but to contaminating cyanate in the preparations used. Cyanate acts by carbamylating the terminal amino groups of both the α- and β-chains and once the cells have been treated, the haemoglobin is permanently changed. Another compound which has been used to carbamylate haemoglobin is carbamyl phosphate (Kraus, Kraus & Grear, 1971). *In vitro* experiments have shown that carbamylation does reduce the propensity of the cells to sickle at a given partial pressure of oxygen; the oxygen affinity of the cells is also raised. This effect is independent of 2,3 DPG in the cell. As treatment of normal red cells with cyanate also raises the oxygen affinity, it is important to know whether the effect is due to direct influence on the sickling process or whether cyanate acts indirectly by changing the oxygen affinity of the haemoglobin, thus decreasing the proportion of deoxyhaemoglobin present at any particular partial pressure of oxygen. Work in our laboratory (May *et al.*, 1972) indicates that it acts solely by changing the oxygen affinity of Hb–S. Other studies show that the red cell survival of *in vitro* treated sickle cells is significantly increased compared to that of untreated cells from the same patient. These results suggest that cyanate may be useful in the long term treatment of sickle cell disease, but there may be certain dangers inherent in its use. One effect of raising the oxygen affinity of sickle cells is to increase the red cell mass, because of the increased erythropoietin drive to the bone marrow (see pages 386 and 393). However, as the sickling process is not primarily affected the cells are still equally liable to sickle if the tissue oxygen tensions fall to sufficiently low levels. As the red cell count rises, the viscosity of the blood increases, particularly when sickling occurs, and widespread sickling might occur in patients treated under certain conditions. In any clinical trials of cyanate this should be borne in mind. Another factor to be taken into account is that although cyanate has a low toxicity when given to animals in the short term (Birch & Schütz, 1946), the long term effect of a substance which reacts with the terminal amino groups of all proteins is as yet completely unknown (see also Ranney, 1972; Segel *et al.*, 1972).

Treatment of complications. A common complication of sickle cell disease is leg ulcers, and the healing of these may be promoted by oral zinc sulphate

(Serjeant, Galloway & Gueri, 1970). Priapism is a serious and painful complication, and, if it does not resolve spontaneously, has to be treated surgically. It often leads to impotence. Oestrogens are useless in the prevention and treatment of this condition.

Management of sickle cell disease during pregnancy and anaesthesia

Patients with one of the sickle cell syndromes present a special problem during pregnancy and surgery. This condition should be screened for by a reliable form of sickling test or by electrophoresis in persons of Negro extraction. If a positive sickling test is found, the condition should be further investigated by electrophoresis of haemoglobin and a full blood count (including reticulocytes) in order to diagnose the exact syndrome present.

In pregnancy, abortion, premature labour and other complications of labour are more common than in normal women. Although there are many patients with sickle cell disease who have had no complications, the outcome in any individual case is always in doubt. The only consistently successful way of reducing the incidence of complications is by regular blood transfusion of the affected patients approximately every six weeks, so that the proportion of Hb–A cells is about 60 per cent of the total. Three to four pints should be given at each transfusion. This regime has two effects. It raises the patient's haemoglobin level to near normal and considerably reduces complications due to the presence of sickle cells. The higher haemoglobin level reduces the erythropoietin drive to the marrow and also the number of (sickle) cells made. So each transfusion lasts longer in terms of replacing sickle cells than might otherwise be expected. In patients with sickle cell trait, no special therapy is indicated, but special care should be taken not to allow them to become anoxic during labour.

The management during surgery and anaesthesia is similar. In sickle cell trait no special preparation by transfusion is necessary except for procedures *likely to involve anoxia of parts of the body.* In such cases it may be positively dangerous, and the author has seen two cases of sickle cell trait who died as a result of massive sickling occuring during cardiac surgery. In the other conditions, pre-operative transfusion so as to have a ratio of 70:30 of normal to sickle cells is aimed for. This can be achieved by two transfusions, one a week before and the other the day before operation. If more urgency is necessary, then an exchange transfusion regime may be used. During anaesthesia it is again important to avoid anoxia of the tissues as well as acidosis and dehydration, as they will make the patient's own remaining cells more liable to sickle.

HOMOZYGOUS HAEMOGLOBINOPATHIES

These have been well described and comprise Hb–C disease, Hb–E disease and Hb–D disease. Hb–O Arab disease has also been described.

There is mild haemolysis which is not fully compensated, leading to haemoglobin levels of 10–12 g/100 ml. The stained blood film shows some hypochromia and target cells. These diseases are found in subjects who are homozygous for any one of the above abnormal haemoglobins, the heterozygous condition being benign. The cause of the haemolysis in these syndromes is not clear but may arise because these haemoglobins show a slight instability

TABLE

HAEMOGLOBINS CAUSING DISEASE

Haemoglobin	Clinical effect PCV per cent	Abnormal haemoglobin per cent	Oxygen dissociation properties, etc.
a. Haemoglobins with a raised oxygen affinity causing polycythaemia, when stable.			
Chesapeake	48–58	20–30	
Capetown	45–52	35	High O$_2$ affinity; almost absent
Yakima	45–55	38	subunit interactions
Kempsey	52–64	37	
Ypsilanti	42–63	c. 40	
Hirose	normal		High O$_2$ affinity, low subunit interactions and Bohr effect
Malmö			High O$_2$ affinity
Rainier	57–59	30	High O$_2$ affinity, almost absent
Bethesda	Hb = 20·5 g/ 100 ml		subunit interactions, normal Bohr effect.
Hiroshima	45–55	50	High O$_2$ affinity; moderate decrease in subunit interaction ('n' = 2); absent Bohr effect
Olympia	c. 60	40	High O$_2$ affinity, normal Bohr, slightly low 'n'
Several unstable haemoglobins referred to in Appendix 2.			
b. Haemoglobins with a low oxygen affinity			
Kansas	Cyanosis due to reduced haemoglobin	50	Very low O$_2$ affinity, absent subunit interactions; dissociates more easily than Hb-A into $\alpha\beta$ dimers
Yoshizuka	Mild anaemia		Low O$_2$ affinity, reduced Bohr effect
Agenogi	None		Low O$_2$ affinity, normal Bohr effect and subunit interactions
Milwaukee	Cyanosis due to met Hb slightly unstable	26–30	Low O$_2$ affinity, normal Bohr effect, reduced subunit interactions
E	Mild anaemia in homozygote	100	Low O$_2$ affinity in red cells of homozygote only
Several unstable haemoglobins referred to in appendix 2			
c. Haemoglobins M			
Boston		22–42	Low O$_2$ affinity, grossly reduced subunit interactions and Bohr effect
Saskatoon		30–40	High O$_2$ affinity, reduced subunit interactions, normal Bohr effect
Iwate	Cyanosis due to Hb–M	30	Low O$_2$ affinity, absent subunit interactions and Bohr effect Molecule fixed in deoxy-conformation
Hyde Park		30–40	Raised O$_2$ affinity, reduced subunit interaction, normal Bohr effect

12.5

Because of Abnormal Function

Electrophoretic mobility	Amino acid substitution	Position in haemo-globin molecule	References
like Hb–J	α92 (FG4) Arg → Leu		1, 2
like Hb–J	α92 (FG4) Arg → Gln		3, 4, 5
cathodal to Hb–A	β99 (G1) Asp → His		6, 7
like Hb–G	β99 (G1) Asp → Asn		8
cathodal to Hb–A multiple "hybrid" and polymer bands	β99 (G1) Asp → Tyr	in α¹β² contact	9, 10
like Hb–A	β37 (C3) Try → Ser		11
Anodal to Hb–A	β97 (FG4) His → Gln		12
like Hb–A	β145 (HC2) Tyr → Cys	Tyr HC2 plays an important role in the	13, 14, 15
	β145 (HC2) Tyr → His	subunit interactions, see text appendix 2.	15
like Hb–J	β146 (H24) His → Asp	C-terminal amino acid known to be concerned in Bohr effect	16, 17, 18
like Hb–A	β20 (B2) Val → Met	surface	103
cathodal to Hb–A	β102 (G4) Asn → Thr	Haem contact also in α¹β² contact	19, 20
Anodal to Hb–A	β108 (G10) Asn → Asp	α¹β¹ contact	21
cathodal to Hb–A	β90 (F6) Glu → Lys	surface of molecule. Lys could form saltbridge with C-terminal carboxyl of the same chain	22
Anodal to Hb–A	β67 (E11) Val → Glu	haem contact	23, 24
like Hb–E	β26 (B8) Glu → Lys	close to α¹β¹ contact	87, 88, 89, 80
Best separated at pH 7·0 after conversion of haemolysate to met form	α58 (E7) His → Tyr		23, 25
	β63 (E7) His → Tyr		23, 26, 27
	α87 (F8) His → Tyr	Haem contact. Tyr forms ionic bond with ferric iron of met haemoglobin	28, 29, 30 31, 32
	β92 (F8) His → Tyr		33, 34

which is not enough to cause disease in the heterozygote when present together with Hb–A. The red cells from patients with Hb–C disease and Hb–D disease have a normal oxygen affinity. The red cells from patients with Hb–E disease and Hb–E–β-thalassaemia have a low oxygen affinity; heterozygote red cells, Hb–A+E and purified Hb–E solutions have a normal oxygen affinity. The reaction of Hb–E with 2,3-DPG is normal.

Haemoglobin J-Tongariki (Gajdusek *et al.*, 1967) is the only α-chain variant which occurs at a measurable frequency, and the homozygous form has been described but is not associated with any pathological effects. This haemoglobin has a normal oxygen affinity.

HAEMOGLOBINS WITH ABNORMAL FUNCTION

Haemoglobins with an increased oxygen affinity

In the family carrying Hb–Chesapeake (Charache, Weatherall & Clegg, 1967) it was noticed that the heterozygotes for the abnormal haemoglobins also had a raised haematocrit. Further investigation showed that this was caused by the high oxygen affinity of the red cells due to the abnormal haemoglobin. Several other abnormal haemoglobins with a raised oxygen affinity leading to polycythaemia have since been reported (see table 12.5). Consideration of the oxygen dissociation curves of the blood from these

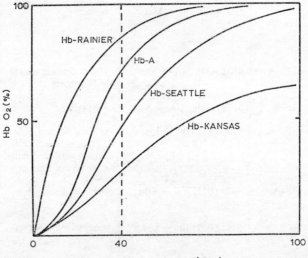

FIG. 12.7. Blood oxygen dissociation curves. As blood passes from the lungs ($P_{O_2}>100$ mmHg) through the tissues (mean venous P_{O_2} c. 40 mmHg) the amount of oxygen given off per gram of haemoglobin is related to oxygen affinity so long as the blood is fully saturated in the arteries. With Hb-Rainier cells with a raised oxygen affinity this will be considerably less than with normal cells; with Hb-Seattle cells with a low oxygen affinity it will be greater than with normal cells. With Hb-Kansas cells there is arterial desaturation, but the delivery capacity per gram haemoglobin is still greater than with normal cells. A normal Bohr effect, blood pH etc. is assumed. (Modified from Stamatoyannopoulos *et al.*, 1971).

patients (Fig. 12.7) shows that for normal oxygen delivery to the tissues there must either be a raised haemoglobin, a low tissue oxygen tension or an increased cardiac output. At normal haemoglobin levels the situation is similar to anaemia in the otherwise normal person. The result would be a low tissue P_{0_2} and/or increased cardiac output. At the same time, increased production of erythropoietin takes place, leading to increased erythropoiesis and an increased red cell mass. This process continues until the whole system is in balance again. At this time, the haemoglobin level is such that the oxygen delivery to the tissues is (near) normal at (near) normal mean venous P_{0_2} and the erythropoietin production will have fallen to a level just sufficient to maintain the balance of red cell destruction and production. As the number of red cells needed for this is only slightly raised above normal, only high normal levels of erythropoietin are found in the steady state. Thus, in this disease the cardiac output and tissue oxygen tension will be normal so long as the red cell mass is raised. However, if it falls, these patients are, in effect, anaemic at normal haemoglobin levels. The physiological aspects of haemoglobins with abnormal function have been reviewed by Stamatoyannopoulos et al. (1971). It has been suggested that the high oxygen affinity of maternal blood would be detrimental to oxygen transport to the foetus. However, it has been pointed out by the above authors that so long as the maternal haemoglobin remains high this is not so. On the other hand, should the maternal haemoglobin fall to anaemic levels due to iron or folate deficiency, the situation is much more serious than in the otherwise normal mother. In those cases which have an abnormal α-chain haemoglobin, the person must have been affected in utero since he would have carried the corresponding α-chain variant of Hb–F; this presumably would also have had a high oxygen affinity. If the control of the level of haemoglobin in the foetus is the same as in the adult then these foetuses would have a very high packed cell volume and might get into difficulty because of the increased blood viscosity.

So far, the reported cases with polycythaemia due to abnormal haemoglobins have been recognised because the abnormal haemoglobin was detected by haemoglobin electrophoresis or, in one case, by alkali denaturation (table 12.5), but it is probable that a neutral amino acid substitution can cause a similar oxygen affinity change of the red cell haemoglobin and to exclude this cause of congenital polycythaemia an oxygen dissociation curve of the red cells should be carried out. In all the reported cases the condition has been benign, and no treatment has been indicated.

Haemoglobins with a low oxygen affinity

Only a few stable haemoglobins with a low oxygen affinity have been described (Table 12.5). A low oxygen affinity of the blood will cause mild anaemia for the same reason that a high oxygen affinity causes polycythaemia. As mild anaemia is common in the population and is in any case associated with a shift in the oygen dissociation curve due to the 2,3-DPG mechanism, this type of haemoglobinopathy presents considerable difficulty in diagnosis, but presumably detailed investigation (oxygen dissociation studies, red cell 2,3-DPG measurement) will bring further cases to light. Haemoglobins with a low oxygen affinity are therefore diagnosed because of some other symptom or sign. This may be cyanosis or concomitant haemolysis due to haemoglobin instability. The latter is discussed in the next section. Hb–Kansas (Table 12.5) (Appendix 2, Fig. 12.18) was diagnosed because the patient had suffered from cyanosis since infancy, and this was caused by the very low oxygen affinity of his haemoglobin. There were no other clinical or haematological abnormalities. The finding of a normal haemoglobin level in the blood rather than the postulated anaemia is explained by the arterial desaturation of Hb–Kansas. Hb–E (see page 386) also has a low oxygen affinity in the red cells.

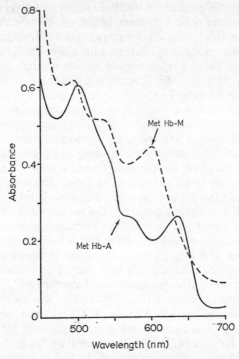

FIG. 12.8. Absorption spectrum at pH 7·0 of methaemoglobin A, compared with methaemoglobin M$_{Saskatoon}$ (from Huehns & Shooter, 1965).

Haemoglobins M

The haemoglobins M are a rare, benign cause of congenital cyanosis (Table 12.5). The differentiation of the biochemical cause of congenital cyanosis from that due to congenital heart disease is important. There are three such conditions. The first of these is congenital methaemoglobinaemia. In these patients there is reduced activity of the enzyme methaemoglobin reductase, and the pigment in the red cells has the spectral characteristics of normal methaemoglobin with an absorption maximum at 632 nm. Measurement of the enzyme will confirm the diagnosis. The second type of biochemical congenital cyanosis is caused by the presence of Hb–M. In these patients the pigment present has a different absorption spectrum from methaemoglobin with the absence of the maximum at 630 nm (Fig. 12.9). Spectral studies of the haemolysate show an abnormal peak at *c*. 600 nm. The diagnosis can be confirmed by electrophoresis in phosphate buffer pH 7·0 of the haemolysate after complete conversion to the methaemoglobin derivative. Under these conditions, the Hb–M's migrate nearer the anode than Hb–A and are characterised by their unusual grey-green colour. The third cause of congenital biochemical cyanosis is the presence of the low oxygen affinity haemoglobins already referred to.

The M haemoglobins were the first abnormal haemoglobins in which it was shown that the abnormality lay in the globin part of the molecule. In each of the four described types one of the two histidines in contact with the haem group in either the α- or β-chain is replaced by tyrosine, and the tyrosine forms an ionic bond with the ferric ion of methaemoglobin, preventing its reduction by methaemoglobin reductase. Although the affected subunit of Hb–M cannot carry oxygen, the normal partner chain can, and the presence of these amino acid substitutions has a marked systematic effect on their oxygen affinity, depending on whether the α- or β-chain is abnormal (see Table 12.5).

Molecular Causes of Changed Oxygen Affinity

The oxygen affinity of haemoglobin depends on the equilibrium between the high affinity (oxy) form of haemoglobin and the low affinity (deoxy) form of the molecule. The detailed description of these two forms has allowed Perutz to compare the probable effect of some amino acid substitutions on this equilibrium (Perutz, 1971a, b). An amino acid substitution which makes the oxy structure the preferred form will cause a high oxygen affinity, while if the deoxy structure is preferred a low affinity results. Another way this equilibrium can be altered is by interaction with neighbouring haemoglobin molecules as occurs in sickle haemoglobin (see page 380).

Interaction with the glycolytic intermediate 2,3-diphosphoglycerate (2,3-DPG) is also important. Increase in 2,3-DPG in the red cell lowers the oxygen affinity while decrease in 2,3-DPG raises it. 2,3-DPG is bound to haemoglobin in the space between the β-chains in the deoxy-form (see Fig. 12.13). In the oxy-form of haemoglobin this space is very much reduced and 2,3-DPG is expelled. Three residues on the β-chains bind 2,3-DPG: histidine β143, lysine β86 and the N-terminal amino group (Perutz, 1970). Anything which interferes with these binding sites reduces the effect of 2,3-DPG on haemoglobin. In Hb–F, histidine β143 is replaced by alanine, and 2,3-DPG binding is reduced. This decreased 2,3-DPG binding explains the higher affinity of foetal red cells compared with adult red cells (Tiyuma & Shimizu, 1970). In Hb–Shepherd's Bush (see later), lysine β86 is indirectly affected, and the 2,3-DPG effect is reduced by one third, resulting in a high oxygen affinity of the red cells. Recent crystallographic work by Arnone has confirmed that these three residues are, in fact, involved and indicates that His β2 also plays a part in 2,3-DPG binding.

Other residues in the haemoglobin molecule have specific functions in relation to the subunit (haem-haem) interactions, the Bohr effect or CO_2 binding (see Perutz, 1970). Abnormal haemoglobins with substitutions affecting these residues have the expected functional change (see Appendix 2).

UNSTABLE HAEMOGLOBINS

Clinical Features

The unstable haemoglobins are one cause of the 'congenital non-spherocytic haemolytic anaemias'. In these conditions, various types of molecular abnormality lead to instability of the haemoglobin molecule and to haemolytic anaemia. The clinical picture varies from patient to patient, some having only slight shortening of red cell life span while in others the degree of haemolysis is much more severe. In the more severely affected patients, there is usually pallor and jaundice as well as splenic enlargement. There is commonly a history of haemolytic crises associated with the ingestion of certain drugs or with infection. As the disease in these patients occurs in the heterozygous condition its occurrence in several generations of the same family may be helpful in distinguishing it from haemolytic disease due to an enzyme deficiency which usually occurs in the homozygous (or hemizygous in the case of G6PD) state. Haematological examination shows a variable anaemia and reticulocytosis. The red cells show variation in size and shape and are usually hypochromic with a low MCHC. In the mildest cases, such as Hb–Seattle (Appendix 2, Table 12.6), the blood film may be normal. Inclusion (Heinz) bodies can occasionally be seen in the film but are usually demonstrated by supravital staining. Often they are found only after incubation without glucose for 24 hours or after splenectomy. Dark urine is found in some cases due to the excretion of dipyrroles of the bilifuscin-mesobilifuscin type. Occasionally, cyanosis is present due to either a low oxygen affinity, as in Hb–Hammersmith (Appendix 2, Table 12.13), or the formation of methaemoglobin. There are no specific physical or haematological signs, and the diagnosis rests on the demonstration of the unstable, abnormal pigment. As most abnormal haemoglobins known do not cause any haemolytic anaemia in the heterozygous state, other possible causes of haemolysis should be carefully excluded. In this connection, examination of other family members is particularly useful as the haemoglobin may be found without haemolysis or vice versa. The biochemical aspects of the unstable haemoglobins have been reviewed (Huehns, 1970).

Detection of Unstable Haemoglobins

One of the reasons why the presence of unstable haemoglobins has often been missed is that they are usually not detected by paper electrophoresis. Nowadays, diagnostic tests utilise more sensitive electrophoretic techniques or depend on demonstrating haemoglobin instability. The demonstration of an abnormal oxygen affinity may be helpful in some cases. Electrophoresis on starch gel, Cellogel or acrylamide gel is a suitably sensitive method, particularly if several different buffer systems at different pH values are used; these supporting media will also separate aggregated haemoglobin molecules. As some haemoglobins separate only in the met-form, this derivative should also be used. Free α- and β-chains should be looked for as these are found in small amounts in some cases. For a description of suitable starch gel electrophoretic methods see Huehns (1968).

Methods based on the stability of the haemoglobin are:

(i) demonstration of inclusion bodies in the cells
(ii) heat denaturation of the haemoglobin
(iii) PCMB precipitation of haemoglobin
(iv) Iso-propanol precipitation.

Inclusion body formation is due to intracellular haemoglobin precipitation. These are demonstrated by supravital staining by, for example, brilliant cresyl blue. They often show up better after splenectomy and in some cases are only detectable after incubation of the cells without glucose for 24 hours.

Another feature of the unstable haemoglobins is their more rapid precipitation than Hb–A on heating of the haemolysate (Fig. 12.10) (Betke *et al.*, 1960; Grimes, Meisler & Dacie, 1964). Again, this test has its drawbacks; if the abnormal haemoglobin is present in only small amounts, or is only mildly unstable, differentiation from the normal may be difficult. We use a dilute haemoglobin solution (*c.* 0·15 g/100 ml) in phosphate buffer pH 6·5, divide this into test and control, incubate at 60°C for half an hour, then add an equal volume of Drabkin's solution and read in a spectrophotometer against suitably diluted Drabkin. Besides this quantitative measure of the amount of haemoglobin lost, a visual estimate of the precipitate should also be made as some of these variants do not carry a haem-group on the affected chain.

Reaction of Hb–A with excess parachloromercuribenzoate (PCMB) causes dissociation into the individual α- and β-chains which can then be separated by starch gel electrophoresis. This technique is useful in scanning for abnormal haemoglobins, but, like all other methods, fails to detect some. PCMB reaction, using strictly controlled conditions (Rosemeyer & Huehns, 1967), with some unstable haemoglobins causes specific precipitation of the abnormal chain, and this may be useful in diagnosis and for the isolation of the abnormal chain. With some electrophoretically inseparable haemoglobins, the dissociated abnormal chain may be seen on electrophoresis. Still other haemoglobins may differ in their dissociation properties, either showing rapid dissociation into subunits, as in Hb–Philly (Appendix 2, Fig. 12.18), or may fail to dissociate (completely) under the usual conditions. More recently, Carrell & Kay (1972) have described a simple test to scan for unstable haemoglobins. The haemolysate is incubated in 17 per cent isopropanol in 0·1M tris buffer pH 7·4 at 37°C for 30 minutes and precipitation looked for.

Finally, a number of the unstable haemoglobins have abnormal oxygen dissociation properties (see Appendix 2), and the finding of a high or low red cell oxygen affinity without the corresponding shift in 2,3-DPG may point to a haemoglobin abnormality.

Molecular Pathology of Unstable Haemoglobins

There are three ways in which the haemoglobin molecule can become unstable. The first is by loss of the haem group, the second by dissociation of the molecule into its separate α- and β-chains, and thirdly, but equally important, by distortion and weakening of the structure of the affected subunit. The last effect often leads to decreased haem-binding by the subunit concerned and also increased dissociation of the molecule. That globin, in contrast to haemoglobin, is very unstable, is a well known observation, and any change of structure in the haem pocket (Appendix 2, Tables 12.10 and 12.11) may lead to lower binding of the haem-group and thus to instability of the molecule (Jacob & Winterhalter, 1970). A number of unstable haemoglobins in which the affected subunit does not bind haem have also been reported. Substitutions at the $\alpha^1\beta^1$ intersubunit contact (Appendix 2, Table 12.12) may cause instability of the haemoglobin molecule if increased dissociation into the individual α- and β-chains is caused, and Hb–Philly is a good example of this. Substitutions involving the $\alpha^1\beta^2$ contact (Appendix 2, Table 12.13) do not have this effect because haemoglobin is normally partially dissociated at this contact into two $\alpha\beta$ dimers. Instability of one of the subunits itself may be caused in various ways. First of all, the new amino acid may be too large to be accommodated in the interior of a subunit, a kind of molecular 'space occupying lesion'. The interior of each subunit consists of apolar or hydrophobic amino acid side chains and the introduction of a polar (charged) amino acid is not possible without distortion of the structure as the hydrophilic group tries to reach the surface of the molecule or draw an oppositely charged side chain near it. A good example of this is Hb–Wien (Appendix 2, Table 12.7). Another way in which the subunit structure may be broken up is the replacement of a helical residue by a prolyl residue. Proline can only be accommodated between helices and at the beginning and end of an helix. Several such substitutions are known (Appendix 2, Table 12.7), all associated with haemoglobin instability and haemolysis. Finally, the subunit structure is held together by a number of bonds between helices, and loss of some of these can lead to instability as, for example, in Hb–Dakar (Appendix 2, Table 12.6). The changes described above lead to instability of the haemoglobin molecule and precipitation of the haemoglobin in the red cell. This process is often associated with methaemoglobin formation or the formation of hemichromes and the blockage of the free sulphydryl groups. The precipitated haemoglobin is removed from the red cell by the pitting phenomenon in the spleen as has been demonstrated by electron microscopy. Consistent with this hypothesis is the finding that inclusion bodies are more easily demonstrated after splenectomy. In many cases the amino acid substitution not only leads to instability of the molecule but also to changes in oxygen affinity, resulting in important physiological consequences, described later. The causes of the change in oxygen affinity have already been discussed (see section on molecular pathology of changes in oxygen dissociation).

Severity of Unstable Haemoglobin Diseases

The degree of haemolysis in these diseases is clearly related to the degree of instability of the haemoglobin involved. Recent studies of a number of unstable β-chain variants have shown that the rate of synthesis of the abnormal chains is the same as that of the corresponding normal chain (except perhaps in exceptional cases, see Huehns, 1970). The amount of abnormal haemoglobin found in the cells is then related to the amount which has already been precipitated. As precipitation followed by pitting causes damage to the red cell membrane it follows that the less abnormal haemoglobin there is in the cell the more cell membrane damage there is and the greater the degree of haemolysis found. Analysis of the published data shows that this is indeed so as there is significant correlation between cell survival and the relative amount of abnormal haemoglobin, a low amount of abnormal haemoglobin (i.e. most precipitation and cell damage) being associated with the shortest cell survival (Fig. 12.9).

Further analyses of the published data on these cases show that there is little correlation between the red cell survival and the packed cell volume or haemoglobin level (Fig. 12.10). If the degree of red cell destruction is not the main determinant of the blood haemoglobin level, then this must be controlled by the erythropoietic response of the marrow. As has already been pointed out, this is closely geared to the oxygen affinity of the red cells (see page 386). Applying similar arguments to the haemolytic states it is found that there is a close correlation between oxygen affinity of the red cells and the

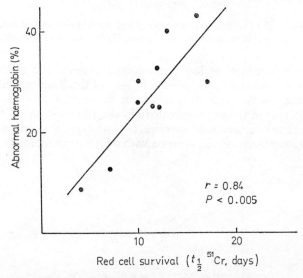

FIG. 12.9. Correlation between red cell survival and per cent abnormal haemoglobin for unstable haemoglobins with aberrant β-chains. (Data from the literature.)

PCV of the peripheral blood (Fig. 12.11). This relationship applies not only to the unstable haemoglobins but also to the sickle cell syndromes and the enzymopathies. In patients where this relationship between packed cell volume and oxygen affinity deviates from that expected from Fig. 12.11, further investigations should be carried out. If the packed cell volume is too low, then the marrow response is lower than expected and some other complicating factor, such as increasing haemolysis, folate deficiency, etc., should be looked for. In one patient with Hb–S+C disease whose packed cell volume was too high for the oxygen affinity, further studies of the patient showed, as expected, a low red cell mass, the relatively high PCV being due to a low plasma volume.

The finding that the packed cell volume (i.e. red cell mass) is closely geared to the oxygen affinity of the red cells means that in haemolytic diseases in the steady state the oxygen delivery capacity of the blood is the same

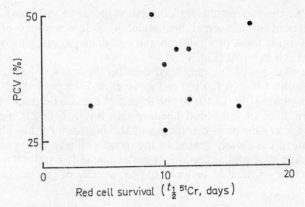

FIG. 12.10. Lack of correlation between red cell survival and packed cell volume (PCV) for unstable haemoglobin diseases. (Data from the literature.)

whether there is a high or low haemoglobin present, and this conclusion accounts for the normal development of many of these patients and the mild nature of the disease. However, it should be noted that although this is undoubtedly true in the uncomplicated disease, in conditions of stress, such as strenuous exercise, increased anaemia, etc., when the tissue oxygen tensions tend to be lower than normal, patients with a high oxygen affinity and a high

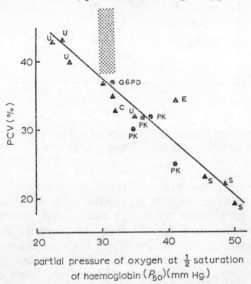

FIG. 12.11. Correlation between the oxygen affinity of red cells with the PCV in patients with chronic haemolytic anaemias in the steady state due to abnormal haemoglobins (▲) and enzyme deficiencies (●), (U) unstable haemoglobins, (S) sickle cell anaemia, (C) haemoglobin C disease, (E) haemoglobin E disease, (PK) pyruvate kinase deficiency, (G6PD) glucose 6-phosphate dehydrogenase deficiency. Normal adults▧. The oxygen affinity was determined on washed red cells suspended in an isotonic phosphate buffer pH 7.1 at 37°C (Bellingham & Huehns, 1968).

PCV are at a distinct advantage compared to those with a low oxygen affinity and a low PCV. This results in part from the position and shape of the oxygen dissociation curve as well as from the higher oxygen capacity of the blood of patients with a high PCV. Another advantage of high oxygen affinity is that the arterial oxygen content is protected against any fall in arterial P_{O_2} due, for example, to respiratory disease. These considerations may explain the finding that among patients who are heterozygous for an abnormal haemoglobin a raised blood oxygen affinity is seen more frequently than a low affinity, and thus accounts for the relative frequency of Hb–Köln. All these factors must be taken into account in the management of these diseases.

Treatment of Diseases Due to the Unstable Haemoglobins

There is no specific treatment for these diseases, but splenectomy is sometimes helpful in patients with severe haemolysis (Hutchison *et al.*, 1964), while in others no improvement can be shown (Cathie, 1952). Each case must therefore be individually assessed by determining the degree of splenic red cell destruction. The increased liability to oxidation of the haemoglobin molecules makes these patients sensitive to the same group of drugs that may cause crises in glucose-6-phosphate dehydrogenase (G6PD) deficiency. In the unstable haemoglobins the molecule is more easily oxidised, while in G6PD deficiency the reductive potential of the cell is reduced. In either case, haemoglobin precipitates in the cell and may lead to haemolytic crises. These drugs (Table 12.4) should therefore be avoided. Another possible line of treatment is by blood transfusions, but these are only occasionally indicated. In assessing the severity of the disease, not only the degree of anaemia but also the oxygen affinity of the red cells should be taken into account (see previous section).

APPENDIX 1

Normal Haemoglobins

Development and genetics

The function of haemoglobin is to transport oxygen to the tissues, and it appears reasonable to expect special pigments for this in the very different conditions which are found *in utero*. There are three stages in haemoglobin development (for review, see Huehns & Beaven, 1971). In the first stage, the embryonic haemoglobins predominate, Hb–Gower 1, Hb–Gower 2 and Hb–Portland 1. These three pigments are rapidly replaced by foetal haemoglobin, Hb–F, and by the 3·5 cm C.R. stage, *c.* 8 weeks' gestation, Hb–F amounts to about 55 per cent. There are only traces of the embryonic haemoglobins after the 5 cm C.R. stage. The functional properties, if any, which distinguish the embryonic haemoglobins from Hb–A and Hb–F are at present unknown. Hb–F is the main pigment of foetal life. It is rapidly replaced by Hb–A and 2–3 per cent Hb–A$_2$ after birth (Fig. 12.12, Table 12.6). Hb–F differs from Hb–A by the replacement of the β-chain by the

γ-chain and has the structure $\alpha_2\gamma_2$. The higher oxygen affinity of foetal red cells compared to that of adult red cells is determined by the different interaction of Hb–F and Hb–A with 2,3-DPG. Whereas 2,3-DPG has a marked effect in lowering the oxygen affinity of Hb–A, the effect on Hb–F is only about half; thus foetal red cells have a higher oxygen affinity than adult red cells (see also page 389).

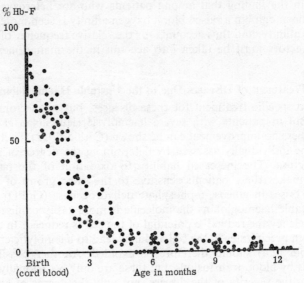

FIG. 12.12. Amounts of Hb-F in the blood of normal infants of various ages to show the wide variation of levels found. (From Huehns & Beaven, 1971).

TABLE 12.6

PROPORTION OF Hb-F FOUND AT VARIOUS AGES

Age	Hb–F per cent
Birth	70–90
1 month	50–75
2 months	25–60
3 months	10–35
4 months	5–20
6 months	< 8
9 months	< 5
1 year	< 2
Adults	not detectable (< 0·4)

Genetically, the synthesis of the various haemoglobin polypeptide chains is controlled by a number of (autosomal) loci, one for each polypeptide chain (for review, see Huehns & Shooter, 1965). The loci for the non-α-chains, the β-, δ- and probably the γ-chains, are linked. There is a common α-chain locus for all the normal haemoglobins, and they are derived from a common metabolic pool. Abnormalities of haemoglobin synthesis of the α-chains, therefore, affect haemoglobins at all stages of development. Besides these loci controlling the synthesis of the globin part of the molecule there are a number of loci for the enzymes involved in the synthesis of haem. Genetic abnormalities of these enzymes give rise to the various kinds of porphyrias (see Rimington, 1959).

Recent structural work on certain γ-chain variants (Schroeder et al., 1968) has shown that there must be two loci controlling the synthesis of γ-chains. The γ-chains made by these loci differ from each other by only a single amino acid substitution. One locus codes for glycine whilst the other codes for the alanine at position 136 of the chain. They have therefore been called the $γ^{gly}$ and $γ^{ala}$ loci.

The suggestion has recently been made that there is more than one locus controlling the synthesis of α-chains (Lehmann & Carrell, 1968). There is as yet very little critical family data, and this is conflicting. In support of the presence of two major α-chain loci is a Hungarian family where some members have three haemoglobins (Hollan et al., 1972): Hb-A, Hb-Gα (αT9 Asp → Asn) and Hb-Jα (α61 Lys → Asn). The presence of three α-chains ($α^A$, $α^G$ and $α^J$) can only be explained by the presence of two structural loci coding for α-chains. Family studies show that the two loci are not (closely) linked. Two α-chain loci have also been reported in the tribal population of Andrhra Pradesh (Bernini et al., 1969). In this case, the second α-locus codes for a minor component with multiple differences from the normal α-chain. The finding that this minor component migrates cathodally to Hb-A_2 on electrophoresis and also gives rise to multiple bands suggests that it may be identical to Hb-Constant Spring with an addition at the C-terminal end (see page 376). If this is so, then this type of α-chain duplication, giving rise to a minor component, may be quite common. Structural studies of Hb-Ho-2 (Ostertag et al., 1971) show that there are two α-Ho-2-chains; both differ from the $α^A$-chain by the substitution α-112 His → Asp and, therefore, have the same electrophoretic mobility. However, fingerprinting of the isolated abnormal haemoglobin shows two abnormal αT-12 peptides. One has the same sequence as the normal αT-12 peptide, except for the substitution His → Asp, while the other has this same substitution as well as two other neutral substitutions. These results indicate the presence of three α-chains in one individual, and can only be explained by a duplicated structural locus for α-chain production. The data further suggest that the second locus is probably a minor locus and is linked to the main α-chain locus.

It is important, in interpreting this evidence for α-chain duplication, to note that it does not follow a uniform pattern; one family shows an unlinked major second locus, while both the others suggest a second minor locus. Against the presence of two α-chain loci are the findings on Hb-J-Tongariki (Abramson et al., 1970; Beaven et al., 1972). These authors have reported several homozygotes for Hb-J-Tongariki, and in each individual no normal α-chains were present. Furthermore, there was no evidence of thalassaemia. As these cases come from widely separated islands in the Pacific, they indicate that no α-chain duplication exists in this population. The finding of

Hb–Gα without any Hb–A in a West African (Shooter *et al.*, 1960) may be another example of a homozygous α-chain abnormality. The data to date therefore indicate that in some populations there is only a single α-chain locus but do not preclude the possibility of duplication, either in particular families, as mentioned above, or in other populations.

Structure and function

Haemoglobin* consists of four polypeptide chains, two α-chains and two β-chains, $\alpha_2\beta_2$. To each polypeptide chain is attached a haem group. Each subunit consists of a long chain of amino acids, 141 for the α-chain and 146 for the β-chain. Each chain is wound up into 8 spiral or helical segments connected to each other by short, non-helical segments to give each subunit a compact (roughly spherical) shape. For descriptive purposes the helices are labelled by the letters A–H starting at the free amino group end, called the N-terminus, the non-helical connecting segments being labelled by the letters of the helices they connect, i.e. the EF segment is the piece of chain connecting the E and F helices; the N-terminal segment is called the NA segment. The haem group in each subunit lies in a deep pocket lined by about 20 hydrophobic (non-polar) residues from the B, C, E, F, G and H helices as well as the CD and FG segment. The iron of the haem group is covalently bonded to histidine F8 (the 8th amino acid of the F helix), while the oxygen molecule is bound to the other side of the iron atom opposite histidine E7. The proprionic side chains of the haem groups make polar contacts with residues CD3 and E10. The structure of each subunit is stabilised by the hydrophobic interactions of the side chains in the interior of each subunit and around the haem group. There are also specific bonds holding the helices together. Interactions between the α- and β-chains are also important.

The four subunits in the haemoglobin molecule lie on the four corners of a tetrahedron (pyramid). There is little contact between like chains (α–α or β–β), while there is close contact between unlike chains. From Fig. 12.13 it can be seen that there are four $\alpha\beta$ contacts: these are of two types called $\alpha^1 \equiv \beta^1$ (or $\alpha^2 \equiv \beta^2$) and $\alpha^1 - \beta^2$ (or $\alpha^2 - \beta^1$). The $\alpha^1 \equiv \beta^1$ contact is firm, while the $\alpha^1 - \beta^2$ contact is relatively weak, and it is at the latter contact that haemoglobin dissociates: $\alpha_2\beta_2 \rightleftharpoons \alpha^1 \equiv \beta^1 + \alpha^2 \equiv \beta^2$.

During oxygenation, the affinity for oxygen increases as the haemoglobin becomes more saturated. This effect is due to the subunit (or haem–haem) interactions, a measure of which is given by the 'n' value of the Hill equation. The basis of the subunit interactions is a dynamic equilibrium between the high affinity and low affinity forms of haemoglobin. In oxyhaemoglobin virtually all the haemoglobin is in the high affinity state, while in deoxyhaemoglobin the vast majority of molecules are in the low affinity state. These two forms, therefore, correspond to the oxy- and deoxy-structural forms of haemoglobins described by Perutz and his co-workers (for refs. see footnote page 398) (Fig. 12.13b). The change from the oxy- to the deoxyform is initiated by a change in the position of the iron relative to the plane of the porphyrin ring and involves the rotation of the $\alpha^1 \equiv \beta^1$ dimers in the

---

* For a detailed description of the haemoglobin molecule see Perutz *et al.* (1968); Muirhead & Greer (1970); Bolton & Perutz (1970); Perutz *et al.* (1969). A short description is given by Perutz (1971a, b).

A.

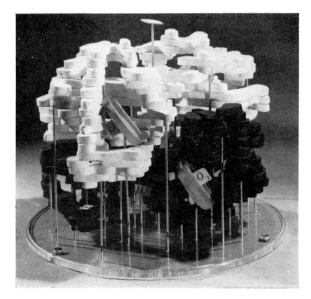

B.

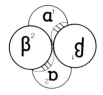

Oxy-haemoglobin

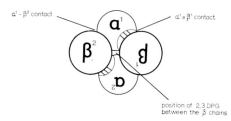

deoxy-haemoglobin

α¹ - β² contact

α¹ ≡ β¹ contact

position of 2,3 DPG
between the β chains

FIG. 12.13. Models of the haemoglobin molecule.

A) Model of haemoglobin at 5 Å resolution. α-chains white, β-chains black.
(Photograph kindly supplied by Dr. M. F. Perutz).
B) Diagrammatic representation of the conformational change of haemo-
globin on oxygenation to show 2,3-DPG binding site between the β-chains.

[*To face p.* 398.

whole (tetramer) molecule over each other at the $\alpha^1 - \beta^2$ contact. This change from the oxy- to the deoxy- form also breaks some salt bridges linking the β-chains to each other and results in an increase in the space between the β-chains. Similarly, salt bridges between the α-chains are also broken but these two chains only move a relatively small distance. The tyrosines HC2 α and β also play an important part in this change of conformation. In the deoxy-form, these residues lie in pockets between the F and H helices, clamping the C-terminal part of the polypeptide chain down; in the oxy-form these tyrosine residues are expelled from their pockets and the C-terminal ends of the haemoglobin chains are freed.

Alteration of the equilibrium mentioned above between the two forms of haemoglobin will decrease or increase the oxygen affinity. A good example of this is the effect of 2,3-DPG, which combines with haemoglobin in the space between the β-chains present only in the deoxy-form (Fig. 12.13b) and pushes the equilibrium to the low affinity state but does not prevent the change to the high affinity state. When this takes place 2,3-DPG is no longer bound at this site. 2,3-DPG therefore lowers the oxygen affinity but does not affect the subunit (haem-haem) interactions. On the other hand, any change, such as an amino acid substitution, which prevents the complete change between the two forms taking place will lower or abolish the subunit (haem-haem) interactions.

Thus, it can be seen that haemoglobin is far from being a passive carrier of oxygen but undergoes radical molecular rearrangement as it takes up oxygen molecules in the lungs and releases them in the tissues, and might well be termed 'the molecular lung' (Perutz, 1971a).

APPENDIX 2

Molecular Pathology of Abnormal Haemoglobins

In Tables 12.5 and 12.7–12.13 the effects on the oxygen dissociation properties and stability of amino acid substitutions in various parts of the molecule are summarised. These results enable the generalisations given in the main text to be made. The detailed atomic interactions of some of these abnormal haemoglobins are given by Perutz & Lehmann, (1968) as well as in the individual paper quoted.

1. Substitutions on the outside of the molecule. Most of these substitutions are relatively benign. Pathological effects only arise if new deleterious interactions occur, such as in sickle cell disease, or if important stabilising bonds are broken, and haemoglobins with such changes are listed in Table 12.7.

2. Substitutions on the interior of a subunit. So far all substitutions described on the interior of a subunit have caused instability of the molecule due to their size, polar character or because they involve the insertion of a proline into a helical part of the polypeptide chain (Table 12.8).

3. Substitutions around the haem groups. Almost all these cause instability of the molecule due to reduced haem binding by the globin part of the

TABLE 12.7

ABNORMAL HAEMOGLOBINS DUE TO REPLACEMENTS AT THE SURFACE OF THE MOLECULE

More than 50 substitutions known without clinical or physiological abnormality: stability and oxygen dissociation studies are not available on most.

Abnormal haemoglobin		Substitution	Comment	Reference
(A) Disease in the homozygote only				
Hb-S	β-6	GLU → VAL	Causes sickle cell disease in the homozygote due to interaction of the new valyl residues with adjacent molecules when in the deoxy form. Low O_2 affinity in cells only, normal subunit interactions. The low oxygen affinity is explained by constraint on the conformational change from the deoxy-to the oxy-form by the sickling process.	35, 36, 37
Hb-C	β-6	GLU → LYS	Mild haemolytic process in homozygote.	38, 39
Hb-D Punjab	β-121	GLU → GLN	No instability or oxygen dissociation abnormality.	40, 41
(B) Disease in the heterozygote only				
Hb-Dakar	α-112	HIS → GLN	Haemolytic anaemia. Interaction between HIS α-112 (G 19) and GLU α-27 (B 8), which helps to hold B and G helices together, is broken, leading to instability.	42
Hb-Hopkins 2	α-112	HIS → ASP	Slight instability, raised O_2 affinity, reduced subunit interaction, no clinical abnormality.	43, 44
Hb-Etobicoke	α-84	SER → ARG	Normal residue stabilizes G and F helices, high O_2 affinity, mild instability.	45
Hb-Hasharon	α-47	ASP → HIS	Mild instability.	46, 47, 48
Hb-L Ferrara	α-47	ASP → GLY	Normal oxygen dissociation.	49
Hb-Seattle	β-76	ALA → GLU	Instability, haemolytic anaemia, low O_2 affinity, near normal subunit interaction. Interaction of new GLU with adjacent HIS occurs.	50, 51
Hb-Hiroshima	β-143	HIS → ASP	Stable, high O_2 affinity, low Bohr effect, slightly low subunit interaction. Polycythaemia.	16, 17, 18
Hb-Agenogi	β-90	GLU → LYS	Low O_2 affinity, normal Bohr effect and subunit interaction.	22
Hb-Porto Alegre	β-9	SER → CYS	No disease, polymer formation by disulphide bond formation.	100
Hb-Olympia	β-20	VAL → MET	Raised O_2 affinity, normal Bohr effect, slightly low 'n'.	103

molecule. The oxygen affinity is usually altered. The haemoglobin M's form a special sub-group (Tables 12.10 and 12.11).

4. **Substitutions in the $\alpha^1\beta^1$ intersubunit contact.** These substitutions are usually benign but may give rise to instability if they cause increased dissociation at this contact (Table 12.12).

TABLE 12.8

ABNORMAL HAEMOGLOBINS DUE TO REPLACEMENTS IN THE INTERIOR OF A SUBUNIT

				Reference
(a) Proline breaks up α-helix				
Genova	β–28	(B 10) (*)	LEU → PRO	52, 53
Perth	β–32	(B 14)	LEU → PRO	54
See also Figs. 12.16 and 12.17.				
(b) Polar residue in non-polar region				
Ann Arbor	α–80		LEU → ARG	55
Sogn	β–14		LEU → ARG	56
Wien	β–130		TYR → ASP	57
Riverdale-Bronx	β–24		GLY → ARG	94
Savannah	β–24		GLY → VAL	95

(*) 10th residue of the B-helix.

5. **Substitutions in the $\alpha^1\beta^2$ intersubunit contact.** The substitutions at this contact do not cause instability because dissociation normally takes place at this contact. As this contact is important in the change from the oxy- to the deoxy- form of haemoglobin, a change of oxygen affinity and subunit (haem–haem-) interactions occurs in almost all abnormal haemoglobin affecting this contact (Table 12.13).

TABLE 12.9

ABNORMAL HAEMOGLOBINS DUE TO DELETIONS

Leiden	GLU at β–6 (or 7) deleted (ref 91)
Freiburg	VAL at β–23 deleted, raised O_2 affinity (92)
Gun Hill	Residues β–93–97 deleted, does not bind haem, leads to high O_2 affinity (93)
Togichi	Residues β–56–59 deleted (101)
Rio de Janeiro (Niteroi)	Residues β–42–44 deleted (102)

All these haemoglobins are unstable and give rise to haemolytic anaemia.

6. **Substitutions in the central cavity and at the β–β intersubunit contact.** Substitutions in this area may affect oxygen affinity by altering DPG binding (see also Hb–ShB, Table 12.11) or by breaking some of the salt bridges maintaining the oxy-structure of haemoglobin. Replacement of histidine β146 by aspartic acid in Hb–Hiroshima reduces the Bohr effect as expected

TABLE 12.10

AMINO ACID SUBSTITUTIONS AT HAEM CONTACTS OF THE α-CHAIN

Position	Amino acid	
32	MET	
39	THR	
42	TYR	
43	PHE → VAL	Torino, unstable. low O_2 affinity (58, 59, 60)
45	HIS	
46	PHE	
58	HIS → TYR	M–Boston, low O_2 affinity, reduced subunit interactions and Bohr effect (23, 25)
61	LYS → ASN	J–Buda, low O_2 affinity, slight instability (96)
62	VAL	
83	LEU	
86	LEU	
87	HIS → TYR	M–Iwate, low O_2 affinity, unstable, absent subunit interaction and Bohr effect (28, 29, 30, 31, 32)
91	LEU	
93	VAL	
97	ASN	
98	PHE	
101	LEU	
129	LEU	
132	VAL	
136	LEU → PRO	Bibba, unstable (61)

(Perutz, 1969). This haemoglobin also has a high oxygen affinity and reduced subunit interaction. Hb–Abruzzo (β143 His → Arg) (Tentori *et al.*, 1971), which causes a well compensated haemolytic anaemia (Hb–12·5 g/100 ml), is of particular interest because His β143 is one of the amino acids binding 2,3-DPG. However, no oxygen dissociation studies have been reported. Hb–Manitoba (Crookston *et al.*, 1969) (α102 Ser → Arg) shows mild heat instability but no disease in the affected individuals. It is difficult to separate on electrophoresis. Oxygen dissociation studies on the red cells show no abnormality. Hb–Singapore (Clegg *et al.*, 1969) (α141 Arg → Pro) is in the α–α contact, but no studies of function have been carried out.

7. **Amino acid deletions and additions.** Amino acid deletions (Table 12.9) have, in every case, caused instability of the molecule. Only two additions to the C-terminal end of the molecule have been described: Hb–Constant Spring, with about 30 extra residues on the α-chain (Milner *et al.*, 1972) and Hb–Tak with 10 extra residues on the β-chain (Flatz *et al.*, 1971). The effect on the function and stability of the molecule has not yet been described.

TABLE 12.11

AMINO ACID SUBSTITUTIONS AT HAEM CONTACTS OF THE β-CHAIN

Position	Amino acid	
31	LEU	
38	THR	
41	PHE	
42	PHE $\nearrow$ SER	Hammersmith, unstable, low O_2 affinity, slightly low subunit interaction (62, 59)
	PHE $\searrow$ LEU	Louisville/Bucaresti, unstable, low oxygen affinity (76)
44	SER	
45	PHE	
63	HIS $\nearrow$ ARG	Zürich, unstable, high O_2 affinity, normal Bohr effect, reduced subunit interaction (63, 64, 65, 66)
	HIS $\searrow$ TYR	M–Saskatoon, unstable, high O_2 affinity, reduced subunit interactions, normal Bohr effect (23, 26, 27)
66	LYS $\rightarrow$ GLU	Toulouse, unstable, normal O_2 dissociation linked to propionic side chain of haem (68)
67	VAL $\nearrow$ ASP	M–Milwaukee, (unstable), low O_2 affinity, normal Bohr effect, reduced subunit interactions (23, 24)
	VAL $\rightarrow$ ALA	Sydney, unstable (69)
	VAL $\searrow$ GLU	Bristol, unstable, low O_2 affinity, normal Bohr effect, slightly decreased subunit interactions (70).
70	ALA	
71	PHE $\rightarrow$ SER	Christchurch, unstable (97)
74	GLY $\rightarrow$ ASP	Shepherd's Bush, unstable, high O_2 affinity, normal Bohr effect, decreased subunit interaction, low 2,3-DPG effect (71, 72)
88	LEU $\nearrow$ PRO	Santa Ana, unstable, no haem group (73)
	LEU $\searrow$ ARG	Boras, unstable, high O_2 affinity (74, 75, 76)
91	LEU $\rightarrow$ PRO	Sabine, unstable, no haem group (77)
92	HIS $\rightarrow$ TYR	M–Hyde Park, unstable, high O_2 affinity, low subunit interaction, normal Bohr shift (33, 34)
96	LEU	
98	VAL $\rightarrow$ MET	Köln, unstable, high O_2 affinity, low subunit interaction, normal Bohr effect, (also in $\alpha^1\beta^2$ contact) (78, 79, 80)
103	PHE	
106	LEU	
137	VAL	
141	LEU	

TABLE 12.12

AMINO ACID SUBSTITUTIONS IN THE $\alpha^1\beta^1$ CONTACT: α-CHAIN RESIDUES ON THE
LEFT, β-CHAIN RESIDUES ON THE RIGHT

	α-chain	β-chain	
Mild anaemia* (81)	G–Chinese α–30 GLU → GLN	Camden β–131 GLN → GLU	No abnormal properties (82)
		Khartoum β–124 PRO → ARG	Probably no abnormal properties* (98)
		New York β–113 VAL → GLU	No abnormal properties (83)
		Hb–P β–117 HIS → ARG	Slightly abnormal red cells* (99)
		Peterborough β–131 VAL → PHE	Unstable, low O₂ affinity, normal Bohr shift and subunit interactions (76)
No abnormal properties (84)	Chiapas α–114 PRO → ARG		
		Yoshizuka β–108 ASN → ASP	Low O₂ affinity, normal subunit interactions, low Bohr shift (21)
		Philly β–35 TYR → PHE	Unstable, increased dissociation into monomers* (85)
		Tacoma β–30 ARG → SER	(86)*
		Hb–E β–26 GLU → LYS	Low O₂ affinity, normal Bohr effect and subunit interactions (87, 88, 89, 80)

* No oxygen dissociation studies.

TABLE 12.13

AMINO ACID SUBSTITUTIONS IN THE $\alpha^1\beta^2$ CONTACT: α-CHAIN RESIDUES ON THE LEFT, β-CHAIN RESIDUES ON THE RIGHT

	α-chain	β-chain	
Stable, high O$_2$ affinity low haem-haem interactions	Chesapeake (1, 2) α–92 ARG $\nearrow$ LEU $\searrow$ GLN J–Capetown (3, 4, 5)		
		Hirose β–37 TRY → SER	High O$_2$ affinity, reduced Bohr effect and subunit interactions (11)
		Malmö β–97 HIS → GLN	High O$_2$ affinity (12)
		Köln β–98 VAL → MET	Unstable, high O$_2$ affinity, low haem-haem interactions (2, 25)
		$\nearrow$ ASN β–99 ASP → TYR $\searrow$ HIS	Kempsey (8) Ypsi (9, 10) Yakima (6, 7) Stable, high O$_2$ affinity, low subunit interactions
		Kansas $\nearrow$ THR β–102 ASN $\searrow$ LYS Richmond	Stable, easily dissociated, low O$_2$ affinity, low haem-haem interactions (19, 20) Stable, normal O$_2$ dissociation, less easily dissociated (90)

References to Text

ABRAMSON, R. R., RUCKNAGEL, D. L., SHREFFLER, D. C. & SAAVE, J. J. (1970). *Science*, **169**, 194.

AKSOY, M. & LEHMANN, H. (1957). *Nature*, **179**, 1248.

ALLISON, A. C. (1964). *Cold Spring Harb. Symp. quant. Biol.*, **29**, 137.

BANNERMAN, R. M. (1972). *Hematologic Reviews*, **3**, 297.

BEAVEN, G. H., HORNABROOK, R. W., FOX, R. H. & HUEHNS, E. R. (1972). *Nature*, **235**, 46.

BELLINGHAM, A. J., DETTER, J. C. & LENFANT, C. (1970). *Trans. Ass. Am. Phys.*, **83**, 113.

BELLINGHAM, A. J. & HUEHNS, E. R. (1968). *Nature*, **218**, 924.

BENNETT, E. & HUEHNS, E. R. (1970). *Lancet*, **2**, 956.

BENSINGER, T. A., MAHMOOD, L., CONRAD, M. E. & McCURDY, P. R. (1972). *Clin. Res.*, in press.

BERNINI, L., DE JONG, W. W. W. & MEERA, KHAM, P. (1969). *Atti. Ass. Genet. Nat.*

BERTLES, J. F. & DÖBLER, J. (1969). *Blood*, **33**, 884.

BETKE, K., MARTI, H. R., KLEIHAUER, E. & BÜTIKOFER, E. (1960). *Klin. Wschr.*, **38**, 529.

BEUTLER, E. (1961). *J. clin. Invest.*, **40**, 1856.

BIRCH, K. M. & SCHÜTZ, F. (1946). *Br. J. Pharmac.*, **1**, 186.

BOLTON, W. & PERUTZ, M. F. (1970). *Nature*, **228**, 551.

BOOKCHIN, R. M. & NAGEL, R. L. (1971). *J. mol. Biol.*, **60**, 263.

CARRELL, R. W. & KAY, R. (1972). *Brit. J. Haemat.* in press.

CARRELL, R. W. & LEHMANN, H. (1969). *Seminars in Hematology*, **6**, 116.

CATHIE, I. A. B. (1952). *Gt. Ormond Str. J.*, **2**, 43.

CERAMI, A. & MANNING, J. M. (1971). *Proc. nat Acad. Sci. U.S.A.*, **68**, 1180.

CHARACHE, S. & CONLEY, C. L. (1964). *Blood*, **24**, 25.

CHARACHE, S., WEATHERALL, D. J. & CLEGG, J. B. (1967). *J. clin. Invest.*, **45**, 813.

CLEGG, J. B., WEATHERALL, D. J. & WONG HOCK BOON. (1969). *Nature*, **222**, 379.

CROOKSTON, J. H., GOLDSTEIN, J., LEHMANN, H. & BEALE, D. (1969). *Can. J. Biochem.*, **47**, 143.

FINK, H. (1969). 2nd Conference on the Problems of Cooley's Anemia. *Ann. N.Y. Acad. Sci.*, **165**, 1.

FLATZ, G., KINDERLEHRER, J., KILMARTIN, J. V. & LEHMANN, H. (1971). *Lancet*, **1**, 732.

GAJDUSEK, D. C., GUIART, J. KIRK, R. L., CARRELL, R. W., IRVINE, D., KYNOCH, P. A. M. & LEHMANN, H. (1967). *J. Med. Genet.*, **4**, 1.

GRIMES, A. J., MEISLER, A. & DACIE, J. V. (1964). *Br. J. Haemat.*, **10**, 281.

HILL, A. V. (1910). *J. Physiol.*, **40**, 4.

HILKOVITZ, G. (1957). *Br. med. J.*, **ii**, 266.

HOLLAN, S. R., SZELENYI, J. G., BRIMHALL, B., DUERST, M., JONES, R. T., KOLER, R. D. & STOCKLEN, Z. (1972). *Nature*, **235**, 47.

HUEHNS, E. R. (1965). *Postgrad. med. J.*, **41**, 718.

HUEHNS, E. R. (1968). *In* 'Chromatographic and Electrophoretic Techniques'. Vol. 2. Ed. I. Smith. p. 291. London: Heinemann.

HUEHNS, E. R. (1970). *Bull. Soc. Chim. biol.*, **52**, 1131.

HUEHNS, E. R. (1971). *Scientific Basis of Medicine Ann. Rev.*, p. 216.

HUEHNS, E. R. & BEAVEN, G. H. (1971). *Clinics Dev. Med.*, **37**, 175.

HUEHNS, E. R. & BELLINGHAM, A. J. (1969). *Br. J. Haemat.*, **17**, 1.

HUEHNS, E. R., FLYNN, F. V., BUTLER, E. A. & SHOOTER, E. M. (1960). *Br. J. Haemat.*, **6**, 388.

HUEHNS, E. R. & SHOOTER, E. M. (1964). *Sci. Prog.*, **52**, 353.

HUEHNS, E. R. & SHOOTER, E. M. (1965). *J. med. Genet.*, **2**, 48.

HUGH-JONES, K., LEHMANN, H. & McALISTER, J. M. (1964). *Br. med. J.*, **ii**, 226.

HUTCHISON, H. E., PINKERTON, P. H., WATERS, P., DOUGLAS, A. S., LEHMANN, H. & BEALE, D. (1964). *Br. med. J.*, **ii**, 1099.

JACOB, H. S. & WINTERHALTER, K. H. (1970). *J. clin. Invest.*, **49**, 2008.

KRAUS, L. M., KRAUS, A. P. & GREAR, J. (1971). *Biochem. biophys. Res. Commun.*, **44**, 1381.

KRAUS, L. M., MIYAJI, T., IUCHI, I. & KRAUS, A. P. (1966). *Biochemistry*, **5**, 370.

LASZLO, J., OBENOUR, W. & SALTZMAN, H. A. (1969). *S. med. J.*, **62**, 453.

LEHMANN, H. (1970). *Lancet*, **2**, 78.

LEHMANN, H. & CARRELL, R. W. (1968). *Br. med. J.*, **4**, 748.

LEVIN, W. C. (1958). *Blood*, **13**, 904.

McCURDY, P. R. & MAHMOOD, L. (1971). *New Engl. J. Med.*, **285**, 992.

McNiel, J. R. (1971). *J. med. Ass. Thailand*, **54**, 153.

Maizels, M., Prankerd, T. A. J. & Richards, J. D. M. (1968). *In* 'Haematology in Diagnosis and Treatment'. London: Ballière, Tindall and Cassell.

May, A., Bellingham, A. J., Huehns, E. R. & Beaven, G. H. (1972). *Lancet*, **i,** 658

Milner, P. F., Clegg, J. B. & Weatherall, D. J. (1971). *Lancet*, **1**, 729.

Milner, P. E., Miller, C., Grey, R., Seakins, M., De Jong, W. W. & Went, L. N. (1970). *New Engl. J. Med.*, **283**, 1417.

Muirhead, H. & Greer, J. (1970). *Nature*, **228**, 516.

Nalbandian, R. M. (ed.) (1971c). *In* 'Molecular Aspects of Sickle Cell Hemoglobin'. Springfield: Charles C. Thomas.

Nalbandian, R. M., Anderson, J. W., Lusher, J. M., Agustsson, A. & Henry, R. L. (1971a). *Am. J. med. Sci.*, **261**, 325.

Nalbandian, R. M., Henry, R., Nichols, B., Kessler, D. L., Camp, F. R. & Vining, K. K. (1970). *Ann. intern. Med.*, **72**, 795.

Nalbandian, R. M., Schultz, G., Lusher, J. M., Anderson, J. W. & Henry, R. L. (1971b). *Am. J. med. Sci.*, **261**, 309.

Na-Nakorn, S., Wasi, P., Pornpatkul, M. & Pootrakul, S. (1969). *Nature*, **223**, 59.

Opio, E. & Barnes, P. M. (1972). *Lancet*, **2**, 160.

Ostertag, W., Von Ehrenstein, G. & Charache, S. (1972). *Nature, New Biology*, **237**, 90.

Perutz, M. F. (1969). *Nature*, **224**, 269.

Perutz, M. F. (1970). *Nature*, **228**, 724.

Perutz, M. F. (1971a). *New Scient. Sci. J.*, **50**, 676.

Perutz, M. F. (1971b). *New Scient. Sci. J.*, **50**, 757.

Perutz, M. F. & Lehmann, H. (1968). *Nature*, **219**, 902.

Perutz, M. F., Muirhead, H., Cox, J. M. & Goaman, L. C. G. (1968). *Nature*, **219**, 131.

Perutz, M. F., Muirhead, H., Mazzarella, L., Crowther, R. A., Greer, J. & Kilmartin, J. V. (1969). *Nature*, **222**, 1240.

Ramot, B., Fisher, S., Remez, D., Schneerson, R., Kahane, D., Ager, J. A. M. & Lehmann, H. (1960). *Br. med. J.*, **ii**, 1262.

Ranney, H. M. (1972). *New Eng. J. Med.*, **287**, 98.

Raper, A. B. (1968). *Ann. Soc. Belge Med. Trop.*, **49**, 207.

Rigas, D. A. & Koler, R. D. (1961). *Blood*, **18**, 1.

Rimington, C. (1959). *Br. med. Bull.*, **15**, 19.

Ringelhann, B., Lewis, R. A., Lorkin, P. A., Kynoch, P. A. M. & Lehmann, H. (1967). *Acta haemat.*, **38**, 324.

Rosemeyer, M. A. & Huehns, E. R. (1967). *J. mol. Biol.*, **25**, 253.

Schroeder, W. A., Huisman, T. H. J., Shelton, J. R., Shelton, J. B., Kleihauer, E. F., Dozy, A. M. & Robberson, B. (1968). *Proc. nat. Acad. Sci.*, (*Wash*), **60**, 537.

Schroeder, W. A. & Jones, R. T. (1965). *Fortschr. Chem. org. NatStoffe.*, **23**, 113.

Seakins, M., Gibbs, W. M., Milner, P. F. & Bertles, J. F. (1972). *N. Engl. J. Med.*, in press.

Segel, G. B., Feig, S. A., Mentzer, W. C., McCaffrey, R. P., Wells, R., Bunn, H. F., Shohet, S. B. & Nathan, D. G. (1972). *New Eng. J. Med.*, **287**, 59.

Serjeant, G. R., Galloway, R. E. & Gueri, C. G. (1970). *Lancet*, **2**, 891.

Shibata, S., Iuchi, I., Miyaji, T., Ueda, S. & Takeda, I. (1963). *Acta haemat. jap.*, **26**, 164.

Shooter, E. M., Skinner, E. R., Garlick, J. P. & Barnicot, N. A. (1960). *Br. J. Haemat.*, **6**, 140.

Sirs, J. A. (1963). *Lancet*, **1**, 971.

STAMATOYANNOPOULOS, G., BELLINGHAM, A. J., LENFANT, C. & FINCH, C. A. (1971). *A. Rev. Med.*, **22**, 221.

TENTORI, L., SORCINI, M. & BUCELLA, C. (1971). In 'Proc. First Meeting Europ. Division, Int. Soc. Haemat.' Abstract Volume, p. 123.

TIYUMA, I. & SHIMIZU, K. (1970). *Fed. Proc.*, **29**, 1112.

WARLEY, M. A., HAMILTON, P. J. S., MARSDEN, P. D., BROWN, R. E., MERSELIS, J. G. & WILKS, N. (1965). *Br. med. J.*, **ii**, 86.

WASI, P. (1970). *J. med. Ass. Thailand*, **53**, 677.

WEATHERALL, D. J. & CLEGG, J. B. (1972). 'The Thalassaemia Syndromes' 2nd edition, Blackwell, Oxford.

YANASE, T., HANADA, M., SEITA, M., OHTA, Y., IMAMURA, T., FUJIMURA, T., KAWASAKI, K. & YAMAOKA, K. (1968). *Jap. J. Hum. Genet.*, **13**, 40.

References to Tables 5, 7, 8, 9, 10, 11, 12, 13

1. CHARACHE, S., WEATHERALL, D. J. & CLEGG, J. B. (1967). *J. clin. Invest.*, **45**, 813.
2. NAGEL, R. L., GIBSON, Q. H. & CHARACHE, S. (1967). *Biochemistry*, **6**, 2395.
3. BOTHA, M. C., BEALE, D., ISAACS, W. A. & LEHMANN, H. (1966). *Nature*, **212**, 792.
4. LINES, J. G. & MCINTOSH, R. (1967). *Nature*, **215**, 297.
5. JENKINS, T., STEVENS, K., GALLO, E. & LEHMANN, H. (1968). *S. Afr. med. J.*, **42**, 1151.
6. JONES, R. T., OSGOOD, E. E., BRIMHALL, B. & KOLER, R. D. (1967). *J. clin. Invest.*, **46**, 1840.
7. NOVY, M., EDWARDS, M. J. & METCALF, J. (1967). *J. clin. Invest.*, **46**, 1848.
8. REED, C. S., HAMPSON, R., GORDON, S., JONES, R. T., NOVY, M. J., BRIMHALL, B., EDWARDS, M. J. & KOLER, R. D. (1968). *Blood*, **31**, 623.
9. GLYNN, K. P., PENNER, J. A., SMITH, J. R. & RUCKNAGEL, D. L. (1968). *Ann. internal Med.*, **69**, 769.
10. RUCKNAGEL, D. L., cited by Stamatoyannopoulos *et al.*, 1971 (ref. 13).
11. YAMAOKA, K. (1971). *Blood*, **38**, 730.
12. LORKIN, P. A., LEHMANN, H., FAIRBANKS, V., BERGLUND, G. & LEONHARDT, T. (1970). *Biochem. J.*, **119**, 68P.
13. STAMATOYANNOPOULOS, G., YOSHIDA, A., ADAMSON, J. & HEINENBERG, S. (1968). *Science*, **159**, 741.
14. STAMATOYANNOPOULOS, G., BELLINGHAM, A. J., LENFANT, C. & FINCH, C. A. (1971). *A. Rev. Med.*, **22**, 221.
15. HAYASHI, A., STAMATOYANNOPOULOS, G., YOSHIDA, A. & ADAMSON, J. (1970). *Nature*, **230**, 264.
16. IMAI, K. (1968). *Archs biochem. Biophys.*, **127**, 543.
17. HAMILTON, H. B., IUCHI, I., MIYAJI, T. & SHIBATA, S. (1969). *J. clin. Invest.*, **48**, 525.
18. PERUTZ, M. F. (1969). *Nature*, **224**, 269.
19. REISSMANN, K. R., RUTH, W. E. & NAMURA, T. (1961). *J. clin. Invest.*, **40**, 1826.
20. BONAVENTURA, J. & RIGGS, A. (1968). *J. biol. Chem.*, **243**, 980.
21. IMAMURA, T., FUJITA, S., OHTA, Y., HANADA, M. & YANANSE, T. (1970). *J. clin. Invest.*, **48**, 2341.
22. IMAI, K., MARIMOTO, H., KOTANI, M., SHIBATA, S., MIYAJI, T. & MATSUMOTO, K. (1970). *Biochem. biophys. Acta*, **200**, 197.
23. GERALD, P. S. & EFRON, M. L. (1961). *Proc. Natn. Acad. Sci. U.S.A.*, **47**, 1758.
24. UDEM, L., RANNEY, H. M., BUNN, H. F. & PISCIOTTA, A. (1970). *J. biol. Chem.*, **48**, 489.

25. SUZUKI, T., HAYASHI, A., YAMAMURA, Y., ENOKI, Y. & TIYUMA, I. (1965). *Biochem. biophys. Res. Commun.*, **19**, 691.
26. MURAWSKI, E., CARTA, S., SORCINI, M., TENTORI, L., VIVALDI, G., ANTONINI, E., BRIMORI, M., WYMAN, J., BUCCI, E. & ROSSI-FANELLI, A. (1965). *Archs biochem. Biophys.*, **111**, 197.
27. SUZUKI, T., HAYASHI, A., SHIMIZU, A. & YAMAMURA, Y. (1966). *Biochem. biophys. Acta*, **127**, 280.
28. MIYAJI, T., IUCHI, I., SHIBATA, S., TAKEDA, I. & TAMURA, A. (1963). *Acta haemat. jap.*, **26**, 538.
29. JONES, R. T., COLEMAN, R. D. & HELLER, P. (1964). *Fed. Proc.*, **23**, 173.
30. HAYASHI, N., MOTOKAWA, Y., KIKUCHI, G. (1966). *J. Biol. Chem.*, **241**, 79.
31. GREER, J., cited in LEHMANN, H. & PERUTZ, M. F. (1968).
32. KIKUCHI, G., HAYASHI, N. & TAMURA, A. (1964). *Biochim. biophys. Acta*, **90**, 199.
33. HELLER, P., COLEMAN, R. D. & YAKULIS, V. J. (1966). *J. clin. Invest.*, **45**, 1021.
34. HAYASHI, A., SUZUKI, T., SHIMIZU, A., IMAI, K., MORIMOTO, H., MIYAJI, T. & SHIBATA, S. (1968). *Archs biochem. Biophys.*, **125**, 895.
35. INGRAM, V. M. (1958). *Biochim. biophys. Acta*, **28**, 539.
36. FRAIMOV, W., RODMAN, T., CLOSE, H. P., CATHCART, R. & PURCELL, M. K. (1958). *Am. J. med. Sci.*, **236**, 225.
37. MAY, A. & HUEHNS, E. R. (1971). International Symposium on Haemoglobin Structure and Function, Bad Nauheim. *Haematologie und Bluttransfusion*, **10**, 279.
38. HUNT, J. A. & INGRAM, V. M. (1960). *Biochim. biophys. Acta*, **42**, 409.
39. RANNEY, H. M., BENESCH, R. E., BENESCH, R. & JACOBS. A. S. (1963). *Biochim. biophys. Acta*, **74**, 544.
40. BAGLIONI, C. (1962). *Biochim. biophys. Acta*, **52**, 437.
41. HUISMAN, T. H. J., STILL, J. & NECHTMAN, C. M. (1963). *Biochim. biophys. Acta*, **74**, 69.
42. ROSA, J., OUDART, J. L., PAGNIER, J., BELKHODJA, O., BOIGNÉ, J. M. & LABIE, D. (1968). Proc. XIIIth Congr. Internat. Soc. Haemat., p. 72.
43. OSTERTAG, W., VON EHRENSTEIN, G. & CHARACHE, S. (1972). *Nature, New Biology*, **237**, 90.
44. CHARACHE, S., OSTERTAG, W. & VON EHRENSTEIN, G. (1972). *Nature, New Biology*, **237**, 88.
45. CROOKSTON, J. H., FARQUHARSON, H. A., BEALE, D. & LEHMANN, H. (1969). *Canad. J. Biochem.*, **47**, 143.
46. HALBRECHT, I., ISAACS, W. A., LEHMANN, H. & BEN-PORAT, F. (1967). *Israel J. med. Sci.*, **3**, 827.
47. SCHNEIDER, R. G., UEDA, S., ALPERIN, J. B., BRIMHALL, B. & JONES, R. T. (1968) *Am. J. Hum. Genet.*, **20**, 151.
48 CHARACHE, S., MONDZAC, A. M., GESSNER, U. & GAYLE, E. E. (1969). *J. clin. Invest.*, **48**, 834.
49. NAGEL, R. L., RANNEY, H. M., BRADLEY, T. B., JACOBS, A. & UDEM, L. (1969). *Blood*, **34**, 157.
50. HUEHNS, E. R., HECHT, F., YOSHIDA, A., STAMATOYANNOPOULOS, G., HARTMAN, J. & MOTULSKY, A. G. (1970). *Blood*, **36**, 209.
51. STAMATOYANNOPOULOS, G., PARER, J. T. & FINCH, C. A. (1969). *New Engl. Engl. J. Med.*, **281**, 915.
52. SANSONE, G. & PIK, C. (1965). *Br. J. Haemat.*, **11**, 511.
53. SANSONE, G., CARRELL, R. W. & LEHMANN, H. (1967). *Nature*, **214**, 877.
54. YATES, A., JACKSON, J. M. & HUEHNS, E. R. unpublished.

55. RUCKNAGEL, D. L., SPENCER, H. H. & BRANDT, N. S. (1968). Proc. XIth Congr. Internat. Soc. Haematology, p. 56 and personal communication.
56. MONN, E., GAFFNEY, P. J. & LEHMANN, H. (1968). *Scand. J. Haemat.*, **5**, 353.
57. PIETSCHMANN, H., LORKIN, P. A., LEHMANN, H. & BRAUNSTEINER, H. cited in PERUTZ & LEHMANN. (1968).
58. PRATO, V. & GALLO, E. (1968). *G. Aciad. Med. Torino*, **131**, 1.
59. BERETTA, A., PRATO, V., GALLO, E. & LEHMANN, H. (1968). *Nature*, **217**, 1016.
60. BELLINGHAM, A. J. & HUEHNS, E. R. (1971). In preparation.
61. KLEIHAUER, E. F., REYNOLDS, C. A., DOZY, A. M., WILSON, J. B., MOORES, R. R., BERENSON, M. P., WRIGHT, C. S. & HUISMAN, T. H. J. (1968). *Biochim. biophys. Acta*, **154**, 220.
62. DACIE, J. V., SHINTON, N. K., GAFFNEY, P. J., CARRELL, R. W. & LEHMANN, H. (1967). *Nature*, **216**, 663.
63. MÜLLER, C. J. & KINGMA, S. (1961). *Biochim. biophys. Acta*, **50**, 595.
64. FRICK, P. G., HITZIG, W. H. & BETKE, K. (1962). *Blood*, **20**, 261.
65. BACHMANN, F. & MARTI, H. R. (1962). *Blood*, **20**, 272.
66. MOORE, W. M. O., BATTAGLIA, F. C. & HELLEGERS, A. F. (1967). *Am. J. Obstet. Gynec.*, **97**, 63.
67. WINTERHALTER, K. H., ANDERSON, N. M., AMICONI, G., ANTONINI, E. & BRUNORI, M. (1969). *Europ. J. Biochem.*, **11**, 435.
68. ROSA, J., LABIE, D., WAJCMAN, H., BOIGNÉ, J. M., CABANNES, R., BIERME, R. & RUFFIE, J. (1969). *Nature*, **223**, 190.
69. CARRELL, R. W., LEHMANN, H., LORKIN, P. A., RAIK, E. & HUNTER, E. (1967). *Nature*, **215**, 626.
70. STEADMAN, J. H., YATES, A. & HUEHNS, E. R. (1970). *Br. J. Haemat.*, **18**, 435.
71. WHITE, J. M., BRAIN, M. C., LORKIN, P. H., LEHMANN, H. & SMITH, M. (1970). *Nature*, **225**, 941.
72. MAY, A. & HUEHNS, E. R. (1972). *Br. J. Haemat.*, **22**, 599.
73. OPFELL, R. W., LORKIN, P. A. & LEHMANN, H. (1968). *J. med. Genet.*, **5**, 292.
74. HALLENDER, A., LORKIN, P. A., LEHMANN, H. & SVENSON, B. (1969). *Nature*, **222**, 953.
75. SVENSON, B. & STRAND, L. (1967). *Scand. J. Haematol.*, **4**, 241.
76. MORIMOTO, H., LEHMANN, H. & PERUTZ, M. F. (1971). *Nature*, **232**, 408.
    KEELING, M. M., OGDEN, L. L., WRIGHTSTONE, R. N., WILSON, J. B., REYNOLDS, C. A., KITCHENS, J. L. & HUISMAN, T. H. J. (1971). *J. clin. Invest.*, **50**, 2395.
77. SCHNEIDER, R. G., UEDA, S., ALPERIN, J. B., BRIMHALL, B. & JONES, R. T. (1969). *New Engl. J. Med.*, **280**, 739.
78. HUTCHISON, H. E., PINKERTON, P. H., WATERS, P., DOUGLAS, A. S., LEHMANN, H. & BEALE, D. (1964). *Br. med. J.*, **ii**, 1099.
79. CARRELL, R. W., LEHMANN, H. & HUTCHISON, H. E. (1966). *Nature*, **210**, 915.
80. BELLINGHAM, A. J. & HUEHNS, E. R. (1968). *Nature*, **218**, 924.
81. SWENSON, R. T., HILL, R. L., LEHMANN, H. & JIM, R. T. S. (1962). *J. biol. Chem.*, **237**, 1517.
82. WADE, P., YATES, A., BELLINGHAM, A. J. & HUEHNS, E. R. (1972). In preparation.
83. RANNEY, H. M., JACOBS, A. S. & NAGEL, R. L. (1967). *Nature*, **213**, 876.
84. JONES, R. T., BRIMHALL, B. & LISKER, R. (1968). *Biochim. biophys. Acta*, **154**, 488.
85. RIEDER, R. F., OSKI, F. A. & CLEGG, J. B. (1969). *J. clin. Invest.*, **48**, 1627.
86. BAUER, E. W. & MOTULSKY, A. G. (1965). *Human Genetik*, **1**, 621.
87. KOLAFAT, T. (1964). *Siriraj Hosp. Gaz.*, **16**, 205.
88. HUNT, J. A. & INGRAM, V. M. (1961). *Biochim. biophys. Acta*, **49**, 520.
89. THOMPSON, R. B., WARRINGTON, R. L. & BELL, W. N. (1965). *Am. J. Physiol.*, **268**, 198.

90. EFREMOV, G. D., HUISMAN, T. H. J., SMITH, L. L., WILSON, J. B., KITCHENS, J. L., WRIGHTSTONE, R. N. & ADAMS, H. R. (1969). *J. biol. Chem.*, **244,** 6105.
91. JONG, W. W. W. DE., WENT, L. N. & BERNINI, L. F. (1968). *Nature*, **220,** 788.
92. JONES, R. T., BRIMHALL, B., HUISMAN, T. H. J., KLEIHAUER, E. & BETKE, K. (1966). *Science*, **154,** 1024.
93. BRADLEY, T. B., WOHL, R. C. & RIEDER, R. F. (1965). *Blood,* **28,** 975.
94. RANNEY, H. M., JACOBS, A. S., ODEM, L. & ZALUSKY, R. (1968). *Biochem. biophys. Res. Commun.*, **33,** 1004.
95. HUISMAN, T. H. J., BROWN, A. K., EFREMOV, G. D., WILSON, J. B., REYNOLDS, C. A., UY, R. & SMITH, L. L. (1971). *J. clin. Invest.*, **50,** 650.
96. BRIMHALL, B., HOLLAN, S., JONES, R. T., KOLER, R. D., STOCKLEN, Z. & SZELENYI, J. G. (1970). *Clin. Res.*, **18,** 184.
97. CARRELL, R. W. & OWEN, M. C. (1971). *Biochim. Biophys. Acta*, **236,** 507.
98. CLEGG, J. B., WEATHERALL, D. J. & WONG HOCK BOON. (1969). *Nature*, **222,** 379.
99. SCHNEIDER, R. G., ALPERIN, J. B., BRIMHALL, B. & JONES, R. T. (1969). *J. Lab. clin. Med.*, **73,** 616.
100. BONAVENTURA, J. & RIGGS, A. (1967). *Science*, **158,** 800.
101. SHIBATA, S., MIYAJI, T., UEDA, S., MATSVOKA, M., IUCHI, I., YAMADA, K. & SHINKAI, N. (1970). *Proc. Jap. Acad.*, **46,** 440.
102. WILTSHIRE, B., PRAXEDES, H. & LEHMANN, K. (1972). *Proc. XIV Int. Cong. Haemat.*
103. STAMATOYANNOPOULOS, G. Personal Communication.

CHAPTER 13

IMMUNOLOGICAL MECHANISMS AND HUMAN DISEASE

W. G. Reeves

Immunology as a discipline has relevance for practically every subdivision of clinical medicine and pathology. The revival of interest in this subject coincided with the advent of tissue transplantation in the late '50s, although gradual progress was also being made in the fields of allergic and auto-immune disease. In addition to classical auto-immune disorders such as Hashimoto's disease and systemic lupus erythematosus, it is now realised that immunological factors may play an important role in many other conditions ranging from farmer's lung to infertility. It now seems that several auto-immune diseases will turn out to be a sequel to some kind of infection although a genetic predisposition may be necessary for their full expression. If syphilis had not been found to be due to treponemal infection early on, it might well have been categorised as an auto-immune disease in view of the abundance of auto-antibodies which may be associated with it. Although the concept of focal sepsis in relation to rheumatoid arthritis finds little support today it makes an intriguing comparison with some of the current work implicating infective causes for this disease. Transplantation and the therapeutic problems it poses have stimulated interest in possible means of abrogating the immune response. This has also led to the closer study of immunological deficiency states both congenital and acquired. Apart from the rare severe deficiencies, minor or localised defects of immunological function may be relatively common and related to the subsequent development of various disorders.

This chapter is not intended to be a comprehensive account of the inter-relationship between immunological factors and disease but an attempt has been made to describe current trends in immunology in relation to a number of topics of major importance. Reference will be made to more specialised sources of information listed at the end of the chapter.

FUNDAMENTAL ASPECTS

Fundamentally, immunology relates to the sequence of events following recognition of a particular unit or moiety as antigenic up to the final expression of an immune (or allergic) response specifically against it via the various mediator cells and substances. This 'immune arc' is diagrammatically represented in Fig. 13.1, with the proviso that 'immune' should not always imply that the response is a beneficial one.

Antigen recognition

Since the work of Landsteiner (1936) it has been realised that units considerably smaller than whole micro-organisms can be recognised as

'foreign' or antigenic. Generally speaking molecules start to become antigenic above a molecular weight of about 5000 although other factors can
modify this threshold. Molecules of a smaller size, e.g. many drugs, require
conjugation to a carrier molecule before they can trigger off an immune
response and are known as haptens. The means whereby an organism is able
to distinguish the most subtle differences between molecules (and can even
recognise a D- from an L-isomer) has to be one of the axioms of any theory of
immunity. The differentiation between 'self' and 'non-self' is of prime
importance and has been extensively discussed by Burnet (1962). Clonal
selection forms the basis of most currently held theories (Burnet, 1969) and a
particularly elegant modification has been proposed by Jerne (1971). The
facility with which antigen is recognised depends very much on its site,
concentration, physical state and persistence within the body. If the dose is
too small or too large immunisation may not occur and a state of tolerance or
paralysis develops (Mitchison, 1968). Further manipulation is usually required to maintain this state indefinitely in the adult animal and once
immunisation has occurred it may be impossible to produce a tolerant state.
Macrophages seem to have a key role in processing antigen and enhancing
the recognition process (Miller, 1968) and many agents used experimentally
to heighten an immune response, e.g. Freund's adjuvant, may act by promot-
ing their activity. During or after processing, antigen becomes localised in
lymphoid organs such as lymph nodes and spleen where it comes into contact
with immunologically competent cells.

Lymphocyte activation

These lymphocytes are of two distinctive kinds although originally they
are all derived from marrow precursors. One variety which has gained its
competence following passage through the thymus, forms the large majority
of circulating lymphocytes in both blood and lymph, and is necessary for the
production of sensitised lymphocytes (Gowans & McGregor, 1965). The
other variety tends to be sessile and reside in the lymphoid follicles of both
lymph nodes and spleen. In the chicken there is good evidence that they
acquire competence in lymphoid tissue associated with the hind-gut and
known as the bursa of Fabricius. The suggestion that the gut-associated
lymphoid tissue plays an identical role in man is still unproven. When
triggered these cells give rise to plasma cells producing specific antibody
(Cooper, et al., 1966). The former kind are known as thymus derived or T
cells, the latter as 'bursa-equivalent' derived or B cells. The thymus and
bursa-equivalent are termed primary lymphoid organs, the lymph nodes and
spleen being categorised as secondary lymphoid organs.

In the secondary lymphoid organs there is considerable opportunity for
intense localisation of antigen and considerable contact with both T and B
cells. Quite what decides which kind of cell will become activated is still not
clear, but there is accumulating evidence that very few immune responses
operate entirely independently of the T cell population even when antibody
is the chief product (Roitt et al., 1969). Co-operation between these two kinds
of lymphocyte may be a basic manoeuvre in the elaboration of an immune
response (Playfair, 1971).

Although both kinds of immunologically competent lymphocyte are morphologically indistinguishable it has recently been possible (in mice) to identify them independently by the use of specific antisera prepared against thymocytes (Raff, 1970). That this is possible is due to the presence of an isoantigen, denoted θ, which is present on thymocytes and to a lesser degree on T cells but which is not represented on B cells. An antiserum has also been developed which will specifically react with B cells (Raff, Nase & Mitchison, 1971) and it is likely that similar reagents for use in human studies will soon become available.

Other studies have shown that a proportion of circulating lymphocytes carry on their surface determinants having some of the characteristics of antibody molecules (Greaves, Torrigiani & Roitt, 1969; Coombs, Feinstein & Wilson, 1969). Macrophages and activated (or 'transforming') lymphocytes also have specific receptors for taking up a special kind of humoral antibody known as cytophilic antibody (Kay, Gurner & Coombs, 1970). From this,

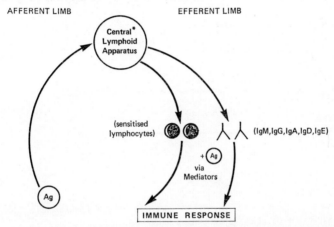

FIG. 13.1. THE IMMUNE ARC. (*The central lymphoid apparatus refers to secondary lymphoid organs e.g. lymph nodes and spleen. Ag = antigen).

and other work describing the production by activated lymphocytes of antigen-specific factors which seem to differ somewhat from conventional antibody molecules and which have an affinity for macrophages (Lachmann, 1971; Feldmann & Basten, 1972) it is obvious that there is considerable potential for intercellular contact and co-operation in the presence of antigen. The complex and previously ill-understood micro-structure of the secondary lymphoid organs thus provides a suitable framework for many of the central events of the immune response.

However obscure these events may be, the initiation of the efferent response coincides with transformation of either or both kinds of immunologically competent cell. They adopt blast cell forms and undergo increased metabolic activity (Ling, 1968). They then proceed to cell division yielding offspring which are either plasma cells manufacturing specific antibody or sensitised lymphocytes capable of reacting in a specific way with the relevant antigen via receptors on their surface but in the absence of free antibody. If the cells appearing in the efferent lymphatics of a regional lymph node undergoing antigenic stimulation are studied it is found that these blast cells have a peak incidence at about four days (Hall & Morris, 1965). One of the attributes of an immunological response is that if the organism should be challenged with the same antigen on a subsequent occasion it will show a brisker and exaggerated response whether it is predominantly mediated by antibody or cells. There is considerable evidence for the existence of 'memory' cells although whether these are identical with the effector cells of the primary response or represent a special category of cell is uncertain (Miller, 1968).

Antibody production

Antibody is synthesised in the highly specialised endoplasmic reticulum of the plasma cell and each cell subserves only a single antigen-combining specificity (Nossal & Makela, 1962) although it seems that plasma cells in culture are able to switch from IgM to IgG production albeit with the same specificity (Nossal *et al.*, 1964). The location of the antibody-producing

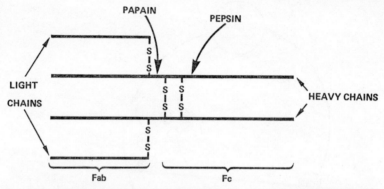

FIG. 13.2. DIAGRAMMATIC STRUCTURE OF AN IMMUNOGLOBULIN MOLECULE (IgG) (after Cohen & Porter).

The sites of cleavage following the action of pepsin or papain and the fragments so produced are indicated.

cells is chiefly determined by the route of administration of the antigen. Following intravenous antigen, antibody is chiefly produced in the spleen, lung and bone-marrow whereas after local instillation antibody is mainly derived from the regional lymph nodes. Occasionally, and particularly when adjuvants are used, local granuloma formation may develop and a significant amount of antibody is then generated by the plasma cells contained within it.

Antibodies or immunoglobulins are now separated into five classes and their contrasting properties are enumerated in Table 13.1. They all have the same basic structure (Fig. 13.2) consisting of four polypeptide chains (two light and two heavy) linked by disulphide bridges (Cohen & Porter, 1964). The classes are distinguished on the basis of major differences in the chemical structure of the heavy chains and they can be readily typed by the use of monospecific antisera.

The structure and function of antibody molecules has been studied by preparing various fragments obtained after treatment with proteolytic enzymes (Cohen & Milstein, 1967) (see Fig. 13.2). The antigen-combining site is located in the Fab fragment (so called because this fragment retains antibody activity) and involves portions of both light and heavy chains. On the other hand the biological activity of these molecules e.g. complement fixation, macrophage attachment, placental transfer, tissue sensitisation etc, is a function of the Fc portion (so called because of its ability to crystallise). It can be seen from the table that not all the classes of heavy chain (i.e. γ, α, μ, δ and ε) or all the sub-classes within a particular class (e.g. γ_1, γ_2, γ_3 and γ_4) have identical properties. Thus there is variation in the structure of the Fc fragment in addition to the very considerable variation in the chemical composition of the Fab fragment which confers specificity for a particular antigen.

TABLE 13.1

PROPERTIES OF THE DIFFERENT CLASSES OF IMMUNOGLOBULIN

(In part from Cohen, 1971)

	IgG	IgA	IgM	IgD	IgE
Heavy chain types	$\gamma_1, \gamma_2, \gamma_3, \gamma_4$	α_1, α_2	μ	δ	ε
Light chain types	κ, λ	κ, λ	κ, λ	κ, λ	κ, λ
Molecular weight	150 000	160 000 (serum) 370 000 (secretory)	900 000	170 000	200 000
Serum level* (mg/100ml)	800–1500	150–400	50–150	c.3	c.0·02
Antibody activity	+	+	+	+	+
Seromucous secretion	−	+ (α_1, α_2)	−	−	
Complement fixation†	+ ($\gamma_1, \gamma_2\ \gamma_3$)	−	+	−	
Macrophage attachment	+ (γ_1, γ_3)	−	−		
Placental transfer	+ ($\gamma_1, \gamma_2, \gamma_3, \gamma_4$)	−	−	−	−
Homologous tissue sensitisation	−§	−	−		+

* The ranges given are for 2 S.D. International standard reference sera have recently been developed with the hope that their wide application will considerably reduce the variation in normal values which exists at present between individual centres (Rowe *et al.*, 1970a, 1970b & 1970c).

† Recent work suggests that some classes of antibody (e.g. γ_1, γ_2, γ_3, α_1 and α_2) may be able to fix complement by an alternative pathway commencing at the C3 stage (Gotze & Müller-Eberhard, 1971).

§ But see page 419.

Immunoglobulin M (IgM) is the characteristic antibody of the primary response and is a much larger molecule than the other classes of antibody, consisting of a polymer of five sub-units each corresponding to the size of an IgG molecule. Within a short time the amount of IgM falls in favour of increasing levels of IgG which predominate in the secondary response to antigen. IgA is chiefly manufactured in plasma cells associated with the gastro-intestinal tract and is secreted in large quantities into its lumen. It is of interest that the increased protection seen with oral live vaccine against poliomyelitis is associated with the development of specific IgA in the gut (Ogra *et al.*, 1968). IgA is also found in saliva, tears, and colostrum, and in the bronchial and urinary tracts. IgD and IgE were both discovered following the characterisation of atypical myeloma proteins (Rowe & Fahey, 1965; Johansson & Bennich, 1967). It was some time before definitive antibody activity could be attributed to IgD but there is now accumulating evidence of its importance (Kantor, Van Herle & Barnett, 1970). IgE is now considered to be identical with reaginic antibody having a considerable facility to sensitise mast cells and basophils (Ishizaka & Ishizaka, 1968). It is of cardinal importance in the production of immediate hypersensitivity reactions. Its value to the organism is still obscure although its presence in the skin and urinary tract would suggest some kind of protective function.

Before any *in vivo* manifestation resulting from the production of antibody (or sensitised lymphocytes) can appear, a second contact with antigen is required. Depending on the class of antibody and its biological function a sequence of events may follow resulting in the release and activation of a number of non-specific factors or mediators which are the final executors of the immune response. The number of substances implicated at this final stage of the immune response is now very large and each pathway may have its own sequence of inter-relating substances (Spector & Willoughby, 1968; Becker, 1969; Lachmann, 1969). Examples include histamine, slow-reacting substance, serotonin, bradykinin and the complement sequence. These in turn may give rise to the involvement of other cells (e.g. polymorphonuclear leucocytes) and factors (e.g. lysosomal enzymes) in the final augmentation of the effect of antigen-antibody combination.

Production of sensitised cells

Sensitised lymphocytes achieve many of their effects independently of the above mechanisms. Contact with antigen is followed by activation of the cell and conversion to a blast form. At about this time a number of soluble factors are released from the cell which have a variety of effects. These are collectively called lymphokines (Dumonde *et al.*, 1969). Recent work suggests that prostaglandins may also be involved (Greaves, Søndergaard & McDonald-Gibson, 1971). (These are a recently delineated group of long-chain fatty acids which occur widely in mammalian tissues and have powerful effects on most organs and tissues in the body (Ramwell & Shaw, 1971).) Two of the most fully studied lymphokines are mitogenic factor and macrophage migration inhibition factor. The former causes non-sensitised lymphocytes to divide and the latter reduces the mobility of macrophages. The blast cells themselves divide to form other sensitised and memory cells. Any of these cells may be directly cytotoxic to target cells (i.e. cells with antigen on their surface). The exact mechanism for this effect is not known although there is evidence that one of the terminal components of the complement sequence may be involved (Perlmann *et al.*, 1969). The relationship of these various factors to the lesions associated with predominantly cell-mediated responses i.e. delayed hypersensitivity, is not yet fully understood although the problem is being actively pursued at the present time (Dumonde & Maini, 1971).

Types of Immune Response

The varieties of immunological response occurring *in vivo* have been classified into four main types (Gell & Coombs, 1968); the first three are mediated by specific antibody, and the last by sensitised lymphocytes alone.

Type I or anaphylactic reactions

Anaphylactic reactions are mediated by reaginic antibody (of class IgE) which passively sensitises tissue cells causing the release of vasoactive substances on contact with antigen. Although IgE is classical reaginic antibody it is still possible that in some circumstances, other classes of antibody (e.g. IgG) may also fulfil similar requirements (Terr & Benz, 1965; Parish, 1970; Stanworth & Smith, 1972).

Type II or cytotoxic reactions

Cytotoxic reactions are mediated by antibody, usually of class IgG or IgM which combines with an antigenic determinant on a cell membrane. Often this event is immediately followed by complement fixation and irreversible damage to the cell. However there are special instances in which damage to the cell membrane may not occur (Fell, Coombs & Dingle, 1966) and the result of antibody combining with a cell membrane can even give rise to stimulation as in the case of the long-acting thyroid stimulator (LATS) (Doniach & Roitt, 1968). Anti-lymphocyte antibody and anti-immunoglobulin sera can also have stimulatory effects on lymphocytes although this does not necessarily represent a 'natural' phenomenon.

Type III or immune complex reactions

Immune complex reactions are mediated by certain combinations of free antigen and antibody. If the size of the complex, its ratio of antigen and antibody, the class of antibody involved and its combining affinity are optimal then such complexes become toxic, producing complement fixation and damage to surrounding structures, usually the small blood vessels in which they lodge (Weigle, 1961). The complement sequence involves at least 13 proteins many of which play an active part in the production of chemotaxis, phagocytosis, inflammation and cell lysis (Lachmann, 1969). Classical serum sickness and the more artificial Arthus reaction are examples of type III reactions.

Type IV or cell-mediated reactions

Cell-Mediated reactions are mediated by sensitised lymphocytes independently of humoral antibody and by the mechanisms outlined above produce the traditional lesions of delayed hypersensitivity e.g. tuberculin sensitivity and homograft rejection.

Inter-relationships

The relationship between cell-mediated and antibody-mediated responses in terms of their relative or mutual usefulness to the organism is poorly understood. It is not uncommon for the two to co-exist during an immune response, having either synergistic or antagonistic effects. Although the concentration of antibody in the circulation may be high it is considerably lower in the extravascular compartment and even at the peak of immunisation it may be insufficient to mount a response outside the blood stream. On the other hand lymphocytes are able to migrate fairly freely and it is possible that one of their chief functions may be to extend the effector arm of the immune response into the tissues (Hall, 1969). In this context it is of interest that homograft rejection is predominantly mediated by lymphocytes although antibody can play a significant part in some situations. However the fact that thymus-derived cells are of such importance in the inductive phase of many antibody responses and that in evolutionary history as well as foetal development effective immune responses and the thymus tend to appear at about the same time suggests more than a booster role for cell-mediated responses (Good & Papermaster, 1964). Indeed Burnet has considered that these cells may have the important function of 'immunological surveillance'; recognising and eliminating host cells which have undergone antigenic alterations due to somatic mutation, physical or chemical damage or virus infection (Burnet, 1969). The correlation between the progressive increase in auto-immune and malignant disease with age gives circumstantial support to the importance of such an 'early warning system' for the detection of 'foreign' (i.e. non-self) antigens. The increased incidence of malignancy following the administration of anti-lymphocyte serum, which acts particularly on thymus-derived cells, is also in keeping with this hypothesis (Allison, 1970).

The relationship between the host and antigenic material appearing within it is obviously complex and involves a number of non-specific as well as specific factors. Their respective contribution to the subsequent immune response has been discussed by Coombs & Smith (1968). Reference for further information on general aspects of immunology is provided in the general reading list at the end of this chapter. It is proposed for the rest of this chapter to consider those areas of clinical medicine in which there has been recent immunological interest and to pin-point the role of immunological mechanisms in the aetiology and pathogenesis of some of these conditions, concluding with a discussion of the therapeutic possibilities which arise.

IMMUNOLOGICAL DEFICIENCY STATES

The varying degrees to which different individuals may be affected by infective disease has often been the source of discussion regarding implied defects of host resistance. A large number of syndromes have now been described but not all involve a defect in immunologically competent cells. Defects in skin and mucous membranes (as in eczema and cystic fibrosis) encourage infection. Quantitative or qualitative disorders of leucocyte function, e.g. neutropenia; chronic granulomatous disease; the Chediak-Higashi syndrome, and myeloperoxidase deficiency may considerably disturb the host's defences (B.M.J., 1969). The abnormal metabolic milieu seen in malnutrition and uncontrolled diabetes also contribute to an increased incidence of infection. Most of the inherited defects in complement so far described do not seem to be associated with infective episodes (Austen, Klemperer & Rosen, 1968) although a familial dysfunction of C5 has been found to give an increased susceptibility to infection with Gram-negative bacteria (Miller & Nilsson, 1970) and a deficiency in K.A.F. (conglutinogen activating factor) has been described in connection with recurrent infection (Abramson et al., 1971). Interferon is known to have effects on a broad spectrum of micro-organisms and it is possible that deficiencies in its production give rise to clinical problems.

Primary Disorders

Setting innate factors aside one is left with those defects involving the immune system itself. The more severe and incapacitating disorders usually manifest themselves in early life and form the majority of those listed in Table 13.2. In essence these disorders fall into three categories: (a) those predominantly affecting antibody production, (b) those predominantly affecting cell-mediated immunity, and (c) those in which both aspects of the immune response are involved. The existence of unilateral defects confirms the validity of compartmenting the immune response into activities subserved by T cells and B cells respectively, as discussed in the previous section.

TABLE 13.2

A CLASSIFICATION OF PRIMARY IMMUNODEFICIENCY
(from W.H.O. Memorandum, 1971)

Type	Suggested cellular defect		
	B cells	T cells	Stem cells
Infantile X-linked agammaglobulinaemia (Bruton type)	+		
Selective immunoglobulin deficiency (IgA)	+*		
Transient hypogammaglobulinaemia of infancy	+		
X-linked immunodeficiency with hyper-IgM	+*		
Thymic hypoplasia (DiGeorge Syndrome)		+	
Episodic lymphopaenia with lymphocytotoxin		+	
Immunodeficiency with normal or hyperimmunoglobulinaemia	+	+†	
Immunodeficiency with ataxia telangiectasia	+	+	
Immunodeficiency with thrombocytopaenia and eczema (Wiskott–Aldrich syndrome)	+	+	
Immunodeficiency with thymoma	+	+	
Immunodeficiency with short-limbed dwarfism	+	+	
Immunodeficiency with generalised haematopoietic hypoplasia	+	+	+
Severe combined immunodeficiency			
(a) autosomal recessive	+	+	+
(b) X-linked	+	+	+
(c) sporadic	+	+	+
Variable immunodeficiency (largely unclassified)	+	+†	

* Involve some but not all B cells.
† Encountered in some but not all patients.

Antibody deficiency

The pattern of infection is often characteristic for the particular immunological deficiency. Patients with a pure but generalised antibody deficiency, e.g. primary sex-linked hypogammaglobulinaemia (Bruton) or the non sex-linked varieties, are especially prone to pyogenic infections e.g. with staphylococci, streptococci, pneumococci and Haemophilus influenzae, although they do not have such an increased susceptibility to infections with viruses and fungi. Selective deficiencies of individual classes of antibodies may also have their own clinical pattern e.g. IgM deficiency predisposes to meningococcal septicaemia (Hobbs, Milner & Watt, 1967) and generalised non-progressive vaccinia (Chandra, Kaveramma & Soothill, 1969). IgM levels are often low in the Wiskott–Aldrich syndrome and this is partly due to a deficiency in IgM antibodies formed against polysaccharide antigens e.g. isoagglutinins; for these patients are able to produce IgM antibody normally against protein antigens (Cooper et al., 1968). This would therefore seem to be an example of a selective deficiency occurring within an individual class of antibody. IgA deficiency is associated with chronic infections of the respiratory tract and disorders of the gastro-intestinal tract (Heremans & Crabbe, 1968). Patients with ataxia telangiectasia are usually deficient in IgA as well as cellular immunity and often have chronic respiratory tract infections but as recent work suggests that they are also deficient in IgE (Biggar et al., 1970) it is not clear which class of antibody is most important in protecting the respiratory tract from infection. The individual role of IgD is still uncertain and no selective deficiency has yet been described.

Cellular deficiency

Patients with predominant T cell defects commonly suffer from viral and fungal infections. Thymic aplasia (the DiGeorge syndrome) is a congenital disorder characterised by failure of development of the third and fourth branchial arches with absence of both thymus and parathyroid glands. The children may present initially with tetany and often have aortic arch abnormalities. Another relatively pure T cell deficiency state is Nezelof's syndrome in which the thymus is hypoplastic but the parathyroids are intact.

Those patients with combined immunodeficiency syndromes e.g. Swiss type agammaglobulinaemia; thymoma with agammaglobulinaemia, and generalised haematopoietic hypoplasia are susceptible to almost every kind of infection and often die in early childhood.

Most of the conditions already discussed are extremely uncommon but it is likely that milder forms of immunodeficiency are more prevalent. Minor forms of primary antibody deficiency have been collectively termed 'dys-gammaglobulinaemia' (Hobbs, 1970) and classified into seven types although several have overlapping characteristics. Localised defects in cellular immunity have been described in chronic mucocutaneous candidiasis (Chilgren et al., 1969; Valdimarsson et al., 1970), and similar findings have recently been found in recurrent herpes (Wilton, Ivanyi & Lehner, 1972). Whether these disturbances antedate the disease has still to be determined. Recenily a condition characterised by recurrent infections has been described in which the patient's monocytes were unresponsive to macrophage migration inhibition factor (see page 418) (Louie & Goldberg, 1972). It seems likely that a number of other abnormal links in the chain will be described in the near future.

Secondary Disorders

There are a large number of disease processes known to impair immune function secondarily (Hobbs, 1968; B.M.J., 1970). Myelomatosis is frequently associated with a polyclonal deficiency of antibody production (Cynarswki & Cohen, 1971), and sarcoidosis, Crohn's disease and lepromatous leprosy are examples of diseases which are associated with impaired cell-mediated immunity (Buckley, Nagaya & Sieker, 1966; Turk & Waters, 1969). Piecemeal removal of various parts of the lymphoid system, e.g. tonsillectomy (Dayton *et al.*, 1971), appendicectomy, block dissection of lymph nodes and splenectomy may be related to subsequent susceptibility to infection. Splenectomy seems to be the most hazardous in this respect and may be followed by septicaemia (Lowdon, Stewart & Walker, 1966, Karatzas, 1966) although the incidence of this complication is not exactly known. However the increased incidence of streptococcal infection and its sequelae in patients with thalassaemia who have had their spleens removed suggests that this may merit further study (Wasi, 1971).

Drug-induced immunodeficiency

Perhaps the commonest type of immunodeficiency seen today is that associated with therapeutic immunosuppression. The use of cytotoxic agents, corticosteroids and anti-lymphocyte serum has become widespread and when used in the dosage required for the control of homograft rejection such measures have often brought a heavy toll of secondary infection. In some series the mortality due to infections has exceeded that due to the primary disease (Crosnier *et al.*, 1970). As has already been seen in connection with those patients suffering from pure T cell deficiencies, a considerable degree of non-specific suppression of cell-mediated immunity (especially relevant to homograft rejection) encourages infection with fungi and viruses in particular, although bacterial infection can also be a problem. Chronic or fulminating infections with aspergillus, candida, pneumocystis, nocardia, herpes, varicella, measles, cytomegalovirus, and other organisms have been described. Immunological studies have confirmed the importance of cell-mediated defences in the development of candida infection in these circumstances (Folb & Trounce, 1970).

Management

Suspicion regarding immunodeficiency is usually aroused by the clinica history. Identification of the type and severity of the defect will require the application of various techniques and a useful approach has been summarised by Soothill (1972).

The measures that are available for the treatment of immunodeficiency states are relatively crude and often ineffective. Prophylactic γ-globulin has been used to reduce the incidence of infections in primary hypogammaglobulinaemia and after studying 176 patients with this condition a Medical Research Council working party recommended a dose of 25 mg per kg per week although this can be exceeded in patients who continue to suffer from severe infections (M.R.C. Working Party on hypogammaglobulinaemia, 1971). The prompt and selective administration of antibiotics (and anti-fungal and anti-viral agents where available) for infective episodes is important but for patients with T cell deficiencies there is little else to offer. In the severe congenital disorders of this kind (e.g. Swiss type of agammaglobulinaemia and the DiGeorge syndrome) attempts have been made at reconstitution with thymus or marrow grafts (de Koning *et al.*, 1969; August *et al.*, 1970). Immunological competence has been established on several occasions following this procedure and may be dramatically effective although the chief hazard is that of a graft-versus-host reaction. This is characterised by a morbilliform rash, fever, diarrhoea, wasting, pancytopænia, splenomegaly and hepatomegaly. It may be transient or may progress to a fatal outcome. Patients with deficient cell-mediated immunity can develop it following conventional blood transfusion. Its severity can be reduced by pretreatment of the donor or donor's cells with immunosuppressive agents and the selection of suitable material by tissue typing.

It is likely that an increasing number of immunodeficiency states will be described during the next few years and although each one may throw new light on a particular aspect of immunological function it is hoped that therapeutic advances will be made *pari passu* to cope with the serious clinical problems that these conditions often present.

INFECTIOUS DISEASES AND AUTOIMMUNITY

At a time when the immunological response to infection was generally considered to be chiefly of protective value to the host Rich postulated that much of the pathology of tuberculous infection was a direct result of immunological factors (Rich & Lewis, 1932; Rich, 1951). His view has largely been borne out with time and it has been shown that caseation and cavity formation will not occur in the absence of tuberculin hypersensitivity (Bloch, 1968). In many instances in the past where toxins liberated by infecting organisms have been invoked as causes of morbidity it is likely that an allergic response may itself be responsible (Gell & Coombs, 1968).

Encephalitis

An interesting animal model in this respect is that of lymphocytic choriomeningitis (LCM) in mice (Hotchin, 1962). If adult mice are infected with the causative virus they develop a severe disease which includes meningitis, encephalitis and myelitis. If infection is introduced in utero the newborn mice do not show any disability and remain well in the short term although they continue to harbour the virus and may later develop chronic renal disease due to the deposition of immune complexes in the glomeruli (Oldstone & Dixon, 1971). If adult mice are given X-irradiation or cytotoxic drugs prior to infection they are less severely affected. This suggests that the immune response plays a major part in the production of the disease. Whether this is chiefly mediated by immune complexes or sensitised cells is debatable although by pre-treatment with anti-lymphocyte serum it has been possible to ameliorate another form of viral encephalitis in mice (Rook & Webb, 1970) and it has been argued that such factors may be important in the development of clinical encephalitis in man (Webb & Smith, 1966). Two examples are subacute sclerosing panencephalitis (Kolar, 1968; Brody & Detels, 1970) and progressive multifocal leucoencephalopathy (Howatson, Nagai & Zuhrhein, 1965).

Pneumonia

The deleterious effect of an immune response to an infective agent has also been demonstrated following immunisation with a killed (inactivated) measles vaccine; the kind used at present in this country is the live attenuated form. If a subject who has received the former kind of vaccine is exposed to a natural measles infection some time later he may develop a severe atypical form of the disease characterised by an unusual rash, myalgia, headache, abdominal pain, pneumonia, pleural effusion and hilar node enlargement, (B.M.J., 1971). This reaction seems to correlate with a heightened cell-mediated response to measles virus in the relative absence of specific antibody (Fulginiti & Arthur, 1969). Another condition which can be aggravated by prior immunisation is that of respiratory syncitial virus infection in childhood and it has been postulated that the morbidity associated with the natural infection may be chiefly a product of the host response, either a type I (anaphylactic) or a type III (immune complex) reaction (Gardner, McQuillin & Court, 1970). Experimental work in mice also emphasises the possibility of immune complex reactions contributing to the pathology of virus pneumonia (Blandford, 1970). An increasingly important group of pulmonary diseases known collectively as extrinsic allergic alveolitis (Pepys, 1969), and exemplified by farmer's lung, is now known to be due to type III, immune complex reactions, occurring in the lung and developed against a number of different fungi and organic dusts.

Hepatitis

A condition which has recently been receiving urgent attention is that of acute viral hepatitis. The discovery of the Australia antigen (Au–Ag) (Blumberg et al., 1967) was a considerable advance and various centres are endeavouring to culture an infective agent in vitro at the present time. The Au–Ag (also called hepatitis-associated antigen (HAA)) is particularly linked with serum hepatitis rather than infectious hepatitis and the development of simple screening tests has enabled its rapid detection in human blood products prior to their administration to patients. The occurrence of a number of serious outbreaks of serum hepatitis in relation to renal dialysis and transplantation programmes has emphasised the importance of the asymptomatic carrier. Many patients on dialysis become antigen-positive without clinical or biochemical evidence of liver disease and may remain so indefinitely. It is likely that this state of lessened reactivity is related to the reduced immunological response seen in uraemia and is reminiscent of the hypo-reactive virus-containing LCM mice described earlier. However in patients who do develop disease there seems to be an interesting correlation between the kind of immune response and the clinical picture (Almeida & Waterson, 1969). With electron-microscopy of sera it has been found that in the carrier state only Au–Ag is seen whereas in acute hepatitis immune complexes of Au–Ag with excess antibody occur and in chronic active hepatitis free antigen as well as complexes may be present suggesting antigen excess. It is likely therefore that the development of hepatitis is associated with a type III immune complex reaction (Zuckerman, Taylor & Bird, 1970). More recent work has demonstrated that the largest of the three varieties of particle seen in Au–Ag positive sera, i.e. the 42 nm Dane particle, can be separated, following detergent treatment, into an outer coat and an inner spherical 27 nm component resembling a rhinovirus (Almeida, Rubinstein & Stott, 1971). This and other work suggests that the infective agent is after all a virus and that the other particles seen under the electron-microscope represent virus-associated protein.

Chronic active hepatitis undoubtedly has a number of causes but evidence is accumulating that some cases which can progress to cirrhosis may develop in association with the presence of Au–Ag in the serum. The frequency with which the antigen is detected in this condition does however relate to the overall prevalence of serum hepatitis in the particular community concerned (Wright, 1971).

Primary biliary cirrhosis also has distinctive immunological features including the presence of a non-organ specific autoantibody reacting with mitochondria (Walker et al., 1965), a generalised impairment of cell-mediated immunity (Fox et al., 1969) and a marked tendency to granuloma formation. A high proportion of these patients have also been found to possess the Au–Ag in their sera and some of them also have the related antibody (Krohn et al., 1970). Once again one returns to considerations of both seed and soil in the genesis of disorders of this kind and the possibility that granuloma formation may occur par excellence when the humoral response greatly exceeds the cell-mediated response. Whether the impaired cell-mediated immunity seen in such conditions as primary biliary cirrhosis, sarcoidosis, Crohn's disease, leprosy and syphilis is present before the infective agent (if any) is acquired has yet to be determined. Au. antigen-antibody complexes have also been implicated in other diseases including polyarteritis nodosa (Gocke et al., 1970), glomerulo-nephritis (Lancet, 1970) and hepatocellular carcinoma (Vogel et al., 1970) and time alone will decide the exact role of this agent in human disease. Certainly the ambiguous value of an immune response towards it make the prospects for a successful vaccine against viral hepatitis relatively unlikely in the near future.

Other infections

These three examples, encephalitis, pneumonia and hepatitis, have been used to illustrate the contribution of the immune response to the pathology of infective disease. Although most of the diseases discussed are of viral origin, this phenomenon is not confined to viral infections and, there are a number of bacterial infections in which a similar contribution from the host to the pathological state occurs (Gell & Coombs, 1968). Patients with sarcoidosis and Crohn's disease show a diminished reactivity to tuberculin although stimulation by other antigens often gives normal results in Crohn's disease. Nevertheless granuloma formation is a constant feature and recent evidence suggests the presence of a transmissible agent in both sarcoid and Crohn's disease tissue of human origin (Mitchell & Rees, 1969, 1970).

Syphilis is a condition with an abundance of immunological features and much of the pathology, especially of the tertiary stage, can be related to the host response. However the specificity of the immune response seems to extend beyond the micro-organism itself for the antibody responsible for the Wasserman reaction can be readily demonstrated by using human tissue as a source of antigen (cardiolipin). This substance is found particularly in mitochondria and more recently a second antibody (cardiolipin fluorescent antibody) has been described in the sera of patients with early syphilis which may be of more use in the diagnosis and management of early syphilis. Although the mitochondrial antibody of primary biliary cirrhosis may give a similar pattern of immunofluorescence it reacts with a different antigen (a lipoprotein) which is also located in the inner membrane of mitochondria (Wright & Doniach, 1971). These antibodies can all be considered as auto-antibodies and it is of interest that the presence of rheumatoid factor, cryoglobulins and cold agglutinins have been described in association with syphilitic infection. However the incidence of thyroid, gastric parietal cell and nuclear antibodies does not seem to be increased in these patients (Wright *et al.*, 1970) and it is likely that especially in the early stages these anti-mitochondrial antibodies do little harm.

Heteroimmunity versus Autoimmunity

In considering the spectrum of diseases characterised by immunological hyper-reactivity, from the classically 'infective' to the classically 'auto-immune' conditions it becomes extremely difficult to decide exactly where the line is to be drawn between heteroimmune and autoimmune disease. By definition, autoimmune reactions occur against host determinants. The classic examples of sympathetic ophthalmia and mumps orchitis have been explained on the basis of sequestered determinants which were not registered as self-components when immunological competence was established but which, following some injury, make contact with host cells and elicit an immune response. It seems unlikely that the majority of autoimmune diseases can be explained on this basis and therefore the phenomena of immunological cross-reactivity or antigenic alteration are invoked. Rheumatic fever is almost certainly an example of the former (Zabriskie *et al.*, 1970) although another sequel to streptococcal infection, acute nephritis, has been shown to be related to immune complex formation rather than being due to anti-glomerular antibodies (Michael *et al.*, 1966). The importance of direct cross-reactions between foreign antigens and self-determinants is largely unknown. The scope for alteration of host components by physical or chemical means or following invasion by micro-organisms, seems more extensive. It is known that viruses are often able to incorporate their own individual chemistry into host cell membranes and nuclei, and micro-organisms may cause chemical alteration by enzyme action. It is also clear that during intra-cellular multiplication certain viruses are able to incorporate host antigens which may persist on the surface of the virus during a subsequent viraemia (Isacson, 1969). Such changes readily lead to an immune response. Whether one calls this hetero- or auto-immunity is largely a semantic problem. Even more subtle alterations in host chemistry may produce a host response and the development of antibodies against reacted complement components (immunoconglutinins) occurs in a variety of clinical situations (Lachmann, 1968) and like rheumatoid factor these can also be regarded as autoantibodies. The other possibility is that the integrity of the host 'self-recognition' system may fail or operate at an inappropriate level. It has been suggested that a gradual failure of this system is an inevitable correlate of the ageing process (Burnet, 1969), and it may be that genetic or environmental factors may hasten the onset of such a failure. There have recently been several suggestions that auto-immunisation may be a frequent occurrence in the normal individual but that it operates at a low level and only produces disease when homoeostatic mechanisms fail (Edgington & Dalessio, 1970; Henriksen, 1970; Field *et al.*, 1970; Micklem *et al.*, 1970).

These and other findings can be explained by accrediting the T cell with controlling as well as co-operating functions in the immune response particularly with regard to the development of auto-immunity (Allison, Denman & Barnes, 1971). Such considerations cut across traditional concepts of immunological tolerance and may lead to a reappraisal of the underlying mechanisms of immunological unresponsiveness (Allison, 1971).

Micro-organisms and autoimmunity

Current evidence suggests that infection with micro-organisms may frequently play a part in the initiation of autoimmune processes in human diseases (Asherson, 1968). Virus-like structures have been detected in the kidney in systemic lupus (Kawano, Miller & Kimmelstiel, 1969) and the NZB/NZW strain of mice which develop a very similar disease are also known to harbour a virus (Lambert & Dixon, 1970). Several micro-organisms have been isolated from the joints of patients with rheumatoid arthritis and recent work suggests that Mycoplasma fermentans may play an important role in the development of this condition (Williams, Brostoff & Roitt, 1970). A number of bacterial antigens have been detected in association with antibody in the affected blood vessels of patients with vasculitis (Parish, 1971) and a recent study implicating the Au–Ag in the pathogenesis of polyarteritis nodosa has already been cited (Gocke *et al.*, 1970). The failure to detect micro-organisms in the relevant tissues of all patients with auto-immune disease induced by such agents should not be surprising, for in experimental virus arthritis it has been shown that virus may only be isolated during the initial stages of the infection (Norton & Storz, 1967).

Constitutional factors

Whether individuals with entirely normal immune systems escape the autoimmune sequelae which may follow infection is not yet clear although evidence from both animal and human studies suggests that an idiosyncratic response may be necessary on the part of the host for such disease to develop. The frequent segregation of auto-immune diseases (especially of the 'organ-specific' kind) within families and within individuals is in keeping with this although the vertical transmission of a virus could also explain such a familial trait. Autoimmune diseases may complicate a number of immunodeficiency syndromes and the near relatives of patients with primary immunoglobulin disorders have an unusually high incidence of autoimmune disease (W.H.O., 1968). Twomey and others have described 10 cases of adult-onset hypogamma-globulinaemia in association with pernicious anaemia in whom cell-mediated immunity seemed to be preserved (Twomey *et al.*, 1969). Autoimmune phenomena have been described following treatment with X-irradiation or alkylating agents in patients with lymphosarcoma and chronic lymphatic leukaemia (Lewis, Schwartz & Damashek, 1966) and it is possible that other physical and chemical agents may precipitate similar events.

Types of Response

Theoretically any of the four types of immunological reaction (see page 419) might operate in autoimmune disease but although there are a number of disorders in which types II, III, and IV are known to take place it is not clear whether anaphylactic responses can occur against host components although host damage may result from an anaphylactic response to extrinsic antigens, and this event is discussed in a later section under the heading of allergy and atopy. It has already been seen that *hetero*-immune type III responses can readily produce host disease and when intravascular immune complexes are formed involving auto-antigens it is logical that the *auto*-immune disease which results should be of the *non-organ specific* kind, e.g. systemic lupus erythematosus and rheumatoid arthritis. The type of fibrosing alveolitis, in which extrinsic allergens are not readily implicated, unlike the extrinsic allergic alveolitis mentioned earlier, tends to be associated with other autoimmune diseases such as rheumatoid arthritis, thyroid disease, Sjögren's syndrome, primary biliary cirrhosis and renal tubular acidosis (Mason *et al.*, 1970). It is possible that this cryptogenic form of fibrosing alveolitis may also develop as a result of immune complex formation and a particularly high incidence of non-organ specific antibodies (notably rheumatoid factor and antinuclear factor) which are uncommon in the extrinsic form, has been demonstrated (Turner-Warwick & Haslem, 1971).

In the organ-specific forms of auto-immune disease, e.g. Hashimoto's disease, pernicious anaemia, idiopathic Addison's disease, etc., both type II and type IV responses occur. Lymphocytic infiltration of the organ concerned is a common finding and either antibodies or lymphocytes from the affected individual may cause damage to the appropriate target cell. Examples of antibodies reacting with host tissues include the long-acting thyroid stimulator of thyrotoxicosis (Doniach & Roitt, 1968), the anti-glomerular basement-membrane antibody of Goodpasture's syndrome (Lerner, Glassock & Dixon, 1967) and the cross-reacting heart-muscle antibody of rheumatic carditis (Zabriskie, Hsu & Seegal, 1970). Specifically sensitised lymphocytes have been shown to be present in idiopathic Addison's disease (Nerup, Anderson & Bendixen, 1970), thyrotoxicosis (Field *et al.*, 1970), ulcerative colitis, (Watson, Quigley & Bolt, 1966), some cases of glomerulonephritis (Rocklin, Lewis & David, 1970), polymyositis (Currie *et al.*, 1971), and experimental allergic encephalomyelitis (Field, 1968). In some instances both humoral and cellular responses may be necessary before the disease is established. Such a possibility has been elegantly demonstrated in an experimental model of allergic orchitis (Brown, Glynn & Holborow, 1967).

It is clear that autoimmunity covers a broad range of immunological reactivity although in many instances knowledge is still fragmentary regarding the specific mechanisms involved. A number of studies utilising recently developed techniques are currently in progress and undoubtedly we will learn much more in the near future about immunological mechanisms in infectious and autoimmune disease. Perhaps the greatest contribution will come from work relating to the development of new antigens within host tissues (Kaplan, 1967) and the importance of infections with viruses or other micro-organisms in this metamorphosis. A clearer understanding of the normal state of immunological unresponsiveness to self antigens and the role of the T cell in maintaining or breaking this control should have far-reaching implications for a number of clinical diseases.

DIABETES

Diabetes mellitus is not usually thought of as an immunological disease and apart from the well-trodden paths of immunoassay and rare examples of insulin allergy and resistance, immunological factors have been given little emphasis. However, there are several other ways in which such factors may be important.

Immune response to insulin

As almost all administered insulin is derived from other species (usually ox or pig) it is not surprising that almost all patients receiving it develop antibodies within a short period of time. In the very large majority this does not seem to cause any short-term problems and resistance or allergy to insulin are both extremely uncommon. Whether the presence of circulating insulin: insulin antibody complexes over a longer period can cause harm is uncertain although there is evidence to suggest that some of the complications of diabetes e.g. retinopathy and nephropathy may be aggravated by such an immune response. The presence of insulin, immunoglobulin and complement within the lesions of diabetic angiopathy has been demonstrated on several occasions (Freedman, Peters & Kark, 1960; Berns et al., 1962; and Coleman et al., 1962) although as small blood vessel walls have an increased permeability in this condition (Ashton, 1963) this uptake could be non-specific. A similar histological picture has been produced in experimental animals following the injection of heterologous insulin (Grieble, 1960). The fact that patients who have never been injected with insulin can develop severe complications indicates that immune complexes cannot be the only cause although it is just possible that complexes of insulin with auto-antibody could be involved.

Although there does not seem to be a close correlation between the amount of insulin antibody present and the insulin requirement of a particular patient, the levels of both free and antibody bound insulin usually rise following the appearance of such antibodies. Insulin: antibody complexes will dissociate when the level of free circulating insulin falls and when antibody levels are high administered insulin can cause hypoglycaemia long after the time of its expected maximal effect (Eskind, Franklin & Lowell, 1953). As hyperinsulinism may be important in the development of atherosclerosis (Sloan, Mackay & Sheridan, 1970; Stout, 1970) and circulating insulin can stimulate the cholesterol synthesis of arterial walls (Stout, 1969) it is possible that the immune response could contribute to the development of atherosclerosis via an enhancing effect on lipid uptake.

Aetiology and pathogenesis of diabetes

Diabetes mellitus is undoubtedly a heterogenous condition with a number of different causes. It is possible that some patients with diabetes, especially the juvenile-onset, insulin-dependent cases, are suffering from an autoimmune disease. Several extensive studies have revealed a significantly increased incidence of autoantibodies of various kinds as well as frequent associations with overt auto-immune disease (Moore, & Neilson, 1963; Ungar *et al.*, 1968; Irvine *et al.*, 1970; Whittingham *et al.*, 1971). Despite this circumstantial evidence most authorities are unable to detect insulin antibodies or anti-pancreatic antibodies in diabetic patients who have never received insulin therapy (Parker *et al.*, 1968; Doniach, 1971).

There are several reasons for suspecting viral infection as a triggering mechanism in the pathogenesis of diabetes although hereditary and other factors are of importance. Viruses have been identified which can directly damage β cells in animals (Taylor, 1969). Gamble & Taylor (1969) found a higher antibody titre to Coxsacke B virus (particularly of type B4) in the sera of insulin-dependent diabetics within three months of onset of their diabetes than was present in the sera of controls. In addition the seasonal variation in the onset of insulin-dependent diabetes in patients under 30 years of age has been shown to have a significant positive correlation with the annual incidence data for infections with Coxsackie virus type B4 but not with other types of virus infection (Gamble & Taylor, 1969). Whether the diabetes which supposedly follows as a sequel to this infection is caused by direct damage due to the virus or develops as the result of autoimmune phenomena which follow the virus infection is debatable. If auto-antibodies or sensitised cells reacting with insulin or β cell components are identified with certainty in these patients then the latter possibility will seem more likely. In the absence of this finding one is more inclined to think in terms of direct viral injury.

ALLERGY AND ATOPY

Allergy, in the sense of an untoward response to an extrinsic agent, can be one of the most vivid and impressive manifestations of immunological processes. Anyone who has witnessed an episode of acute anaphylaxis will be in no doubt as to the potential for harm as well as benefit which these processes can offer the host. Such a response usually follows the parenteral administration of antigen and the commonest agent known to do this at the present time is penicillin. Less severe symptoms may follow oral or bronchial challenge although pronounced symptoms of such an immediate hyper-sensitivity (type I) reaction have been recorded in which a patient was found to react against a glycoprotein present in her husband's seminal fluid (Halpern & Robert, 1967). Fortunately this problem is a very unusual one.

Here, in contrast with many of the phenomena described in the previous section, there is no doubt that we are dealing with hetero-immune responses. Such allergic responses can be one of the four classic kinds of immune response enumerated on page 419 although more than one type can co-exist at the same time.

Type 1 *reactions* may vary considerably in their severity and any of the following features may develop: pruritis, flushing, pallor, cyanosis, dyspnoea, wheezing, tightness in the chest, abdominal pain, vomiting, hypotension, circulatory failure, unconsciousness and death. In man, unlike the guinea-pig, bronchospasm is not the commonest disturbance following an 'anaphylactic' reaction to substances administered via the parenteral route. In mild cases urticaria may be the main feature and may persist for several days. The antigens (or allergens) most commonly involved are drugs (especially penicillin), foreign sera, contrast media and insect bites. The routine prophylactic administration of horse anti-tetanus serum to patients with superficial wounds was abandoned because the mortality rate from anaphylactic reactions was overtaking that due to tetanus in untreated cases (Adams, Laurence & Smith, 1969). Many of the features of atopic disease, e.g. allergic hay-fever and asthma, are also caused by type I reactions to the common allergens, e.g. grass pollen, house dust, animal dander etc., and the comparatively localised route of antigen challenge is related to the localisation of the clinical manifestations. Atopy is considered in more detail shortly.

Type II reactions against foreign antigens are less evident because of the necessity for the antigen to be situated on a cell surface. The classic example, of course, is the incompatible blood transfusion, although drugs may often adsorb to the formed elements of the blood giving rise to drug-induced haemolysis, agranulocytosis or thrombocytopenia. Whether primary combination occurs between drug and blood cell followed by reaction with antibody or whether immune complexes secondarily attach to blood cells involving them as 'innocent bystanders' is debated (Ackroyd & Rook, 1968) and it is likely that several mechanisms operate respectively in different instances (Carstairs, 1968). Drugs which readily produce this type of reaction include quinine, phenacetin, para-aminosalicylic acid, penicillin and sedormid (now withdrawn).

Type III reactions are more common and variable in their manifestations. The classical syndrome is that of serum sickness. About eight days after the administration of foreign serum fever develops accompanied or followed by lymphadenopathy, splenomegaly, polyarthritis and often a generalised urticaria. Both a neutrophil and eosinophil leucocytosis and transient proteinuria may coincide with the clinical symptoms. Dixon's group have reproduced this condition in rabbits following the injection of bovine serum albumin and have shown that the time of maximum formation of immune complexes coincides with the peak of the illness (Dixon *et al.*, 1958). However, as with acute systemic anaphylaxis, this typical syndrome is usually only seen after the parenteral administration of antigen and here drugs and foreign sera are again top of the list of causes. In some instances fever may be the chief feature and this is not infrequently seen in association with drug therapy (Cluff & Johnson, 1964). Localised forms of type III reactions occur following localised introduction of antigen e.g. extrinsic allergic alveolitis in the lung (discussed briefly on page 425) and the Arthus reaction in the skin. Challenge by the oral route can be followed by truncated forms of serum sickness, e.g. 'Furadantin lung' and penicillamine nephropathy. More generalised and chronic examples of immune complex disease are disseminated lupus erythematosus and polyarteritis nodosa and their chronicity is presumably related to the continuing presence of antigen. Polyarteritis nodosa has been recorded in association with serum sickness and following the administration of a number of therapeutic agents (Symmers, 1958) and disseminated lupus can be triggered, if not caused, by drug therapy (Holborow, 1969).

Type IV or cell-mediated reactions are traditionally distinguished from those due to humoral antibody by their prolonged time course, hence the term '*delayed hypersensitivity*'. The commonest clinical example is contact dermatitis which can be caused by a wide range of allergens, from heavy metals to plants and organic chemicals (Calnan, 1968). Type IV reactions in addition to type I reactions may play a part in the allergic response of some individuals to insect bites and the relative contributions of these two types of allergic response may vary during the natural history of an individual's hypersensitivity state (Frankland, 1968).

Predisposing factors

Allergic disease is a common, and often serious, problem. Apart from the 'atopic' allergens, therapeutic agents are the most important cause of allergic disorders, and are often responsible for serious disability and death (Reeves & Trounce, 1971). Why some people experience allergic reactions, often repeatedly throughout their lives, and others do not, is obscure. It is likely that the pattern of contact with the particular substance is often important, for as has already been discussed on page 414, variations in the dose, time sequence, and route of administration may decide whether immunisation does, or does not, take place. An allergic response is most likely to occur after a second challenge with the substance, there having been an interim period in which there was no contact with the substance concerned. The reason why the very large majority of insulin-treated diabetics do not develop insulin resistance due to antibody formation may be related to the regular frequent administration of the antigen. In those rare cases where insulin resistance is a problem there is often a history of a break in insulin therapy. Even so, almost all patients who are treated with insulin, penicillin or a number of other antigenic substances make antibodies against the antigen concerned and therefore other factors such as the kind of antibody produced, its specificity, affinity, amount and the balance between the four types of allergic response may be significant in determining the presence of an untoward reaction in a particular patient.

The presence of other factors having adjuvant activity may also be important. Long-acting preparations, e.g. of penicillin, are notorious for the allergic reactions which they may produce. This may be partly due to the presence of other moieties which confer an adjuvant effect and also the fact that in such a depot preparation one may administer both the primary sensitising dose as well as the secondary challenging dose at one and the same time. A coincidental infection may also provide an adjuvant effect and the considerably exaggerated incidence of hypersensitivity to penbritin seen in patients with glandular fever is well documented (Pullen, Wright & Murdoch, 1967).

Constitutional abnormalities may also encourage allergic reactions. Patients with thyroid disease in association with antithyroid antibodies more frequently develop allergy to penicillin (Blizzard *et al.*, 1959) and those with an atopic trait have a heightened ability to develop type I reactions to foreign material and often have a family as well as a personal history of allergy. Patients with urticaria pigmentosa also have an increased tendency to show this kind of reaction (Frankland, 1968). Individual biochemical idiosyncrasies may also explain variations in susceptibility, e.g. the rate of metabolism and excretion of a drug as well as the avidity with which host proteins bind to it may prove to be key factors.

The Atopic Trait

The term atopy was introduced by Coca (Coca & Cooke, 1923) to describe a particular type of clinical hypersensitivity characterised by the immediate hypersensitivity (type I) wheal-and-flare reaction and occurring in association with hay-fever and asthma. The atopic trait or syndrome has since been extended to include the following conditions: atopic dermatitis, allergic rhinitis (hay-fever), allergic (extrinsic) asthma, and allergic gastroenteropathy. The gastroenteropathy is the least recognised of these disorders occurring in young children who may present with oedema, hypoproteinaemia, anaemia, eosinophilia and retarded growth (Waldman *et al.*, 1967). Their protein-losing gastroenteropathy is aggravated by milk and examination of their sera has revealed the presence of milk antibodies. It is usually associated with asthma, eczema and hay-fever and shows a favourable response to corticosteroid therapy. Proteinuria leading to a typical nephrotic syndrome has also been described in relation to atopic hypersensitivity (Wittig & Goldman, 1970). Recent studies in a small group of patients with 'minimal change' nephrotic syndrome in association with a relatively localised grass-pollen allergy and an atopic trait have demonstrated a seasonal rise in serum levels of reaginic antibody (IgE) against grass-pollen which coincides with the rise in pollen count, the onset of their hay-fever and the relapse of their proteinuria (Reeves, Cameron & Ogg, 1971). Although the exact mechanism of production of the proteinuria is obscure it is possible that careful skin-testing of all minimal change nephrotics as well as urine-testing of all atopic patients during their seasonal relapse may show that this relationship is more common than was formerly supposed. Migraine has often been linked with atopic disease but apart from the presence of dietary factors which may aggravate it and the occasional coincidental finding of other atopic features in a particular patient there is little to suggest a direct relationship.

For many years the antibodies which mediate type I reactions were known to be non-precipitating, skin-sensitising and heat-labile. In the early part of the last decade it was thought most likely that they belonged to the immuno-globulin class IgA. However, after painstaking work on the reaginic antibody present in association with ragweed hypersensitivity (Ishizaka, Ishizaka & Hornbrook, 1968) and following the discovery of a new immunoglobulin class present in high concentration in the blood of a patient with myelomatosis (Johansson & Bennich, 1967) it became clear that reaginic antibody was identifiable with this new class of antibody, IgE. Nevertheless as mentioned earlier (page 419) it is still possible that in some circumstances other classes of antibody may show reaginic behaviour. Several techniques have now been developed for measuring serum levels of IgE (originally called IgND) and raised levels have been detected in patients with allergic asthma, atopic dermatitis and parasitic infestations (Johansson, 1969). It is not entirely certain that the process of atopic sensitisation lies completely within the domain of humoral reaginic antibody. It has been considered, particularly by dermatologists, that cell-mediated immunity may be of importance in atopic dermatitis and cellular hypersensitivity to grass pollen has been detected in patients with summer hay-fever (Brostoff and Roitt, 1969); it being suggested that this is a reflection of co-operation between T and B cells in the production of IgE by the latter.

Role of Reaginic Antibody in the Normal State

None of the information we have to date offers a satisfactory explanation for the raison d'etre of reaginic antibody (IgE). Most of its apparent effects seem to cause the organism more harm than good, at least in those individuals who display immediate hypersensitivity responses. It may have quite a different function in the normal non-atopic individual in whom its presence can also be detected but in reduced amounts. It has been suggested that it may have an important role in protection against parasitic infestation and the pheno-menon of 'self-cure' seen in Nippostrongylus brasiliensis infection in the rat affords a possible example (Jones & Ogilvie, 1967). The fact that some of the highest serum levels of IgE recorded in man have been found in people with parasitic disease is also of interest. Yet this still seems to be an unlikely reason for the presence of reaginic antibody responses in normal people to a wide variety of antigens but in the absence of any clinical disturbance (Humphrey & White, 1970).

It has already been stated that antibody concentrations tend to be ex-tremely low in the extravascular compartment. IgE, sitting as it does via its Fc fragment (see Fig. 13.2) on the surface membrane of tissue mast cells, is in an ideal position to supervise extravascular immunity. Should antigen appear in this situation and make contact with a suitable IgE molecule then vaso-active amines and other substances including heparin are released from the mast cell granules. In the skin this is seen as a wheal and flare response which is largely due to the marked increase in capillary permeability that follows the release of these substances. This will allow a considerable amount of serum protein including antibody to pass into the extravascular tissue in this local site in addition to polymorphonuclear leucocytes and monocytes. Thus it is possible that effective concentrations of other antibody classes may be achieved outside the circulation setting in train a number of defence mechanisms e.g. opsonisation, phagocytosis and complement fixation, otherwise reserved for the intravascular compartment. Cochrane has demonstrated experimentally a direct correlation between immune complex localisation in vessel walls and IgE-mediated vasoactive amine release from basophils (Cochrane, 1971) and it seems likely that the amine release from extravascular mast cells will have a similar effect. This hypo-thesis finds circumstantial confirmation in the observation that it is un-common to see, after suitable challenge, a type III response in the skin in the complete absence of a type I response (Hargreave et al., 1966; Pepys et al.,

1968). Those patients who show marked type III responses, as in pulmonary aspergillosis or bird fancier's lung, usually have a detectable type I response in addition.

It has been suggested that there is a negative association between allergic and atopic conditions on the one hand and cancer on the other (Ure, 1969). This observation requires confirmation on a much more extensive epidemiological basis but it is conceivable that reaginic antibody itself provides an alternative surveillance system to that often attributed to sensitised lymphocytes, which could offer some protection against the establishment of aberrant cell clones.

The preponderance of IgE production in the skin is in keeping with the idea that it may act locally by boosting effective antibody concentrations in tissues. IgA seems to predominate in the gut and as this antibody is secreted into its lumen it may offer protection even before the antigenic material has entered the tissues. For this reason secretory IgA may be much more useful here than tissue IgE. In the respiratory tract also IgA seems to be as much in evidence as IgE (Ishizaka, 1971; Tomasi, 1971) and this may reflect a similar contribution from intra-luminal immunity in addition to tissue defences. In the skin, tissue reponses are the first line of defence in view of its dessicated exterior and constant exposure to foreign material. The urinary tract seems to be more like the bronchial tree in that it has considerable numbers of both IgA and IgE producing cells (Kaufman & Hobbs, 1970; Turner et al., 1970).

Atopy as a Form of Immunodeficiency

It seems clear that individuals displaying the atopic trait have some kind of constitutional defect which renders them prone to the excessive production of reaginic antibody. There are a number of reports describing atopic features in association with antibody deficiency states, e.g. sex-linked hypogammaglobulinaemia, the Wiskott–Aldrich Syndrome and selective immunoglobulin deficiencies (Peterson, 1965; Berglund et al., 1968; Kaufman & Hobbs, 1970). The latter study has shown that 7 per cent of an atopic population had a deficiency of IgG, IgM or IgA (i.e. the serum level of one or more of these classes was more than 2 s.D. below the limits of normal for age). The commonest deficiency was of IgA and a further 20 per cent of these patients had immunoglobulin levels around the lower limits of normality. It is possible that a relative failure of antibody production of other classes, especially IgA, may place undue pressure on tissue antibody (i.e. IgE) which after prolonged stimulation may increase in amount sufficiently to produce atopic manifestations. Normal IgA production tends to be sub-maximal before adulthood is reached and some atopic patients may be late developers in this respect. The fact that a reasonable proportion of atopic children lose their symptoms as they grow up would tie in with a delay in the maturity of humoral responses of this kind. The production of 'blocking' antibodies following a course of desensitisation may be a means of overcoming this state of relative immunodeficiency by massive and sustained antigenic stimulation. The greater chances of success when desensitising against a single agent e.g. grass-pollen, as opposed to a batch of antigens may reflect a limitation on the number of cells available for the production of blocking antibody.

MALIGNANT DISEASE

Antigenicity

If tumours are not antigenic to their hosts then immunological factors can play little part in their development and subsequent growth. Although there may be some loss of tissue-specific antigens with the development of malignancy it was clear from the pioneer work of Gorer on transplantation immunity that tumour tissue was capable of being recognised as foreign after transfer to another animal (Gorer, 1961). Since then it has been realised that many tumours also acquire new tumour-specific antigens and that for virally induced neoplasms these antigens are identical for each primary tumour produced by the same virus, whereas with chemically or physically induced tumours each primary tumour (even in the same host) will have a unique antigenic structure (Old & Boyse, 1964 and 1965). These antigens vary greatly in their potency but an immune response has been demonstrated in a number of human neoplasms (Klein, 1970). These include leukaemia, Burkitt's lymphoma, nasopharyngeal carcinoma, osteogenic sarcoma, neuroblastoma and malignant melanoma (Hellstrom *et al.*, 1968; Morton *et al.*, 1969, Fass, Herberman & Ziegler, 1970; Fairley, 1970; Powles *et al.*, 1971). Although choriocarcinoma has a number of immunological features it is not certain how they correlate with the behaviour of the tumour (Bagshawe, 1970). A likely reason for the infrequent detection of tumour-specific antibody in some other malignancies is their transient nature due, at least, in part, to adsorption by the growing tumour (see page 441) (Odili & Taylor, 1971). Surgical removal is often associated with a rise in titre of such antibody. From this evidence it is clear in some instances at least, that there must be a failure of the host's immunological detection and defence mechanisms.

Reasons for Failure of the Immune Response

The successful development of an aberrant population of cells can be subdivided into two stages: (*a*) initial escape, and (*b*) failure of the host to reject the established tumour (Alexander, 1969). There are a number of possible ways in which the immune response may be compromised. These are outlined in Fig. 13.3 (a modified from of Fig. 13.1) and the numbers mentioned in the text refer to it. Although some tumour-specific antigens may be too weak to elicit a potent response in other cases insufficient antigenic material may be released to cause stimulation (**1**). If the growth of an abnormal clone is rapid it may outstrip the developing immune response. Several animal tumours bearing distinctive antigens are capable of transfer to another normal animal by the inoculation of a very small number of cells (Alexander, 1969) and it is possible that the growth threshold for escape may often be quite low. Certainly it seems that for each individual tumour and host there is a critical tumour size beyond which the immune response is ineffective.

Central defects

Other factors may operate at the central part of the immune arc (**2, 3** and **4**). If the neoplasm is caused by a virus that has been present from birth (i.e. vertically transmitted) then a state of specific immunological tolerance may exist and the tumour-specific antigens will be recognised as self (**2**). This has been demonstrated in a number of animal tumours (Harris & Sinkovics, 1970) and may occur in man. It is also possible that specific tolerance could be related to the particular amount and pattern of antigen release by the developing tumour as in the case of experimental 'low' and 'high' zone tolerance described earlier (Mitchison, 1968). The chemical form in which antigen is presented to the immune apparatus may also be relevant. It has been shown that extracts from certain organs (e.g. liver) may be more 'tolerogenic' than extracts prepared from other organs of the same animal (e.g. kidney) (Brent, Hansen & Kilshaw, 1971). That the immune response can become suppressed

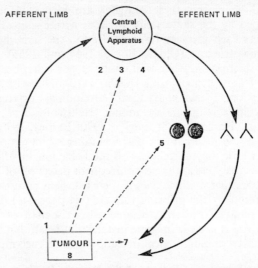

Fig. 13.3. MECHANISMS BY WHICH THE IMMUNE RESPONSE AGAINST MALIGNANT TISSUE MAY BE BLOCKED IN THE PATIENT WITH ESTABLISHED CANCER. 1. Insufficient release of antigen. 2. Specific tolerance. 3. Specific suppression of the release of immunoblasts. 4. Generalised paralysis. 5. Impaired activity of sensitised lymphocytes. 6. Immunological enhancement. 7. Mediator inhibition. 8. Immunoadsorbent effect of the tumour itself. (Broken lines indicate the possible sites of action of non-antigen factors which may be released by some malignant tissues). For explanation see text.

while a tumour remains *in situ* has been demonstrated by Mikulska, Smith & Alexander (1966). They found that after removal of a primary tumour a state of immunity developed which made it more difficult to re-establish the tumour in the same animals. When chemically induced sarcoma cells possessing tumour specific-antigens are inoculated into the tissues of an animal the blast response seen in the efferent lymphatics draining the appropriate area is similar to the response following any other type of antigenic stimulation (Alexander *et al.*, 1969). However, once a tumour has become established the cellular response fails although this suppression can be reversed within 24 hours by removal of the tumour. Examination of the regional lymph nodes has shown that even in the presence of the tumour there is considerable transformation into blast cells within the node but that their release into the efferent lymphatics seems to be arrested. This effect is a local one and is also specific for the particular antigens of the individual tumour and does not compromise other immune responses (3). What relationship this phenomenon bears to the traditional forms of immunological tolerance is uncertain. Recently it has been suggested that human tumours may themselves produce a substance which inhibits lymphocyte migration so that although sensitisation may have occurred the expression of cell-mediated immunity is prevented (Wolberg & Goelzer, 1971). Specific non-reactivity of patients with malignant melanoma has been demonstrated when tested with autologous tumour extracts although patients with localised tumours did respond (Fass, Herbermann & Ziegler, 1970a). A similar non-reactivity has also been found in patients with Burkitt's lymphoma which reverted to normal when in clinical remission (Fass *et al.*, 1970b).

In other situations there is a more general impairment of the immune response (4) and it has been a frequent observation that patients with malignant disease tend to give inferior responses to a number of different test antigens (Lytton, Hughes & Fulthorpe, 1964; Hughes & Mackay, 1965; Solowey & Rapaport, 1965; Southam, 1968). Generally the degree of impairment correlates with the extent of the neoplasm; those patients with well-localised lesions having responses very similar to normal controls. Often those reactions mediated by sensitised lymphocytes are more severely affected than those due to antibody and this disparity is particularly marked in Hodgkin's disease (Leibowitz, 1966). Whether these defects precede or succeed the development of neoplasia is uncertain. Patients with various immunological deficiencies, e.g. hypogammaglobulinaemia; ataxia-telangiectasia and the Wiskott–Aldrich syndrome, are known to have an increased incidence of malignancy although the majority of the tumours that they develop arise in the reticulo-endothelial system (Doll & Kinlen, 1970). Recently several groups have described associations between histocompatibility antigen (HL-A) types and susceptibility to malignant disease (Walford *et al.*, 1970; Ellman, Green & Martin, 1970; Forbes & Morris, 1970). HL-A types are also related to immune reactivity although susceptibility to viruses and other factors may explain this association.

It is being increasingly realised that patients who have received therapeutic immunosuppression are more prone to develop tumours (Doll & Kinlen, 1970; Allison, 1970; Schneck & Penn, 1971). The effect of non-specific suppression of the immune response on the growth of a malignant neoplasm in man has been demonstrated by the unwitting transplantation of donor malignant cells along with a kidney transplant. After a tumour had developed in the recipient immunosuppressive therapy was stopped and regression of the neoplasm as well as rejection of the kidney followed (Wilson *et al.*, 1968). In this case the presence of transplantation antigens in addition to tumour-specific antigens will have promoted the rejection process.

Tumour factors

In those instances where a fairly generalised depression of immune reactivity is seen in the presence of a tumour and before a state of general debility has developed, it is possible that factors elaborated by the tumour itself (apart from antigen) may give rise to this anergic state. It is well known that a number of human neoplasms are able to synthesise various ectopic factors which may affect normal physiology elsewhere in the body (Azzopardi. Freeman & Poole, 1970 (see Chapter 1) and cells which have undergone a considerable degree of dedifferentiation may produce a variety of irrelevant molecules. Restoration of immune reactivity following irradiation or therapy with cytotoxic drugs (Sokal & Primikirios, 1961; Aisenberg, 1962) suggest that similar factors may affect immune mechanisms. Whether the general impairment of reactivity occurs centrally or at a peripheral level is not clear although the failure to transfer tuberculin sensitivity to patients with Hodgkin's disease by the transfer of sensitised lymphocytes (Kelly *et al.*, 1960) suggests a peripheral defect in this particular form of neoplasia. The fact that *in vitro* lymphocyte transformation to phytohaemagglutinin, impaired in patients with breast cancer can be restored by the use of homologous instead of autologous serum (Whittaker, Rees & Clark, 1971) also suggests the presence of inhibiting serum factors (5). Whether this represents a form of antibody or another kind of factor, possibly elaborated by the tumour itself, is not clear.

Role of cell-mediated immunity

The relative efficacy of humoral and cellular immunity against neoplastic growth varies from tumour to tumour. Cytotoxic antibodies have been found in association with various neoplasms, including malignant melanoma in man (Fairley, 1970) and there is some indication that their presence may be associated with a more favourable prognosis. It is unlikely that they can have much effect on an established solid tumour but they may be active against blood-borne cancer cells which are known to circulate in association with various human tumours and thus prevent or delay the development of metastases. Such a possibility has been established for an animal model (Alexander & Hall, 1970). In most examples of malignant disease however. cellular immunity seems to be more relevant to the rate of tumour growth. In several human tumours including carcinomas of breast and stomach and Hodgkin's disease the degree of lymphocytic infiltration of the primary lesion has been correlated with prognosis (Black & Speer, 1958; Hamlin. 1968; Lukes, 1964; Bloom, Richardson & Field, 1970) and enlargement of the regional nodes when not due to the spread of tumour has been similarly associated (Cutler, Zippin & Asire, 1969; Crile, 1965). Much animal and human work supports the importance of cellular mechanisms (Harris & Sincovics, 1970) and in animals the passive transfer of sensitised lymphocytes has caused complete regression of primary tumours (Alexander, Delorme & Hall, 1966). Transfer of homologous immunologically competent cells can produce graft-versus-host disease and for this reason the use of irradiated cells or cell-free extracts is preferred (Alexander *et al.*, 1967; Alexander & Hall, 1970). It is too early to comment on the application of this work to the management of solid tumours in man although it is likely that such measures may be of use in the future if only as adjuvants.

Peripheral blockade

At one time it was thought that antisera raised in animals against human tumour extracts might be of use in the treatment of malignant disease. It is now realised that immune sera can cause increased growth of a tumour rather than regression, by a process known as immunological enhancement (6) (Gorer, 1960; Milner, Evans & Weiser, 1964). This effect is probably achieved by competition for antigenic sites on the tumour cells between blocking antibody and sensitised lymphocytes and if such antisera are administered then the cell-mediated responses of the host may be effectively blocked. This phenomenon has been put to good effect to prevent the rejection of organ transplants (French & Batchelor, 1969). Endogenous blocking factors are currently being described in a wide variety of clinical situations and notably in several forms of malignant disease e.g. hypernephroma (Horn & Horn, 1971), malignant melanoma (Hellstrom & Hellstrom, 1971) and adenocarcinoma (Hellstrom et al., 1969).

It is possible that mechanisms **2, 3, 4, 5** and **6** all represent different aspects of the same fundamental process and a clearer understanding of the cellular and chemical basis of immunological unresponsiveness (see page 450) will illuminate this presently confused field.

Other mechanisms

The remaining stages at which the immune arc may be modified in the presence of a tumour are at the mediator level (7) and at the tumour itself (8). Anti-inflammatory factors have been identified in association with injury and inflammation (Billingham, Robinson & Robson, 1969) and the elaboration of such an agent by a tumour itself or following necrosis and infection could explain some of the non-specific effects on immune responses already described (7) (Johnson, Maibach & Salmon, 1971). If a tumour itself is sufficiently large it may function as an immunoadsorbent and mop up all the available antibody so that none can be detected in the peripheral blood (8). This is one possible explanation for the disappearance of tumour-specific antibody with progression of the tumour (Fairley, 1970).

A cell which has not been mentioned so far in relation to tumour immunity is the macrophage. There is evidence that in some situations, and in the presence of cytophilic antibody, these cells can be cytotoxic for tumour cells (Alexander, 1970). Other work in the rat has shown that non-specifically activated macrophages can kill tumour cells in *vitro* and that this effect can be blocked by a particular subclass of IgG antibody (IgG_2) (Keller & Jones, 1971). Whether this has any relevance for man is not yet apparent.

Immunotherapy

Immunotherapy can be envisaged in a number of ways. *Passive immunisation* can be attempted with either immune serum or sensitised cells. Both these approaches and their potential hazards have been already discussed. *Active immunisation* can be specific or non-specific. In the former case irradiated autologous tumour cells or their extracts are administered to enhance the immune response. This can be effective if the amount of residual tumour is small (Haddow & Alexander, 1964) and its success may be the result of systemic immunisation bypassing the failure of the local nodes to discharge immunoblasts (Alexander, 1970). However initial attempts to improve the prognosis in malignant melanoma by this means have not been successful although in some cases the immune response appears to have been boosted (Ikonopisov *et al.*, 1970; Currie, Lejeune & Fairley, 1971).

Non-specific stimulation seems to be rather more effective although it is not clear why this should be so. Live B.C.G. and corynebacterium parvum have both been shown to aid the inhibition of growth of grafted tumours if given prior to implantation (Halpern *et al.*, 1966). Mathé (1970) has found that these agents are also of therapeutic use after a tumour has become established and has used a combination of irradiated autologous cells with B.C.G. in the management of acute leukaemia. This is only instituted after intensive efforts at reduction of the number of leukaemic cells with chemotherapy, for it is only when the total number is down to the order of 10^5 cells that an effect can be achieved. Local inoculation with viruses has also been used and can produce regression of intradermal lesions in malignant melanoma (Hunter-Craig *et al.*, 1970) but this approach seems to be of limited application at present. The beneficial effect of natural measles infection on the course of acute lymphoblastic leukaemia and Burkitt's lymphoma which has been recently suggested is also of interest in this context (Bluming & Ziegler, 1971).

Knowledge concerning immunological mechanisms in malignant disease is steadily growing and it is likely that a more complete understanding of the reasons for the subjugation of the immune response which occurs in malignancy will provide more effective measures to combat this disease process.

TRANSPLANTATION

There are a number of clinical situations in which almost total failure of a single organ may occur in the presence of satisfactory function of the rest of the body. When this occurs in a relatively young person and in the absence of any prospect of improvement, e.g. as in acute hepatic necrosis, renal failure, emphysema, ischaemic heart failure, etc., transplantation offers dramatic possibilities. With tissues such as cartilage and bone immunological rejection does not seem to be a major problem due in part to their relatively poor state of vascularisation. Corneal grafts which were earlier thought to share this inert quality have recently been shown to be subject to immunological rejection especially if the diseased cornea is vascularised prior to operation (Casey, 1972). Apart from the above the only human tissue homografts which have become established in the transplantation repertoire are those of kidney liver and bone marrow. Human pancreas and kidney have been transplanted together in patients with severe diabetic nephropathy but the results to date have not been particularly encouraging (Lillehei *et al.*, 1971). Heart and lung transplantation still present formidable problems and skin has proved to be one of the most immunogenic tissues when transferred as a homograft (Rapaport & Dausset, 1968).

The reasons for this wide variation in organ susceptibility are complex. Kidney homografts may do best because they undergo 'adaptation' (Woodruff, 1960); they constantly release antigen into the circulation (Lawrence, 1968); they are transferred into hosts with impaired immune responses (Dammin, Couch & Murray, 1957); the functional damage incurred prior to transfer into the host is often extremely mild; dialysis allows the recipient to be made relatively fit prior to organ transfer, and because there are relatively sensitive clinical indices of rejection. Despite these advantages, impressive results have only followed the advent of sensitive techniques for tissue typing of both donor and host material. There are now a number of different techniques available and most of them show general agreement regarding the major differences within the human histocompatibility antigen (HL-A) system (Van Rood, 1969; Terasaki, 1970).

Mechanisms of rejection

In most situations cell-mediated immunity seems to be of paramount importance in homograft rejection although experimentally immune sera when transferred to a prospective host can cause prompt rejection (Rapaport & Converse, 1958) and the late failure of kidney homografts may sometimes be related to the accumulation of IgM and complement on the glomerular basement membrane (McKenzie & Whittingham, 1968). Conversely antibody may operate to good effect via the phenomenon of immunological enhancement already discussed on page 441.

By competition with sensitised lymphocytes for the same antigenic receptors in the graft such 'enhancing' antibody may abrogate the effective immune response. Enhancement has been used experimentally to prolong the life of kidney grafts (French & Batchelor, 1969), and attempts have been made to achieve this in man (Batchelor et al., 1970). A wide variety of other measures have been attempted to suppress the host response and these are discussed in more detail in the following section.

Immunosuppression and infection

Most 'immuno-suppressive' agents, including cytotoxic drugs, corticosteroids and antilymphocyte serum, have the serious defect of non-specifically suppressing cell-mediated immunity with the result that a number of viruses, fungi and protozoa (see page 423) may become pathogenic and cause serious problems which may prove fatal. Immunological tolerance and immunological enhancement are both antigen-specific forms of immunosuppression and although it is not yet clear what relationship they have to each other, concerted efforts are being made to apply them to the practical problem of homograft rejection (Batchelor et al., 1970; Brent, Hansen & Kilshaw, 1971). They are discussed more fully in the next section.

Other complications

Two other complications may ensue following successful transplantation. Firstly the disease which affected the original diseased organ may appear in the homograft with equally unfortunate results (Glassock et al., 1968; Merrill, 1969) and secondly the transfer of donor malignant cells along with the homograft may allow the successful development of a tumour in an immunosuppressed host (Wilson et al., 1968). There is now abundant evidence that the non-specific suppression of cell-mediated immunity is associated with an increased incidence of host malignancy especially affecting the reticuloendothelial tissues , brain and skin (Allison, 1970; Doll & Kinlen, 1970; Schneck & Penn, 1971; Walder, Robertson & Jeremy, 1971). Another problem which may follow the transfer of allogeneic tissue (i.e. from a non-identical member of the same species) is that of graft-versus-host disease—a condition already mentioned on page 424. This is most commonly a sequel to marrow transfer and if severe can have fatal results.

In vitro tests for rejection

At present the success of organ and tissue transfer which may stimulate a powerful immune response depends very much on the availability of relatively swift, sensitive and specific laboratory tests to aid the diagnosis of clinical rejection episodes. This enables the dose of immunosuppressive drugs to be kept to a minimum and thus reduces the risk of complications arising from such therapy itself. A number of *in vitro* tests purported to reflect cell-mediated immunity are currently in use, e.g. lymphocyte transformation, leucocyte or macrophage migration inhibition and immunocytoadherence. Some of these techniques have already proved to be of value and analysis of the mechanisms and specificity of these reactions continues (Smith *et al.*, 1969; Falk *et al.*, 1970; *British Medical Journal*, 1971b; Melnick & Friedman, 1971; Munro *et al.*, 1971; Parker & Mowbray, 1971).

HL-A antigen preparation

With a large amount of work currently in progress on the chemical separation, characterisation and preparation of the HL-A antigens (Davies *et al.*, 1971; Etheridge & Najarian, 1971) it is hoped that it will not be long before such refined preparations can be used in these *in vitro* studies of homograft rejection. They will also be of use for raising monospecific antisera for use in tissue typing and may be of particular value in producing states of clinical tolerance and enhancement.

THERAPEUTIC ASPECTS

In the last few years the term 'immunosuppression' has been incorporated into general usage to describe almost any procedure which may cause some reduction in the clinical disturbance and/or pathological lesions of conditions in which immunological factors are assumed to play an important part. However, it is important to realise that in many of the human (as opposed to animal) situations in which 'immunosuppressive' agents have been used there is often inadequate information regarding the pathogenesis of the disease and that very few of these agents do in fact have an effect specifically related to the immune response. It was in association with transplantation that the most urgent need for potent means of inhibiting immunity arose and most of the agents used have been cytotoxic drugs originally introduced for cancer therapy. Soon after the introduction of corticosteroids into clinical use it was realised that they had a potential for dealing with a broad spectrum of chronic inflammatory diseases. However, the exact mode of action of these and a number of other substances in current use is still unclear.

When powerful drugs are used in an attempt to blot out immune reactivity two main problems arise: (*a*) toxic side-effects of the drug itself, and (*b*) infective disease which may be caused by normal pathogens or organisms which are not pathogenic to a normal host but which become so following the development of an iatrogenic immunological deficiency state (see page 423). It is now also realised that generalised immunosuppression may be followed by an increased incidence of malignant disease.

In order to assess the potential value and specificity of the various agents currently available one can consider their effects in relation to the four classical kinds of allergic or immune response described on pages 419 and 431–3; and a somewhat dogmatic and incomplete summary of their relative effects is set out in Fig. 13.4. Inflammation is considered separately because substances which seemingly affect immune responses may only have their effect at this terminal mediator stage without having any effect on specific immunity itself. Some of the evidence has been obtained in animal studies which are not always analagous to the human situation and methods of assessing the response may vary wildly. The dosage, timing and frequency of administration of the agents concerned may cause considerable variation in their effects and in animal studies the timing of the drug in relation to the timing of antigen challenge is of crucial importance. When more than one agent is given at a time, interaction may occur between them resulting in antagonistic or synergistic effects. This has been demonstrated for prednisolone and cyclophosphamide in the rat and may apply to man (Hayakawa *et al.*, 1969). For a more detailed discussion of the rationale for, and actions of, these various therapeutic measures the reader is referred to reviews by Berenbaum (1967); Kantor (1968); Schwartz & Borel (1968), and Schwartz (1969).

X-rays and Cytotoxic Drugs

Sub-lethal irradiation is the traditional way to produce depletion of antibody responses in animals but has only infrequently been used for this purpose in man in view of its toxic, mutagenic and leukaemogenic effects. The effect on humoral immunity is greater before antigen administration but either way it has very little effect on cell-mediated responses. Cytotoxic drugs which function non-specifically as anti-proliferative agents are more effective in inhibiting cell-mediated responses although some, e.g. cyclophosphamide have quite a powerful anti-inflammatory effect. Some inhibition of antibody production can be achieved when higher doses are used and the secondary response (IgG antibody) tends to be more readily suppressed than the primary response (IgM antibody) (Santos & Owens, 1966; Rowley, MacKay & McKenzie, 1969). This may explain the finding, mentioned in the previous section, that kidney homografts which fail after a long period of function often show accumulation of IgM on the glomerular basement membrane (McKenzie & Whittingham, 1968). The drugs most frequently used have been azathioprine and cyclophosphamide although 6-mercaptopurine, chlorambucil and methotrexate have also been tried.

Azathioprine has given beneficial results in the management of diseases such as rheumatoid arthritis (Mason *et al.*, 1969), systemic lupus (Corley, Lessner & Larsen, 1966; Michael *et al.*, 1967; Kaplan, Sztejnbok & Chase, 1968; Drinkard *et al.*, 1970), chronic hepatitis (MacKay, 1968), Crohn's disease (Brooke, Hoffman & Swarbrick, 1969; Jones *et al.*, 1969), ulcerative colitis (MacKay & Wall, 1968; Arden-Jones, 1969), auto-immune haemolytic anaemia (Worlledge *et al.*, 1968), idiopathic thrombocytopenic purpura

(Bouroncle & Doan, 1969) and pemphigus and pemphigoid (Greaves *et al.*, 1971). However, very few of these studies have used methods which permit an accurate and unbiased evaluation; the study by Mason *et al.* (1969) being one of the notable exceptions. Most of these assessments have been made on highly selected groups of patients (often the most severely affected) and side-effects have been common. In general, it is recommended that the maintenance dose of azathioprine should not exceed 3 mg kg^{-1} d^{-1} and that blood counts should be performed at frequent intervals especially during the initial period.

Very few useful comparisons have been made between different anti-proliferative agents but it seems that cyclophosphamide is at least as effective and in some instances, e.g. 'minimal change' nephrotic syndrome (Moncrieff *et al.*, 1969) and renal lupus (Cameron *et al.*, 1970) may be superior. Impressive results were obtained when NZB/NZW mice were treated with cyclophosphamide (Russell & Hicks, 1968). These animals (page 428) provide a useful model of systemic lupus and in those that were treated the incidence of renal disease fell from 100 per cent to 6·7 per cent. Cyclophosphamide has given striking results in rheumatoid arthritis (American Rheumatism Association, 1970) and a particularly impressive feature was the reduction in joint erosions seen on X-ray. However, these results were only achieved at the cost of a high incidence of side-effects although most of them were reversed on stopping the cytotoxic agent. Clinical improvement has also been recorded following its use in uveitis and Wegener's granulomatosis (Buckley & Gills (1969); Novack & Pearson (1971)), and in organ transplantation (Starzl *et al.* (1971)). Cyclophosphamide is most effective in doses which produce leucopenia and the maintenance dose required to keep the leucocyte count at between 3000 and 4000 per mm$_3$ is usually about 3 mg kg^{-1} d^{-1}.

Three valuable studies in rodents have scientifically contrasted the therapeutic and toxic effects of different cytotoxic drugs in relation to their immunosuppressive effect (Berenbaum & Brown (1964); Floersheim (1970) and Currie (1971)). In each of these investigations cyclophosphamide gave a more favourable therapeutic/toxic ratio than other drugs such as: azathioprine, chlorambucil, 6-mercaptopurine and methotrexate, and its significant anti-inflammatory activity was noted. It is obvious that there is an urgent need for further human investigations in which the disease states are clearly defined, the drugs are given in a controlled double-blind manner, and objective methods of evaluation are used. There is a vast amount of published work relating to the immunosuppressive treatment of disease which is impossible to interpret and almost entirely valueless. Individual patients often require individual decisions but before generalisations can be made objective data must be produced. Although something is known about the specificity of action of the anti-proliferative agents, knowledge is still fragmentary and until the types of immunological reaction taking place in these various diseases are clearly identified it will be difficult to match the drug to the disease.

Anti-lymphocyte Serum

Anti-lymphocyte serum (ALS) can non-specifically blot out cell-mediated immunity (Woodruff, 1967). It is therefore considered suitable for the control of homograft rejection and this has been its main application. The disadvantages of this non-specific blockage have already been stressed and although it is now used in many different centres it should only be considered as a holding measure until more specific approaches are available. Depression of interferon production following treatment with ALS has been described and may play a part in the increased susceptibility to infection and neoplasia (Barth, Friedman & Malmgren, 1969). ALS has the added problem that being a foreign protein patients become immunised against it and may respond with anaphylactic or immune complex disturbances (e.g. renal damage) although the induction of tolerance to it by the initial administration of a single

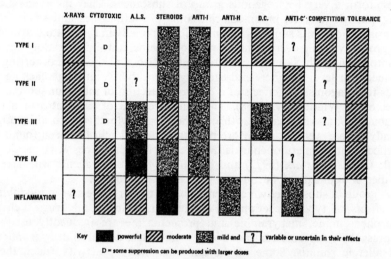

FIG. 13.4. THE RELATIVE EFFECTS OF VARIOUS IMMUNOSUPPRES-SIVE MEASURES ON THE FOUR TYPES OF IMMUNE REACTION AND ON INFLAMMATION. (Cytotoxic = cytotoxic drugs; ALS = anti-lymphocyte serum; Anti-I = anti-inflammatory agents; Anti-H = anti-histamines; DC = disodium cromoglycate; Anti-C = complement inhibitors). For discussion see text.

(Type I = anaphylactic; type II = cytotoxic; type III = immune complex, and type IV = cell-mediated reactions).

massive dose intravenously has been successful (Taub *et al.*, 1969). As anti-glomerular basement membrane antibody has been detected in certain batches of ALS (Fortner *et al.*, 1971) renal damage could also develop due to a type II mechanism.

There is evidence to suggest that some anti-lymphocyte sera may inhibit type III responses as well (Turk & Polak, 1969) and it has also been shown recently that some sera contain an anti-inflammatory protein (Billingham, Robinson & Gaugas, 1970). Both these effects may therefore contribute towards its therapeutic effect.

Corticosteroids

These are the most powerful anti-inflammatory agents known. They also have a stabilising action on membrane permeability, which amongst other things reduces the release of lysosomal enzymes (Weissman & Thomas, 1964). Large doses can have a lympholytic effect and for this reason may be of use in the suppression of acute homograft rejection episodes (Bell *et al.*, 1971). Corticosteroids have a modifying effect on all of the four types of immune response and it is uncertain which of its various actions are most important. The clinical impression is that type III reactions are most susceptible and the administration of steroids can have a dramatic effect on the symptomatology of serum sickness as well as other disorders mediated by complex formation.

Anti-inflammatory Agents and Mediator Antagonists

These form a very heterogenous group of substances. They include; salicylates, phenylbutazone, indomethacin, some phenothiazines and some antimalarials. Gold salts suppress inflammation especially in rheumatoid arthritis but probably act in a very different way to the other anti-inflammatory agents (Kantor, 1968). The latter are able to inhibit various phenomena occurring at the mediator level e.g. increased capillary permeability, although each agent tends to antagonise the effects of a different selection of mediator substances (Spector & Willoughby, 1968). The clinical effects of salicylates in acute rheumatism and rheumatoid arthritis, and of phenylbutazone in ankylosing spondylitis are well known. More recently indomethacin has been found to be effective in glomerulonephritis (Michielsen, Verberckmoes & Hemerijckx, 1970; Clarkson *et al.*, (1972) and it is likely that these agents will have a number of applications beyond the field of rheumatology.

A group of substances which seem to be particularly effective at modifying the effects of type I reaction are the anti-histamines, and drugs such as chlorpheniramine, mepyramine and promethazine are frequently used to suppress the symptoms associated with insect bites, urticarial drug eruptions and allergic rhinitis. Some of the anti-inflammatory activity which these drugs possess may be independent of their ability to antagonise histamine and those with a phenothiazine structure in particular, may be achieving part of their therapeutic effect via a stabilising effect on membranes in general. Yet it is realised that several mediators other than histamine may be released during type I reactions (e.g. slow-reacting substance, serotonin and bradykinin) and it is probably for this reason that antihistamines are largely ineffective in controlling allergic asthma. It is worth noting in passing that the most effective inhibitor of an acute type I reaction such as anaphylaxis is adrenaline which acts by a different mechanism to the antihistamines and when given subcutaneously is the only therapeutic measure which may prevent its dire consequences. Studies in the rat (Orange, Valentine & Austen, 1968) and in man (Mallen, 1965) have suggested that diethylcarbamazine (a standard treatment for filariasis) may be an effective inhibitor of slow-reacting substance. Serotonin antagonists are also known e.g. methysergide, but it seems that in man, unlike certain experimental animals, serotonin is not a common product of immune reactions (Spector & Willoughby, 1968).

Recently a remarkable advance in the control of type I responses has been made. Disodium cromoglycate has been shown to be able to inhibit the release of histamine from mast cells even in the presence of both antibody and its corresponding antigen (Orr & Cox, 1969). This can only be achieved if the drug is administered *before* antigen is introduced (Pepys *et al.*, 1968) and prophylactic treatment can be of considerable benefit to patients with allergic asthma and rhinitis. As yet this drug cannot be given systemically but it is hoped that in the future, preparations of similar substances will be produced which can be used for other examples of immediate hypersensitivity reactions.

Inhibitors of various steps in the complement sequence might be expected to abort both type II and type III phenomena. A cobra venom inactivator of C3 and a shark serum inactivator of C4 have been described but they are both antigenic and are therefore of little clinical value. Nevertheless suitable complement inhibitors may become available in the future and would be particularly useful in the management of such conditions as auto-immune haemolytic anaemia and systemic lupus.

Antigen-specific Immunosuppression

Finally, there are antigen-specific forms of immunosuppression. They include immunological enhancement and immunological tolerance and they probably represent the ultimate in therapeutic manipulation of the immune response. Their superiority lies in the fact that the organism behaves entirely normally to any antigen other than the one in question and therefore problems of iatrogenic infection and neoplasia do not arise. Enhancement is best considered under the general heading of *competition* (see Fig. 13.4) between the various types of reactivity. A well-established form of immunological competition is that which is produced between blocking antibody (usually IgG) and reaginic antibody (Ige) during a course of desensitisation. Enhancement refers to the successful competition of non-cytotoxic antibody with sensitised lymphocytes reacting against foreign tissue such as a homograft or a tumour. In this situation the antibody may coat the antigenic sites on the surface of the tissue so masking them from cellular attack. The application of immunological enhancement to the control of homograft rejection and the potential enhancing ability of antisera raised against tumour antigens have already been discussed in previous sections. The passive administration of specific antibody can also be used to prevent immunization taking place as in the prevention of Rhesus haemolytic disease (A combined study from centres in England and Baltimore, 1971). It is likely that other forms of competition occur between antibodies of different classes and Centifanto & Kaufman (1971) describe the inhibitory effect of IgG on the neutralizing activity of IgA antibody against Herpes simplex virus.

Immunological tolerance is that situation where there is a specific failure of the immune system to respond to a particular antigen. Tolerance is specific for the particular antigen concerned and presupposes the presence of an otherwise intact immune apparatus. However it begins to look as if some situations in which tolerance has been described may operate via some kind of immunological competition akin to enhancement (Levey, 1971; Mitchison, 1971) and the term 'specific non-reactivity' may then only apply to a particular segment of the immune response. Tolerance can readily be induced in the adult by administration of the antigen when the organism is immunologically immature so that it becomes incorporated into the definition of 'self' (Billingham, Brent & Medawar, 1955). In the adult relatively short-lived states of tolerance can be produced by giving particularly small or large doses of antigen (Mitchison, 1968) although other factors may considerably affect this double threshold (Gowland, 1965). Drug induced tolerance has frequently been described although there are some contrasting features with classical acquired tolerance (Many & Schwartz, 1970). The combination of an anti-proliferative agent with antigen can produce a state of specific un-responsiveness despite the use of a dose of antigen that would normally give rise to antibody synthesis.

One of the recurring problems in auto-immune disease is that the antigen has usually been present for a considerable time and the prospects of inducing a tolerant state seem extremely remote. However it has recently been shown that the administration of nucleic acid followed by cyclophosphamide to NZB/NZW mice with active lupus can produce a greater reduction in the level of auto-antibodies than cyclophosphamide alone (Steinberg & Talal, 1970). The induction of a tolerant state can also be encouraged by the co-administration of ALS and antigen (Lance & Medawar, 1969) although if foreign lymphoid cells are used as antigen, graft-versus-host disease may develop. Sub-cellular extracts have been used also in conjunction with ALS to study the prolongation of skin-graft survival and it has been shown for spleen extracts that the time interval between giving the extract and the antiserum is of particular importance (Brent & Kilshaw, 1970); the greatest effect being seen when the extract was given well before skin grafting and ALS treatment. It is argued that this may be because antigen mobilises the relevant population of host lymphocytes which are then eliminated by the ALS. A similar process may operate in drug-induced tolerance. A further development of considerable interest is that liver extracts have an even greater ability to induce tolerance in a similar experimental system (Brent, Hansen & Kilshaw, 1971). This is in keeping with the findings of Calne that a pig liver homograft can prolong the survival of skin, renal and cardiac homografts from the same animal (Calne et al., 1969).

The exact relationship between tolerance and enhancement is currently debated but studies on classical neonatally-induced tolerance in animals have revealed the presence of serum factors which play a major part in maintaining unresponsiveness (Hellström, Hellström & Allison, 1971) and it may be that they each represent opposite sides of the same coin. More recently another specific form of immunosuppression has been described which involves the use of antibody directed against the antigen recognition sites on the host's lymphocytes (Ramseier & Lindenmann, 1969; Davies, 1971). The extent to which these different phenomena may be exploited with regard to clinical problems such as homograft rejection, allergy and auto-immune disease are problems for the future.

CONCLUSION

A number of clinical topics have been discussed in the light of current immunological ideas. Discussion concerning the possible immunological mechanisms that may operate has been based on the principle that immunologically competent cells fall into two main categories: thymus derived or T cells which give rise to sensitised lymphocytes and bursa equivalent-derived or B cells which give rise to antibody-producing plasma cells. Although these two populations of cells may co-operate in various ways the reality of such a distinction is demonstrated by an analysis of the various forms of immunological deficiency states; by studying the pattern of response in infections, 'auto-immune' and allergic disease, and by the action of certain therapeutic agents e.g. ALS. Another point in favour of this compartmentation is shown by the existence of neoplasia affecting these two progenies of cell. Myelomatosis and macroglobulinaemia with their autonomous productions of monoclonal antibody are examples of B cell tumours whereas there is evidence to suggest that the predominant cell in acute lymphatic leukaemia has the characteristics of a T cell (Yata *et al.*, 1970; Moore & Minowada, 1972). Chronic lymphatic leukaemia behaves rather differently and most of the current data supports a B cell origin (Papamichail, Brown & Holborow, 1971; Wilson & Nossal, 1971).

The final outcome of an immune response will always depend on the balance between the various classes of antibody elaborated as well as the relative degree of production of sensitised cells, although none of these can function without involving a number of different but often inter-related mediator substances. The respective roles of the different classes of antibody in defence against infection is only partially understood for although the function of IgM, IgG and IgA antibody is fairly clear the exact role of IgE in non-atopic subjects is still uncertain and that for IgD it is largely unknown. Sensitised lymphocytes seem particularly suited to detecting the appearance of antigens in extra-vascular sites and may thus be ideally suited to detecting antigenic alterations in host material. This is in keeping with the finding that cell-mediated immunity is of particular importance in the response to neoplastic cells.

Although the future may provide a number of relatively sophisticated ways of manipulating the immune response as a means of controlling diseases of various kinds the most promising direction may be towards identifying those individuals who are constitutionally at risk. The classical forms of immunodeficiency are fortunately rare and easily recognised, but minor forms are probably much more common and may be easily missed. However in autoimmune disease, allergy and possibly some cases of malignant disease there are implied constitutional abnormalities and the prompt recognition of these defects may become as important as early diagnosis is now in metabolic disorders such as phenylketonuria and galactosaemia, once suitable means of management become available.

ACKNOWLEDGEMENTS

I am particularly grateful to Professor S. Cohen, Professor P. J. Lachmann, Dr. S. Leibowitz and Professor M. H. Lessof for discussion and advice and to the department of medical illustration, Guy's Hospital Medical School for their help with the figures.

Bibliography

BURNET, F. M. (1969). 'Cellular immunology'. Melbourne University Press. Cambridge University Press.

CALNE, R. Y. (1971). 'Clinical organ transplantation'. Oxford: Blackwell.

GELL, P. G. H. & COOMBS, R. R. A. (Eds) (1968). 'Clinical aspects of immunology'. Second edition. Oxford: Blackwell.

GLYNN, L. E. & HOLBOROW, E. J. (1965). 'Autoimmunity and disease'. Second edition. Oxford: Blackwell.

HERBERT, W. J. & WILKINSON, P. C. (Eds) (1971). 'A dictionary of immunology'. Oxford: Blackwell.

HUMPHREY, J. H. & WHITE, R. G. (1970). 'Immunology for students of medicine'. Oxford: Blackwell.

MIESCHER, P. A. & MULLER-EBERHARD, H. J. (Eds) (1968 Vol. I) and (1969 Vol. II). 'Textbook of immunopathology'. New York and London: Grune and Stratton.

ROITT, I. M. (1971). 'Essential immunology'. Oxford: Blackwell.

W.H.O. (1968). Technical report series No. 402. 'Genetics of the immune response'.

W.H.O. (1970). Technical report series No. 448. 'Factors regulating the immune response'.

References

ABRAMSON, N., ALPER, C. A., LACHMANN, P. J., ROSEN, F. S. & JANDL, J. H. (1971). *J. Immunol.*, **107**, 19.

ACKROYD, J. F. & ROOK, A. J. (1968). *In* 'Clinical Aspects of Immunology'. Eds. P. G. H. Gell & R. R. A. Coombs, p. 693. 2nd Ed. Oxford: Blackwell.

A Combined Study from Centres in England and Baltimore. (1971). *Br. med. J.*, **2**, 607.

ADAMS, E. B., LAURENCE, D. R. & SMITH, J. W. G. (1969). 'Tetanus'. Oxford: Blackwell.

AISENBERG, A. C. (1962). *J. clin. Invest.*, **41**, 1964.

ALEXANDER, P. (1969). *In* 'Fifth Symposium in Advanced Medicine', p. 194. London: Pitman.

ALEXANDER, P. (1970). *Br. med. J.*, **4**, 484.

ALEXANDER, P., BENSTED, J., DELORME, E. J., HALL, J. G. & HODGETT, J. (1969). *Proc. R. Soc. B.*, **174**, 237.

ALEXANDER, P., DELORME, E. J. & HALL, J. G. (1966). *Lancet*, **1**, 1186.

ALEXANDER, P., DELORME, E. J., HAMILTON, L. D. G. & HALL, J. G. (1967). *Nature, Lond.*, **213**, 569.

ALEXANDER, P. & HALL, J. G. (1970). *Adv. Cancer Res.*, **13**, 1.

ALLISON, A. C. (1970). *Br. med. J.*, **4**, 419.

ALLISON, A. C. (1971). *Lancet*, **2**, 1401.

ALLISON, A. C., DENMAN, A. M. & BARNES, R. D. (1971). *Lancet*, **2**, 135.

ALMEIDA, J. D., RUBINSTEIN, D. & STOTT, E. J. (1971). *Lancet*, **2**, 1225.

ALMEIDA, J. D. & WATERSON, A. P. (1969). *Lancet*, **2**, 983.

AMERICAN RHEUMATISM ASSOCIATION. (1970). *New Engl. J. Med.*, **283**, 883.

ARDEN-JONES, R. (1969). *Proc. R. Soc. Med.*, **62**, 499.

ASHERSON, G. L. (1968). *Prog. Allergy*, **12**, 192.

ASHTON, N. (1963). *Br. J. Ophthal.*, **47**, 511.

AUGUST, C. S., LEVEY, R. H., BERKEL, A. I., ROSEN, F. S. & KAY, H. E. M. (1970). *Lancet*, **1**, 1080.

AUSTEN, K. F., KLEMPERER, M. R. & ROSEN, R. S. (1968). *In* 'Birth Defects Original Article Series', Vol. 4, Eds. D. Bergsma & R. A. Good, p. 418. New York: The National Foundation.

AZZOPARDI, J. G., FREEMAN, E. & POOLE, G. (1970). *Br. med. J.*, **4**, 528.

BAGSHAWE, K. D. (1970). *Br. med. J.*, **4**, 426.

BARTH, R. F., FRIEDMAN, R. M. & MALMGREN, R. A. (1969). *Lancet*, **2**, 723.

BATCHELOR, J. R., ELLIS, F., FRENCH, M. E., BEWICK, M., CAMERON, J. S. & OGG, C. S. (1970). *Lancet*, **2**, 1007.

BECKER, E. L. (1969). *Proc. R. Soc. B.*, **173**, 383.

BELL, P. R. F., BRIGGS, J. D., CALMAN, K. C., PATON, A. M., WOOD, R. F. M., MACPHERSON, S. G. & KYLE, K. (1971). *Lancet*, **1**, 876.

BERENBAUM, M. C. (1967). *Symp. Tissue Org. Transplant.* (*Suppl., J. Clin. Path.*), **20,** 471.

BERENBAUM, M. C. & BROWN, I. N. (1964). *Immunology,* **7,** 65.

BERGLUND, G., FINNSTROM, O., JOHANSSON, S. G. O. & MOLLER, K. L. (1968). *Acta pediat. Scand.,* **57,** 89.

BERNS, A. W., OWENS, C. T., HIRATA, Y. & BLUMENTHAL, H. T. (1962). *Diabetes,* **11,** 308.

BIGGAR, D., LAPOINTE, N., ISHIZAKA, K., MEUWISSEN, H., GOOD, R. A. & FROMMEL, D. (1970). *Lancet,* **2,** 1089.

BILLINGHAM, R. E., BRENT, L. & MEDAWAR, P. B. (1955). *Ann. N.Y. Acad. Sci.,* **59,** 409.

BILLINGHAM, M. E. J., ROBINSON, B. V. & GAUGAS, J. M. (1970). *Nature, Lond.,* **227,** 276.

BILLINGHAM, M. E. J., ROBINSON, B. V. & ROBSON, J. M. (1969). *Br. med. J.,* **2,** 93.

BLACK, M. M. & SPEER, F. D. (1958). *Surg. Gyn. Obstet.,* **106,** 163.

BLANDFORD, G. (1970). *Br. med. J.,* **1,** 758.

BLIZZARD, R. M., HAMWI, G. J., SKILLMAN, T. G. & WHEELER, W. E. (1959). *New Engl. J. Med.,* **260,** 112.

BLOCH, H. (1968). *In* 'Textbook of Immunopathology', Vol. 1, Eds. P. A. Miescher & H. J. Muller-Eberhard, p. 302. New York: Grune & Stratton.

BLOOM, H. J. G., RICHARDSON, W. W. & FIELD, J. R. (1970). *Br. med. J.,* **3,** 181.

BLUMBERG, B. S., GERSTLEY, B. J. S., HUNGERFORD, D. A., LONDON, W. T. & SUTNICK, A. I. (1967). *Ann. Int. Med.,* **66,** 924.

BLUMING, A. Z. & ZIEGLER, J. L. (1971). *Lancet,* **2,** 105.

BOOTH, L. J. & ABER, G. M. (1970). *Lancet,* **2,** 1010.

BOURONCLE, B. A. & DOAN, C. A. (1969). *J. Am. Med. Ass.,* **207,** 2049.

BRENT, L., HANSEN, J. A. & KILSHAW, P. J. (1971). *Transp. proc.,* **3,** 684.

BRENT, L. & KILSHAW, P. J. (1970). *Nature, Lond.,* **227,** 898.

BRITISH MEDICAL JOURNAL. (1969). Editorial, **4,** 317.

BRITISH MEDICAL JOURNAL. (1970). Editorial, **4,** 573.

BRITISH MEDICAL JOURNAL. (1971a). Editorial, **2,** 235.

BRITISH MEDICAL JOURNAL. (1971b). Editorial, **4,** 316.

BRODY, J. A. & DETELS, R. (1970). *Lancet,* **2,** 500.

BROOKE, B. N., HOFFMAN, D. C. & SWARBRICK, E. T. (1969). *Lancet,* **2,** 612.

BROSTOFF, J. & ROITT, I. M. (1969). *Lancet,* **2,** 1269.

BROWN, P. C., GLYNN, L. E. & HOLBOROW, E. J. (1967). *Immunology,* **13,** 307.

BUCKLEY, C. E. & GILLS, J. P. (1969). *Archs intern. Med.,* **124,** 29.

BUCKLEY, C. E., NAGAYA, H. & SIEKER, H. O. (1966). *Ann. Int. Med.,* **64,** 508.

BURNET, F. M. (1962). 'The integrity of the body'. Harvard University Press.

BURNET, F. M. (1969). 'Cellular Immunology'. Melbourne University Press.

CALNAN, C. D. (1968). *In* 'Clinical Aspects of Immunology', Eds. P. G. H. Gell & R. R. A. Coombs, p. 756. 2nd Edn. Oxford: Blackwell.

CALNE, R. Y., SELLS, R. A., PENA, J. R., DAVIS, D. R., MILLARD, P. R., HERBERTSON, B. M., BINNS, R. M. & DAVIES, D. A. L. (1969). *Nature, Lond.,* **223,** 472.

CAMERON, J. S., BOULTON-JONES, M. ROBINSON, R. & OGG, C. S. (1970). *Lancet,* **2,** 846.

CARSTAIRS, K. (1968). *Proc. R. Soc. Med.,* **61,** 1309.

CASEY, T. A. (1972). *Trans. Ophthal. Soc. U.K.* (In the press).

CENTIFANTO, Y. M. & KAUFMAN, H. E. (1971). *In* 'The secretory immunologic system'. Eds. D. H. Dayton, P. A. Small, R. M. Chanock, H. E. Kaufman & T. B. Tomasi, p. 331. Bethesda, Maryland: National Institute of Child Health and Human Development.

CHANDRA, R. K., KAVERAMMA, B. & SOOTHILL, J. F. (1969). *Lancet,* **1,** 687.

CHILGREN, R. A., MEUWISSEN, H. J., QUIE, P. G., GOOD, R. A. & HONG, R. (1969). *Lancet*, **1**, 1286.

CLARKSON, A. R., MACDONALD, M. K., CASH, J. D. & ROBSON, J. S. (1972). *Br. med. J.*, **3**, 255.

CLUFF, L. E. & JOHNSON, J. E. (1964). *Prog. Allergy*, **8**, 149.

COCA, A. F. & COOKE, R. A. (1923). *J. Immunol.*, **8**, 163.

COCHRANE, C. G. (1971). *J. exp. Med.*, **134**, 75s.

COHEN, S. (1971). *In* 'Excerpta Medica I.C.S. No. 232: New concepts in allergy and clinical immunology', p. 22.

COHEN, S. & MILSTEIN, C. (1967). *Adv. Immunol.*, **7**, 1.

COHEN, S. & PORTER, R. R. (1964). *Adv. Immunol.*, **4**, 287.

COLEMAN, S. L., BECKER, B., CANAAN, S. & ROSENBAUM, L. (1962). *Diabetes*, **11**, 375.

COOMBS, R. R. A., FEINSTEIN, A. & WILSON, A. B. (1969). *Lancet*, **2**, 1157.

COOMBS, R. R. A. & GELL, P. G. H. (1968). *In* 'Clinical Aspects of Immunology', Eds. P. G. H. Gell & R. R. A. Coombs, p. 575. 2nd Edn. Oxford: Blackwell.

COOMBS, R. R. A. & SMITH, H. (1968). *In* 'Clinical Aspects of Immunology', Eds. P. G. H. Gell & R. R. A. Coombs, p. 423. 2nd Edn. Oxford: Blackwell.

COOPER, M. D., CHASE, H. P., LOWMAN, J. T., KRIVIT, W. & GOOD, R. A. (1968). *In* 'Birth Defects Original Article Series', Vol. 4, Eds. D. Bergsma & R. A. Good, p. 378. New York: The National Foundation.

COOPER, M. D., PETERSEN, R. D. A., SOUTH, M. A. & GOOD, R. A. (1966). *J. exp. Med.*, **123**, 75.

CORLEY, C. C., LESSNER, H. E. & LARSEN, W. E. (1966). *Am. J. Med.*, **41**, 404.

CRILE, G. (1965). *Surg. Gyn. Obstet.*, **120**, 975.

CROSNIER, J., LESKI, M., KREIS, H. & DESCAMPS, B. (1970). *Proc. 4th int. Congr. Nephrol. Stockholm*, **3**, 270.

CURRIE, G. A., LEJEUNE, F. & FAIRLEY, G. H. (1971). *Br. med. J.*, **2**, 305.

CURRIE, H. L. F. (1971). *Clin. exp. Immunol.*, **9**, 879.

CURRIE, S., SAUNDERS, M., KNOWLES, M. & BROWN, A. E. (1971). *Q. J. Med.*, **XL**, 63.

CUTLER, S. J., ZIPPIN, C. & ASIRE, A. J. (1969). *Cancer*, **23**, 243.

CYNARSWKI, M. T. & COHEN, S. (1971). *Clin. exp. Immunol.*, **8**, 237.

DAMMIN, G. J., COUCH, N. P. & MURRAY, J. E. (1957). *Ann. N.Y. Acad. Sci.*, **64**, 967.

DAVIES, D. A. L. (1971). *In* 'Immunological tolerance to tissue antigens'. Eds. N. W. Nisbet & M. W. Elves. (In the press.)

DAVIES, D. A. L., COLOMBANI, J., VIZA, D. C. & HAMMERLING, U. (1971). *Clin. exp. Immunol.*, **8**, 87.

DAYTON, D. H., SMALL, P. A., CHANOCK, R. M., KAUFMAN, H. E. & TOMASI, T. B. (Editors). (1971). 'The secretory immunologic system', p. 274. Bethesda, Maryland: National Institute of Child Health and Human Development.

DEVEY, M., SANDERSON, C. J., CARTER, D. & COOMBS, R. R. A. (1970). *Lancet*, **2**, 1280.

DIXON, F. J., VASQUEZ, J. J., WEIGLE, W. O. & COCHRANE, C. G. (1958). *Archs. Path.*, **65**, 18.

DOLL, R. & KINLEN, L. (1970). *Br. med. J.*, **4**, 420.

DONIACH, D. (1971). Personal communication.

DONIACH, D. & ROITT, I. M. (1968). *In* 'Clinical aspects of Immunology'. Eds. P. G. H. Gell & R. R. A. Coombs, p. 933. 2nd Edn. Oxford: Blackwell.

DRINKARD, J. P., STANLEY, T. M., DORNFELD, L., AUSTIN, R. C., BARNETT, E. V., PEARSON, C. M., VERNIER, R. L., ADAMS, D. A., LATTA, H. & GONICK, H. C. (1970). *Medicine, Baltimore*, **49**, 411.

DUMONDE, D. C. & MAINI, R. N. (1971). *Clin. Allergy*, **1**, 123.

DUMONDE, D. C., WOLSTENCROFT, R. A., PANAYI, G. S., MATTEW, M., MORLEY, J. & HOWSON, W. T. (1969). *Nature, Lond.*, **224**, 38.

EDGINGTON, T. S. & DALESSIO, D. J. (1970). *J. Immunol.*, **105**, 248.

ELLMAN, L., GREEN, I. & MARTIN, W. J. (1970). *Lancet*, **1**, 1104.

ESKIND, I. B., FRANKLIN, W. & LOWELL, F. C. (1953). *Ann. intern. Med.*, **38**, 1295.

ETHERIDGE, E. E. & NAJARIAN, J. S. (1971). *Transp. proc.*, **3**, 224.

FAIRLEY, G. H. (1970). *Br. med. J.*, **4**, 483.

FALK, R. E., THORSBY, E., MÖLLER, E. & MÖLLER, G. (1970). *Clin. exp. Immunol.*, **6**, 445.

FASS, L., HERBERMAN, R. B. & ZIEGLER, J. (1970a). *New Engl. J. Med.*, **282**, 776.

FASS, L., HERBERMAN, R. B., ZIEGLER, J. L. & KIRYABWIRE, J. W. M. (1970b). *Lancet*, **1**, 116.

FELDMANN, M. & BASTEN, A. (1972). *J. exp. Med.*, **136**, 49.

FELL, H. B., COOMBS, R. R. A. & DINGLE, J. T. (1966). *Int. Arch. Allergy*, **20**, 146.

FIELD, E. J. (1968). *In* 'Clinical Aspects of Immunology'. Eds. P. G. H. Gell & R. R. A. Coombs, p. 1063. 2nd Edn. Oxford: Blackwell.

FIELD, E. J., CASPARY, E. A., HALL, R. & CLARK, F. (1970). *Lancet*, **1**, 1144.

FLOERSHEIM, G. L. (1970). *Clin. exp. Immunol.*, **6**, 861.

FOLB, P. I. & TROUNCE, J. R. (1970). *Lancet*, **2**, 1112.

FORBES, J. F. & MORRIS, P. J. (1970). *Lancet*, **2**, 849.

FORTNER, J. G., SHIU, M. H., BALNER, H., WILSON, C. B., SICHUK, G., KAWANO, N., HOLMES, J. T. & BEATTIE, E. J. (1971). *Transp. Proc.*, **3**, 383.

FOX, R. A., JAMES, D. G., SCHEVER, P. J., SHARMA, O. & SHERLOCK, S. (1969). *Lancet*, **1**, 959.

FRANKLAND, A. W. (1968). *In* 'Clinical Aspects of Immunology'. Eds. P. G. H. Gell & R. R. A. Coombs, p. 633. 2nd Edn. Oxford: Blackwell.

FREEDMAN, P., PETERS, J. H. & KARK, R. M. (1960). *Archs. intern. Med.*, **105**, 524.

FRENCH, M. E. & BATCHELOR, J. R. (1969). *Lancet*, **2**, 1103.

FULGINITI, V. A. & ARTHUR, J. H. (1969). *J. Pediat.*, **75**, 609.

GAMBLE, D. R., KINSLEY, M. L., FITZGERALD, M. G., BOLTON, R. & TAYLOR, K. W. (1969). *Br. med. J.*, **3**, 627.

GAMBLE, D. R. & TAYLOR, K. W. (1969). *Br. med. J.*, **3**, 631.

GARDNER, P. S., McQUILLIN, J. & COURT, S. D. M. (1970). *Br. med. J.*, **1**, 327.

GELL, P. G. H. & COOMBS, R. R. A. (1968). *In* 'Clinical aspects of immunology'. Ed. P. G. H. Gell & R. R. A. Coombs, p. XXI. 2nd Edn. Oxford: Blackwell.

GLASSOCK, R. J., FELDMAN, D., REYNOLDS, E. S., DAMMIN, G. J. & MERRIL, J. P. (1968). *Medicine, Baltimore*, **47**, 411.

GOCKE, D. J., HSU, K., MORGAN, C., BOMBARDIERI, S., LOCKSHIN, M. & CHRISTIAN, C. L. (1970). *Lancet*, **2**, 1149.

GOOD, R. A. & PAPERMASTER, B. W. (1964). *Adv. Immunol.*, **4**, 1.

GORER, P. A. (1960). *In* 'Cellular aspects of immunity'. Eds. G. E. W. Wolstenholme & M. O'Connor, p. 330. London: Churchill.

GORER, P. A. (1961). *Adv. Immunol.*, **1**, 345.

GÖTZE, O. & MÜLLER-EBERHARD, H. J. (1971). *J. exp. Med.*, **134**, 90s.

GOWANS, J. L. & McGREGOR, D. D. (1965). *Prog. Allergy*, **9**, 1.

GOWLAND, G. (1965). *Br. med. Bull.*, **21**, 123.

GREAVES, M. W., BURTON, J. L., MARKS, J. & DAWBER, R. P. R. (1971). *Br. med. J.*, **1**, 144.

GREAVES, M. W., SØNDERGAARD, J. & McDONALD-GIBSON, W. (1971). *Br. med. J.*, **2**, 258.

GREAVES, M. F., TORRIGIANI, G. & ROITT, I. M. (1969). *Nature, Lond.*, **222**, 885.

GRIEBLE, H. G. (1960). *J. Lab. Clin. Med.*, **56**, 819.

HADDOW, A. & ALEXANDER, P. (1964). *Lancet*, **1**, 452.

HALL, J. G. (1969). *Lancet*, **1**, 25.

HALL, J. G. & MORRIS, B. (1965). *J. exp. med.*, **121**, 901.

HALPERN, B. N., BIOZZI, G., STIFFLE, C. & MOULTON, D. (1966). *Nature, Lond.*, **212**, 853.

HALPERN, B. N., KY, T. & ROBERT, B. (1967). *Immunology*, **12**, 247.

HAMLIN, I. M. E. (1968). *Br. J. Cancer*, **22**, 383.

HARGREAVE, F. E., PEPYS, J., LONGBOTTOM, J. L. & WRAITH, D. G. (1966). *Lancet*, **1**, 445.

HARRIS, J. E. & SINKOVICS, J. G. (1970). 'The immunology of malignant disease'. St. Louis: C. V. Mosby.

HASHEM, N. & CARR, D. H. (1963). *Lancet*, **2**, 1030.

HAYAKAWA, T., KANAI, N., YAMADA, R., KURODA, R., HIGASHI, H. MOGAMI, H. & JINNAI, D. (1969). *Biochem. Pharmacol.*, **18**, 129.

HELLSTRÖM, I. & HELLSTRÖM, K. E. (1971). *Transp. Proc.*, **3**, 721.

HELLSTRÖM, I., HELLSTRÖM, K. E. & ALLISON, A. C. (1971). *Nature, Lond.*, **230**, 50.

HELLSTRÖM, I., HELLSTRÖM, K. E., EVANS, C. A., HEPPNER, G. H., PIERCE, G. E. & YANG J.P. S. (1969) *Proc. Nat Acad. Sci. U.S.A.*, **62**, 362.

HELLSTRÖM, I., HELLSTRÖM, K. E., PIERCE, G. E. & YANG, J. P. S. (1971). *Nature, Lond.*, **220**, 1352.

HEREMANS, J. F. & CRABBÉ, P. A. (1968). *In* 'Birth Defects Original Article series', Vol. 4. Ed. D. Bergsma & R. A. Good, p. 298. New York: The National Foundation.

HOBBS, J. R. (1968). *Proc. R. Soc. Med.*, **61**, 883.

HOBBS, J. R. (1970). *In* 'Immunology and Development'. Ed. M. Adinolfi, p. 114. London: Heinemann.

HOBBS, J. R., MILNER, R. D. G. & WATT, P. J. (1967). *Br. med. J.*, **4**, 583.

HOLBOROW, E. J. (1969). *Proceedings of the European Society for the Study of Drug toxicity*, **10**, 7.

HORN, L. & HORN, H. L. (1971). *Lancet*, **2**, 466.

HOTCHIN, J. (1962). *Cold Spring Harb. Symp. quant. Biol.*, **27**, 479.

HOWATSON, A. F., NAGAI, M. & ZURHEIN, G. M. (1965). *Canad. med. Ass. J.*, **93**, 379.

HUGHES, L. E. & MACKAY, W. D. (1965). *Br. med. J.*, **2**, 1346.

HUMPHREY, J. H. & WHITE, R. G. (1970). *In* 'Immunology for students of Medicine', 3rd Edn., p. 444. Oxford: Blackwell.

HUNTER-CRAIG, I., NEWTON, K. A., WESTBURY, G. & LACEY, B. W. (1970). *Br. med. J.*, **2**, 512.

IKONOPISOV, R. L., LEWIS, M. G., HUNTER-CRAIG, I. D., BODENHAM, D. C., PHILLIPS, T. M., COOLING, C. I., PROCTOR, J., FAIRLEY, G. H. & ALEXANDER, P. (1970). *Br. med. J.*, **2**, 752.

IRVINE, W. J., CLARKE, B. F., SCARTH, L., CULLEN, D. R. & DUNCAN, L. J. P. (1970). *Lancet*, **2**, 163.

ISACSON, P. (1969). 'Pathogenesis and etiology of demyelinating diseases'. *Add. ad. Int. Arch. Allergy*, **36**, 139.

ISHIZAKA, K. & ISHIZAKA, T. (1968). *J. Allergy*, **42**, 330.

ISHIZAKA, K., ISHIZAKA, T. & HORNBROOK, M. M. (1968). *J. Immunol.*, **97**, 840.

ISHIZAKA, K., ISHIZAKA, T., TAD, T. & NEWCOMB, R. W. (1971). *In* 'The secretory immunologic system'. Ed. D. H. Dayton, P. A. Small, R. M. Chanock, H. E. Kaufman & T. B. Tomasi, p. 71. Bethesda, Maryland: National Institute of Child Health and Human Development.

JERNE, N. K. (1971). *Europ. J. Immunol.*, **1**, 1.

JOHANSSON, S. G. O. (1969). *Proc. R. Soc. Med.*, **62**, 975.

JOHANSSON, S. G. O. & BENNICH, H. (1967). *Immunology*, **13**, 381.

JOHNSON, M. W., MAIBACH, H. I. & SALMON, S. E. (1971). *New Engl. J. Med.*, **284**, 1255.

JONES, F. A., BROWN, P., LENNARD-JONES, J. F., JONES, J. H. & MILTON-THOMPSON, G. J. (1969). *Lancet*, **2**, 795.

JONES, V. E. & OGILVIE, B. M. (1967). *Immunology*, **12**, 583.

KANTOR, T. G. (1968). *In* 'Textbook of Immunopathology', Vol. 1. Eds. P. A. Miescher & H. J. Muller-Eberhard, p. 217. New York & London: Grune & Stratton.

KANTOR, G. L., VAN HERLE, A. J. & BARNETT, E. V. (1970). *Clin. exp. Immunol.*, **6**, 951.

KAPLAN, M. H. (1967). *In* 'Cross-reacting antigens and neoantigens'. Ed. J. J. Trentin, p. 48. Baltimore: Williams & Williams.

KAPLAN, D. A., SZTEJNBOK, M. & CHASE, P. H. (1968). *Arthr. Rheum.*, **11**, 490.

KARATZAS, N. B. (1966). *Br. med. J.*, **2**, 1500.

KAUFMAN, H. S. & HOBBS, J. R. (1970). *Lancet*, **2**, 1061.

KAWANO, K., MILLER, L. & KIMMELSTIEL, P. (1969). *New Engl. J. Med.*, **218**, 1228.

KAY, A. B., GURNER, B. W. & COOMBS, R. R. A. (1970). *Int. Arch. Allergy*, **37**, 113.

KELLER, R. & JONES, V. E. (1971). *Lancet*, **2**, 847.

KELLY, W. D., LAMB, D. L., VARGO, R. L. & GOOD, R. A. (1960). *Ann. N.Y. Acad. Sci.*, **87**, 187.

KLEIN, G. (1970). *Br. med. J.*, **4**, 418.

KOLAR, O. (1968). *Lancet*, **2**, 1242.

DE KONING, J., DOOREN, L. J., VAN DEKKUM, D. W., VAN ROOD, J. J., DICKE, K. A. & RÁDL, J. (1969). *Lancet*, **1**, 1223.

KROHN, K., FINLAYSON, N. D. C., JOKELAINEN, P. T., ANDERSON, K. E. & PRINCE, A. M. (1970). *Lancet*, **2**, 379.

LACHMANN, P. J. (1968). *In* 'Clinical Aspects of Immunology'. Eds. P. G. H. Gell & R. R. A. Coombs, p. 401. 2nd Edn. Oxford: Blackwell.

LACHMANN, P. J. (1969). *Proc. R. Soc. B.*, **173**, 371.

LACHMANN, P. J. (1971). *Proc. R. Soc. B.*, **176**, 425.

LAMBERT, P. H. & DIXON, F. J. (1970). *Clin. exp. Immunol.*, **6**, 829.

LANCE, E. M. & MEDAWAR, P. B. (1969). *Proc. R. Soc. B.*, **173**, 447.

LANCET. (1970). Editorial, **2**, 347.

LANDSTEINER, K. (1936). 'The Specificity of Serological Reactions'. Springfield: Thomas.

LAWRENCE, H. S. (1968). *In* 'Human transplantation'. Eds. F. T. Rapaport & J. Dausset, p. 11. New York: Grune & Stratton.

LEIBOWITZ, S. (1966). *Guy's Hosp. Rep.*, **115**, 341.

LERNER, R. A., GLASSOCK, R. J. & DIXON, F. J. (1967). *J. exp. Med.*, **126**, 989.

LEVEY, R. H. (1971). *Transp. Proc.*, **3**, 41.

LEWIS, F. B., SCHWARTZ, R. S. & DAMASHEK, W. (1966). *Clin. exp. Immunol.*, **1**, 3.

LILLEHEI, R. C., SIMMONS, R. L., NAJARIAN, J. S., KJELLSTRAND, C. M. & GOETZ, F. C. (1971). *Transp. Proc.*, **3**, 318.

LING, N. R. (1968). 'Lymphocyte stimulation'. Amsterdam: North-Holland.

LOUIE, J. S. & GOLDBERG, L. S. (1972). *Clin. exp. Immunol.*, **11**, 469.

LOWDON, A. G. R., STEWART, R. H. M. & WALKER, W. (1966). *Br. med. J.*, **1**, 446.

LUKES, R. J. (1964). *J. Am. med. Ass.*, **190**, 914.

LYTTON, B., HUGHES, L.E. & FULTHORPE, A. J. (1964). *Lancet*, **1**, 69.

MACKAY, I. R. (1968). *Q. J. Med.*, **37**, 379.

MACKAY, I. R. & WALL, A. J. (1968). *Am. J. Dig. Dis.*, **13**, 850.

MALLÉN, M. S. (1965). *Ann. Allergy*, **23**, 534.

MANY, A. & SCHWARTZ, R. S. (1970). *Clin. exp. Immunol.*, **6**, 87.

MASON, A. M. S., MCILLMURRAY, M. B., GOLDING, P. L. & HUGHES, D. T. D. (1970). *Br. med. J.*, **4**, 596.

MASON, M., CURREY, H. L. F., BARNES, C. G., DUNNE, J. F., HAZLEMAN, B. L. & STRICKLAND, I. D., (1969). *Br. med. J.*, **1**, 420.

MATHÉ, G. (1970). *Br. med. J.*, 4, 487.

McKENZIE, I. F. C. & WHITTINGHAM, S. (1968). *Lancet*, 2, 1313.

MELNICK, H. D. & FRIEDMAN, H. (1971). *Transp. Proc.*, 3, 465.

MERRILL, J. P. (1969). *Transp. Proc.*, 1, 994.

MICHAEL, A. F., DRUMMOND, K. N., GOOD, R. A. & VERNIER, R. L. (1966). *J. clin. Invest.*, 35, 237.

MICHAEL, A. F., VERNIER, R. L., DRUMMOND, K. N., LEVITT, J. I., HERDMAN, R.C., FISH, A. J. & GOOD, R. A. (1967). *New Engl. J. Med.*, 276, 817.

MICHIELSEN, P., VERBERCKMOES, R. & HEMERIJCKX, W. (1970). *Proc. 4th int. Congr. Nephrol., Stockholm*, 3, 92.

MICKLEM, H. S., ASFI, C., STAINES, N. A. & ANDERSON, N. (1970). *Nature, Lond.*, 227, 947.

MIKULSKA, Z. B., SMITH, C. & ALEXANDER, P. (1966). *J. Nat. Cancer Inst.*, 36, 29.

MILLER, M. E. & NILSSON, U. R. (1970). *New Engl. J. Med.*, 282, 354.

MILLER, J. F. A. P. (1968). *In* 'Clinical aspects of immunology'. Eds. P. G. H. Gell & R. R. A. Coombs, p. 289. 2nd Edn. Oxford: Blackwell.

MILNER, J. E., EVANS, C. A. & WEISER, R. S. (1964). *Lancet*, 2, 816.

MITCHELL, D. N. & REES, R. J. W. (1969). *Lancet*, 2, 81.

MITCHELL, D. N. & REES, R. J. W. (1970). *Lancet*, 2, 168.

MITCHISON, N. A. (1968). *Immunology*, 15, 509.

MITCHISON, N. A. (1971). *Transp. Proc.*, 3, 953.

MONCRIEFF, M. W., WHITE, R. H. R., OGG, C. S. & CAMERON, J. S. (1969). *Br. med. J.*, 1, 666.

MOORE, G. E. & MINOWADA, J. (1972). *Lancet*, 1, 38.

MOORE, J. M. & NEILSON, J. McE. (1963). *Lancet*, 2, 645.

MORTON, D. L., MALMGREN, R. A., HALL, W. T. & SCHIDLOVSKY, G. (1969). *Surgery*, 66, 152.

M.R.C. Working Party. (1971). *Br. med. J.*, 2, 239.

M.R.C. Working party on Hypogammaglobulinaemia. (1971). Spec. Rep. Ser. med. Res. Counc., 310, London: H.M.S.O.

MUNRO, A., BEWICK, M., MANUEL, L., CAMERON, J. S., ELLIS, F. G., BOULTON-JONES, M. & OGG, C. S. (1971). *Br. med. J.* 3, 271.

NERUP, J., ANDERSON, V. & BENDIXEN, G. (1970). *Clin. exp. Immunol.*, 6, 733.

NORTON, W. L. & STORZ, L. (1967). *Arthr. & Rheum.*, 10, 1.

NOSSAL, G. J. V. & MÄKELÄ, O. (1962). *Ann. Rev. Microbiol.*, 16, 53.

NOSSAL, G. J. V., SZENBERG, A., ADA, G. L. & AUSTIN, C. M. (1964). *J. exp. Med.*, 119, 485.

NOVACK, S. N. & PEARSON, C. M. (1971). *New Engl. J. Med.*, 284, 938.

ODILI, J. L. & TAYLOR, G. (1971). *Br. med. J.*, 4, 584.

OGRA, P. L., KARZON, D. T., RIGHTHAND, F. & MacGILLIVRAY, M. (1968). *New Engl. J. Med.*, 279, 893.

OLD, L. J. & BOYSE, E. A. (1964). *Ann. Rev. Med.*, 15, 167.

OLD L. J. & BOYSE, E. A. (1965). *Fed. Proc.*, 24, 1009.

OLDSTONE, M. B. A. & DIXON, F. J. (1971). *In* 'Immunopathology VI'. Ed. P. A. Miescher, p. 391. Basel: Schwabe.

ORANGE, R. P., VALENTINE, M. D. & AUSTEN, K. F. (1968). *Proc. Soc. Exp. Biol. Med.*, 127, 127.

ORR, T. S. C. & COX, J. S. G. (1969). *Nature, Lond.*, 223, 197.

PAPAMICHAIL, M., BROWN, J. C. & HOLBOROW, E. J. (1971). *Lancet*, 2, 850.

PARISH, W. E. (1970). *Lancet*, 2, 591.

PARISH, W. E. (1971). *Clin. Allergy*, 1, 97.

PARKER, J. R. & MOWBRAY, J. F. (1971). *Transplantation*, 11, 201.

PARKER, M. L., PILDES, R. S., CAHO, K. L., CORNBLATH, M. & KIPNIS, D. M. (1968). *Diabetes*, 17, 27.

PEPYS, J. (1969). 'Hypersensitivity diseases of the lungs due to fungi and organic dusts'. Monographs in Allergy, No. 4. Basel: Karger.

PEPYS, J., HARGREAVE, F. E., CHAN, M. & McCARTHY, D. S. (1968). *Lancet*, **2**, 134.

PERLMANN, P., PERLMANN, H., MÜLLER-EBERHARD, H. J. & MANNI, J. A. (1969). *Science*, **163**, 937.

PETERSON, R. D. (1965). *J. Pediat.*, **66**, 226.

PLAYFAIR, J. H. L. (1971). *Clin. exp. Immunol.*, **8**, 839.

POWLES, R. L., BALCHIN, L. A., FAIRLEY, G. H. & ALEXANDER, P. (1971). *Br. med. J.*, **1**, 486.

PULLEN, H., WRIGHT, N. & MURDOCH, J. McC. (1967). *Lancet*, **2**, 1176.

RAFF, M. C. (1970). *Immunology*, **19**, 637.

RAFF, M. C., NASE, S. & MITCHISON, N. A. (1971). *Nature, Lond.*, **230**, 50.

RAMSEIER, H. & LINDENMANN, J. (1969). *Pathologia Microbiol.*, **34**, 374.

RAMWELL, P. & SHAW, J. E. (Editors). (1971). 'Prostaglandins'. *Ann. N.Y. Acad. Sci.*, **180**, 1–568.

RAPAPORT, F. T. & CONVERSE, J. M. (1958). *Ann. Surg.*, **147**, 273.

RAPAPORT, F. T. & DAUSSET, J. (Editors). (1968). *In* 'Human Transplantation'. New York & London: Grune & Stratton.

REEVES, W. G. & TROUNCE, J. R. (1971). *Guy's Hosp. Rep.*, **120**, 245.

REEVES, W. G., CAMERON, J. S. & OGG, C. S. (1971). *Lancet*, **1**, 1299.

RICH, A. R. (1951). 'The pathogenesis of tuberculosis'. Springfield: Thomas.

RICH, A. R. & LEWIS, M. R. (1932). *Bull. Johns Hopkins Hosp.*, **50**, 115.

ROCKLIN, R. E., LEWIS, E. J. & DAVID, J. R. (1970). *New Engl. J. Med.*, **283**, 497.

ROITT, I. M., GREAVES, M. F., TORRIGIANI, G., BROSTOFF, J. & PLAYFAIR, J. H. L. (1969). *Lancet*, **2**, 367.

VAN ROOD, J. J. (1969). *Lancet*, **1**, 1142.

ROOK, G. A. W. & WEBB, H. E. (1970). *Br. med. J.*, **4**, 210.

ROWE, D. S., ANDERSON, S. G. & GRAB, B. (1970a). *Bull. Wld. Hlth. Org.*, **42**, 535.

ROWE, D. S., ANDERSON, S. G. & TACKETT, L. (1970b). *Bull. Wld. Hlth. Org.*, **43**, 607.

ROWE, D. S. & FAHEY, J. L. (1965). *J. exp. Med.*, **121**, 185.

ROWE, D. S., TACKETT, L., BENNICH, H., ISHIZAKA, K., JOHANSSON, S. G. O. & ANDERSON, S. G. (1970c). *Bull. Wld. Hlth. Org.*, **43**, 609.

ROWLEY, M. J., MACKAY, I. R. & McKENZIE, I. F. C. (1969). *Lancet*, **2**, 708.

RUSSELL, P. J. & HICKS, J. D. (1968). *Lancet*, **1**, 440.

SANTOS, G. W. & OWENS, A. H. (1966). *Nature, Lond.*, **209**, 622.

SCHNECK, S. A. & PENN, I. (1971). *Lancet*, **1**, 983.

SCHWARTZ, R. B. & BOREL, Y. (1968). *In* 'Textbook of Immunopathology', Vol. 1. Ed. P. A. Miescher & H. J. Müller-Eberhard, p. 227, New York & London: Grune & Stratton.

SCHWARTZ, R. S. (1969). *New Engl. J. Med.*, **280**, 367.

SLOAN, J. M., MACKAY, J. S. & SHERIDAN, B. (1970). *Br. med. J.*, **4**, 586.

SMITH, M. G. M., EDDLESTON, A. L. W. F., DOMINGUEZ, J. A., EVANS, D. B., BEWICK, M. & WILLIAMS, R. (1969). *Br. med. J.*, **4**, 275.

SOKAL, J. E. & PRIMIKIRIOS, N. (1961). *Cancer*, **14**, 597.

SOLOWEY, A. C. & RAPAPORT, F. T. (1965). *Surg. Gyn. Obstet.*, **121**, 756.

SOOTHILL, J. F. (1972). *In* 'Textbook of Paediatrics'. Ed. J. O. Forfar & G. C. Arneil. London and Edinburgh: Churchill-Livingstone. (In the press.)

SOUTHAM, C. M. (1968). *Cancer Res.*, **28**, 1433.

SPECTOR, W. G. & WILLOUGHBY, D. A. (1968). 'The pharmacology of inflammation'. London: E.U.P.

STANWORTH, D. R. & SMITH, A. K. (1972). *Lancet*, **2**, 491.

STARZL, T. E., HALGRIMSON, C. G., PENN, I., MARTINEAU, G., SCHROTER, G., AMEMIYA, H., PUTNAM, C. W. & GROTH, C. G. (1971). *Lancet*, **2**, 70.

STEINBERG, A. D. & TALAL, N. (1970). *Clin. exp. Immunol.*, **1**, 687.

STOUT, R. W. (1969). *Lancet*, **2**, 467.

STOUT, R. W. (1970). *Br. med. J.*, **3**, 685.

SYMMERS, W. St. C. (1958). *In* ' Sensitivity Reactions to Drugs ', Ed. M. L. Rosenheim & R. Moulton, p. 209. Oxford: Blackwell.

TAUB, R. N., KOCHWA, S., BROWN, S. M., RUBIN, A. D. & DAMASHEK, W. (1969). *Lancet*, **2**, 521.

TAYLOR, K. W. (1969). *J. clin. Path. suppl.* (*Ass. clin. Path.*), **2**, 76.

TERASAKI, P. I. (1970). *In* 'Histocompatibility Testing 1970'. Copenhagen: Munksgaard.

TERR, A. I. & BENZ, J. D. (1965). *J. Allergy*, **36**, 433.

TOMASI, B. T., BULL, D., TOURVILLE, D., MONTES, M. & YURCHAK, A. (1971). *In* 'The secretory immunologic system'. Ed. D. H. Dayton, P. A. Small, R. M. Chanock, H. E. Kaufman & T. B. Tomasi, p. 41. Bethesda, Maryland: National Institute of Child Health and Human Development.

TURK, J. L. & POLAK, L. (1969). *Lancet*, **1**, 130.

TURK, J. L. & WATERS, M. F. R. (1969). *Lancet*, **2**, 243.

TURNER, M. W., JOHANSSON, S. G. O., BARRATT, T. M. & BENNICH, H. (1970). *Int. Arch. Allergy*, **37**, 409.

TURNER-WARWICK, K. & HASLAM, P. (1971). *Clin. Allergy*, **1**, 83.

TWOMEY, J. J., JORDAN, P. H., JARROLD, T., TRUBOWITZ, S., RITZ, N. D. & CONN, H. O. (1969). *Am. J. Med.*, **47**, 340.

UNGAR, B., STOCKS, A. E., MARTIN, F. I. R., WHITTINGHAM, S. & MACKAY, J. R. (1968). *Lancet*, **2**, 415.

URE, D. M. J. (1969). *Scott. med. J.*, **14**, 51.

VALDIMARSSON, H., HOLT, L., RICHES, H. R. C. & HOBBS, J. R. (1970). *Lancet*, **1**, 1259.

VOGEL, C. L., ANTHONY, P. P., MODY, N. & BARKER, L. F. (1970). *Lancet*, **2**, 621.

WALDER, B. K., ROBERTSON, M. R. & JEREMY, D. (1971). *Lancet*, **2**, 1282.

WALDMANN, T. A., WOCHNER, R. D., LASTER, L. & GORDON, R. S. (1967). *New Engl. J. Med.*, **276**, 761.

WALFORD, R. L., FINKELSTEIN, S., NEERHOUT, R., KONRAD, P. & SHANBROM, E. (1970). *Nature, Lond.*, **225**, 461.

WALKER, J. G., DONIACH, D., ROITT, I. M. & SHERLOCK, S. (1965). *Lancet*, **1**, 827.

WASI, P. (1971). *Lancet*, **1**, 949.

WATSON, D. W., QUIGLEY, A. & BOLT, R. J. (1966). *Gastroenterology*, **51**, 985.

WEBB, H. E. & SMITH, C. E. G. (1966). *Br. med. J.*, **2**, 1179.

WEIGLE, W. O. (1961). *Adv. Immunol.*, **1**, 283.

WEISSMAN, G. & THOMAS, L. (1964). *Recent Prog. Horm. Res.*, **20**, 215.

WHITTAKER, M. G., REES, K. & CLARK, C. G. (1971). *Lancet*, **1**, 892.

WHITTINGHAM, S., MATHEWS, J. D., MACKAY, I. R., STOCKS, A. E., UNGAR, B. & MARTIN, F. I. R. (1971). *Lancet*, **1**, 763.

WILLIAMS, M. H., BROSTOFF, J. & ROITT, I. M. (1970). *Lancet*, **2**, 277.

WILSON, J. D. & NOSSAL, G. J. V. (1971). *Lancet*, **2**, 1153.

WILSON, R. E., HAGER, E. B., HAMPERS, C. L., CORSON, J. M., MERRILL, J. P. & MURRAY, J. E. (1968). *New Engl. J. Med.*, **278**, 479.

WILTON, J. M. A., IVANYI, L. & LEHNER, T. (1972). *Br. med. J.* **1**, 723.

WITTIG, H. J. & GOLDMAN, A. S. (1970). *Lancet*, **1**, 542.

WOLBERG, W. H. & GOELZER, M. L. (1971). *Nature, Lond.*, **229**, 632.

WOODRUFF, M. F. A. (1960). *In* 'The transplantation of Tissues and Organs', p. 96, Springfield: Thomas.

WOODRUFF, M. F. A. (1967). *Symp. Tissue Org. Transplant.* (*suppl. J clin. Path.*), **20**, 466.

World Health Organization Memorandum. (1971). *Bull. Wld. Hlth. Org.*, **45**, 125.

World Health Organization Technical Report Series, 402. (1968). p. 34. 'Genetics of the Immune Response'.

WORLLEDGE, S. M., BRAIN, M. C., COOPER, A. C., HOBBS, J. R. & DACIE, J. V. (1968). *Proc. R. Soc. Med.*, **61**, 1312.

WRIGHT, D. J. M. & DONIACH, D. (1971). *Proc. R. Soc. Med.*, **64**, 419.

WRIGHT, D. J. M., DONIACH, D., LESSOF, M. H., TURK, R. L., GRIMBLE, A. S. & CATTERALL, R. D. (1970). *Lancet*, **1**, 740.

WRIGHT, R. (1971). *Proc. R. Soc. Med.*, **64**, 276.

YATA, J., KLEIN, G., KOBAYASHI, N., FURUKAWA, T. & YANAGISAWA, M. (1970). *Clin. exp. Immunol.*, **7**, 781.

ZABRISKIE, J. B., HSU, K. C. & SEEGAL, B. C. (1970). *Clin. exp. Immunol.*, **7**, 147.

ZUCKERMAN, A. J., TAYLOR, P. E. & BIRD, R. G. (1970). *Clin. exp. Immunol.*, **7**, 439.

CHAPTER 14

THE CARDIOMYOPATHIES

CELIA OAKLEY

Cardiomyopathy is defined as heart muscle disease of unknown cause or association.

Cardiomyopathies can be divided into two major categories and one sub-group (Table 14.1). The two big classes which have clinical, functional and pathological distinction are recognised by *systolic pump failure* which has been called congestive cardiomyopathy (COCM) and *diastolic compliance failure* which is the hall-mark of hypertrophic cardiomyopathy (HOCM).

In congestive cardiomyopathy (COCM) the left ventricular cavity is dilated secondary to inadequacy of contractile function and hypertrophy is secondary. In hypertrophic cardiomyopathy (HOCM) the hypertrophy appears to be a primary characteristic of the abnormal myocardial cell and

TABLE 14.1

HEART MUSCLE DISEASE

SYSTOLIC PUMP FAILURE	Primary congestive cardiomyopathy
	Secondary
	    Heart muscle disease of known
	    cause or association

DIASTOLIC COMPLIANCE FAILURE	Hypertrophic cardiomyopathy
	    With obstruction
	    Without obstruction

OBLITERATIVE CARDIOMYOPATHY	Endomyocardial Fibrosis Löffler's Disease

obstruction to left ventricular ejection is now realised to be an inconstant feature.

A small third category, Obliterative Cardiomyopathy, is appended by common usage rather than of right. In endomyocardial fibrosis which is endemic in certain tropical areas, and in Löffler's disease of temperate regions gradual fibrotic obliteration of the ventricular cavity is frequently associated with atrio-ventricular valve regurgitation. A fundamental difference from other cardiomyopathies is the lack of evidence of a generalised impairment of myocardial function, the haemodynamic dysfunction being a consequence of cavity obliteration and structural damage to the atrioventricular valves.

Three categories of cardiomyopathy are thus identified (Fig. 14.1) and it can be seen from Table 14.2 that among patients with heart muscle disorder who were investigated at the Royal Postgraduate Medical School a cause was found only in a minority of patients. All the secondary heart muscle disorders were of the congestive variety and nearly all the familial ones were of the hypertrophic type.

Any generalised damage to the myocardium whether it be from toxic, infective, metabolic or unknown cause results in reduction of contractile force and if sufficiently severe leads to left ventricular dilatation and congestive heart failure. Only when the cause cannot be found should this failure of systolic pump function be called congestive cardiomyopathy. Before this diagnosis of exclusion is reached, all known causes and associations of left ventricular failure must be eliminated. A list of secondary heart muscle disorders is shown in Table 14.3. When heart muscle disorder is either of

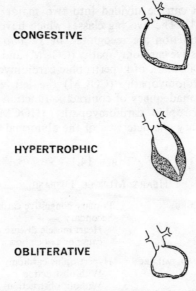

CONGESTIVE

HYPERTROPHIC

OBLITERATIVE

Fig. 14.1. Systolic pump failure results in left ventricular dilatation, Congestive Cardiomyopathy (COCM). Diastolic compliance failure results from abnormal myocardial growth, hypertrophic cardiomyopathy (HOCM) and is not associated with cavity dilatation. The third group is numerically very small, characterised by gross structural changes.

known cause, known association or occurs with involvement of other organs it is preferable that it should be so described, e.g. sarcoid heart disease, pregnancy heart disease or cardiac haemochromatosis rather than as a cardiomyopathy.

The word cardiomyopathy has previously been used to describe any 'acute, subacute or chronic disorder of heart muscle often involving endocardium and pericardium of unknown or unusual aetiology but not secondary to structural deformity of the heart, systemic or pulmonary hypertension or coronary atheroma'. (Goodwin, 1964).

Others have broadened the definition to include myocardial disorders stemming from congenital or acquired defects of coronary blood flow or associated with rheumatic valvular disease (Hudson, 1970). Although it is

TABLE 14.2

RELATIVE INCIDENCE OF THE DIFFERENT TYPES OF HEART MUSCLE
DISORDER
Seen in the Clinical Cardiology Unit of the Royal Postgraduate Medical School, London,
over one decade 1960 to 1970:

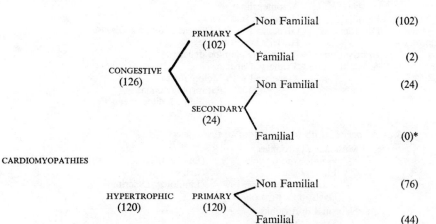

* No patients with familial haemochromatotic cardiomyopathy or glycogen storage
(Pompe's disease) happened to enter the series during this period.

TABLE 14.3

CLASSIFICATION OF HEART MUSCLE DISORDER

I PRIMARY CARDIOMYOPATHY

Systolic Pump Failure	Congestive Cardiomyopathy
	Endocardial fibroelastosis
Diastolic Compliance Failure	Hypertrophic Cardiomyopathy
Obliterative	Endomyocardial fibrosis
	Löffler's Disease
	('Endocarditis parietalis fibroplastica')

II HEART MUSCLE DISEASE OF KNOWN CAUSE OR ASSOCIATION

1. *Infective*   Viral (post myocarditic)
Bacterial (diphtheria toxin)
Protozoal (schistosoma cruzi, Chagas' Disease)

TABLE 14.3—*(cont.)*

CLASSIFICATION OF HEART MUSCLE DISORDER—*(cont.)*

II HEART MUSCLE DISEASE OF KNOWN CAUSE OR ASSOCIATION—*(cont.)*

2. *Metabolic*

Pregnancy	Peripartal and puerperal
Endocrine	Thyrotoxic
	Hypothyroid
	Acromegalic
Familial	Haemochromatosis
Disorders	Glycogen Storage Disease (Pompe's Disease)
	Hurler's syndrome
Deprivation	Beri beri (Thiamine deficiency)
Amyloid	'Primary' Cardiac
	Associated with Melomatosis
	Paraproteinaemias
	Familial Mediterranean Fever
	Chronic Sepsis

3. Associated with NEUROMUSCULAR DISORDERS

(*a*) Muscular dystrophies

Pseudohypertrophic	(Duchenne's)
Limb girdle	(Erb's)
Facioscapulohumoral	(Landouzy-Déjerine)
Dystrophia myotonica	

(*b*) Neuronal dystrophies

Friedrich's Ataxia

4. Associated with GENERAL SYSTEM DISEASES

Systemic lupus erythematosus
Polyarteritis nodosa
Rheumatoid arthritis
Dermatomyositis and polymyositis
Scleroderma
Sarcoidosis
Leukaemia

5. SENSITIVITY PHENOMENA

Serum sickness
Post vaccinial
Sulphonamides

6. TOXIC (due to specific myocardial poisons)

Heavy metals
  Antimony (Stilbamidine)
  Arsenic
  Cobalt
Emetine
Alcohol
Phenothiazines and tricyclic antidepressants
Anaesthetics
  Chloroform
  Cyclopropane
  Halothane

7. Due to PHYSICAL AGENTS

Radiation fibrosis
Heat stroke

8. SENILE

true that myocardial dysfunction may become important in almost any kind of heart disease, confusion rather than clarification results from this usage.

Some of the conditions listed in Table 14.3 do not ordinarily present with the cardiac disorder but if cardiomegaly or heart failure is a known mode of presentation the condition has been included. Most of the toxic agents (including diphtheria toxin) do not give rise to a permanent or progressive left ventricular disorder after removal of the cause but since they can cause death from dysrhythmia or be the occult cause of congestive heart failure the list of drugs is particularly important.

This chapter will be concerned mainly with primary congestive cardiomyopathy and with hypertrophic cardiomyopathy.

PRIMARY CONGESTIVE CARDIOMYOPATHY

In this disorder left ventricular contractile force is impaired (pump failure), blood is incompletely ejected from the ventricles and the heart dilates. Although death may follow within weeks of the first symptoms of heart failure, many patients live for years with slowly deteriorating left ventricular function whilst others seem to achieve a stable state with modest ventricular dilatation and considerable compensatory hypertrophy of the left ventricular wall.

Geographical Incidence

Primary congestive cardiomyopathy is seen in all parts of the world. The disease is common but the real incidence is poorly known. Only since 1967 has there existed a special category for cardiomyopathies in the international classification of diseases (Fejfar, 1968). Most of the data on cardiomyopathies comes from hospitals but the clinical signs are mundane and it is uncertain what proportion of cases are recognised and documented. Data from the few population surveys which have been done suggest that primary cardiomyopathy is commoner in certain under-developed and tropical countries than it is in Great Britain or the U.S.A. Myocardial disorder seems particularly common in Jamaica where coronary atheroma is rare, evidence of abnormality being found in 36 per cent of 269 males and in 43 per cent of 279 females who were examined clinically and by electrocardiograms and chest radiographs. (Fodor, et. al. 1964.) In Great Britain and the U.S.A. where coronary artery disease is common, diagnosis is more difficult as ischaemic heart disease is often the preferred diagnosis in older patients dying from primary cardiomyopathy and the frequency of heart muscle disorder has understandably been underrated.

Age and Sex Incidence

No age is immune and the sexes are equally affected, but children are less often affected than adults.

Pathology

Although the aetiology is unknown and may be diverse, few pathological distinctions can be made between different cases except for those which seem to correlate with the duration of the disorder prior to death.

The ventricles are dilated and the papillary muscles and trabeculae are flattened. The left ventricular wall is pale, soft and of normal thickness in fulminating cases but firm, fibrous and hypertrophied in longstanding cases. Antemortem thrombus is commonly present on the endocardium of the ventricles. The coronary arteries are usually rather free from atheroma even in elderly subjects.

Light microscopy

This may reveal remarkably little abnormality. In fulminating cases some necrosis and round cell infiltration may be visible but the profuse inflammatory cell infiltrates and haemorrhagic necrosis seen in virus myocarditis are absent. Excess myocardial lipid is present and probably accounts for the pallor and flabbiness of the gross specimen. In longstanding cases there is some myocardial cell hypertrophy and scattered fibrosis. Abnormalities in the small coronary arteries are infrequent and mainly confined to intimal proliferation in areas of fibrosis.

Electron-microscopy and histochemical studies

These have so far been even more disappointing. No infective bodies or evidence of virus infection have been found. Necrosis of myofibrils, proliferation of mitochondria, an excess of lysosymes and of lipofuscin granules are non-specific changes.

Clinical Features

The clinical picture depends on the stage at which the disorder is detected and on its severity. Sometimes a large heart is found on a routine chest radiograph in an asymptomatic patient and there is no evidence that the disorder is always progressive. In other instances the cardiac problem seems to start abruptly with a brisk febrile illness of influenzal type after which left ventricular failure develops and may be either severe, permanent and progressive or it may improve and stabilise. The relevance of this premonitory illness may be more apparent than real because early left ventricular failure is still frequently mistaken for bronchitis or 'virus pneumonia' and cardiac patients frequently tend to date the onset of chronic disability from an intercurrent illness.

The symptoms are those of left ventricular failure and vary from acute pulmonary oedema to fatigue and dyspnoea on effort. About 10 per cent of patients describe typical ischaemic cardiac pain. Congestive features with hepatic pain on effort or stooping, leg oedema and ascites may follow but are occasional presenting symptoms in patients whose left ventricular failure has not brought about noticeable shortness of breath.

A small subgroup of patients present with dysrhythmias, often ventricular in origin, extremely recalcitrant, sometimes fatal and often seeming to occur at a stage of the disease when left ventricular function is still reasonably good.

Sinus rhythm is usual but atrial fibrillation often develops in the more severely affected or older patients. The pulse volume is small, pulsus alternans is occasionally a striking feature but may often be found if sought while taking the blood pressure. Mild pulsus paradoxus is common in patients with congestive failure but disappears with diuretic therapy.

The jugular venous pressure is initially normal, later on it is high and shows either a dominant *a* wave in patients who have developed pulmonary hypertension or increased amplitude with a prominent y descent and trough in patients with congestive failure. The onset of tricuspid regurgitation is accompanied by an expansile v wave.

The left ventricular impulse is displaced, and often diffuse. An almost constant feature of the disease is a left ventricular third heart sound which occurs at the moment of completion of left ventricular filling. This may be palpable and can be recorded easily on the impulse cardiogram. The timing of the third sound is earliest in patients with the poorest left ventricular function. In patients with a less dilated left ventricle, a fourth sound due to an augmented atrial contribution to ventricular filling can often be heard.

The second heart sound may be 'single' or there may be paradoxical splitting but is sometimes perfectly normal; pulmonary valve closure may be accentuated.

Systolic murmurs due to functional mitral regurgitation or to tricuspid regurgitation may develop. Occasionally these are prominent enough to arouse suspicion of organic mitral valve disease.

The electrocardiogram is never normal in symptomatic patients and can show almost any abnormality or combination of abnormalities. A pattern of left ventricular hypertrophy with prolongation and distortion of the qRS complex in left ventricular leads and abnormal T waves is most common. Left bundle branch block or hemiblock is frequent, so is right bundle branch block but complete atrioventricular block is rare except in Chagas' disease. A pattern resembling anteroseptal infarction can be misleading (Fig. 14.2a). Evidence of left atrial enlargement is early and right atrial P waves may follow. The total voltage may be increased or low.

The chest radiograph (Fig. 14.3a) shows an enlarged left ventricle with a normal aortic shadow. Generalised chamber enlargement occurs later (Fig. 14.3b).

Evidence of a raised pulmonary venous pressure with dilated upper zone veins is followed by Kerley B lines at the costophrenic angles and pulmonary artery dilatation at the roots of the lungs. Shadows of pulmonary infarction and pleural effusion may be seen.

Haemodynamics

Systolic pump failure is usually advanced by the time a patient seeks advice and is submitted to cardiac catheterisation so that the earliest changes are poorly documented. Reduction in the rate of rise of pressure in the left ventricle before the aortic valve opens (iso-volumic period) and reduction in the ejection velocity are early features. Reduction in stroke volume is at first compensated by an increase in heart rate which maintains minute output. Failure of the left ventricle to empty leads to an increase in residual volume which is responsible for an abnormally high end-diastolic pressure. The high pulmonary venous pressure which follows left ventricular failure gives rise in the milder and more longstanding cases to considerable pulmonary arterial hypertension, but in other instances right ventricular failure seems to be a result of the same myocardial damage which affects the left ventricle; congestive features with a high jugular venous pressure and hepatomegaly then occur with a *low* right ventricular systolic pressure. Mitral and tricuspid regurgitation are common. They result initially from over distension of the ventricles with distraction of the subvalvar apparatus but later there is also dilatation of the fibrous ring of the valves with permanent failure of apposition of the valve cusps. An increase in wall tension for the same systolic pressure is a consequence of an increase in cavity size and this is one of the major determinants of myocardial metabolic demand. Dilatation, tachycardia, reduced diastolic time and increased myocardial muscle mass may be responsible for relative ischaemia. Myocardial oxygen extraction is ordinarily almost complete so that very little extra oxygen is available unless coronary blood flow increases. Whether ischaemia plays a part in advancing the functional derangement at a late stage in the disease is not yet known but it is likely to explain the angina which develops in some patients with very large hearts.

Left ventricular cine angiography best reveals the diminished contractile activity which is seen to involve all parts of the ventricle. The cavity is dilated but of normal shape (Fig. 14.4). The dilatation which results from accumulation of blood in the ventricle provides an automatic compensatory mechanism whereby the amount of shortening of each myocardial fibre may be severely curtailed yet still result in the delivery of a near normal stroke volume. Increased myocardial fibre length at the onset of contraction is also important in the genesis of increased contractile force through the Frank–Starling mechanism but this is relevant in the regulation of the stroke output of the normal heart and has not been shown to have any role in the regulation of the failing heart. There is no evidence that changes in ventricular filling pressure materially influence stroke output in these patients. Diuretics can therefore be prescribed with relief of symptoms caused by pulmonary venous hypertension but without important loss of forward output. Even in patients with advanced myocardial failure the intracardiac pressures may fall to normal or near normal after vigorous diuretic therapy and wrong inferences may be made unless the stroke output is carefully noted and cine angiography of the left ventricle carried out.

Non-invasive methods of investigation have advanced considerably in the last few years and now provide sensitive means of following the progress of patients with heart muscle disease; the combination of phonocardiography, arterial and praecordial impulse recording and echocardiography provide the most valuable information. Measurement of systolic time intervals by simultaneous fast-speed recordings of the electrocardiogram, the phonocardiogram and the external carotid arterial pulse provides an easily repeated measure of left ventricular performance (Fig. 14.5). Total electromechanical systole is measured from the onset of ventricular depolarisation Q to the aortic component of the second heart sound, $(Q - S_2)$, the systolic ejection time (SET) is the interval from the beginning of the upstroke of the carotid pulse to the notch of the incisura and the pre-ejection period (PEP) is the interval from onset of ventricular depolarisation to the beginning of left ventricular ejection and derived by subtracting systolic ejection time from $Q - S_2$; systolic ejection time and pre-ejection period measured in this way vary no more than 3 m.sec from the same intervals recorded by E.C.G. and by a catheter tip micromanometer in the ascending aorta. In myocardial disease pre-ejection period is prolonged and systolic ejection time is abbreviated when $Q - S_2$ is still within normal limits. The ratio of pre-ejection

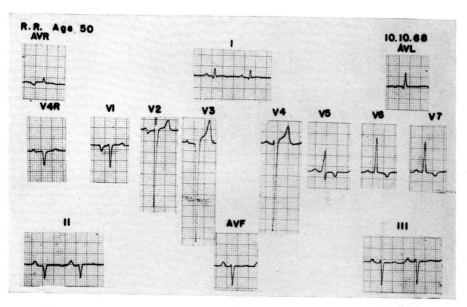

FIG. 14.2. (a) Pseudo-infarct pattern on ECG of patient with COCM whose selective coronary angiograms are shown in Figs. 2b and 2c. The ECG shows left anterior hemiblock and suggests anteroseptal infarction.

[To face p. 470.

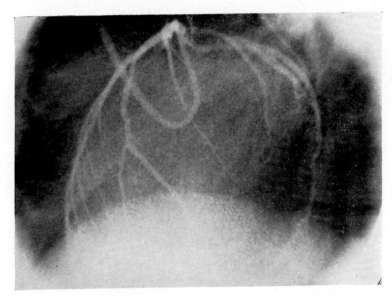

FIG. 14.2. (*b*) Normal left coronary artery seen in left lateral projection.

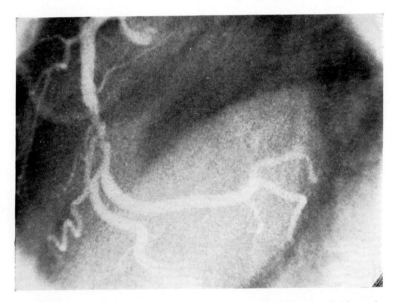

FIG. 14.2. (*c*) Abnormal right coronary artery, also left lateral view. An atheromatous plaque is seen just before the origin of the posterior descending branch but the stenosis was not critical and did not hold up blood flow when viewed on the original cine nor are there any collateral vessels to the distal part of the right coronary. No focal fibrosis was found at autopsy. (Reproduced by courtesy of *Brit. Heart J.* (1971) **33**, Suppl. VI, 179).

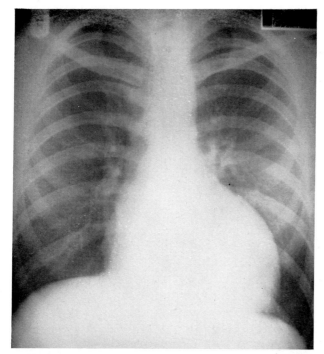

a.

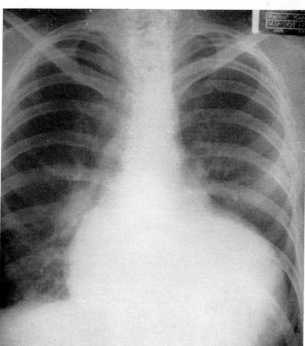

b.

FIG. 14.3. Progressive cardiac enlargement is seen in the same patient. Fig. 3a shows considerable dilatation of the left ventricle and slight enlargement of the left atrium. Fig. 3b shows pulmonary congestion and gross cardiac dilatation which now involves all the chambers; it was taken 2 years after Fig. 3a and 4 months before the patient's death.

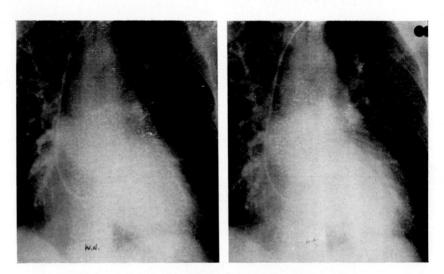

Fɪɢ. 14.4. Angiographic appearance of the left heart chambers after contrast injection into the main pulmonary artery in COCM. There is little visible difference between diastole on the left and systole on the right. The wall of the left ventricle is only moderately thickened.

period: systolic ejection time is relatively constant at 0.35 in health and the increased value of pre-ejection period: systolic ejection time in myocardial disease provides a sensitive indicator of reduced left ventricular function which can be used also to follow progress. This ratio has also been correlated with stroke volume, left ventricular end-diastolic pressure, left ventricular end-diastolic volume and most closely with the ejection fraction of the left ventricle. Since the left ventricular ejection fraction VED — VES/VED* (Miller & Swan, 1964) is one of the most generally accepted measures of left ventricular function these changes in systolic time intervals can be regarded as valid indicators of changes in myocardial performance (Weissler, Harris & Schoenfeld 1968, 1969; Martin *et al.*, 1971).

Analysis of the rate and amplitude of left ventricular wall movement by means of reflected ultrasound is rapidly establishing itself as another non-invasive means of measuring left ventricular performance. An indication of the ejection fraction of the left ventricle can be obtained by measuring the maximum and minimum distance between the posterior and septal walls of the left ventricle in diastole and in systole from the reflected echoes (Fig. 14.6) (Fogenbaum, Zaky & Nasser, 1967; Popp & Harrison, 1970). Ultrasound records of the movement of the anterior cusp of the mitral valve can yield information about the speed of left ventricular filling and the left atrial pressure (Fig. 14.7).

Differential Diagnosis of Congestive Cardiomyopathy

The main differential diagnoses of congestive cardiomyopathy are listed in Table 14.4 together with the more important distinguishing features.

Constrictive pericarditis

Myocardial disease and constrictive pericarditis can occasionally be difficult to distinguish. Fortunately it is more common for a false diagnosis of constrictive pericarditis to be made than for the opportunity of a curative pericardectomy to be missed because myocardial disease has been assumed. The similarities are usually more superficial than real and a correct clinical diagnosis can be reached. Less often the distinction is not made without laboratory studies. Only in exceptional cases should exploratory thoracotomy be necessary.

A clinical similarity with constrictive pericarditis is most likely in the following conditions:

1. Cases of secondary myocardial disease with extensive myocardial infiltration, classically *amyloid heart disease*, because the heart remains relatively small.
2. Congestive cardiomyopathy with endocardial involvement, particularly polyarteritis nodosa and related systemic disorders with eosinophilia. In these ill understood general systemic disorders, it should be remembered that *constrictive pericarditis can also occur* and may even be commoner than a constrictive form of cardiomyopathy.

* Where VED = Volume at end-diastole and VES = Volume at end-systole.

3. *Löffler's Disease*—another disorder with a blood eosinophilia, but very rare.
4. Advanced cases of *hypertrophic cardiomyopathy* (see section on HOCM) with greatly raised left ventricular filling pressure and no obstruction to left ventricular outflow.

TABLE 14.4

DIFFERENTIAL DIAGNOSIS OF CONGESTIVE CARDIOMYOPATHY

Disease	*Differential Features*	
	Relative	*Absolute*
Ischaemic heart disease	Angina E.C.G. Lipid Abnormality	Selective Coronary Angiography
Hypertensive Heart Failure	Renal Disease History of High B.P.	None
Chronic Pericardial Effusion	Relatively few symptoms No gallop	Normal E.C.G.
Obliterative Pulmonary Hypertension with Severe Right Heart Failure	E.C.G. X-ray Pulmonary Systolic Click Early A_2 Late P_2 Pulmonary Regurgitation	No pulmonary venous congestion Normal left sided pressures Normal LV angio
Aortic Stenosis with Severe Congestive Failure	Murmur. Soft A_2 Pulse	Calcified Aortic Valve
Constrictive Pericarditis	Heart not enlarged Calcified Pericardium No Pulmonary Hypertension Equal left and right sided ventricular filling pressures	No LV Dilatation Normal LV Angiogram
Right Atrial Myxoma	Syncope Tricuspid Murmurs Constitutional Signs	Angiographic
Isolated Tricuspid Stenosis	Venous *a* No ventricular enlargement Disproportionate Right Atrial Enlargement	Carcinoid Syndrome
Left Atrial Myxoma	Syncope Mitral Murmurs Constitutional Signs Severe Pulmonary Hypertension	Angiographic

It must be emphasised that 'constrictive' features in primary congestive cardiomyopathy are a direct consequence of incomplete systolic emptying of the ventricles so that the atrio-ventricular valves open when the ventricular

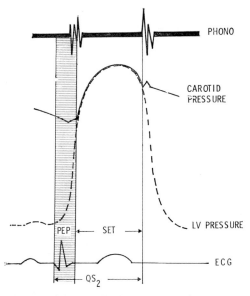

FIG. 14.5. The division of the systolic time intervals (after Weissler *et al.*, 1968).

ULTRASOUND ASSESSMENT OF VENTRICULAR WALL MOVEMENT

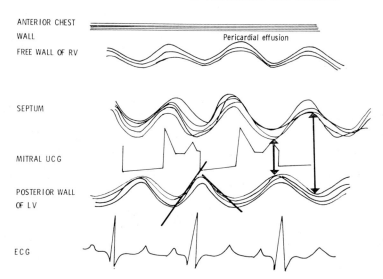

FIG. 14.6. Diagram of the structures from which ultrasound reflections can be recorded to aid recognition of left ventricular dysfunction in cardiomyopathies. The mitral valve echo is shown between the septal and posterior wall echoes; the vertical arrows show the measurements which are taken to obtain an estimate of left ventricular ejection fraction.

The oblique lines on the posterior wall echoes show how measurements of the rate of systolic (inward) and diastolic (outward) movement of the left ventricle can be made. Scale: vertical, cm, horizontal, seconds (not shown).

[*To face p.* 472.

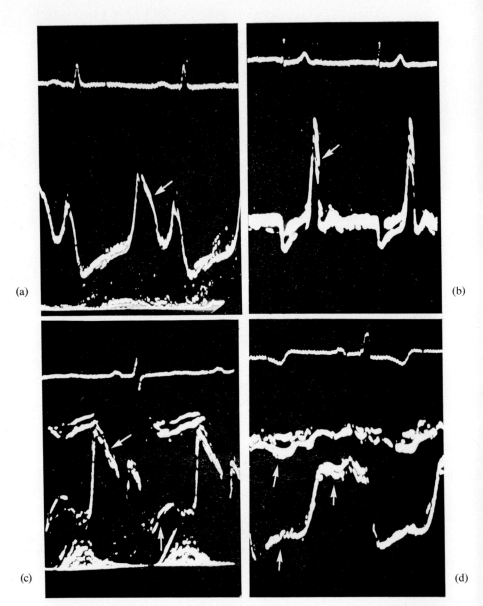

Fig. 14.7. (*a*) Normal mitral echocardiogram (UCG) for comparison with typical
appearance in COCM shown in Fig. 7b. The much more rapid and complete
diastolic closure slope in COCM is obvious (arrowed). Fig. 7c shows a
typical record from a patient with HOCM. The diastolic closure slope
(arrowed) is slower than normal, but of even greater diagnostic specificity is
the systolic re-opening movement (upward arrow). The proximity of the
septal echoes to the mitral anterior cusp is also clearly seen. In Fig. 7d is
shown the record of another patient with HOCM whose diastolic closure
slope is even slower (arrowed). This patient had no obstruction and the much
less obvious systolic re-opening movement is apparent (arrowed). Septal
echoes are shown and arrowed. (Time scale horizontal. The dots are $\frac{1}{2}$ sec.
apart. Vertical dots are 1 cm apart).

cavities are still partially full of blood. The result is reduced and rapidly completed diastolic inflow and a high left atrial pressure. Evidence of pulmonary venous hypertension is nearly always present in cardiomyopathy but is rare in constrictive pericarditis.

Arterial pulsus paradoxus is common in constrictive pericarditis, rarer in COCM but when *pulsus alternans* is found it excludes constrictive pericarditis from the differential diagnosis.

The *praecordial impulse* is usually systolic and active in COCM with a displaced left ventricular apex as well as a parasternal heave. Praecordial pulsation is quiet or absent in constrictive pericarditis. When palpable at all the thrust is diastolic and coincides with the third heart sound.

The *third heart sound* is earlier in constrictive pericarditis than in cardiomyopathy. In the most severe cases it may fall only 0·04 to 0·06 seconds after aortic valve closure and be mistaken for a delayed pulmonary valve closure sound or even for a mitral opening snap. In COCM the third sound is later, rarely less than 0·1 seconds and usually 0·12 to 0·16 seconds after aortic valve closure.

The *electrocardiogram* in constrictive pericarditis shows only low voltage, a shift of the transition zone of the QRS to the left in the praecordial leads and ST − T wave changes. IN COCM the E.C.G. almost invariably gives clear evidence of myocardial disease with widening, deformity and often increased voltage of the qRS. Atrial fibrillation can occur in either disorder.

The *heart size* is always increased in COCM but is frequently normal in constrictive pericarditis. An exception is active tuberculous pericarditis in which epicardial fibrosis and constriction can co-exist with a persisting pericardial effusion.

Finally *haemodynamic study* usually reveals high but bilaterally equal ventricular end-diastolic pressures in the two ventricles in constrictive pericarditis and equal left and right atrial pressures. In COCM the left ventricular end-diastolic pressure and the left atrial pressure are usually higher than the corresponding pressures on the right side of the heart. The relatively milder elevation in left sided filling pressures in constrictive pericarditis accounts for the rarity of pulmonary venous congestion and of pulmonary arterial hypertension in this condition.

Left ventricular angiography in constrictive pericarditis reveals normal systolic contraction and no increase in residal volume. The total dimensions of the chamber are on the small side of normal, and the coronary arteries lie inside the outer border of the heart shadow. In COCM the systolic emptying of the left ventricle is seen to be incomplete, the residual volume is increased.

Right atrial contrast injection for the detection of a gap between the edge of the right atrial chamber and the right hand border of the heart can be misleading because a pericardial effusion is common in COCM with congestive heart failure and a high venous pressure. Echocardiography can be used to distinguish between pericardial thickening and pericardial effusion.

Ischaemic heart disease

Left ventricular power failure secondary to coronary atheroma can be clinically impossible to distinguish from COCM and the final arbiter is selective coronary angiography. In the majority of patients there are sufficient clues to one or other diagnosis to permit reasonably accurate clinical diagnosis, but until the coronary arteries have been seen, a diagnosis of COCM should be considered as tentative rather than proven. Left ventricular failure from occlusive coronary disease can occur without a history of angina or infarction. Normal coronary arteries may be found in obese middle aged men with angina whose left ventricular failure has then to be attributed to cardiomyopathy. Abnormal plasma lipids and a family history of coronary artery disease do not exclude a cardiomyopathy but are clinically significant.

A history of angina was obtained in 10 per cent of patients with COCM and was the presenting symptom in 5 of these. Angina was only seen in those patients who had considerable left ventricular enlargement.

E.C.G. changes suggestive of focal infarction were present in 5 out of 30 consecutive patients with COCM who were seen at the Royal Postgraduate Medical School over a two year period and in whom no coronary abnormality, focal wall thinning, ventricular dyskinesia or focal myocardial necrosis or fibrosis were found. Four of these patients had left anterior hemiblock with changes suggestive of antero-septal or apical infarction (Fig. 14.2). Hollister and Goodwin (1963) pointed out that complete left bundle branch block in a patient presenting with left ventricular failure makes it more likely that the patient has a cardiomyopathy than coronary artery disease.

Distortion of the left ventricular cavity seen on cine angiography with aneurysm formation, localised poverty of movement (dyskinesia) or focal absence of movement (akinesia) makes cardiomyopathy unlikely. In COCM it is usual to see generalised poverty of movement with a cavity which is enlarged but of normal shape whereas in ischaemic heart failure the base of the heart often contracts unduly briskly in sharp contrast to the body and apex. Filling defects due to endomural thrombus and mild mitral reflex may be seen in either condition.

Selective coronary angiography invariably shows occlusion or critical (>90 per cent) narrowing of two or more major coronary branches in patients with heart failure of ischaemic origin. There is usually generalised irregularity of lumen, multiple occlusions and an extensive collateral circulation. Patients with COCM by contrast are mostly strikingly free from atheroma even when in the coronary age group. It is tempting to speculate whether ventricular hypokinesia and enlargement may not protect the coronary arteries from intimal fractures consequent upon the acute angulation which occurs with every systole in the normally active heart. Single plaques do not of course permit a diagnosis of left ventricular failure due to atheroma to be entertained (Fig. 14.2c).

Ischaemic heart disease also arises in the differential diagnosis of patients with hypertrophic cardiomyopathy (qv).

Relation Between Systemic Hypertension and Congestive Cardiomyopathy

Systemic hypertension was a feature in 18 out of 102 patients with congestive cardiomyopathy who were studied. Of great interest were four other patients in whom sustained hypertension only developed after the initial presentation in normotensive left ventricular failure and the blood pressure did not rise until left ventricular function had improved. In these patients the provisional diagnosis of congestive cardiomyopathy had to be relinquished in favour of hypertensive heart disease. If left ventricular function had not improved the diagnosis of congestive cardiomyopathy would have remained. It is common

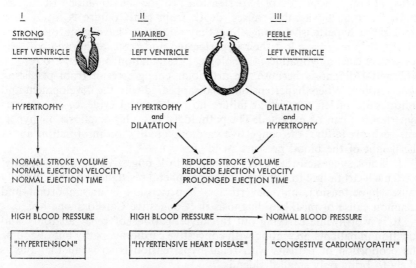

POSSIBLE RESPONSES TO A HIGH PERIPHERAL VASCULAR IMPEDANCE

I	II	III
STRONG	IMPAIRED	FEEBLE
LEFT VENTRICLE	LEFT VENTRICLE	LEFT VENTRICLE
HYPERTROPHY	HYPERTROPHY and DILATATION	DILATATION and HYPERTROPHY
NORMAL STROKE VOLUME NORMAL EJECTION VELOCITY NORMAL EJECTION TIME	REDUCED STROKE VOLUME REDUCED EJECTION VELOCITY PROLONGED EJECTION TIME	
HIGH BLOOD PRESSURE	HIGH BLOOD PRESSURE ⟶ NORMAL BLOOD PRESSURE	
"HYPERTENSION"	"HYPERTENSIVE HEART DISEASE"	"CONGESTIVE CARDIOMYOPATHY"

FIG. 14.8. Schema to show how hypertensive heart disease could masquerade as cardiomyopathy.

to see patients with established hypertension in whom the size of the left ventricle, the degree of failure or the electrocardiographic abnormality seem to be out of proportion to the height of the blood pressure. In most of these it seems that the blood pressure may have fallen with the onset of left ventricular contractile failure. In left ventricular failure with a normal blood pressure the calculated systemic vascular resistance is frequently higher than it is in patients with well preserved left ventricular function and grossly elevated blood pressures. The blood pressure will only be high when the volume and velocity of ejection of blood from the left ventricle is sufficient to bring this about. (Fig. 14.8.) In other words patients with 'Hypertensive Heart Disease' and failure differ only in being hypertensive from patients with 'Congestive Cardiomyopathy' and the latter will also become hypertensive if left ventricular performance improves without reciprocal release of peripheral vasoconstrictor forces.

Observation of hypertensive patients with left ventricular failure suggests that if the peripheral vascular resistance goes up rather suddenly and then remains up, the left ventricle may either recover, in which case the blood pressure will go up, or remain in failure in which case the blood pressure may remain within or close to normal limits. In the former case the diagnosis is likely to be hypertensive heart disease and in the latter congestive cardiomyopathy (Oakley, 1971).

A further piece of circumstantial evidence in favour of a hypertensive basis for so-called congestive cardomyopathy lies in the frequency of hypertensive disease and congestive cardiomyopathy in a population. In Uganda and Jamaica great attention has been paid to the incidence of heart disease with extensive clinical, epidemiological and pathological surveys (Stuart, et al., 1962, Stuart & Hayes, 1963; Fodor et al., 1964; Fejfar, 1968). In these areas, although accidents of hypertension provide the commonest cause of death from cardiovascular causes, death from heart failure is rarely seen among the hypertensive, suggesting that once they have gone into heart failure, they may have lost their hypertension and been categorised with the congestive cardiomyopathies. Pathological examination is unlikely to resolve differential diagnosis because the arteriolar changes result from persisting hypertension. Where hypertension has disappeared with the development and continuance of left ventricular failure no pathological evidence of previous hypertension can be expected. The pathologist bases his diagnosis of 'hypertensive heart failure' or 'congestive cardiomyopathy' on information about the height of the blood pressure in life.

It is not suggested that every patient with 'Congestive Cardiomyopathy' owes his heart failure to a change in the peripheral resistance which ordinarily causes hypertension, but, nevertheless hypertension is an important and common cause of mistaken diagnosis in 'Congestive Cardiomyopathy'.

It is worthwhile carrying out full investigations of renal anatomy and function in patients presenting with congestive cardiomyopathy but of course the proportion of patients with renal hypertension is so small that this is likely to bring only small dividends.

Relation between Hypertrophy and Prognosis in Congestive Cardiomyopathy

The prognosis in congestive cardiomyopathy is very variable. In some patients cardiomegaly has been well documented over as long as ten to twenty years before heart failure and death occur. In others the duration of illness between the onset of symptoms and death is a few months. The relation between the duration of the disease, the severity of the functional impairment, the amount of hypertrophy, the existence of persisting or antecedent hypertension and the prognosis have been studied (Kristinsson et al., 1968; Oakley, 1971). Left ventricular volumes were measured by a modification of Arvidsson's angiographic method and left ventricular mass was calculated by Rackley's method (Arvidsson, 1961; Rackley et al., 1964). Normal data were obtained from patients without disorders of the left ventricle who were undergoing diagnostic catheterisation but were found either to have abnormalities which only affected the right ventricle or normal hearts.

Studies were carried out comparing those patients with congestive cardio-myopathy who had died with those who had survived.

Prolonged survival was unusual in patients in whom the absolute end-diastolic volume of the left ventricle exceeded 200 ml/m² or two and a half times the maximal diastolic volume found in the normal controls. Prolonged survival was also unusual in patients with an ejection fraction of less than 20 per cent (compared with over 60 per cent in normal patients). Patients with a less dilated left ventricular cavity also failed to survive if the left ventricular wall remained thin. The absolute muscle mass did not seem to be relevant but a longer survival time in congestive cardiomyopathy was asso-ciated with a higher wall thickness to cavity ratio. The prognosis therefore seemed to be better when wall hypertrophy matched the severity of the left ventricular contractile failure. Survival in congestive cardiomyopathy seems to be related to the ability of the heart to hypertrophy as well as to the severity of the contractile failure.

Viruses and the Heart: Post-myocarditis Cardiomyopathy

Acute viral myocarditis with pericarditis are well substantiated. All the Coxsackie B viruses have been incriminated but also Echo 9, Echo 6, Echo 30 and Influenza A₂ (Bell & Grist, 1970). During the illness there is often evi-dence of multisystem involvement with pneumonia, myalgia and encephalitis or meningitis. The clinical importance of widespread myalgia in providing a clue to the presence of myocarditis in a patient with a virus illness has been stressed (Lewes, D. 1970, personal communication).

Death due to myocardial failure during the acute illness is not uncommon, but only a minority of patients seem to develop a chronic myocardial disorder although this has been well documented (Saikani et al., 1968; Bengtsson, 1970). It is uncertain in what proportion of patients previous virus infection accounts for the development of chronic congestive cardiomyopathy because no trace of previous infection, viral, bacterial or protozoal is to be found in the myocardia of such patients either in biopsy specimens or after death.

Alcohol and the Heart

Alcohol has been incriminated as a cause of myocardial disease in three ways:—

1. *Cobalt* poisoning in heavy beer drinkers in Quebec.
2. *Thiamine Deficiency* in alcoholics who take grossly inadequate diets (beri-beri heart disease).
3. Cardiomyopathy caused by *alcohol itself*.

The first two are of course only accompaniments of alcoholism. Chronic cobalt poisoning can lead to heart failure in the absence of alcohol and protein malnutrition sensitises the myocardium to the effect of the cobalt. The cause and effect relationship of the cobalt has now been amply proven in experimental studies. The cobalt additive was included in the formula of the brewers as a stabiliser of the froth on the beer, and the uncovering of its role in the causation of an epidemic of heart failure among Quebec beer drinkers is a fascinating story. (Kasteloot et al., 1966; Mercier & Patry,

1967; Morin, 1967). Whether 'beer-drinker's heart' in this country could ever have had a similar basis is uncertain, but cobalt is said not to have been a constituent of English beer. The concentration of cobalt in the Quebec beer was within permitted limits and it was only by the ingestion of such huge quantities of beer that virtually no other source of calories was taken and protein intake was inadequate that the total quantity of cobalt became important.

Beri-beri heart disease is virtually non-existent in this country as it is difficult to avoid the ingestion of adequate amounts of thiamine even on the meanest diets. Thiamine deficiency leads to a high output state and heart failure with a bounding pulse, hot hands and a large dilated heart—quite different from either cobalt intoxication, COCM, alcoholic or other aetiology.

Although strong views are held in many quarters, it is still uncertain if excessive consumption of alcohol can cause congestive cardiomyopathy. The protagonists (Brigden & Robinson, 1964; Burch & De Pasquale, 1968) note a high incidence of heavy drinking in patients with COCM; they state that some patients improve when they abstain from alcohol but that few can be so persuaded and that most alcoholic patients lie about their drinking habits. Certain shapes of the ST segment and T wave of the E.C.G. have been noted in cases of alcoholic cardiomyopathy (Evans, 1959). Histochemical studies have shown heavy deposits of neutral lipids throughout the myocardium and some characteristic electron microscopic appearances have been described with the formation of dense mitochondrial inclusions (Hibbs, Ferrans & Black, 1965; Alexander, 1966, 1967).

Others doubt the connection between alcohol and heart muscle disease. At Royal Postgraduate Medical School no difference was found in the drinking habits of patients with COCM compared with patients with other heart diseases nor haemodynamic improvement after carefully monitored ceasation of alcohol intake over a period of months. The E.C.G.'s have not differed between the alcoholic and abstemious patients with COCM, and finally, it is now agreed that *no* specific light microscopic, ultrastructural or histochemical changes distinguish alcoholic from non-alcoholic cardiomyopathies (Mitchell & Cohen, 1970).

An acute depressant effect of alcohol on left ventricular dynamics has been shown beyond doubt (Riff, Jain & Doyle 1969) but provides no evidence that acohol may cause permanent and irreversible systolic pump failure and experimental rats who daily ingested vast amounts of ethyl alcohol ('a quarter of their weight for a quarter of their lives') failed to develop a cardiomyopathy (Burch, 1971).

The mechanism by which alcohol may cause a cardiomyopathy is quite unknown but it has been suggested that acetaldehyde, the principal metabolite of alcohol stimulates the release of noradrenaline from nerve endings within the myocardium and that this could lead eventually to depletion of myocardial noradrenaline stores (James & Bear, 1967).

The non-selective deterrant effect of alcohol on enzyme induction in the liver may be mirrored in similar actions within the myocardium but the controversy over the role of alcohol in the genesis of cirrhosis of the liver is also still unsettled. (See page 211.)

Alcohol may be one of several toxins which sensitise the myocardium of susceptible subjects to damage by viral or other toxic agents as yet unknown but the case against it remains unproven.

Cardiomyopathy Associated with Neuromuscular Disorders

Heart muscle disease is common in association with heredofamilial myopathic and neuromyopathic disease. In the non-myotonic progressive muscular dystrophies it is an important cause of death. It is an occasional presenting problem in dystrophia myotonica as well as a cause of death and it occurs most frequently of all in a neuronal dystrophy, Friedreich's ataxia.

Progressive Muscular Dystrophy

Cardiac involvement is most prominent in the classic pseudohypertrophic dystrophy of Duchenne, least frequent and more difficult to detect in the limb-girdle and facio-scapulo-humoral dystrophies (Perloff, DeLeon & O'Doherty, 1966).

Clinical detection of cardiac involvement in Duchenne's dystrophy is often not easy because of the effort required for simple tasks, diaphragmatic dystrophy or thoracic deformity but there is a distinctive electrocardiographic pattern that is related specifically to this dystrophy. The right-sided precordial leads show tall R waves or occasionally RSr' or polyphasic R waves. Deep Q waves may be seen in the lateral praecordial leads (Perloff, Roberts & DeLeon, 1967). Abnormal E.C.G.'s have also been seen in asymptomatic female carriers (Mann, DeLeon & Perloff, 1968).

These E.C.G. patterns do not have a clear pathological basis. They have been shown not to be due to thoracic deformity, right ventricular hypertrophy, pulmonary hypertension, conduction disturbances or coronary artery anomaly. It has been suggested that they may reflect dystrophic lesions in the posterobasal portion of the left ventricle.

Plasma enzymes may permit recognition of cardiac involvement if cardiac enzymes are separated from the skeletal muscle enzymes which are more copiously liberated into the plasma. A raised plasma creatine kinase occurs in the unaffected female carriers.

In the more chronic muscular dystrophies of later onset, cardiac involvement may occasionally be a presenting feature and in some instances the evidence for a co-existing skeletal myopathy is hard to find. It is therefore worth seeking out evidence of skeletal myopathy in any patient with a cardiomyopathy particularly the rare patients with COCM and a family history of heart disease. Creatine kinase estimation and electromyography may be used to pick out these cases.

Dystrophia myotonica

Cardiac enlargement, dysrhythmias and electrocardiographic abnormalities have long been known to occur in dystrophia myotonica. Conduction disturbances with atrioventricular block, Adams-Stokes attacks and sudden death have been reported (Cannon, 1962).

Friedreich's ataxia

Electrocardiographic abnormalities have been found in over 90 per cent of cases but heart failure is rare under the age of ten (Perloff, 1971).

The heart shows muscle fibre hypertrophy, interstitial fibrosis and focal necrosis (Hewer, 1969). There is also said to be obliterative disease of small intramural coronary arteries (Ivemark & Thorén, 1964) but angina is rare.

The relationship between the neurological disorder, the myocardial disease and the coronary artery pathology is totally obscure.

Treatment of Congestive Cardiomyopathy

There have been no advances in treatment. The mainstay is still rest, digitalis and diuretics. The worth of digitalis has been measured in serial improvement in the systolic time intervals with relapse after withdrawal of the drug. Burch has advocated prolonged bed rest for up to a year (Burch, Walsh & Black, 1963). In advanced cases the reduction in venous return and heart rate may be followed by shrinkage of the heart and a reduction in ventricular end-diastolic pressures but there is no evidence of improvement in myocardial performance or of permanent benefit as in most cases relapse promptly follows resumption of activity. Nevertheless a wheel chair life may prolong survival and should at least be considered in patients with advanced disease.

Pericardectomy has been tried but the rationale is obscure because an increase in cardiac size following pericardial release is hardly to be welcomed and the Frank-Starling mechanism is usually regarded as inapplicable in these diseased over-stretched hearts. Perhaps the reported benefit (Barnard, 1971) comes from release of excess pericardial fluid which is commonly present and may create a vicious circle of increasing right atrial pressure and increasing transudation of oedema fluid into the pericardium. It is important to look for evidence of a pericardial effusion in patients with a very high venous pressure in cardiomyopathy because striking improvement can follow its removal and initiate an overdue diuresis with a further fall in venous pressure on both sides of the heart.

When the problems of rejection and infection can be better combated, cardiac transplantation will provide the only real means of achieving worthwhile improvement in cardiovascular performance in advanced congestive cardiomyopathy.

HYPERTROPHIC CARDIOMYOPATHY (HOCM)

The first known description of this disorder is that of Dittrich in 1852 (cited by Hudson, 1970). In 1907 Schmincke wrote his account and was soon followed by Bernheim (1910) who probably also described patients with HOCM when he reported obstruction within the right ventricular cavity caused by a bulging and hypertrophied interventricular septum. This was a syndrome which thereafter went by Bernheim's name but its existence was doubted until HOCM was rediscovered half a century later. Modern recognition of the disorder followed the description of Brock in 1957 and of Teare in 1958. Since then intensive studies in major cardiac centres on both sides of the Atlantic have gradually brought better appreciation of the functional abnormality, the broad clinical spectrum and the natural history. Since the disorder was first named, we have learned that obstruction to left ventricular emptying is an inconstant feature and prefer 'Hypertrophic Cardiomyopathy' to our earlier name 'Hypertrophic Obstructive Cardiomyopathy' (Cohen et al., 1964). Idiopathic Hypertrophic Subaortic Stenosis' of the American literature (Braunwald *et al.*, 1964) or 'Muscular Subaortic Stenosis' (Wigle, Marquis & Alger, 1967) in Canada seem to be inappropriate also. 'HOCM' is a fairly euphonius contraction with a not inappropriate meaning in 1920's theatrical slang.*

In some patients with HOCM, obstruction to left ventricular emptying remains unchanged through the years; in others it disappears spontaneously and in still others obstruction may never occur at all. The disorder may take the same or different forms in members of the same family but the pathological appearances do not differ nearly as markedly as the numerous clinical guises and it is frequently difficult to distinguish at necropsy between patients with obstruction and those without obstruction during life.

It now seems that the fault in the myocardial cell is one of increased bulk and decreased diastolic distensibility. Electrophysiological abnormalities recently reported by Coltart and Meldrum (1970) hint at an underlying metabolic fault but so far none has been discovered. The wide spectrum of clinical features and variable prognosis between patients may depend on the geographical location and the number and degree of affliction of abnormal myocardial cells within the hearts of affected subjects.

It is still not known for certain whether HOCM is a single disorder or a series of related disorders. It may be compared to the skeletal muscle dystrophies in which the distribution of affected muscle groups, time of onset and speed of progression determine disability and prognosis. As in the muscular dystrophies some patients seem to have forms of the disease which eventually cease to progress.

Incidence

The true incidence of HOCM is unknown. Certainly it is much more common than used to be thought (Table 14.2). Clinical under-diagnosis is still prevalent and the signs may be attributed to a congenital septal defect or rheumatic valvular disease according to the age of the patient. The reputed rarity of the disorder in tropical countries can possibly be explained by a low incidence of hospital admission because urgent symptoms such as congestive failure are rare.

Inheritance

A familial incidence has been found in nearly one-third of the patients seen at the Royal Postgraduate Medical School. The true incidence may be even higher but recognition of this would depend on examination of first cousins, aunts and uncles of all diagnosed patients in addition to the first degree relatives who have been examined so far.

Pathology

The left ventricular muscle is usually asymmetrically hypertrophied with the septum thicker than the free wall as originally described by Teare, but gross thickening of the free wall may also be seen particularly in the hearts of children. The left ventricular cavity is usually of normal size but may appear to be diminished by protruberance of enlarged papillary muscles into it. The cavity of the right ventricle sometimes appears slit like, wrapped

* HOCUM: hoax . . . (O.E.D.).

around the bulging interventricular septum. The free wall of the right ventricle is either normal or slightly thickened. The valves are normal and the coronary arteries are of larger calibre than in the normal heart.

Light microscopy

Light microscopy reveals grossly hypertrophied myocardial fibres which are often several times thicker as well as shorter than hypertrophied myo-cardial fibres from the left ventricle in fixed outflow tract obstruction. Fibres average up to 90μm in HOCM, 20μm in ordinary hypertrophy and 5 to 12μm in normal hearts. Many of the nuclei are very large and of abnormal appearance with a characteristic glycogen inclusion body with 'perinuclear halo'. The disposition of the myocardial fibres often appears to be disorganised with characteristic 'whorling' (Van Noorden, Olsen & Pearse, 1971). This disarrangement may result from hyperplasia or from profuse fibre branching. A variable amount of interstitial fibrosis is present but no inflammatory infiltrate.

Electron microscopy and histochemical studies

Ultrastructural and histochemical studies have not assisted towards our understanding of the structural or functional basis of the disorder but HOCM can be distinguished from other types of left ventricular hypertrophy by these techniques (Van Noorden, Olsen & Pearse, 1971). Ferrans (1971) has described interdigitating branching of myofibrils in HOCM and although such branching is seen in other hypertrophied myocardia, the branching in HOCM is much more profuse and might account for the development of abnormal isometric tensions during shortening as well as impede diastolic compliance.

It is disappointing that the changes differ quantitatively rather than qualitatively from those in left ventricular hypertrophy due to other causes and Pearse's (1964) earlier suggestion of an excess of nerve fibres and noradrenaline has not been confirmed. Nevertheless the ability to distinguish HOCM fibres from normal or 'normally hypertrophied' fibres (fibres which have undergone normal secondary hypertrophy) *in the same heart* is an interesting development. The shape of the fibres and the appearance of their nuclei allow the distribution of HOCM fibres to be mapped out within the myocardium. This permits the formulation of the 'geographical' hypothesis that variation in the placement and number of these fibres as well as in the time of onset and speed of progression of their functional deficiency could permit almost limitless variations in the end result. This may explain the 'gross' similarity but wide clinical differences between patients with HOCM.

Clinical Features

Early phase

The clinical features depend on the location and severity of the hypertrophy as well as on the state of advancement of the disorder. Cardiac abnormality has not been recognised in the early phases of the disease when symptoms are absent and murmurs presumably clinically inconspicuous or

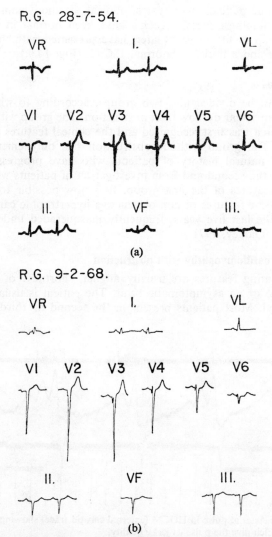

R.G. 28-7-54.

VR   I.   VL

VI V2 V3 V4 V5 V6

II.   VF   III.

(a)

R.G. 9-2-68.

VR   I.   VL

VI V2 V3 V4 V5 V6

II.   VF   III.

(b)

FIG. 14.9. (a) Normal ECG in patient with HOCM, 4 years before presentation in pulmonary oedema with ECG shown in (b). The 1968 ECG shows a left anterior hemiblock and pseudo septal infarct patterns similar to that of the patient with COCM shown in Fig. 2.

absent. There is circumstantial evidence that the visible and functional abnormality is usually acquired although the predisposition is congenital. A very few fatal cases have been seen in infancy. These may have been hearts populated almost completely by HOCM cells. Early HOCM is probably quite unrecognisable clinically and would need more sophisticated haemo-dynamic, angiocardiographic and perhaps electrocardiographic techniques of investigation for its detection than are available today. The electrocardio-gram is not a sensitive indicator of early HOCM, for it has been normal in a number of our patients with typical clinical, haemodynamic and angio-cardiographic findings. Early E.C.G.'s have been normal in some of our patients who, up to fifteen years later, have presented with the fully developed disorder and a floridly abnormal E.C.G. (Fig. 14.9.)

Developed disease

Patients can be divided into two groups, according to whether or not there is left ventricular outflow tract obstruction. The group with obstruction is the one which was first recognised and the clinical features are now very well known. The group without obstruction has only emerged through following the natural history of patients who have progressed from the first group to the second and from investigation of patients whose relatives have typical features of the first group. It is now possible to describe the often unobtrusive features of non-obstructive hypertrophic cardiomyopathy which, until the last five years, frequently masqueraded under all manner of diagnoses. (Oakley, 1971.)

Hypertrophic cardiomyopathy with obstruction

The presenting features are usually angina, shortness of breath, exertional syncope or an asymptomatic bruit. The patient is usually physically well developed. Most patients present in the second or third decades but

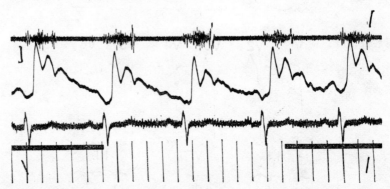

FIG. 14.10. Arterial pulse in HOCM (external carotid trace) showing the systolic dip which give the pulse its jerky quality.

typical features can be present at almost any age. The arterial pulse is strikingly ill-sustained but the pulse volume is not increased (Fig. 14.10). The venous pressure is normal or may show a flicking *a* wave. A presystolic atrial filling beat is nearly aways palpable at the apex (Fig. 14.11a). Sometimes a second systolic outward thrust can be felt after the systolic beat and although rare it is a virtually diagnostic sign of the disorder. The left atrial filling beat (fourth heart sound) is usually of too low frequency to be audible although it can always be recorded on a phonocardiogram (Fig. 14.11b). A systolic murmur follows the first heart sound after a short silent interval. This systolic murmur often starts rather abruptly and is decrescendo up to the aortic closure sound (Fig. 14.12a). The systolic murmur is usually maximal at or inside the apex but is often transmitted to the axilla. It is usually less well heard in the aortic area and is poorly transmitted up the carotids. An apical third heart sound is occasionally heard and is said to be commoner in the patients with mitral regurgitation (Schlesinger, F. 1971, personal communication). Sometimes a short mid-diastolic murmur can be heard. A non-specific

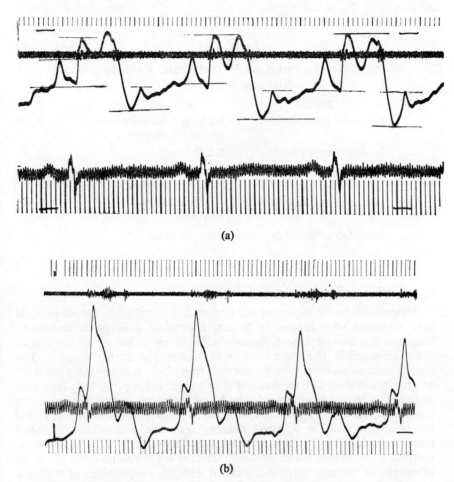

(a)

(b)

Fig. 14.11. (a) Impulse record before and (b) after treatment with propranolol in a patient with HOCM.

diamond shaped ejection murmur may be heard at the left sternal edge and is produced in the right ventricular outflow tract. The apical asymmetrical systolic murmur has been shown in haemodynamic studies to be produced at the site of the outflow tract gradient. It is thus a clinical indicator of the presence of left ventricular outflow tract obstruction.

A murmur of similar shape has been recorded in the left atrium from the same patients. Since the outflow tract obstruction and the mitral regurgitation have similar timing and usually occur together, the murmurs due to these two haemodynamic faults cannot easily be separated one from the other by external auscultation. The ejection murmur at the left sternal edge is frequently associated with the presence of a small gradient in the ventricular cavity attributable to encroachment of the septum upon this cavity (Bernheim Effect). The second heart sound frequently shows reversed splitting with P_2 preceding A_2 on expiration. The differential diagnosis is summarised in Table 14.5.

TABLE 14.5

DIFFERENTIAL DIAGNOSIS OF HYPERTROPHIC CARDIOMYOPATHY
WITHOUT OBSTRUCTION

Disease	Differential Features
Congestive Cardiomyopathy	3rd heart sound more common Angina less common
Ischaemic Heart Disease	E.C.G. usually
'Silent' Mitral Stenosis	Calcification of the mitral valve Pulmonary hypertension
Left Atrial Myxoma	Constitutional signs Murmurs
Constrictive Pericarditis	Early 3rd sound E.C.G. Sometimes calcification

Hypertrophic cardiomyopathy without obstruction

Dyspnoea is by far the commonest presenting symptom but other patients have presented with congestive failure, abdominal swelling or embolism. Murmurs are usually absent. Sinus rhythm is usual but atrial fibrillation is not uncommon. The pulse is of small volume and normal contour. The jugular venous pressure may be normal, may show a dominant *a* wave or be grossly elevated. The cardiac impulse is quiet but a presystolic beat may be felt. The second heart sound may be rather widely split due to an early aortic component and sometimes the delayed pulmonary valve closure sound has been mistaken for a mitral opening snap and a diagnosis of mitral stenosis made (Fig. 14.12b). A third heart sound or short mid-diastolic murmur is sometimes heard. Systolic murmurs are uncommon but the onset of congestive features may be associated with the development of tricuspid regurgitation and a pansystolic murmur.

Atrial fibrillation is uncommon until the disease had advanced to a stage where the left ventricular end diastolic pressure is extremely high. The loss of the atrial contribution to left ventricular filling associated with an irregular rate with many diastolic intervals of inadequate length for optimal filling of the incompliant left ventricle usually results in severe clinical deterioration from a fall in output. Nevertheless many patients stabilise and can continue many years after the onset of the dysrhythmia.

Embolism is a common complication of atrial fibrillation in HOCM and should be combated by anticoagulant therapy on a permanent basis. It is not possibe to distinguish from the electrocardiogram or from the

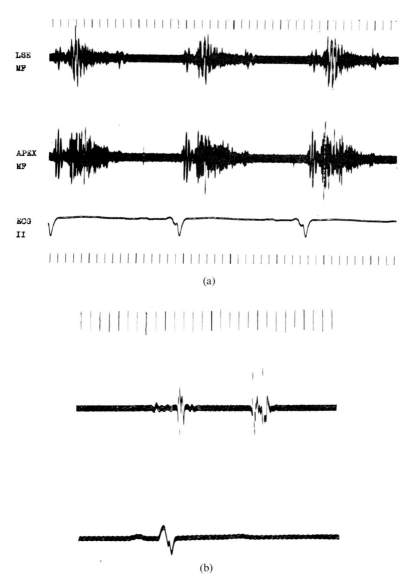

FIG. 14.12. (a) Typical phonocardiogram (PCG) in HOCM with outflow obstruction.

(b) PCG in HOCM without obstruction to show presystolic (atrial) sound and widely split second heart sound.

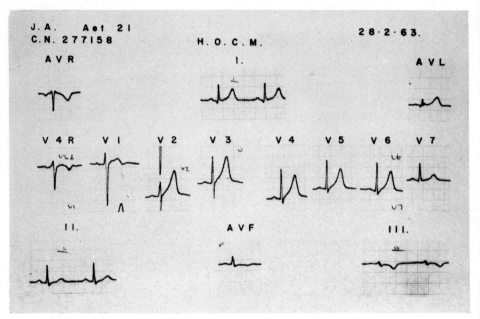

FIG. 14.13. ECG's in HOCM.

(a) Only mildly abnormal ECG (very tall T waves) from a 21 year old man who dropped dead in a fight. Autopsy showed typical and floridly severe HOCM confirming the clinical and laboratory findings in life.

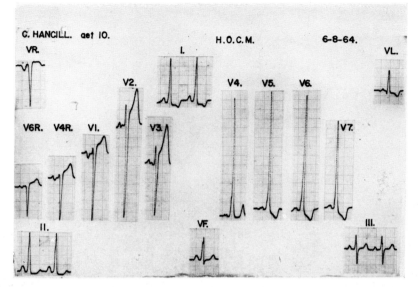

FIG. 14.13. ECG's in HOCM.

(b) Typical psuedo pre-excitation pattern from a boy with severe distinctive HOCM. Note short P-R, absent q and widened qRS with suspicion of a delta wave in V4-7.

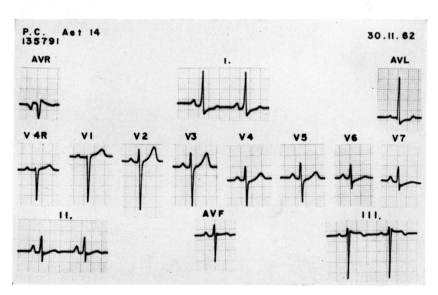

(c) ECG from a 14 year old girl, a member of a family with a high incidence of sudden death from HOCM. It shows a less dramatic version of the ECG shown in Fig. 14b but the PR interval is within normal limits.

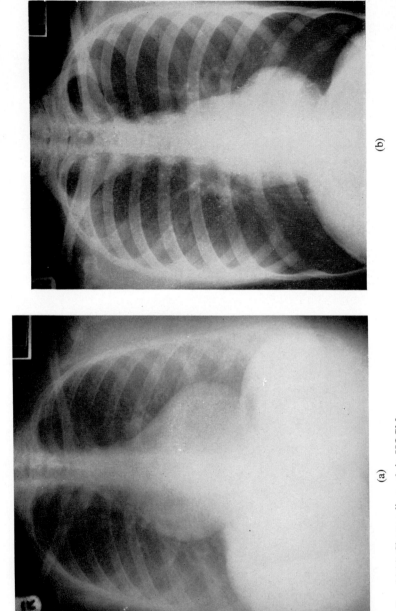

(a)

(b)

FIG. 14.14. Chest radiograph in HOCM.

(a) globular heart in patient whose ECG was shown in Fig. 14.13c. (b) normal appearance apart from 'squared off' apex from a 17 year old girl with severe HOCM.

cardiac silhouette between patients with obstruction and those without it. Table 14.6 summarises the differential diagnosis in HOCM without obstruction. The *Electrocardiogram* can be normal or bizarrely abnormal (Fig. 14.13). While certain features and combinations hint strongly at the diagnosis of HOCM, the abnormality can be quite mundane and suggest ischaemic or rheumatic heart disease. In contrast to COCM a normal E.C.G. does not weigh strongly against a diagnosis of HOCM particularly if the patient is young. Rarely the E.C.G. can be near to normal even in patients who die suddenly.

E.C.G. features which suggest HOCM in a child are a very high voltage qRS but otherwise normal complexes. Deep but narrow *q* waves in lateral, mid or even in right praecordial leads, or an appearance similar to that in ventricular pre-excitation with a somewhat short P–R interval, absence of the normal septal *q* waves and a prolonged high voltage qRS may be seen.

TABLE 14.6

DIFFERENTIAL DIAGNOSIS OF HYPERTROPHIC CARDIOMYOPATHY
WITH OBSTRUCTION

Disease	Differential Features
Aortic Stenosis	Sustained pulse Click or valve calcification E.D.M. common Post-stenotic dilatation
Discrete Subaortic Stenosis	Pulse may be small Soft A₂ E.D.M. common
Rheumatic Mitral Regurgitation	AF common. Big LA Pansystolic murmur Response to drugs
Non-rheumatic Mitral Regurgitation	Sometimes midsystolic click 3rd heart sound
Small Ventricular Septal Defect	Pansystolic or early systolic murmur No atrial beat

Common E.C.G. features are signs of left and/or right ventricular hypertrophy, diffuse repolarisation changes and very rarely complete left or right bundle branch block.

When an E.C.G. with any such abnormalities in ventricular depolarisation or repolarisation is seen the presence of disproportionate left atrial, right atrial or biatrial P waves should immediately support HOCM. They reflect the high end-diastolic pressures in the ventricles.

The *Chest Radiograph* is also much more variable in appearance in HOCM than it is in COCM (Fig. 14.14). This is because increased muscle bulk has to be very gross to deform the cardiac outline and dilatation of chambers upstream from the left ventricle in HOCM depends on multiple factors such as the severity of the impediment to ventricular filling, age and duration of disease. A completely normal cardiac silhouette does not exclude a diagnosis of HOCM. In general the heart is usually less enlarged than in COCM. The aorta is not dilated. Sometimes the left border of the left ventricle below the left atrium shows a prominence due to muscular hyper-trophy and this can give an otherwise normal cardiac silhouette a charac-teristic square outline.

Very often the heart is a little bulky but of normal shape. In more severe cases the left atrium is dilated and there may be evidence of pulmonary venous hypertension mimicking mitral valve disease. When the left atrium dilates in HOCM it usually dwarfs the left ventricle whereas the reverse is true in COCM.

In cases with congestive failure the heart usually remains relatively small and it is this which often raises the question of constrictive peri-carditis. In rare instances marked cardiac enlargement is associated with the development of a pericardial effusion or with dilatation of the right heart chambers.

Haemodynamics

The diagnostic feature is the finding of a raised left ventricular end-diastolic pressure (LVEDP) in association with an increase in the thickness of the left ventricular wall and in the absence of discernible cause (Fig. 14.15a).

This pressure is sometimes at the upper limit of normal at rest but shows an enhanced atrial 'kick'. It continually rises briskly on exercise or after intravenous isoprenaline (2 to 4 μg are sufficient) and this response greatly aids recognition of the disease in mild cases in which normality is the alterna-tive diagnosis. The normal heart usually shows a fall or no change in the pressure after exercise or isoprenaline.

A systolic pressure drop between the cavity and vestibule of the left ventricle is not invariable in HOCM nor can a gradient aways be induced pharmacolo-gically. Provocation of outflow tract obstruction is better achieved by inhala-tion of amyl nitrite (Fig. 14.15a) than with isoprenaline as the latter can cause a spurious gradient due to overshoot or catheter-trapping associated with enhanced left ventricular emptying. A gradient is often first seen after diagnostic LV angiography and the effect of this obligatory provocation can be assessed prior to the introduction of other agents. If the aortic pulse fails to show a systolic dip in a patient with a gradient, artefact (due to catheter trapping) should be suspected.

In patients with obstruction to left ventricular ejection the aortic pressure pulse shows a rapid upstroke and an equally rapid fall off to a systolic dip followed by a delayed tidal wave associated with prolonged left ventricular ejection. It is this ill-sustained percussion wave which gives the pulse its cha-racteristic jerky quality to palpation. The commencement of the systolic dip coincides with the onset of obstruction following early unimpeded ejection of blood from the ventricle (Fig. 14.15a). The velocity of left ventricular ejection is suddenly curtailed and a notch marks the left ventricular pressure pulses at the commencement of mitral reflux coincident with the onset of obstruction. At the same time murmurs can be recorded from the left ventricular outflow tract and from within the left atrium showing their dual origin in these patients (Fig. 14.15b and 14.15c). The gradient can be completely abolished with phenylephrine in HOCM but not in fixed organic stenosis and 0·3 to 0·5 mg of phenylephrine should be administered in any patient in whom organic

B.F. AMYL NITRITE

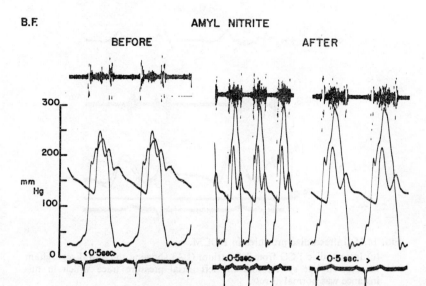

FIG. 14.15. Intracardiac pressures in HOCM.

(a) Simultaneous LV and central aorta showing high LVEDP, rising further after amylnitrite which has induced obstruction and typical change in the arterial pulse.

H.M. INTRA-CARDIAC P.C.G. L.V. OUTFLOW

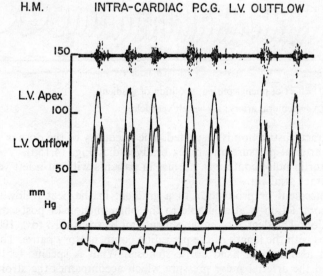

(b) Intracardiac PCG showing the origin of the murmur in the outflow tract of the left ventricle (LV). The pressure difference between the apex and outflow portion of the LV is seen in the simultaneously inscribed traces.

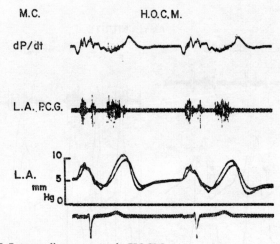

FIG. 14.15. Intracardiac pressures in HOCM.

(c) Intracardiac PCG from left atrium (LA) showing the mitral regurgitant murmur in late systole and the left atrial pressure trace which in this instance was normal at rest.

HYPERTROPHIC CARDIOMYOPATHY WITH OBSTRUCTION.

EFFECT OF I.V. PHENYLEPHRINE 0·3mgm.

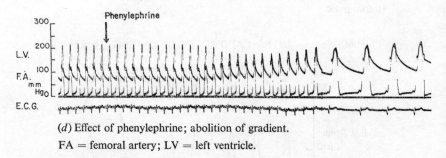

(d) Effect of phenylephrine; abolition of gradient.

FA = femoral artery; LV = left ventricle.

outflow tract obstruction is suspected. The adequacy of the dose is shown by a rise in arterial pressure and reflex bradycardia (Fig. 14.15d).

The aortic pulse contour is normal in patients without a left ventricular outflow tract gradient.

Enhancement or production of a gradient in the beat following a premature contraction is attributable to the phenomenon of post-extrasystolic potentiation. The degree of enhancement can be from zero to >100 mm Hg and varies with the length of the preceding compensatory pause. This phenomenon is also seen in fixed aortic stenosis. What is specific to HOCM is the fall in the arterial pulse pressure which accompanies the stronger beat. (Brockenbrough, Braunwald & Morrow, 1961). Absence of the post-ectopic beat phenomena in HOCM patients without outflow tract obstruction does not preclude the diagnosis but its absence in patients with a gradient at rest or after provocation by other means is against a diagnosis of HOCM.

Left atrial hypertension can be absent at rest or very marked and the pulmonary artery pressure also may be normal but it can be considerably elevated in severe cases. A gradient within the right ventricular cavity can often be recorded and is attributable to encroachment of the hypertrophied septum on the right ventricular cavity. The right atrial pressure pulse often shows an augmented *a* wave in such cases in the absence of pulmonary hypertension (Bernheim Effect). A high right ventricular end-diastolic pressure is common and is associated with cavity restriction in some cases and to right ventricular pump failure in rare instances with advanced disease.

The cardiac output may be normal or low at rest but it fails to rise normally on exercise. In severe cases the tachycardia of exercise is associated with a fall in stroke volume and a rise in left atrial pressure and in left ventricular end-diastolic pressure.

Selective left ventricular angiography is best carried out as a ciné study in the right anterior oblique projection which best reveals cavity size and shape in systole and diastole, the anatomy of the outflow tract and the presence and timing of any mitral regurgitation (Fig. 14.16a). Although systolic deformation of the cavity caused by hypertrophied papillary muscles and a bulging septal wall is common these features are not always present. The diagnosis is based only on proof of left ventricular hypertrophy after exclusion of any known cause. A normally shaped left ventricular cavity does not preclude the diagnosis; it may be seen in patients without outflow tract obstruction and particularly in children who frequently show no obstruction but have a particularly severe form of the disease.

The coronary arteries are of unusually wide calibre in HOCM and it is common to see a profusion of small vessels which in normals are too small to be visible. Differentiation of left ventricular muscle thickening from pericardial effusion can usefully be made by looking at the position of the coronary arteries in relation both to the cavity and to the outer border of the cardiac shadow. When excess pericardial fluid is present the coronaries lie inside the outer cardiac border but a normal distance from the cavity. When excess muscle is present the distance from cavity to coronaries is increased but the coronaries lie on the outer cardiac border.

The site of obstruction to left ventricular outflow lies at the point of apposition of the anterior mitral cusp to the bulging septal wall during systole (Fig. 14.16a). The anterior cusp is visible in good quality angiograms as a thin line which is bent in an L shape instead of showing as a straight line between the free border and the point of attachment to the aortic root. The anterior mitral cusp is thus dislocated anteriorly into an open position during systole (Pridie & Oakley, 1970) and this is why mitral reflux tends to occur in those patients who have outflow obstruction but not as often in those without outflow tract obstruction.

It has often been thought that the obstruction lies further down in the ventricle at the point where the cavity often shows marked 'waisting' during systolic ejection (Fig. 14.16b) but the true point of obstruction has been established beyond doubt not only by visualisation of the abnormally positioned anterior cusp but also by the fact that a transseptal catheter passed from the left atrium into the left ventricle invariably finds the high pressure part of the left ventricle with the first ventricular beat on entry. Since the transseptal catheter must enter the left ventricle below the anterior mitral cusp but above this muscular waist the site of obstruction must lie above the muscular waist. This point is stressed because the anterior mitral cusp is harder to see than the obvious muscular indentation below it.

Mitral regurgitation is seen as a late systolic event which often looks more severe than it is because the regurgitated contrast is not spread throughout systole and because the left atrium is of normal size or at least not of the proportions found in rheumatic valve disease. The volume of regurgitation is rarely large or of haemodynamic importance. This explains the lack of a dominant *v* wave in the left atrial pulse of patients with HOCM despite easily seen mitral regurgitation. Severe mitral regurgitation is rare, poorly tolerated and usually of sudden onset during infective endocarditis.

The left ventricular volume in HOCM is usually normal. The ejection fraction is often abnormally high—0·8 or even more—in patients with obstruction but normal, 0·5 to 0·7 in patients with slight or absent obstruction. In advanced cases the ejection fraction may be low. The end-diastolic volume is within normal limits. This means that advanced cases can have severely reduced stroke volumes. An increased left ventricular end-diastolic pressure is very rare in HOCM and advanced HOCM does *not* become COCM with dilated cavity compensating for greatly reduced contractile function even though clinical heart failure with oedema is present.

Echocardiography

Techniques using the ultrasound cardiogram (U.C.G.) have proved to be useful both in the diagnosis of patients with HOCM and in the elucidation of the haemodynamic abnormality.

Systolic re-opening of the anterior cusp of the mitral valve in HOCM was first observed by Pridie (1968) at Royal Postgraduate Medical School and was subsequently reported by others (Shah, Gramiak & Kramer, 1969; Popp & Harrison, 1969, Pridie & Oakley, 1970). The abnormal anterior movement in late systole is greatest in patients with marked left ventricular outflow tract obstruction and can be augmented or provoked by amyl nitrite. The echocardiographic phenomenon fits in with the angiographically de-monstrated systolic opening movement of the anterior mitral cusp in patients with obstruction and lends weight to the belief in its importance in producing outflow obstruction. The U.C.G. frequently shows late systolic apposition of the anterior mitral cusp and septal echoes in such cases.

The systolic re-opening movement of the mitral valve in HOCM seen on ultrasound records is virtually diagnostic of the disorder.

Systolic re-opening is most marked in patients who have the least free wall hypertrophy but marked asymmetrical hypertrophy of the septum. In these patients there may be increased shortening of the less afflicted muscle of the free wall and anterior papillary muscle which results in excessive pull on the anterior cusp towards the poorly contracting septal wall. An alterna-tive explanation is that diminished longitudinal shortening of the left ventricle in systole observed in some patients with HOCM results in abnormal traction on the valve cusps with consequent systolic re-opening of the mitral valve. (Klein, Gordon & Lane, 1970).

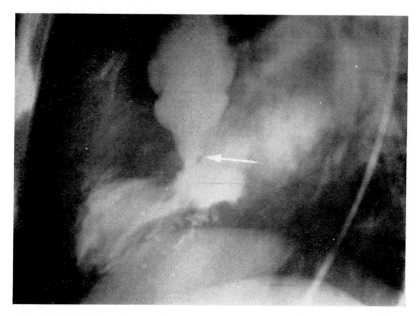

Fig. 14.16. (*a*) LV angiogram in left lateral projection in HOCM with obstruction (systolic phase). The point where the anterior cusp meets the septum during systolic re-opening of the mitral valve is clearly seen and at the same time mitral regurgitation occurs. (arrow).

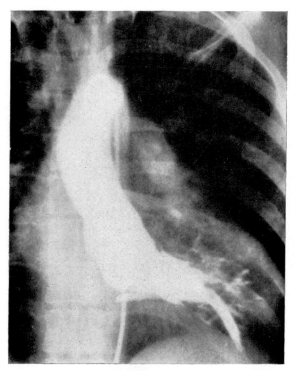

(*b*) Frontal view of LV angiogram in HOCM. The thickness of the LV free wall is well shown but the site of outflow obstruction cannot be seen in this projection.

[*To face p.* 492

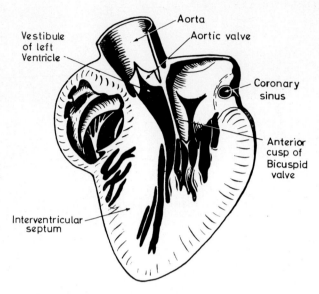

FIG. 14.17. Diagrammatic longitudinal section through heart to show the relationship of the mitral (bicuspid) valve anterior cusp to the ventricular septum (after Tandler, *Textbook of Anatomy*, 1926).

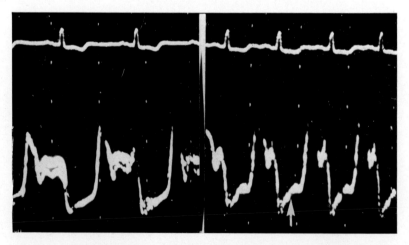

FIG. 14.18. UCG to show appearance of mitral systolic re-opening after amylnitrite. (arrowed).

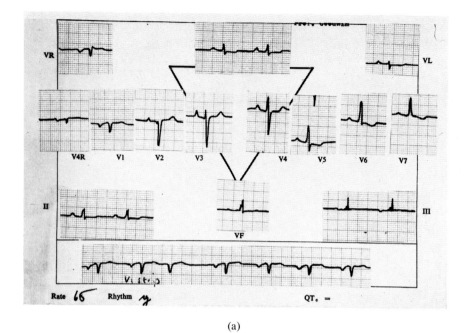

(a)

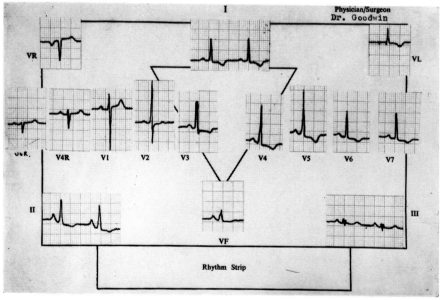

(b)

FIG. 14.20. (a) ECG taken in 1958 in patient with intermittent AF. (b) shows the very similar ECG of her daughter in 1963.

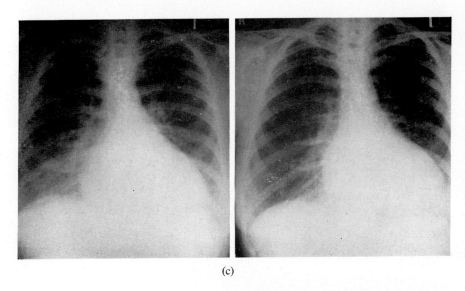

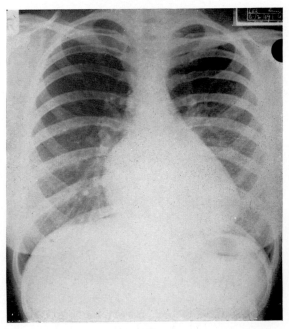

FIG. 14.20 (*c*) shows her chest radiographs taken in 1959 and 1969 compared with that of her daughter (*d*).

(c)

(d)

In addition to systolic re-opening the U.C.G. in HOCM shows abnormal proximity of the septal echoes to the anterior mitral cusp during systole and a reduced diastolic closure rate of the mitral valve. These form a diagnostic triad (Figs. 14.7 and 14.18); although the first is the most specific the last two on their own are highly suggestive or even diagnostic of HOCM in patients without an outflow tract gradient in whom diagnoses of constrictive pericarditis, COCM or ischaemic heart disease may have been considered. A similar slow diastolic closure slope is seen in mitral stenosis but there are no septal echoes and the valve cusp is usually thickened.

Natural History

Long term follow up of patients with HOCM reveals various patterns. Patients may seem to remain unchanged for many years. Sudden death may occur out of the blue or occasionally after a period of deterioration. Infective endocarditis (Vecht & Oakley, 1968), systemic embolisation, atrial fibrillation and congestive failure have all been seen. Patients of particular interest are the children of affected parents in whom the course of the disorder may be followed from the time that it first becomes discernible. It has also been instructive to see members of the same family in whom the disorder appears to be taking different forms or is at a different stage of advancement. Our knowledge of the later progress of the disease comes from a small group of patients who have been closely documented through a process of continuous haemodynamic change over the years. Observations on these three groups provide the basis for our knowledge of the natural history of HOCM. (Table 14.7.)

There is no doubt that the disorder tends to be progressive. The onset and progression of electrocardiographic abnormality has been documented the most frequently. Study of the symptomatic course and prognosis of HOCM by Swan et al., (1971) revealed that disability and sudden death in HOCM were associated with a higher left ventricular end-diastolic pressure than in patients who survived and who had less disability. Left ventricular outflow tract obstruction is revealed as an earlier or less severe form of the disorder when the left ventricular end-diastolic pressure may be lower than it is in patients without an outflow tract obstruction. Sudden death was rather uncommon among their patients with obstruction but infective endocarditis was seen in four such patients and probably may affect either the regurgitant mitral valve or the left ventricular outflow tract. Infective endocarditis has not been seen in patients with non-obstructive HOCM.

Spontaneous progressive decrease in outflow tract obstruction was noted in eight patients. In these patients disappearance of the murmur was associated with increasing effort dyspnoea in all and progressive cardiac enlargement in five. Evidence of a progressively rising left ventricular end-diastolic pressure was seen from the increase in left atrial size and the development of pulmonary venous congestion. Atrial fibrillation has developed in fifteen patients and systemic embolisation has been seen in nine patients. Loss of the atrial contribution to left ventricular filling is associated with a serious deterioration in most instances with evidence of a fall in cardiac output and sometimes with the onset of congestive failure. Pulmonary oedema was seen in three patients of whom two were in sinus rhythm. Congestive heart failure was seen in twelve patients. (Table 14.8.)

TABLE 14.7

NATURAL HISTORY AND PROGRESSION IN HOCM
PROGRESSIVE HYPERTROPHY AND DETERIORATING FUNCTION
FROM PHASES I TO V

I	Mode of Onset	Unknown Rarely present at birth
II	Obstruction and Mitral Regurgitation	Risk of infective endocarditis Risk from surgical treatment Sudden death uncommon
III	Loss of Obstruction	Diagnosis frequently incorrect Heart disease often not detected at all Risk of sudden death
IV	More severe Compliance Failure	High risk of sudden death Increase in disability Risk of atrial fibrillation Embolism Heart failure
V	Loss of Ejectile Force	

N.B. Many patients never enter phase II and others never leave it. Death is usually in phase III or IV and few survive to phase V.

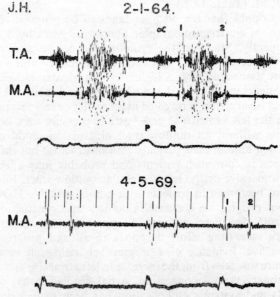

FIG. 14.19. PCG's 5 years apart to show spontaneous loss of atrial presystolic filling murmur and loss of murmurs of outflow tract obstruction in a boy who died in 1970 at the age of 18.

TABLE 14.8

HYPERTROPHIC OBSTRUCTIVE CARDIOMYOPATHY

100 *Patients*

76 treated medically, 24 treated surgically

26 DEATHS

'Sudden' death	10*
Operative death	7
Congestive failure	3
Pulmonary oedema	2
Embolism	2*
Infective endocarditis	2*

Progression in 76 medically treated patients

Loss of murmurs	8
Atrial fibrillation	15
Embolism	9
Heart failure	12

* Includes 4 late post-operative deaths; 2 sudden deaths,
1 from embolism and 1 from infective endocarditis.

Considering the relatively small proportion of patients in this series with HOCM who have been followed for more than five years the high proportion of such patients who have shown dramatic haemodynamic change is impressive and suggests that this is the usual expectation of patients during twenty or more years with the disorder. The similarity of electrocardiogram and chest radiographs of a mother and daughter with entirely different clinical features of HOCM provides a striking illustration of the probable natural history (Fig. 14.20). The mother presented in 1958 with atrial fibrillation, congestive failure and systemic embolism without murmurs. She is still alive today and virtually unchanged. The daughter presented with typical murmurs of HOCM with obstruction and this diagnosis was subsequently proved by haemodynamic studies. The mother and daughter have a closely similar angiographic appearance except that the mother has no outflow tract gradient either at rest or on provocation. It should be noted that the mother still has no left ventricular cavity dilatation despite the onset of congestive failure in 1958; clinical congestive failure in HOCM results from progression of the diastolic fault rather than from the acquisition of systolic failure. It is tempting to think that the mother resembled the daughter thirty years ago and that the daughter will go on to lose her murmurs and will develop congestive features in the years ahead.

Haemodynamic study in patients who have lost outflow tract obstruction or who are first studied in the non-obstructive phase suggests that loss of obstruction results from commencing loss of contractile function so that systolic cavity size becomes bigger and the anterior mitral cusp no longer approaches the septum. Alternative explanations could be progressive fibrosis of the anterior papillary muscle which limits its ability to dislocate the anterior cusp into the ventricle or even a loss of muscle bulk in the septum. An impressive demonstration of the last hypothesis was seen in a patient who suffered an occlusion of the anterior descending branch of the left coronary artery due to dissection by catheter during selective coronary angiography. Infarction of the anterior wall of the heart was followed by sudden and permanent loss of all bruits with loss of the systolic re-opening movement previously seen on her U.C.G.

Disorder in Childhood

Children under ten years old who have presented on account of symptoms or the discovery of a murmur (rather than because of the possession of a relative with the disease) have shown several special features which are worthy of mention. They have usually presented with syncopal attacks or breathlessness; they have unimpressive murmurs but a prominent left atrial filling beat; they show marked hypertrophy of the free wall of the heart as well as the septum, little or no outflow tract obstruction or mitral reflux but very high left ventricular filling pressures. They have fared poorly with a high incidence of sudden death and autopsy has showed particularly florid generalised left ventricular hypertrophy in addition to massive septal involvement.

Because of the lack of prominent murmurs the existence of heart disease is often missed in these children. Despite massive hypertrophy of the left ventricle the E.C.G. and chest radiograph may sometimes be only minimally abnormal although more often the increased muscle bulk is sufficient to cause characteristic globular enlargement of the heart on X-ray.

These children seem to suffer from a particularly severe and fatal form of the disorder due possibly to a high proportion of abnormal cells within the myocardial population. This leads to early death from compliance failure associated with inability to maintain left ventricular filling at high heart rates, inability to maintain adequate coronary perfusion to meet the increased metabolic costs of exercise and a tendency to sudden fatal dysrhythmia.

Probable Aetiology

The cause of HOCM is quite unknown. It is probably inherited as a dominant in some afflicted families and as a recessive trait in others. (Emanuel, Withers & O'Brien, 1971.) Meerschwam in 1969 produced evidence of skeletal muscle abnormality in some of his patients with HOCM who showed raised serum levels of muscle enzymes and abnormal electromyograms. Swan et al., have so far been unable to confirm this observation in our patients.

Electrophysiological abnormalities have been shown by Coltart & Meldrum (1970) in studies on single myocardial fibres excised at operation for relief of outflow tract obstruction in patients with HOCM. There has been a slow rate of development of the action potential from a normal resting potential, prolonged repolarisation and a decreased rate of follow on rapid stimulation.

No biochemical or enzymatic fault has yet been found and present knowledge of the cause of mechanism of HOCM is as limited as it is in the skeletal progressive muscular dystrophies. It is possible that a disorder of myocardial fibre growth determines the myocardial disarray with progressive hypertrophy resultant upon isometric stresses set up during contraction but if so we still lack a reason for the failure of normal myocardial cellular geometry.

Treatment

The aims of treatment are to relieve symptoms, to slow down the rate of progression and to reduce the risk of sudden death (Table 14.9). Measurable criteria of benefit are a reduction in left ventricular end-diastolic pressure and the relief of outflow tract obstruction.

TABLE 14.9

AIMS OF TREATMENT IN HOCM

I	Relief of Symptoms	Dyspnoea
		Angina
		Syncope
II	Improvement of Haemodynamic fault	Raised ventricular filling pressure
		Obstruction to left ventricular ejection
		Low cardiac output
III	Improvement of Prognosis	
IV	Delay in Progression of the Disorder	
V	Eugenic	Family counselling

Surgical resection can remove the obstruction to outflow (Bentall *et al.*, 1965, Morrow *et al.*, 1968) but it is not yet known whether the other more important objectives are achieved—the spontaneous loss of obstruction is accompanied by a rise in left ventricular end-diastolic pressure and deterioration rather than improvement. Surgical treatment carries an appreciable mortality and has not been followed by any evident improvement in the long term natural history in our series although Morrow *et al.* report a better experience. (Table 14.6.) Beta-adrenergic blocking drugs had been used in HOCM for more than 5 years without any firm conclusions emerging. Although they alleviate angina if present, outflow tract obstruction is influenced only to a small extent. At the Royal Postgraduate Medical School the effects of β-adrenergic blockade on left ventricular end-diastolic pressure in HOCM has been examined both acutely and during chronic oral administration. Heart rate, cardiac output, left ventricular and aortic pressure were measured at rest, during exercise and after 20 to 40 mg of practolol.

Practolol caused a reduction in the pressure at rest and a much more striking reduction during exercise (it fell from $34 \pm 4 \cdot 1$ to $25 \pm 3 \cdot 0$ mmHg in nine patients) even though left ventricular stroke work simultaneously increased slightly. Subsequent work has shown a similar reduction in left ventricular end-diastolic pressure both at rest and during exercise following propranolol. Outflow tract obstruction was variably affected but fell only in a few patients.

Acute studies on a bicycle ergometer have shown the effect of propranolol on exercise capacity, heart rate and stroke output. These studies also carried out at Royal Postgraduate Medical School showed that the physical working capacity of patients with HOCM is significantly lower than normal, even in patients who claim to be asymptomatic. After propranolol the same exercise was achieved at a slower heart rate than before (Edwards *et al.*, 1970).

The effects of chronic oral administration of β-adrenergic blocking drugs have been judged by a double blind study using non-invasive means of assessment with apex cardiography and mitral echocardiography as well as conventional and auscultatory criteria. A reduction or even total abolition of the atrial beat of the impulse cardiogram was observed in the patients while taking either practolol (80 mg twice daily) or propranolol (80 mg three times a day) but not while they were on the placebo. U.C.G.'s showed improvement in the filling of the left ventricle with increase in the speed of the diastolic closure slope suggesting improvement in the rate of filling of the left ventricle.

General measures

Patients with outflow obstruction and mitral regurgitation should be protected from infective endocarditis as in valvular heart disease (Vecht and Oakley, 1970). The development of atrial fibrillation should be treated with anticoagulents to prevent systemic embolisation and by electrical reversion to sinus rhythm as often as this is followed by a worthwhile period of sinus rhythm. When permanent fibrillation becomes unavoidable the ventricular rate should be controlled and this may often be achieved by β-adrenergic blocking drug alone but if this is unsuccessful the addition of digoxin is not contra-indicated. Diuretics may be needed in advanced cases.

Treatment of HOCM in pregnancy

Pregnancy in women with HOCM has pursued a reasonably tranquil course. It has been our policy to administer propranolol throughout pregnancy, to give it intramuscularly (10 mg) at the commencement of labour and to ensure a fast second stage. Caesarean section has not been practised except for obstetric reasons. (Turner, Oakley & Dixon, 1968.)

References

ALEXANDER, C. S. (1966). *Am. J. Med.*, **41**, 213.
ALEXANDER, C. S. (1967). *Br. Heart J.*, **29**, 200.
ARVIDSSON, H. (1961). *Acta radiol.*, **56**, 321.
BARNARD, P. (1971). Proceedings of International Symposium on Cardiomyopathies and Cardiac Metabolism, Bellville, South Africa. October 1971. In the press.
BELL, E. & GRIST, N. R. (1970). *Lancet*, **1**, 326.
BENGTSSON, E. (1968). *Cardiologia*, **52**, 97–108.
BENTALL, H. H., CLELAND, W. P., OAKLEY, C. M., SHAH, P. M., STEINER, R. E. & GOODWIN, J. F. (1965). *Br. Heart. J.*, **27**, 585.
BERNHEIM, P. I. (1910). *Rev. Med.*, **30**, 785.
BRAUNWALD, E., LAMBREW, C. T., ROCKOFF, S. D., ROSS, J. JR. & MORROW, A. G. (1964). *Circulation, Suppl. IV*, **30**, 3.
BRIGDEN, W. W. & ROBINSON, J. F. (1964). *Br. med. J.*, **2**, 1283.
BROCK, R. C. (1957). *Guys Hosp. Rep.*, **106**, 221.
BROCKENBROUGH, E. C., BRAUNWALD, E. & MORROW, A. G. (1961). *Circulation*, **23**, 189.
BURCH, G. E., WALSH, J. J. & BLACK, W. L. (1963). *J. Am. Med. Ass.*, **183**, 81.
BURCH, G. E. & DePASQUALE, N. P. (1968). *Cardiologia*, **52**, 48.

BURCH, G. E. (1971). Proceedings of International Symposium on Cardiomyopathies and Cardiac Metabolism. Bellville, South Africa. October 1971. In the press.

CANNON, P. J. (1962). *Am. J. Med.*, **42**, 765–775.

COHEN, J., EFFAT, H., GOODWIN, J. F., OAKLEY, C. M. & STEINER, R. E. (1964). *Br. Heart J.*, **26**, 16–32

COLTART, D. J. & MELDRUM, S. J. (1970). *Br. med. J.*, **4**, 217.

CONNOR, D. H., SOMERS, K., HUTT, M. S. R., MANION, W. C. & D'ARBELA, P. G. (1967). *Am. Heart J.*, **74**, 687.

CONNOR, D. H., SOMERS, K., HUTT, M. S. R., MANION, W. C. & D'ARBELA, P. G. (1968). *Am. Heart J.*, **75**, 107–124.

EDWARDS, R. H. T., KRISTINSSON, A., WARRELL, D. A. & GOODWIN, J. F. (1970). *Brit. Heart J.* **32**, 219.

EMANUEL, R., WITHERS, R. & O'BRIEN, K. (1971). *Lancet*, **2**, 1065.

EVANS, W. (1959). *Br. Heart J.*, **21**, 445.

FOGENBAUM, H., ZAKY, A. & NASSER, W. K. (1967). *Circulation*, **35**, 1092.

FEJFAR, Z. (1968). *Cardiologia*, **52**, 9–19.

FERRANS, V. (1971). Proceedings of International Symposium on Cardiomyopathies and Cardiac Metabolism. October 1971. In the press.

FODOR, J., MIALL, W. E., STANDARD, K. L., FEJFAR, Z. & STUART, K. L. (1964). *Bull. Wld. Hlth. Org.*, **31**, 321.

GOODWIN, J. F. (1964). *Br. med. J.*, **1**, 1527–1595.

GOODWIN, J. F. (1970). *Lancet*, **1**, 731–739.

HEWER, R. (1969). *Br. Heart J.*, **31**, 5–14.

HIBBS, R. G., FERRANS, V. J. & BLACK, W. C. (1965). *Am. Heart J.*, **69**, 766.

HOLLISTER, R. M. & GOODWIN, J. F. (1963). *Br. Heart J.*, **25**, 357.

HUDSON, R. E. B. (1970). *In* 'Cardiovascular Pathology'. Vol. 3, pp. 474, 546. London: Edward Arnold.

IVEMARK, B. & THOREN, C. (1964). *Acta med. scand.*, **175**, 227–237.

JAMES, T. N. & BEAR, E. S. (1967). *Am. Heart J.*, **74**, 243.

KASTELOOT, H., TERRYN, R., BOSMANS, P. & JOOSSENS, J. V. (1966). *Acta Cardiol.*, **21**, 341.

KLEIN, M. D., LANE, F. J. & GORLIN, R. (1965). *Am. J. Cardiol.*, **15**, 773–781.

KRISTINSSON, A. CROXSON, R. S., EVERSON PEASE, A. G., OAKLEY, C. M. & GOODWIN J. F. (1968). *Proceedings of the Vth European Congress of Cardiology*, (Athens, Sept. 1968).

LÖFFLER, W. (1936). *Schweitz Med. Wshcr.*, **66**, 817.

MCDERMOTT, P. H., DELANIE, A. L., EAGAN, J. D. & SULLIVAN, J. F. (1966). *J. Am. Med. Ass.*, **198**, 253.

MANN, O., DELEON, A. C. JR. & PERLOFF, J. K. (1968). *Am. J. Med. Sci.*, **255**, 376–381.

MARTIN, C. E., SHAVER, J. A., THOMPSON, M. E., REEDY, P. S. & LEONARD, J. J. (1971). *Circulation*, **44**, 419.

MEERSCHWAMM, I. S. (1969). *In* 'Hypertrophic Obstructive Cardiomyopathy'. p. 129. Amsterdam.

MERCIER, G. & PATRY, G. (1967). *Canad. Med. Ass. J.*, **97**, 884.

MILLER, G. A. H. & SWAN, H. J. C. (1964). *Circulation*, **30**, 205.

MITCHELL, J. H. & COHAN, L. S. (1970). *Mod. Concepts cardiovasc. Dis.*, **39**, 109.

MORIN, Y. L. P. (1967). *Canad. Med. Ass. J.*, **97**, 901.

MORROW, A. G., FOGARTY, T. J., HANNAH, H. III, & BRAUNWALD, E. (1968). *Circulation*, **37**, 589.

OAKLEY, C. M. (1971). *Br. Heart J. Suppl. VI*, **33**, 179.

OAKLEY, C. M. (1971). *In* 'Hypertrophic Obstructive Cardiomyopathy', Ciba Foundation Study Group No. 37, p. 9. London: Churchill.

PEARSE, A. G. E. (1964). *In* 'Cardiomyopathies', p. 132. A Ciba Foundation Symposium. London: Churchill.

PERLOFF, J. K., DELEON, A. C. JR. & O'DOHERTY, D. (1966). *Circulation*, **33**, 625.

PERLOFF, J. K., ROBERTS, W. C. & DELEON, A. C. JR. (1967). *Am. J. Med.*, **42**, 179.

PERLOFF, J. K. (1971). *Mod. Concepts cardiovasc. Dis.*, **40**, 23.

POPP, R. L. & HARRISON, D. C. (1970). *Circulation*, **41**, 493.

PRIDIE, R. B. & TURNBULL, T. A. (1968). *Proceedings of the Vth European Congress of Cardiology* (Athens, September 1968), p. 263.

PRIDIE, R. B. & OAKLEY, C. M. (1970). *Br. Heart J.*, **32**, 203–208.

RACKLEY, C. E., DODGE, H. T., COBLE, Y. D. JR. & HAY, R. E. (1964). *Circulation*, **29**, 666.

RIFF, D. P., JAIN, A. C. & DOYLE, J. T. (1969). *Am. Heart J.*, **78**, 592.

SAINANI, G. S., KROMPOTIC, E. & SLODKIL, S. J. (1968). *Medicine*, **47**, 133–147.

SCHMINCKE, A. (1907). *Dt. med. Wschr.*, **33**, 2082.

STUART, K. L., MIALL, W. E., TULLOCH, J. A. & CHRISTIAN, D. E. (1962). *Br. Heart J.*, **34**, 455.

STUART, K. L. & HAYES, J. A. (1963). *Q. J. Med.*, **32**, 99.

SWAN, D. A., BELL, B., OAKLEY, C. M. & GOODWIN, J. F. (1971). *Br. Heart J.*, **33**, 671.

TEARE, R. D. (1958). *Br. Heart J.*, **20**, 1–8.

TURNER, G. M., OAKLEY, C. M. & DIXON, H. G. (1968). *Br. med. J.*, **4**, 1–11.

WEISSLER, A. M., HARRIS, W. S. & SCHOENFELD, C. D. (1968). *Circulation*, **37**, 149–159.

VAN NOORDEN, S., OLSEN, E. G. J. & PEARSE, A. G. E. (1971). *Cardiovasc. Res.*, **5**, 118.

VECHT, R. J. & OAKLEY, C. M. (1968). *Br. med. J.*, **1**, 455.

WEBB-PEPLOE, M. M., CROXSON, R. S., OAKLEY, C. M. & GOODWIN, J. F. (1971). *Postgrad. J. Med.*, **47**, (Suppl.) 93.

WIGLE, E. D., MARQUIS, Y. & AUGER, P. (1967). *Circulation*, **35**, 1100.

INDEX

PRINTED IN GREAT BRITAIN BY THE WHITEFRIARS PRESS LTD.
LONDON AND TONBRIDGE